Malaria

Biology in the Era of Eradication

A subject collection from *Cold Spring Harbor Perspectives in Medicine*

OTHER SUBJECT COLLECTIONS FROM *COLD SPRING HARBOR PERSPECTIVES IN MEDICINE*

Antibiotics and Antibiotic Resistance

The p53 Protein: From Cell Regulation to Cancer

Aging: The Longevity Dividend

Epilepsy: The Biology of a Spectrum Disorder

Molecular Approaches to Reproductive and Newborn Medicine

The Hepatitis B and Delta Viruses

Intellectual Property in Molecular Medicine

Retinal Disorders: Genetic Approaches to Diagnosis and Treatment

The Biology of Heart Disease

Human Fungal Pathogens

Tuberculosis

The Skin and Its Diseases

MYC and the Pathway to Cancer

Bacterial Pathogenesis

Transplantation

Cystic Fibrosis: A Trilogy of Biochemistry, Physiology, and Therapy

Hemoglobin and Its Diseases

Addiction

Parkinson's Disease

Type 1 Diabetes

Angiogenesis: Biology and Pathology

SUBJECT COLLECTIONS FROM *COLD SPRING HARBOR PERSPECTIVES IN BIOLOGY*

Cilia

Microbial Evolution

Learning and Memory

DNA Recombination

Neurogenesis

Size Control in Biology: From Organelles to Organisms

Mitosis

Glia

Innate Immunity and Inflammation

The Genetics and Biology of Sexual Conflict

The Origin and Evolution of Eukaryotes

Endocytosis

Mitochondria

Signaling by Receptor Tyrosine Kinases

Malaria

Biology in the Era of Eradication

A subject collection from *Cold Spring Harbor Perspectives in Medicine*

EDITED BY

Dyann F. Wirth
Harvard T.H. Chan School of Public Health

Pedro L. Alonso
World Health Organization, Global Malaria Programme

COLD SPRING HARBOR LABORATORY PRESS
Cold Spring Harbor, New York • www.cshlpress.org

Malaria: Biology in the Era of Eradication

A subject collection from *Cold Spring Harbor Perspectives in Medicine*
Articles online at www.perspectivesinmedicine.org

Executive Editor	Richard Sever
Managing Editor	Maria Smit
Senior Project Manager	Barbara Acosta
Permissions Administrator	Carol Brown
Production Editor	Diane Schubach
Production Manager/Cover Designer	Denise Weiss
Publisher	John Inglis

Front cover artwork: Concept of malaria parasites and their mosquito vector, with tools for understanding and controlling the disease. (Image adapted from iStock.com/nongpimmy.)

Library of Congress Cataloging-in-Publication Data

Names: Wirth, Dyann Fergus, editor. | Alonso, Pedro L., editor.
Title: Malaria biology in the era of eradication / edited by Dyann F. Wirth, Harvard T.H. Chan School of Public Health and Pedro L. Alonso, University of Barcelona.
Description: Cold Spring Harbor, New York : Cold Spring Harbor Laboratory Press, 2017 | A subject collection from Cold Spring Harbor Perspectives in Medicine | Includes bibliographical references and index.
Identifiers: LCCN 2016016648 | ISBN 9781621821229 (hardback)
Subjects: LCSH: Malaria--Molecular aspects. | Host-parasite relationships. | Malaria--Treatment. | BISAC: MEDICAL / Diseases. | MEDICAL / Immunology. | MEDICAL / Infectious Diseases.
Classification: LCC QR201.M3 M332 2016 | DDC 614.5/32--dc23
LC record available at https://lccn.loc.gov/2016016648

10 9 8 7 6 5 4 3 2 1

All World Wide Web addresses are accurate to the best of our knowledge at the time of printing.

For a complete catalog of all Cold Spring Harbor Laboratory Press publications, visit our website at www.cshlpress.org.

Contents

Contents

Preface

THIS BOOK FOCUSES ON THE FUNDAMENTAL SCIENTIFIC KNOWLEDGE OF MALARIA BIOLOGY that will inform the worldwide elimination campaign. Malaria remains a major global health problem and, over the past decade, there has been a focus on reducing the burden of the disease. This is a historical inflection point—knowledge about the parasite, the insect vector, and the human host is rapidly expanding and the challenge now is to translate this knowledge into tools that can be used to impact the disease and its transmission. At the same time, exploration of these fundamental systems is generating new and interesting basic biological questions. The human host, insect vector, and parasite are interacting in a complex systems ecology. We can see the evolution of both the parasite and the mosquito vector occurring in real time—the emergence of drug and insecticide resistance are prime examples.

The chapters in this book focus on the last decade of research. This is a period when the focus of malaria research shifted from pathogenesis and disease mechanism to interrupting transmission. This change in emphasis was, in part, the result of a set of high-level decisions led by Bill and Melinda Gates and their foundation to focus on malaria elimination and eradication. During this same period, there have been technological advances that have greatly enhanced fundamental science investigation, advances in genomics, systems biology, cell biology and imaging, and, most recently, advanced genetic engineering, including gene drive approaches to modify mosquito populations.

Perhaps most important from the perspective of the editors are the remaining gaps in our knowledge and the gaps in the translation of that knowledge for public health impact. Rather than reiterating what is covered in the book, we identify here key knowledge gaps that need to be addressed as we begin to translate the basic science discoveries to the problem of elimination and eradication of malaria. First is understanding the course of natural infection as transmission is decreasing, including understanding relevant vector biology, identifying key determinants of immunity, and deciphering the differences in infections of the five *Plasmodium* species that cause human disease. Understanding the biology of the *Plasmodium vivax* liver stage is critical. Second is understanding the emergence and spread of insecticide resistance in mosquitoes and drug resistance in parasite populations. The selective force of interventions generates population bottlenecks and understanding these dynamics is now within technical reach with a renewed emphasis on surveillance and molecular epidemiology. Third is a renewed focus on vector competence, including fundamentals of vector biology and the interaction of the parasite with its mosquito vector. The enabling technology of gene drives now makes intervention at the level of mosquito populations possible and understanding the implications is the next opportunity and challenge.

Regardless of the current successes in reducing transmission and resulting decreases in cases and mortality, there is constant evolution of the parasite, the vector, the human host, and the environment and a fundamental understanding of malaria biology is key to the next generation of interventions. Enabling technologies now make it possible to interrogate parasite and vector biology to understand key liabilities for targeting future interventions. Host–parasite and vector–parasite interactions are the next frontier in our understanding of disease progression and transmission. The microbiomes of the human and the mosquito are likely to play key roles, and we are just beginning to understand their interplay with immunity and nutrition.

We are deeply grateful to our colleagues who have authored chapters in this collection for their thoughtful exploration of these and other critical themes in the biology of malaria eradication. The next decade promises great advances in our understanding of malaria biology and the translation of that knowledge to inform elimination and eradication, surely with significant contributions by the authors of this book. Additionally, we are thankful to Dr. Bronwyn MacInnis for her steadfast efforts on spearheading this project, and to Lucia Ricci for her help and creativity with artwork. We are also indebted to Project Manager Barbara Acosta and her colleagues at Cold Spring Harbor Laboratory Press for their professionalism and patience in seeing this ambitious and important volume through to its impressive completion.

DYANN WIRTH
PEDRO ALONSO

Malaria Transmission and Prospects for Malaria Eradication: The Role of the Environment

Marcia C. Castro

Department of Global Health and Population, Harvard T.H. Chan School of Public Health, Boston, Massachusetts 02115

Correspondence: mcastro@hsph.harvard.edu

Environmental factors affect the transmission intensity, seasonality, and geographical distribution of malaria, and together with the vector, the human, and the parasite compose the malaria system. Strategies that alter the environment are among the oldest interventions for malaria control, but currently are not the most prominent despite historical evidence of their effectiveness. The importance of environmental factors, the role they play considering the current goals of malaria eradication, the different strategies that can be adopted, and the current challenges for their implementation are discussed. As malaria elimination/eradication takes a prominent place in the health agenda, an integrated action, addressing all elements of the malaria system, which contributes to improved knowledge and to building local capacity and that brings about positive effects to the health of the local population has the greatest chance to produce fast, effective, and sustainable results.

"Like chess, (malaria) is played with a few pieces, but is capable of an infinite variety of situations" (Hackett 1937). Four pieces comprise the malaria system: the vector, the parasite, the human, and the environment (Table 1). The triad human–vector–parasite exists within (and interacts with) the environment, resulting in a variety of unique local patterns of malaria transmission that have been associated with specific definitions (e.g., forest malaria, urban malaria, frontier malaria). Each of these unique transmission patterns present distinct challenges, requiring a tailored package of control interventions.

A multitude of factors impact each of the four pieces in the malaria system, adding complexity to the proper understanding and control of malaria (Singer and Castro 2011). The vector is shaped by the type of *Anopheles* species and associated feeding, resting, biting, and breeding behavior, flight range, vectorial capacity, mortality and reproduction rate, mosquito resistance to insecticides, and larval resistance to larvicides. Important issues regarding the parasite include the type and strain, resistance to antimalarial drugs, and duration of infection. The human component is shaped by several factors including genetic and acquired immunity, behavior, demographics, culture, socioeconomic characteristics, and politics. Last, the environment component depends both on the natural environment—temperature, humidity, rainfall, soil quality, elevation/slope, land cover, hydrography, presence of natural enemies of

Table 1. A systemic view of malaria: Factors, control strategies, and challenges

Elements	Factors	Control strategies	Challenges
Vector	Species; feeding, resting, biting, host, and breeding preference; flight range; life span; vectorial capacity; reproduction rate; resistance	Insecticide-treated nets; indoor residual spraying; larval source management; fogging or area spraying	Mosquito behavior change; insecticide resistance; novel vector control (traps, engineered mosquitoes); genetic differences
Parasite	Type and strain; resistance to antimalarials; duration of infection	Case management; malaria seasonal chemoprevention; intermittent presumptive treatment; mass drug administration	New diagnostic tools; sub-microscopic parasitemia; asymptomatic infections; gametocyte cycle; genetic diversity; hypnozoites; drug resistance; vaccines
Human	Genetic/acquired immunity; knowledge (transmission, prevention, treatment); age; migratory pattern; occupation; education; cultural beliefs; behavior; access to care; population density; political context (public health interventions, support and infrastructure, construction of major development projects, implementation of foreign assistance, political stability, and governance); globalization (market pressures, choice of crops, exploitation of natural resources); environmental change	Personal protection (repellents, protective clothing); behavior change communication	Community participation; adherence to control; risk perception; behavior change; human mobility; forced mobility (climate, conflicts); malaria in pregnancy Scale-up; sustainability of recent achievements; funding (donor fatigue); political commitment; intersectoral collaboration; strong health system; surveillance; counterfeit drugs; affordable drugs; supply chain management
Environment	Natural: temperature, rainfall, humidity; elevation/slope; soil quality; vegetation; hydrology; presence of natural enemies of mosquitoes and larvae; natural disasters Human-made: urbanization; land change/use; housing type; deforestation; infrastructure (water, waste collection, sanitation); development projects (dams, roads, oil pipelines, mining, railways, irrigation, resettlement); disasters facilitated by human change	Environmental management; house improvement	Infrastructure projects; environmental change; extreme climatic events

 Cite this article as *Cold Spring Harb Perspect Med* doi: 10.1101/cshperspect.a025601

mosquitoes and larvae, and natural disasters—and the human-made environment—land use, land change, deforestation, housing type, infrastructure (water, sanitation, and waste collection), urbanization, development projects (e.g., roads, railways, dams, irrigation, mining, resettlement projects, and oil pipelines), and disasters facilitated by human-made changes.

Each of these factors may affect malaria positively or negatively, and effects can be modified depending on how they interact with each other. In addition, many of these factors are not static, but rather change/adapt to pressure or novel local conditions, bringing about additional challenges for malaria control. Examples include the development of drug and insecticide resistance, changes in vector (Chinery 1984; Sattler et al. 2005; Awolola et al. 2007) and human behavior (Maheu-Giroux and Castro 2013), and environmental changes (Keiser et al. 2004; Gething et al. 2010; Castro and Singer 2011; Yamana and Eltahir 2013; Hahn et al. 2014). Therefore, although specific interventions target each of the four pieces that compose the malaria system, two equally important issues deserve special attention. First, efforts to control (and eventually eradicate) malaria must address all four components of the malaria system. Second, the implementation of a package of interventions must be accompanied by a surveillance effort that allows fine tuning strategies in the event of changing local conditions.

This article focuses on the environmental component of the malaria system, considering (1) its interactions with other elements in the system, (2) the ways through which control strategies could address environmental determinants, and (3) if and why considering the environmental component is crucial for current goals of malaria eradication.

ENVIRONMENTAL DETERMINANTS OF MALARIA TRANSMISSION

Several environmental factors impact mosquito and parasite vital rates, and thus affect the transmission intensity, seasonality, and geographical distribution of malaria. These factors fall into two broad categories: natural and human-made environment, as detailed next.

Natural Environment

Climate-based factors, temperature and precipitation, are the primary environmental determinants of malaria. Temperature impacts vector and parasite development and thus is an important constraint on the geographical suitability to malaria (Gething et al. 2011). The extrinsic development of the parasite is constrained within a certain temperature range (Macdonald 1957), extremely high temperatures are likely to produce smaller and less fecund mosquitoes (Warrell and Gilles 2002), and increasing temperatures reduce the time for mosquito maturation (from larva to adult form) and increase the feeding frequency (Service 1980; Martens et al. 1999). Recent models indicate that malaria transmission (as measured by the R_0) is constrained to temperatures between 16°C and 34°C, with optimal transmission at 25°C (Mordecai et al. 2013), ~6°C lower than previously estimated (Martens et al. 1997; Craig et al. 1999; Parham and Michael 2010).

The frequency, duration, and intensity of precipitation contribute to the formation of suitable water habitats for mosquito breeding. Although water pools must persist for a long enough time for mosquito development, heavy precipitation has been associated with immature mortality (Paaijmans et al. 2007). Because *Anopheles* mosquitoes have different breeding preferences, and other natural conditions such as water temperature and quality, soil characteristics, and vegetation cover (Yamana and Eltahir 2013) can modify the suitability of the aquatic habitat for mosquito development, the relationship between rainfall and malaria has produced contrasting results, with some studies reporting positive impacts (Loevinsohn 1994; Kilian et al. 1999; Lindblade et al. 1999), and others finding negative or nonsignificant ones (Lindsay et al. 2000; WHO 2000; Singh and Sharma 2002).

Extreme weather events (e.g., tropical storms, droughts, hurricanes, cyclones, typhoons) often have the most dramatic impacts on human health (Kovats et al. 1999). The El

Niño Southern Oscillation (ENSO) is a phenomenon often associated with extreme weather events across the globe, with significant impacts in malaria transmission (Kovats et al. 2003). Although the periodicity of ENSO varies, early warning systems (some up to 1 year ahead) that monitor sea surface temperature facilitate the adoption of measures in anticipation of the consequences of extreme weather events (Ludescher et al. 2014).

Local hydrography, hydrology, and topography affect the water flow and collection, and the formation of water pools (Bomblies et al. 2008; Yamana and Eltahir 2013). For example, in the Amazon region the water level of the rivers increases dramatically during the rainy season, flooding the areas immediately proximal to the margins. When the rainy season is ending the water level decreases, and pools of water suitable for mosquito breeding appear because of the irregularity of the terrain (Peixoto 1917).

The presence of natural predators of mosquito larvae can contribute to control the population size of malaria vectors, depending on the physicochemical properties of the water habitat (Dida et al. 2015). Humidity affects mosquito survival, because under very dry conditions mosquitoes will desiccate (Jawara et al. 2008). Last, natural disasters can also result in increased malaria transmission (Watson et al. 2007) through population displacement, and habitat change after an earthquake and flooding that facilitate the proliferation of mosquito breeding habitats (Sáenz et al. 1995; Gagnon et al. 2002). In contrast to the ENSO phenomenon, natural disasters often happen without warning, leaving little room to plan in anticipation of their negative impacts.

Human-Made Environment

Human-made transformations of the natural environment serve many purposes and can result in reductions or increases in malaria transmission. The implementation of development projects, such as roads, railways, dams, irrigation, mining, population resettlement, and oil extraction, to name a few, often result in social and environmental impacts that, if not properly assessed and mitigated, bring about negative effects on people's health. Such impacts are associated with, for example, deforestation that can create ideal breeding grounds for mosquitoes; migration of naive populations to malaria-endemic areas, or migration of infected people to areas where the malaria vector is present and transmission, albeit absent or very low, is suitable; a large concentration of workers living in poor housing and thus highly exposed to the vector; and creation of ideal water habitats for mosquito breeding, such as artificial lakes associated with dam construction. These and other consequences of development projects, as well as the negative impacts on health, have been well documented for more than a century (e.g., Cruz 1972; Ghebreyesus et al. 1999; Lerer and Scudder 1999; Jackson and Sleigh 2000; Keiser et al. 2005a; Knoblauch et al. 2014). Nevertheless, they continue to happen and to threaten the lives of many in malaria-endemic areas, exposing major flaws in the transparency and execution of environmental impact assessments (Erlanger et al. 2008).

The massive deforestation observed in the Brazilian Amazon in the 1970s and 1980s (driven by large cattle-ranching and human settlement efforts) was associated with a major increase of malaria, and brought about a new definition to describe the dynamics of transmission in the region: frontier malaria (Sawyer and Sawyer 1987; Castro et al. 2006). It has been hypothesized that extensive deforestation and disorganized occupation could be indirectly responsible for modifications in mosquito behavior (outdoor biting), subtracting its former sources of food (wild animals, who were scared away by the new settlers) and bringing man closer to its breeding places (Deane 1988).

Regarding agriculture, the impact on malaria depends on the type of crop, the planting system, the irrigation practice, and the characteristics of the local *Anopheles* (Yasuoka and Levins 2007). Without proper management of irrigation, rice fields often provide ideal grounds for mosquito breeding (International Rice Research Institute and Joint WHO/FAO/UNEP Panel of Experts on Environmental Management for Vector Control 1988). Specifically related to

Cite this article as *Cold Spring Harb Perspect Med* doi: 10.1101/cshperspect.a025601

maize, it has been shown that its pollen is a nutritious food for the larvae of the most common malaria vector in Ethiopia, contributing to increasing vector density, mosquito longevity, and malaria infection (Ye-Ebiyo et al. 2000; Kebede et al. 2005). Also, the practice of cultivating crops such as sweet potato and beans, among others, using raised planting beds interspaced by channels that naturally provide irrigation result in highly productive breeding habitats for *Anopheles* (Dongus et al. 2009).

The availability of basic infrastructure (water, sanitation, waste collection) in residential areas is another factor that can modify human exposure to a malaria infection, depending on the characteristics of local malaria vectors. The need to collect water from streams or closer to areas where mosquito density is higher, to bathe in rivers, and to defecate and urinate near forested areas around villages are associated with a higher human–vector contact (Castro et al. 2006; Gryseels et al. 2015). Also, the accumulation of waste that can block the water flow of drains contribute to the formation of water pools ideal for mosquito breeding (Castro et al. 2010).

The process of urbanization is expected to contribute to lower malaria transmission through better health care, improved house construction, and a reduced number of breeding habitats for *Anopheles* mosquitoes caused by water pollution and large areas of impervious surface (Castro et al. 2004; De Silva and Marshall 2012). However, declining economies, uncontrolled urban growth (with large fractions of the population living under slum-like conditions lacking proper infrastructure), and adaptation of malaria vectors to the urban environment bring additional challenges to urban malaria control (Chinery 1984; Keiser et al. 2004).

Another important aspect of the human-made environment is the housing quality and the extent to which it offers a barrier against the malaria vector. In malaria-endemic areas, houses with open eaves, without screens, and without doors and/or windows offer higher risk of human–vector contact and are associated with higher malaria transmission (Sawyer and Sawyer 1987; Gamage-Mendis et al. 1991; Tusting et al. 2015).

ENVIRONMENT-BASED INTERVENTIONS FOR MALARIA CONTROL

Strategies that alter the environmental characteristics associated with malaria transmission are among the oldest interventions for malaria control (Stromquist 1920). They can be grouped into three types of activities, aiming to reduce the number of breeding habitats for malaria vectors or to reduce the human–vector contact. First, a permanent modification of the environment, such as drainage, filling, and land leveling; these activities often demand large-scale engineering work. Second, a manipulation of the environment that demands recurrent activities, such as regulation of water level in reservoirs, intermittent irrigation, afforestation/deforestation, and vegetation removal from water bodies. Third, modification of human habitation through resettlement or improved housing (WHO 1982).

Environmental management was crucial for the elimination of malaria in European countries and in the United States and to reduce the burden of the disease in many other locations (Pomeroy 1920; Boyd 1926; Neiva 1940). Important endeavors, including the construction of the Panama Canal (Gorgas 1915), copper mining in Zambia, former Rhodesia (Watson 1953; Utzinger et al. 2002), and rubber production in Malaysia (Watson 1921), were unlikely to have the same outcome if environmental management was not adopted as part of the package of interventions for malaria control. Malaria transmitted by a bromeliad-breeding mosquito was eliminated from the South of Brazil through removal of bromeliads from urban areas and introduction of eucalyptus trees (on which bromeliads do not grow) in forested areas (Pinotti 1951; Deane 1988). Housing improvement, first introduced by the Italian hygienist Angelo Celli at the end of the 19th century, was a crucial intervention in Europe, in the United States, and during wars (screening barracks) (Carter and Mendis 2002; Lindsay et al. 2002). The use of intermittent irrigation strategies for control of rice-field malaria has been and continues to be an important strategy in China (Baolin 1988; Singer and Castro 2011).

The historical examples of the successful use of environmental management are many, both in urban and rural settings, and they proved to be cost effective (Konradsen et al. 2004; Keiser et al. 2005b). A few lessons learned include the combination of control strategies (with environment management playing a central role) idiosyncratic to each locality, the multidisciplinary nature of the control staff (entomologist, epidemiologist, ecologist, hydrologist, physician, and engineer), the importance of surveillance to inform the need to fine-tune the package of interventions, and the recognition that about 3 years would be necessary to obtain expected results (B Singer, unpubl.).

Lessons from contemporary environmental management for malaria control are twofold. First, it should be established with the participation of the community, which contributes to the sustainability of the activity and promotes a sense of ownership and empowerment (Fillinger et al. 2008; Castro et al. 2009). Second, multisectoral collaboration should be pursued, integrating health actions with sectors responsible for agriculture, urban planning, transportation, education, and finance (United Nations Development Programme and Roll Back Malaria Partnership 2013).

Currently, environmental management has very low priority, maybe as a result of the urgent desire for novel technologies that could quickly resolve the malaria problem (Lindsay et al. 2002). The opportunity, however, not only exists but is unique at a time when malaria eradication is back to the health agenda, as detailed in the next section.

FUTURE PERSPECTIVES

Inspired by the 2007 Gates Malaria Forum, malaria eradication came back to the global health agenda. Malaria-endemic countries intensified control measures, particularly indoor residual spraying, use of artemisinin combination therapy for treatment, and distribution of insecticide treated nets. Significant progress has been achieved, and since the year 2000, the average prevalence of malaria infection in children aged 2–10 has declined by 47%, and an increasing number of countries are moving toward malaria elimination. Despite these achievements, there are still 198 million cases of malaria, about 584,000 deaths annually (WHO 2014), and challenges abound (Table 1).

Specifically related to the environment, existing unfavorable conditions as well as ongoing and projected environmental changes must be analyzed considering the interactions between the different elements in the malaria system. For example, environmental transformations may result in vector behavior change, imposing constraints on vector control interventions (Ferguson et al. 2010). This complexity of the system deserves more careful attention by malaria control programs, as exemplified next.

Housing improvements that could help reduce malaria transmission include screening of doors, windows, and eaves, closing eaves, installing ceilings, improving roofs, sealing cracks in walls, using higher quality building materials, creating new housing designs, and installing eave tubes (Lindsay et al. 2002; Ogoma et al. 2009; Tusting et al. 2015). Those are applicable in areas where conditions leave inhabitants highly exposed to contact with malaria vectors, such as urban and rural areas where poor housing prevails, and in refugee camps. The increase in conflicts that force populations into refugee camps (Rowland and Nosten 2001) and the increase in the frequency and intensity of natural disasters (IPCC 2013), demanding quick housing solutions, are two examples of current and future threats to malaria eradication efforts that could be mitigated with housing improvement, combined with other interventions.

In addition, current patterns of urban growth that result in concentration of poor housing and lack of infrastructure can facilitate the vector adaptation to water habitats that traditionally would not be suitable for mosquito breeding, and the creation of pockets of malaria infection among worse off areas. In this regard, recent population trends show that although currently Africa is the least urbanized region (40% of the population living in urban areas), it shows the fastest pace of urbanization and by 2050, 56% of its population will be living in urban areas (United Nations et al. 2015). Thus, in anticipation of major changes, intersectoral collaboration becomes crucial. Environmental management strategies should be implemented concurrently with city growth, minimizing the negative effects commonly associated with rapid and unplanned urbanization (United Nations et al. 2015).

Also, environmental management is likely to increase the return of other malaria control interventions. For example, in Dar es Salaam, a third of all anopheline-positive water habitats were found in drains (Castro et al. 2010). Considering that the city has included larval control in the package of interventions, the cost and effort invested in that activity could be reduced if drains were regularly maintained to prevent water stagnation. The initial cost of cleaning drains may be high, given the massive accumulation of waste materials after years of lacking proper maintenance. However, in the long run, costs of keeping drains clean are lower than the resources needed to acquire and apply larvicides in the drains (UMCP et al. 2007; Castro et al. 2009). In addition, the use of environmental management strategies is likely to impact other vector-borne diseases (e.g., dengue and lymphatic filariasis), contributing to a much broader health improvement.

Although expanding areas protected under environmental conservation policies would be beneficial to prevent an increase in malaria transmission (Bauch et al. 2015), current trends make it reasonable to expect that deforestation will continue to be a reason for concern, particularly in the Amazon forest, driven by cattle ranching, agriculture, mining, large-scale development projects, and land invasions. When deforestation is planned and/or anticipated because of a specific activity that is implemented through legally approved mechanisms (e.g., development projects), there is an opportunity to adopt mitigation strategies to prevent increases in vector density and in malaria transmission. To be successful, however, these strategies must be closely monitored. In contrast, when deforestation results from illegal operations there is

no planning, no warning, and thus no opportunity to counteract the impacts on malaria. In such a scenario, outbreaks are often observed, and responses only happen after a major health problem has already happened.

Considered as the biggest global health threat of the 21st century (Costello et al. 2009; WHO 2009; Watts et al. 2015), climate change is a significant environmental change currently unfolding, with worldwide consequences. Climatic effects on vector-borne diseases can occur directly, through extreme events (e.g., drought, flooding), increases in average temperature, and changes in precipitation patterns, but also indirectly, by population displacement and water and food insecurity, which impact individuals' exposure and vulnerability to infections.

Despite the uncertainty embedded in climate change scenarios (IPCC 2013), malaria burden is likely to be impacted by climate change. The magnitude of the impact will depend on many issues, such as (1) the pattern of variability in temperature (Paaijmans et al. 2010); (2) how countries are planning in anticipation of future changes; (3) how adaptation strategies are adopted at varied scales (individual, community, institutional); (4) the combination of malaria control strategies in place; (5) the extent to which the risk of infection determined by local characteristics can be augmented by climatic changes; and (6) the level of clinical immunity (Laneri et al. 2015). Such complexity is reflected by contrasting results of global models on the impact of climate change on malaria (Martens et al. 1999; Rogers and Randolph 2000; Pascual et al. 2006; Gething et al. 2010; Yamana and Eltahir 2013; Laneri et al. 2015). The impacts and the responses are unlikely to be uniform across and within regions (Takken et al. 2005), and this adds another layer of complexity to the efforts of malaria eradication.

CONCLUDING REMARKS

Environmental factors affect malaria transmission in different ways depending on the local ecosystem and on the transformations it has suffered through human action. They also interact with other elements of the malaria system, resulting in a variety of local transmission profiles. This is a characteristic of malaria that adds complexity to disease control and elimination. There is no unique combination of control strategies that works in every setting, and each must be tailored to address local characteristics of transmission.

As malaria-endemic countries embrace elimination goals, focus has been given to testing, treatment, and vector control by indoor residual spraying and insecticide treated nets. Overall, environmental aspects have not received much attention by malaria control programs. One could argue that potential reasons include (1) limited financial and human resources; (2) lack of local expertise integrating health, hydrology, and engineering; (3) restricted knowledge on the additional benefit of adopting environmental management in different settings in combination with other interventions already in place; and (4) the desire to find a new technological solution.

It is unquestionable that progress in reducing cases and deaths has been achieved in the past decade, although not uniformly across and within countries. Although significant reductions can be achieved without control strategies that focus on the environment, the assumption that a fully successful control program can exist while neglecting environmental issues is naïve, and a mistake from a programmatic point of view.

Arguments favoring environmental interventions are threefold. First, by targeting all elements of the malaria system progress toward elimination can be faster and more cost effective. Because the elements of the system interact with each other, the returns from interventions can be maximized by concurrently addressing all elements, for example, human behavior affects the impact of other interventions (such as bednet use). Thus, by including behavior change campaigns in the control package it is possible to maximize local acceptance and updates of other interventions; also, environmental management can contribute to reducing the costs of other interventions, such as use of larviciding. Second, gains are likely to be sustainable. Because environmental strategies target

the source of the problem (from a vector point of view) and have a long-term impact (if properly maintained), it is expected that the direct benefits, and interactions with other elements in the malaria system, will last longer. Third, environmental management benefits go beyond malaria and are expected to also affect the incidence of dengue, lymphatic filariasis, and other vector-borne diseases. Thus, by promoting a healthier environment, these interventions make an important contribution to the overall improvement of local health conditions, probably reaching out to populations that are not directly benefited by other malaria control interventions.

Environmental management strategies have been successfully implemented in malaria-endemic settings in the past (Keiser et al. 2005b). The knowledge regarding what/how to do is available, and so is the evidence regarding its impact. Considering the current scenario, where (1) changes to the environment are fast, often unplanned, significantly favoring vector breeding, and thus should be mitigated, (2) extreme weather events are more frequent and intense, and therefore adaptation strategies are urgently needed, and (3) vectors adapt to urban ecologies, breeding in places previously considered to be unsuitable for larval development, failing to introduce environmental strategies into the package of malaria control interventions is a missed opportunity with implications for the success and sustainability of other control efforts. However, the adoption of environmental strategies demands local knowledge and expertise: knowledge to identify places where targeting the environment is feasible and beneficial to the reduction of malaria transmission; entomological knowledge on vector species composition and behavior; and expertise to plan, implement, maintain, and monitor the activities.

Realistically, it is probably the case that most malaria control programs do not have the proper knowledge and expertise to effectively account for the local environment in control efforts, and maybe do not even have comprehensive entomological information (Ulrich et al. 2013). Thus, filling in these gaps is imperative, and the task could be better accomplished by fostering an integrated collaboration between donors, the industry, academia, and different sectors of the government (United Nations Development Programme and Roll Back Malaria Partnership 2013).

One of the challenges for incorporating environmental interventions is funding. Most resources are placed on interventions that have shown to be effective in bringing about significant declines in transmission in high-endemic countries (bednets, indoor residual spraying, and treatment). However, if a plateau is achieved, and those interventions are not able to promote further declines, what is the next step? Incorporation of other well-known but currently less used interventions, such as environmental management, may lack the political and financial support because funding agencies might not be willing to sponsor them on the grounds that (1) they are not novel, (2) they are not a priority, or (3) the country has no knowledge and expertise to implement them. Depending on the local characteristics of malaria transmission, such a scenario may hamper attempts to quickly move toward elimination.

As elimination/eradication takes a prominent place in the health agenda of malaria-endemic countries; an integrated action, addressing all elements of the malaria system, which contributes to improve knowledge and to build local capacity, and that brings about positive effects to the health of the local population, has the greatest changes to produce fast, effective, and sustainable results.

REFERENCES

Awolola TS, Oduola AO, Obansa JB, Chukwurar NJ, Unyimadu JP. 2007. *Anopheles gambiae s.s.* breeding in polluted water bodies in urban Lagos, southwestern Nigeria. *J Vector Borne Dis* **44:** 241–244.

Baolin L. 1988. Environmental management for the control of ricefield-breeding mosquitoes in China. Vector-borne disease control in humans through rice agroecosystem management. *Proceedings of the Workshop on Research and Training Needs in the Field of Integrated Vector-Borne Disease Control in Riceland Agroecosystems of Developing Countries.* March 9–14, 1987 (ed. IRR Institute), pp. 111–121. International Rice Research Institute in collaboration with the WHO/FAO/UNEP Panel of Experts on Environmental Management for Vector Control, Manila, Philippines.

Bauch SC, Birkenbach AM, Pattanayak SK, Sills EO. 2015. Public health impacts of ecosystem change in the Brazilian Amazon. *Proc Natl Acad Sci* **112:** 7414–7419.

Bomblies A, Duchemin JB, Eltahir EAB. 2008. Hydrology of malaria: Model development and application to a Sahelian village. *Water Resources Res* **44:** W12445.

Boyd MF. 1926. The influence of obstacles unconsciously erected against anophelines (housing and screening) upon the incidence of malaria. *Am J Trop Med Hyg* **6:** 157–160.

Carter R, Mendis KN. 2002. Evolutionary and historical aspects of the burden of malaria. *Clin Microbiol Rev* **15:** 564–594.

Castro MC, Singer BH. 2011. Malaria in the Brazilian Amazon. In *Water and sanitation related diseases and the environment: Challenges, interventions and preventive measures* (ed. Selendy J), pp. 401–420. Wiley, Hoboken, NJ.

Castro MC, Yamagata Y, Mtasiwa D, Tanner M, Utzinger J, Keiser J, Singer BH. 2004. Integrated urban malaria control: A case study in Dar es Salaam, Tanzania. *Am J Trop Med Hyg* **71:** 103–117.

Castro MC, Monte-Mór RL, Sawyer DO, Singer BH. 2006. Malaria risk on the Amazon frontier. *Proc Natl Acad Sci* **103:** 2452–2457.

Castro MC, Tsuruta A, Kanamori S, Kannady K, Mkude S. 2009. Community-based environmental management for malaria control: Evidence from a small-scale intervention in Dar es Salaam, Tanzania. *Malaria J* **8:** 57.

Castro MC, Kanamori S, Kannady K, Mkude S, Killeen GF, Fillinger U. 2010. The importance of drains for the larval development of lymphatic filariasis and malaria vectors in Dar es Salaam, United Republic of Tanzania. *PLoS Negl Trop Dis* **4:** e693.

Chinery WA. 1984. Effects of ecological changes on the malaria vectors *Anopheles funestus* and the *Anopheles gambiae* complex of mosquitoes in Accra, Ghana. *J Trop Med Hyg* **87:** 75–81.

Costello A, Abbas M, Allen A, Ball S, Bell S, Bellamy R, Friel S, Groce N, Johnson A, Kett M, et al. 2009. Managing the health effects of climate change. *Lancet* **373:** 1693–1733.

Craig MH, Snow RW, le Sueur D. 1999. A climate-based distribution model of malaria transmission in sub-Saharan Africa. *Parasitol Today* **15:** 105–111.

Cruz OG. 1972. Madeira-Mamoré Railway Company: Considerações gerais sobre as condições sanitárias do rio Madeira. 1910 [Madeira Mamoré Railway Company: Overall assessment of the sanitary conditions of the Madeira River. 1910]. In *Opera ominia* (ed. Cruz OG), pp. 564–624. Instituto Oswaldo Cruz, Rio de Janeiro.

Deane LM. 1988. Malaria studies and control in Brazil. *Am J Trop Med Hyg* **38:** 223–230.

De Silva PM, Marshall JM. 2012. Factors contributing to urban malaria transmission in sub-Saharan Africa: A systematic review. *J Trop Med* **2012:** 819563.

Dida G, Gelder F, Anyona D, Abuom P, Onyuka J, Matano AS, Adoka S, Kanangire C, Owuor P, Ouma C, et al. 2015. Presence and distribution of mosquito larvae predators and factors influencing their abundance along the Mara River, Kenya and Tanzania. *SpringerPlus* **4:** 136.

Dongus S, Nyika D, Kannady K, Mtasiwa D, Mshinda H, Gosoniu L, Drescher AW, Fillinger U, Tanner M, Killeen GF, et al. 2009. Urban agriculture and *Anopheles* habitats in Dar es Salaam, Tanzania. *Geospatial Health* 3: 189–210.

Erlanger TE, Krieger GR, Singer BH, Utzinger J. 2008. The 6/94 gap in health impact assessment. *Environ Impact Assess Rev* 28: 349–358.

Ferguson HM, Dornhaus A, Beeche A, Borgemeister C, Gottlieb M, Mulla MS, Gimnig JE, Fish D, Killeen GF. 2010. Ecology: A prerequisite for malaria elimination and eradication. *PLoS Med* 7: e1000303.

Fillinger U, Kannady K, William G, Vanek MJ, Dongus S, Nyika D, Geissbuhler Y, Chaki P, Govella NJ, Mathenge E, et al. 2008. A tool box for operational mosquito larval control: Preliminary results and early lessons from the urban malaria control programme in Dar es Salaam, Tanzania. *Malaria J* 7: 20.

Gagnon AS, Smoyer-Tomic KE, Bush ABG. 2002. The El Niño southern oscillation and malaria epidemics in South America. *Int J Biometeorol* 46: 81–89.

Gamage-Mendis AC, Carter R, Mendis C, De Zoysa AP, Herath PR, Mendis KN. 1991. Clustering of malaria infections within an endemic population: Risk of malaria associated with the type of housing construction. *Am J Trop Med Hyg* 45: 77–85.

Gething PW, Smith DL, Patil AP, Tatem AJ, Snow RW, Hay SI. 2010. Climate change and the global malaria recession. *Nature* 465: 342–346.

Gething P, Van Boeckel T, Smith D, Guerra C, Patil A, Snow R, Hay S. 2011. Modelling the global constraints of temperature on transmission of *Plasmodium falciparum* and *P. vivax*. *Parasit Vectors* 4: 92.

Ghebreyesus TA, Haile M, Witten KH, Getachew A, Yohannes AM, Yohannes M, Teklehaimanot HD, Lindsay SW, Byass P. 1999. Incidence of malaria among children living near dams in northern Ethiopia: Community based incidence survey. *BMJ* 319: 663–666.

Gorgas GWC. 1915. *Sanitation in Panama*. Appleton, New York.

Gryseels C, Durnez L, Gerrets R, Uk S, Suon S, Set S, Phoeuk P, Sluydts V, Heng S, Sochantha T, et al. 2015. Re-imagining malaria: Heterogeneity of human and mosquito behaviour in relation to residual malaria transmission in Cambodia. *Malaria J* 14: 165.

Hackett L. 1937. *Malaria in Europe: An ecological study*. Oxford University Press, London.

Hahn MB, Gangnon RE, Barcellos C, Asner GP, Patz JA. 2014. Influence of deforestation, logging, and fire on malaria in the Brazilian Amazon. *PLoS ONE* 9: e85725.

International Rice Research Institute, Joint WHO/FAO/UNEP Panel of Experts on Environmental Management for Vector Control. 1988. *Vector-borne disease control in humans through rice agroecosystem management. Proceedings of the Workshop on Research and Training Needs in the Field of Integrated Vector-Borne Disease Control in Riceland Agroecosystems of Developing Countries*. March 9–14, 1987. International Rice Research Institute in collaboration with the WHO/FAO/UNEP Panel of Experts on Environmental Management for Vector Control, Manila, Philippines.

IPCC. 2013. *Final draft underlying scientific-technical assessment. IPCC 5th assessment report "Climate change 2013: The physical science basis," Working Group I—12th Session*. Stockholm, September 23–26, 2013, www.ipcc.ch/report/ar5/wg1/#.UkveNn_gFTU.

Jackson S, Sleigh A. 2000. Resettlement for China's Three Gorges Dam: Socio-economic impact and institutional tensions. *Communis Post-Commun* 33: 223–241.

Jawara M, Pinder M, Drakeley CJ, Nwakanma DC, Jallow E, Bogth C, Lindsay SW, Conway DJ. 2008. Dry season ecology of *Anopheles gambiae* complex mosquitoes in The Gambia. *Malaria J* 7: 156.

Kebede A, McCann JC, Kiszewski AE, Ye-Ebiyo Y. 2005. New evidence of the effects of agro-ecologic change on malaria transmission. *Am J Trop Med Hyg* 73: 676–680.

Keiser J, Utzinger J, Castro MC, Smith T, Tanner M, Singer BH. 2004. Urbanization in sub-Saharan Africa and implications for malaria control. *Am J Trop Med Hyg* 71: 118–127.

Keiser J, Castro MC, Maltese MF, Bos R, Tanner M, Singer BH, Utzinger J. 2005a. Effect of irrigation and large dams on the burden of malaria on global and regional scale. *Am J Trop Med Hyg* 72: 392–406.

Keiser J, Singer BH, Utzinger J. 2005b. Reducing the burden of malaria in different eco-epidemiological settings with environmental management: A systematic review. *Lancet Infect Dis* 5: 695–708.

Kilian AH, Langi P, Talisuna A, Kabagambe G. 1999. Rainfall pattern, El Niño and malaria in Uganda. *Trans R Soc Trop Med Hyg* 93: 22–23.

Knoblauch A, Winkler M, Archer C, Divall M, Owuor M, Yapo R, Yao P, Utzinger J. 2014. The epidemiology of malaria and anaemia in the Bonikro mining area, central Cote d'Ivoire. *Malaria J* 13: 194.

Konradsen F, van der Hoek W, Amerasinghe FP, Mutero C, Boelee E. 2004. Engineering and malaria control: Learning from the past 100 years. *Acta Tropica* 89: 99–108

Kovats RS, Bouma MJ, Haines A. 1999. *El Niño and health*. World Health Organization, Geneva.

Kovats RS, Bouma MJ, Hajat S, Worrall E, Haines A. 2003. El Niño and health. *Lancet* 362: 1481–1489.

Laneri K, Paul RE, Tall A, Faye J, Diene-Sarr F, Sokhna C, Trape JF, Rodó X. 2015. Dynamical malaria models reveal how immunity buffers effect of climate variability. *Proc Natl Acad Sci* 112: 8786–8791.

Lerer LB, Scudder T. 1999. Health impacts of large dams. *Environ Impact Assess Rev* 19: 113–123.

Lindblade KA, Walker ED, Onapa AW, Katungu J, Wilson ML. 1999. Highland malaria in Uganda: Prospective analysis of an epidemic associated with El Niño. *Trans R Soc Trop Med Hyg* 480–487: 480–487.

Lindsay SW, Bodker R, Malima R, Msangeni HA, Kisinza W. 2000. Effect of 1997–98 El Niño on highland malaria in Tanzania. *Lancet* 355: 989–990.

Lindsay SW, Emerson PM, Charlwood JD. 2002. Reducing malaria by mosquito-proofing houses. *Trends Parasitol* 18: 510–514.

Loevinsohn ME. 1994. Climatic warming and increased malaria incidence in Rwanda. *Lancet* 343: 714–718.

Ludescher J, Gozolchiani A, Bogachev MI, Bunde A, Havlin S, Schellnhuber HJ. 2014. Very early warning of next El Niño. *Proc Natl Acad Sci* 111: 2064–2066.

 Cite this article as *Cold Spring Harb Perspect Med* doi: 10.1101/cshperspect.a025601

Macdonald G. 1957. *The epidemiology and control of malaria*. Oxford University Press, London.

Maheu-Giroux M, Castro MC. 2013. Do malaria vector control measures impact disease-related behaviour and knowledge? Evidence from a large-scale larviciding intervention in Tanzania. *Malaria J* **12:** 422.

Martens WM, Jetten T, Focks D. 1997. Sensitivity of malaria, schistosomiasis and dengue to global warming. *Climatic Change* **35:** 145–156.

Martens P, Kovats RS, Nijhof S, Vries Pd, Livermore MTJ, Bradley DJ, Cox J, McMichael AJ. 1999. Climate change and future populations at risk of malaria. *Global Environ Change* **9:** S89–S107.

Mordecai EA, Paaijmans KP, Johnson LR, Balzer C, Ben-Horin T, Moor E, McNally A, Pawar S, Ryan SJ, Smith TC, et al. 2013. Optimal temperature for malaria transmission is dramatically lower than previously predicted. *Ecol Lett* **16:** 22–30.

Neiva A. 1940. Profilaxia da malária e trabalhos de engenharia: Notas, comentários, recordações. *Revista Clube Engenharia* **VI:** 60–75.

Ogoma S, Kannady K, Sikulu M, Chaki P, Govella N, Mukabana W, Killeen G. 2009. Window screening, ceilings and closed eaves as sustainable ways to control malaria in Dar es Salaam, Tanzania. *Malaria J* **8:** 221.

Paaijmans KP, Wandago MO, Githeko AK, Takken W. 2007. Unexpected high losses of *Anopheles gambiae* larvae due to rainfall. *PLoS ONE* **2:** e1146.

Paaijmans KP, Blanford S, Bell AS, Blanford JI, Read AF, Thomas MB. 2010. Influence of climate on malaria transmission depends on daily temperature variation. *Proc Natl Acad Sci* **107:** 15135–15139.

Parham PE, Michael E. 2010. Modeling the effects of weather and climate change on malaria transmission. *Environ Health Perspect* **118:** 620–626.

Pascual M, Ahumada JA, Chaves LF, Rodó X, Bouma M. 2006. Malaria resurgence in the East African highlands: Temperature trends revisited. *Proc Natl Acad Sci* **103:** 5829–5834.

Peixoto A. 1917. *O problema sanitário da Amazônia*, p. 28. Officinas Graphicas da Bibliotheca Nacional, Rio de Janeiro, Brazil.

Pinotti M. 1951. The biological basis for the campaign against the malaria vectors in Brazil. *Trans R Soc Trop Med Hyg* **44:** 663–682.

Pomeroy AWJ. 1920. The prophylaxis of malaria in Dar es Salaam, East Africa. *J Royal Army Med Corps* **35:** 44–63.

Rogers DJ, Randolph SE. 2000. The global spread of malaria in a future, warmer world. *Science* **289:** 1763–1766.

Rowland M, Nosten F. 2001. Malaria epidemiology and control in refugee camps and complex emergencies. *Ann Trop Med Parasitol* **95:** 741–754.

Sáenz R, Bissell RA, Paniagua F. 1995. Post-disaster malaria in Costa Rica. *Prehosp Disaster Med* **10:** 154–160.

Sattler MA, Mtasiwa D, Kiama M, Premji Z, Tanner M, Killeen GF, Lengeler C. 2005. Habitat characterization and spatial distribution of *Anopheles* sp. mosquito larvae in Dar es Salaam (Tanzania) during an extended dry period. *Malaria J* **4:** 4.

Sawyer DR, Sawyer DO. 1987. *Malaria on the Amazon frontier: Economic and social aspects of transmission and control*. CEDEPLAR, Belo Horizonte, Brazil.

Service MW. 1980. *A guide to medical entomology*. Macmillan, London.

Singer BH, Castro MC. 2011. Reassessing multiple-intervention malaria control programs of the past: Lessons for the design of contemporary interventions. In *Water and sanitation related diseases and the environment: Challenges, interventions and preventive measures* (ed. Selendy J), pp. 151–166. Wiley, Hoboken, NJ.

Singh N, Sharma VP. 2002. Patterns of rainfall and malaria in Madhya Pradesh, central India. *Ann Trop Med Parasitol* **96:** 349–359.

Stromquist WG. 1920. Malaria control from the engineering point of view. *Am J Public Health* **10:** 497–501.

Takken W, Vilarinhos PTR, Schneider P, Santos F. 2005. Effects of environmental change on malaria in the Amazon region of Brazil. In *Environmental change and malaria risk: Global and local implications* (ed. Takken W, Martens P, Bogers R), pp. 113–123. Wageningen University, The Netherlands.

Tusting L, Ippolito M, Willey B, Kleinschmidt I, Dorsey G, Gosling R, Lindsay S. 2015. The evidence for improving housing to reduce malaria: A systematic review and meta-analysis. *Malaria J* **14:** 209.

Ulrich JN, Naranjo DP, Alimi TO, Müller GC, Beier JC. 2013. How much vector control is needed to achieve malaria elimination? *Trends Parasitol* **29:** 104–109.

UMCP, IMCP, NMCP, JICA, HSPH. 2007. *Assessment of the impact of environmental management on larval presence and prevalence of malaria infection in Dar es Salaam, Tanzania. Survey description and standard operational procedures*. Urban Malaria Control Programme (UMCP), Integrated Malaria Control Project (IMCP), Tanzania National Malaria Control Programme (NMCP), Japan International Cooperation Agency (JICA), Harvard School of Public Health (HSPH), Dar es Salaam, Tanzania.

United Nations, Department of Economic and Social Affairs, Population Division. 2015. *World urbanization prospects: The 2014 revision*, ST/ESA/SER.A/366. United Nations, New York.

United Nations Development Programme, Roll Back Malaria Partnership. 2013. *Multisectoral action framework for malaria*. United Nations Development Programme (UNDP) and Roll Back Malaria Partnership (RBM), Geneva.

Utzinger J, Tozan Y, Doumani F, Singer BH. 2002. The economic payoffs of integrated malaria control in the Zambian copperbelt between 1930 and 1950. *Trop Med Int Health* **7:** 657–677.

Warrell DA, Gilles HM. 2002. *Essential malariology*. Arnold, New York.

Watson JT, Gayer M, Connolly MA. 2007. Epidemics after natural disasters. *Emerg Infect Dis* **13:** 1–5.

Watson M. 1921. *The prevention of malaria in the Federated Malay States: A record of twenty years' progress*. J. Murray, London.

Watson M. 1953. *African highway: The battle for health in Central Africa*. J. Murray, London.

Watts N, Adger WN, Agnolucci P, Blackstock J, Byass P, Cai W, Chaytor S, Colbourn T, Collins M, Cooper A, et al. 2015. Health and climate change: policy responses to protect public health. *Lancet* **386:** 1861–1914.

WHO. 1982. Manual on environmental management for mosquito control: With special emphasis on malaria vectors. World Health Organization, Geneva.

WHO. 2000. El Niño and its health impact. World Health Organization (WHO Fact Sheet No. 192 rev.), Geneva.

WHO. 2009. Protecting health from climate change: Global research priorities. World Health Organization, Geneva.

WHO. 2014. World malaria report 2014. World Health Organization, Geneva.

Yamana TK, Eltahir EAB. 2013. Projected impacts of climate change on environmental suitability for malaria transmission in West Africa. *Environ Health Perspect* **121:** 1179–1186.

Yasuoka J, Levins R. 2007. Impact of deforestation and agricultural development on anopheline ecology and malaria epidemiology. *Am J Trop Med Hyg* **76:** 450–460.

Ye-Ebiyo Y, Pollack RJ, Spielman A. 2000. Enhanced development in nature of larval *Anopheles arabiensis* mosquitoes feeding on maize pollen. *Am J Trop Med Hyg* **63:** 90–93.

Cite this article as *Cold Spring Harb Perspect Med* doi: 10.1101/cshperspect.a025601

Determinants of Malaria Transmission at the Population Level

Teun Bousema[1,2] and Chris Drakeley[2]

[1]Department of Medical Microbiology, Radboud University Medical Center, Nijmegen 6525 GA, The Netherlands

[2]Department of Immunology & Infection, London School of Hygiene & Tropical Medicine, London WC1E 7HT, United Kingdom

Correspondence: teun.bousema@radboudumc.nl; chris.drakeley@lshtm.ac.uk

Transmission of malaria from man to mosquito defines the human infectious reservoir of malaria. At the population level this is influenced by a variety of human, parasite, and mosquito vector factors some or all of which may vary depending on the epidemiological setting. Here, we review our current state of knowledge related to human infectiousness to mosquitoes and how current malaria control strategies might be adapted to focus on reducing this. While much progress has been made in malaria control, we argue that an improved understanding of human infectivity will allow more effective use of current control tools and make elimination a more feasible goal.

Considerable progress has been made in our understanding of the production and maturation of *Plasmodium falciparum* gametocytes and associated factors related to the biology of malaria transmission at the level of the individual malaria-infected patients (Meibalan and Marti 2016). In this review, we examine how these individual factors combine with epidemiological and entomological elements to define transmission at the population level. The premise is that if we are able to better understand transmission, we can then more effectively target malaria transmission stages in the fraction of the human population that is most important for onward malaria transmission to mosquitoes. Moreover, improving our understanding of malaria transmission at the population level will also allow more accurate monitoring of the effects of control and elimination programs to specifically counter the likelihood of resurgence of malaria in areas that remain receptive to malaria.

THE HUMAN PARASITE RESERVOIR: A MATTER OF SENSITIVITY

Community estimates of parasite carriage by microscopy (as parasite prevalence) are the most widely available malaria metrics and are commonly used to compare malaria transmission intensity between areas (Hay et al. 2009) and compare infection burden between different populations within malaria-endemic regions (Smith et al. 2005). Routine microscopy has a sensitivity in the range of $50-100$ parasites/μL of blood (Okell et al. 2012). Rapid diagnostic tests (RDTs), lateral flow devices that are based on histidine-rich protein 2 (HRP2) or *Plasmodium* lactate dehydrogenase (pLDH) and aldolase (Bell et al. 2006), achieve a similar sensitivity ~100 parasites/μL (Banoo et al. 2006) and are increasingly widely used for routine malaria diagnosis and epidemiological surveys (Bastiaens et al. 2014). Estimates of parasite prevalence from RDTs are often slightly higher than microscopy because of the persistence of antigen after infection has been cleared (Wu et al. 2015). Molecular methods for malaria detection and species identification include nested polymerase chain reaction (nPCR) (Snounou et al. 1993), quantitative PCR (qPCR), quantitative reverse transcription (qRT)-PCR, and nucleic acid sequence-based amplification (NASBA), and invariably detect a larger number of infections. nPCR, for which most data is available, in conjunction with microscopy data, detects approximately twice as many infections as microscopy (Okell et al. 2012), but the fraction of infections that is undetectable by microscopy varies considerably between endemic areas and population groups. Although parasite prevalence overall is lower, the proportion of infections present at submicroscopic parasite densities is largest in low-endemic areas (Fig. 1). This may reflect the lower density of malaria parasites in low transmission settings that may, in turn, be explained by a lower likelihood of superinfection and a large fraction of monoclonal infections, which are better controlled by the human immune system (Okell et al. 2012). In all areas in which transmission intensity is sufficiently high to elicit an age-dependent acquisition of immunity, adults are more likely to carry submicroscopic infections (Proietti et al. 2011; Nguyen et al. 2012; Mosha et al. 2013). The role of antimalarial immunity in determining the density and detectability of infections is currently incompletely understood. In the context of malaria-elimination initiatives, it is of great relevance to understand the influence of waning residual immunity (that follows successful malaria control) on the likelihood that malaria infections elicit malaria symptoms and reach densities that are detectable by currently available diagnostics (Wu et al. 2015).

GAMETOCYTE PRODUCTION AND THE HUMAN INFECTIOUS RESERVOIR

Not surprisingly, in a similar way that molecular diagnostics have identified increased number of malaria infections, molecular assays for the sexual-stage gametocytes have unveiled a previously unappreciated pool of low-density gametocyte carriers (Bousema and Drakeley 2011). The detection of gametocyte-specific mRNA, primarily based on Pfs25 mRNA (Bousema and Drakeley 2011; Wampfler et al. 2013), pfg377, or Pfs230 (Nwakanma et al. 2008), has shown that mature gametocytes can be detected in the majority of symptomatic (Nassir et al. 2005; Nwakanma et al. 2008; Sawa et al. 2013; Eziefula et al. 2014) and asymptomatically *P. falciparum*–infected individuals (Ouedraogo et al. 2007; Shekalaghe et al. 2007; Nwakanma et al. 2008), even if densities of asexual parasites are below the microscopic threshold for detection (Ouedraogo et al. 2007; Shekalaghe et al. 2007; Wampfler et al. 2013).

The presence of an undetectable gametocyte fraction was assumed before the advent of molecular gametocyte diagnostics as a result of observations of successful mosquito infections from individuals who had no gametocytes detected by microscopy (Boudin et al. 1993b; Bousema et al. 2012a). The proportion of mosquitoes that becomes infected after feeding on these submicroscopic, and therefore low-density, gametocyte carriers is typically two- to fivefold lower than on microscopy-positive gametocyte carriers (Coleman et al. 2004; Schneider et al. 2007; Ouedraogo et al. 2009, 2015; Bousema et al. 2012a; Churcher et al. 2013). However, the high number of these individuals in many endemic settings makes submicroscopic gametocyte carriers potentially significant contributors to malaria transmission (Bousema et al. 2014).

It would seem important that from a public health perspective, a better understanding of the detectability of malaria infections that infect mosquitoes and quantification of the relative contribution of patent and subpatent infections to the human infectious reservoir is required. As examples, two recent studies that determined

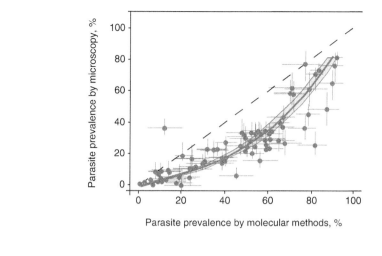

Figure 1. Submicroscopic parasite carriage as a function of malaria transmission intensity. Prevalence of *Plasmodium falciparum* infections detected by nested polymerase chain reaction (nPCR, *x*-axis) or microscopy (*y*-axis) in the same individuals. Each data point and associated confidence intervals represent data from one cross-sectional survey. The dotted line shows the correlation that would be expected if the prevalence of infection detected by both methods was the same. The solid line with shaded area represents the best fit to the data and confidence interval (Okell et al. 2012). (Panel from Okell et al. 2012; adapted, with permission, from the authors.) The shaded arrows in the panel below shows (*top*) the intensity of malaria transmission, which is typically defined by microscopy and ranges from low to high transmission intensity; (*middle*) the average parasite density in infections that increases with transmission intensity; and (*bottom*) the proportion of infections that is submicroscopic. While the proportion of the population that is malaria-infected is lowest in low-endemic settings, the fraction of these infections that is submicroscopic (undetectable by microscopy and rapid diagnostic tests [RDTs]) (Wu et al. 2015) is largest in low-endemic settings.

infectivity in community surveys indicate that onward transmission to mosquitoes is possible from infections that have no detectable gametocytes or asexual parasites by microscopy. In a moderate transmission setting in Senegal, 8% (2/25) of infectious individuals had no parasites detected by microscopy, yet were responsible for 18.2% (12/66) of all mosquito infections. A similar study in a high-endemic setting in Burkina Faso found that 28.7% (25/87) of infectious individuals were parasite-free by microscopy, yet responsible for 17.0% (145/855) of all infected mosquitoes (Ouedraogo et al.

2015). The latter study was the first to use molecular assays in combination with mosquito feeding assays and confirmed that all infectious individuals had parasites detected by RNA-based diagnostics (Ouedraogo et al. 2015). In a setting of intense malaria transmission in Burkina Faso, a substantial proportion of infectious individuals harbored parasite densities below 100 parasites/μL, the density realistically detected by microscopy and RDTs (Fig. 2). These and other findings from transmission studies (Stone et al. 2015) would suggest two relatively clear and distinct paths for diagnostics for re-

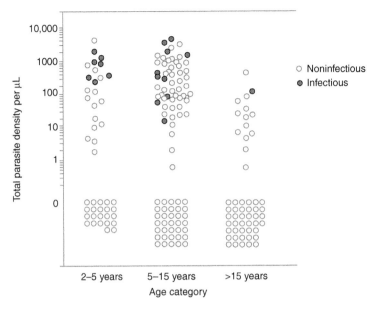

Figure 2. Parasite density and infectivity in relation to age in an area of intense malaria transmission. Each dot represents an individual in which parasite carriage was determined and quantified by a quantitative polymerase chain reaction (qPCR) (Hermsen et al. 2001) and onward malaria transmission was determined by membrane feeding assays. Open dots represent uninfected individuals (parasite density equals zero) or malaria-infected individuals who are not infectious to mosquitoes. Closed circles indicate infectious individuals. Parasite density and the likelihood of infecting mosquitoes are highest in children; onward transmission to mosquitoes is commonly observed at densities below the microscopic threshold for detection (Slater et al. 2015).

search and public health settings. First, more detailed research studies aiming to quantify the human infectious reservoir or quantify the impact of transmission-blocking interventions would benefit from the use of sensitive, quantitative molecular tools to detect asexual parasite populations and gametocytes. In contrast, outside research settings, malaria surveillance and surveys to support and evaluate community interventions would not require gametocyte-specific diagnostics but instead rely on sensitive methods to detect all stages of infection on the assumption that all parasite infections are viable sources of gametocytes and therefore potentially infectious (Bousema et al. 2014).

DEMOGRAPHIC AND ENVIRONMENTAL FACTORS INFLUENCING MALARIA TRANSMISSIBILITY

Many previous studies aiming to determine the human infectious reservoir often selected individuals with microscopically detected gametocytes for transmission experiments (Stone et al. 2015) and, as discussed above, it is now clear that this approach will have missed individuals who harbor submicroscopic gametocyte densities and who are potentially infectious. However, even if individuals are selected randomly from a population to assess their infectivity, these infectivity assessments do not allow drawing firm conclusions on the relative importance of different populations for onward transmission. The selection of study participants often does not take into account the demographic structure of populations. All available studies on the human infectivity to mosquitoes that included a wide age range, observed that the proportion of mosquitoes that become infected in mosquito feeding assays is higher in children, because they have higher gametocyte densities than adults (Muirhead-Thomson 1957; Graves et al. 1988; Githeko et al. 1992; Boudin et al. 1993a; Bonnet et al. 2003; Gaye et al. 2015). Yet, when estimates are adjusted for the demographic composition of the population, the importance of older individuals becomes clearer and in many settings adults comprise >20% of the human infectious reservoir (Muirhead-Thomson 1957; Graves et al. 1988; Githeko et al. 1992; Bonnet et al. 2003; Stone et al. 2015). This contribution may be increased further if, in addition to demographic composition, both accessibility and attractiveness of humans to mosquitoes are also considered. These factors have never been directly incorporated in assessments of the human infectious reservoir, although it is well known that the number of mosquito bites a person experiences is highly variable. This is mostly driven by human behavior and use of protective measures. In areas with good bednet coverage because of the specific targeting of children and pregnant women, net use is highest in young children (<5 years) and lowest in older children and adolescents (Baume and Marin 2007; Bernard et al. 2009; Matovu et al. 2009; Kulkarni et al. 2010). Moreover, older individuals also tend to spend more evening hours awake, unprotected by a net and sometimes outdoors where a relevant, and potentially increasing, proportion of bites of malaria-transmitting mosquitoes occurs (Braimah et al. 2005; Reddy et al. 2011; Moiroux et al. 2012). Adults are also more likely to attract mosquitoes (Muirhead-Thomson 1951; Thomas 1951; Clyde and Shute 1958; Carnevale et al. 1978; Port et al. 1980), a phenomenon probably associated with their larger body weight and surface area (Port et al. 1980) and possibly with body temperature and chemical cues that change with increasing age (Knols et al. 1995; Mukabana et al. 2002; Qiu et al. 2006). The lower intervention use, shorter sleeping times, and increased attractiveness to mosquitoes all make older children and adults considerably more likely to be fed on by anopheline vectors and thereby increase their plausible contribution to the human infectious reservoir for malaria if they are infectious to mosquitoes (Fig. 3).

By their nature, cross-sectional surveys are typically time-dependent and reflect a relatively short period or snapshot of population infectivity to mosquitoes. This creates challenges for extrapolating single time-point measurements of infectivity to an overall contribution to transmission. It is clear that infections have differing dynamics in different hosts, which will depend on both intrinsic (e.g., age and immunity as a result of local malaria endemicity) and extrinsic factors (e.g., treatment seeking behavior and treatment). There are very limited data on longitudinal infectiousness of individuals or populations following natural infections. Malaria therapy studies have shown that individuals can be infected for up to a year and be infectious to mosquitoes at multiple time points during this period (Jeffery and Eyles 1955). In the absence of sufficiently detailed data from natural infections, the malaria therapy data form a key component of infectiousness in malaria mathematical models (Ross et al. 2006; Okell et al. 2012; Johnston et al. 2013). However, as discussed above, continual exposure to parasites and the acquisition of immunity will influence asexual and, consequently, sexual parasite levels, which together with factors such as human genetics, exposure to other infections, and nutrition and the restricted demographic range of the participants in the malaria therapy studies limits interpretation from these studies. One of the important suggestions from malaria therapy data that requires further studies in natural infections concerns temporal fluctuations in the infectivity of gametocytes during an infection (Johnston et al. 2013). This corroborates anecdotal reports from natural infections that the likelihood of mosquito infection at a given gametocyte density may fluctuate between seasons and potentially with the duration of malaria infections (Ouedraogo et al. 2015) and would clearly be a very important factor to parametrize malaria transmission models. A recent analysis of case reports and infections post-blood-transfusion has suggested that infections with *P. falciparum* may last for up to 13 years (Ashley and White 2014). No data on gametocyte carriage or infectivity are available for these and other chronic infections, yet such data may be vitally important in managing malaria resurgence in areas of low transmission.

Broadly speaking, two types of infection scenario can be seen as bookends with individ-

A Age-stratified population

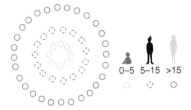

0–5 5–15 >15

B Proportion of individuals with gametocytes

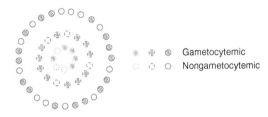

⊛ ❋ ◎ Gametocytemic
○ ○ ○ Nongametocytemic

Contribution to the human infectious reservoir

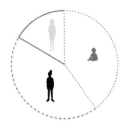

C Proportion of individuals infective to mosquitoes

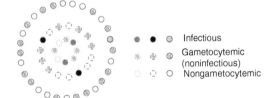

● ● ◎ Infectious
❋ ⊛ ◎ Gametocytemic (noninfectious)
○ ○ ○ Nongametocytemic

Contribution adjusted for body size and relative exposure

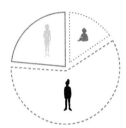

Figure 3. The human infectious reservoir for malaria. Individuals in the figure are represented by circles in three age groups: <5 (dark gray), 5–15 (black), and >15 years (light gray). The age-stratified population (*A*) reflects the abundance of individuals in each group based on a simplified population age structure in sub-Saharan Africa. (*B*) Speckling within circles represents the presence of *Plasmodium falciparum* gametocytes by molecular methods. (*C*) Solid filled circles represent who are infectious to mosquitoes in membrane feeding assays. Many gametocytemic individuals are not infectious to mosquitoes at the moment of sampling. The *top* pie chart presents the proportional contribution of each age group to the human infectious reservoir for malaria after taking into account the demographic distributions in the population. The *bottom* pie chart presents the same contribution to the human infectious reservoir for malaria, taking into account differences in mosquito-biting frequency that are related to differences in behavior, protective measures, and attractiveness to mosquitoes because of body size and other host characteristics. (From data in Stone et al. 2015; adapted, with permission, from Elsevier © 2015.)

uals transitioning from one to the other as immunity develops. Initially, acute infections in individuals with limited immunity would be expected to result in higher parasite and gametocyte densities infecting high numbers of mosquitoes. These infections would be of relatively short duration curtailed by drugs or, in a worst-case scenario, death. Eventually, infections in immune individuals will achieve low parasite densities and consequently infect few mosquitoes and only sporadically. These infections, however, might be expected to last for several weeks and months as infections are asymptomatic. The infectiousness of any subsequent or superinfection may also depend on when in a transmission season this occurs. Ouédraogo

Cite this article as *Cold Spring Harb Perspect Med* doi: 10.1101/cshperspect.a025510

et al. (2015) showed that as parasite and gametocyte densities declined during a transmission season in Burkina Faso, so did infectiousness to mosquitoes. The decline was more pronounced in the youngest age groups, which was hypothesized to be a result of transmission-blocking immunity (discussed below), while the infectiousness of adults remained consistent and low. Longitudinal data such as these need to be interpreted in the context of the likelihood of the infected host being sampled by a mosquito. In Burkina Faso, where malaria transmission vector densities are highly seasonal and in the dry season infectious individuals may rarely be bitten and mosquitoes that do bite may not survive to transmit malaria. Counts of infected mosquitoes can be used to estimate indirect measures of population infectiousness or k (Killeen et al. 2006; Tusting et al. 2014). These measures are perhaps of more use for evaluating entomological factors than for characterizing the human infectious reservoir for malaria as individual human or age-specific contributions cannot be derived. Additionally, there are inconsistencies in methodological approaches used to calculate k, including variation in mosquito trapping techniques that only sample a subset of available mosquitoes, limiting the broader relevance of any estimates.

HUMAN IMMUNE RESPONSES INFLUENCING MALARIA TRANSMISSIBILITY

Human immune responses can influence malaria transmission in several ways. Immune responses that reduce or prevent the establishment of blood-stage parasitemia or reduce the multiplication of the asexual will reduce malaria transmission potential by simply reducing the number of parasites that become gametocytes. Immune responses may also directly target gametocytes or their infectivity to mosquitoes. As described in detail in Meibalan and Marti (2016), early-stage gametocytes of *P. falciparum* sequester primarily in the bone marrow (Sinden and Smalley 1979). There is incomplete evidence for immune recognition of proteins that are present on the surface of erythrocytes that contain developing gametocytes

and may influence gametocyte sequestration (Hayward et al. 1999; Rogers et al. 2000) and maturation (Sutherland 2009; Tonwong et al. 2012). Similarly, naturally acquired antibody responses have been described that recognize erythrocytes containing mature, infectious gametocytes and these antibodies have been hypothesized to play a role in the immune clearance of circulating gametocytes (Saeed et al. 2008). However, experimental evidence for these immune responses to gametocyte-infected erythrocytes is difficult to show and a functional phenotype is only speculative. By comparison, the natural acquisition of antibody responses that influence the infectivity of gametocytes/gametes in mosquitoes is well established. Gametocytes circulate for an average of 4 to 7 days (Bousema et al. 2010), after which gametocytes are removed from the bloodstream in the spleen and gametocyte proteins become accessible to the human immune system. Proteomic analysis has identified >2000 proteins that are expressed in gametocytes of which several hundred that are specific to stage IV and V gametocytes (Lasonder et al. 2002, 2016; Le Roch et al. 2004; Silvestrini et al. 2010). Immune recognition and the functionality of immune responses have been described for only a handful of these proteins. This is due, in part, to a lack of specific reagents to examine immune recognition, which is in turn influenced by the fact that several protein families have complicated tertiary structure. The limited immune responses to gametocyte antigens may be a result of reproductive restraint in which the parasite produces low levels of gametocytes to avoid the induction of effective immunity (Taylor and Read 1997).

The functionality of antibody responses to gametocyte and gamete antigens can be most convincingly assessed in in vitro experiments in which purified IgG is mixed with cultured gametocytes and offered to mosquitoes in the standard membrane feeding assay (SMFA) (Ponnudurai et al. 1989). The SMFA has revealed that naturally acquired antibodies to sexual-stage malaria parasites may inhibit fertilization in the mosquito midgut by inhibiting gamete mobility, reducing contact between male and female gametes or complement-mediated gamete lysis (Vermeulen et al. 1985; Grotendorst et al. 1986; Kaslow et al. 1992; Ranawaka et al. 1994). At present, the most convincing evidence for naturally acquired transmission-reducing immunity (TRI) has been associated with the presence of antibodies to proteins Pfs230 and Pfs48/45 (Rener et al. 1983), which are present on the surface of gametocytes/gametes and play an important role in male microgamete fertility (van Dijk et al. 2001; Eksi et al. 2006). Pfs25 and Pfs28 (Duffy and Kaslow 1997) are candidate proteins for the development of vaccines that elicit TRI but play no relevant role in naturally acquired TRI because these genes are posttranscriptionally repressed until the parasite's development in the mosquito midgut (Pradel 2007) and proteins are therefore not exposed to the human immune system (Miura et al. 2013). Antibody responses to Pfs8/45 and Pfs230 have been detected in numerous malaria-endemic settings and have been associated with TRI (Premawansa et al. 1994; Healer et al. 1999; Bousema et al. 2006, 2010; Drakeley et al. 2006; Jones et al. 2015) and monoclonal antibodies against several epitopes of these proteins reproducibly inhibit parasite fertilization. However, the role of Pfs45/48 and Pfs230 antibodies in natural malaria transmission remains to be quantified and a possible role of antibody responses to other sexual-stage antigens has been hypothesized but remains to be proven. Despite the need for more research in this area, it is evident that human immune responses can reduce the transmissibility of gametocytes in many African settings (Bousema et al. 2011) and that a fraction of gametocyte carriers, estimated at ~5%, is capable of completely preventing mosquito infection (Bousema et al. 2006, 2007; Drakeley et al. 2006).

CONSIDERATIONS FOR THE DEPLOYMENT OF TRANSMISSION-REDUCING INTERVENTIONS

Key considerations for any intervention that aim to reduce transmission are intervention coverage and the duration of the transmission-reducing effects. Coverage is essential in light of the discussion above about the relatively high prevalence of potentially infectious individuals who would be missed by current diagnostics. Recent work on trial design for transmission-blocking vaccines (TBVs) suggests that coverage of 80% is required for a viable vaccine effect (Delrieu et al. 2015) with efficacy further enhanced if the immunity induced lasts for 12 months or longer. This latter point has implications for choice of vaccine antigen and immunization strategies. The impact of all TBV will be dependent on their ability to induce long-lasting TRI. Vaccines based on prefertilization antigens such as Pfs48/45 and Pfs230 may benefit from natural boosting of immune responses because these proteins are expressed in gametocytes and thereby naturally presented to the immune system. TBV based on postfertilization antigens (e.g., Pfs25) would not be boosted as the immune system is not exposed to these antigens and are thereby fully dependent on the immunization approach (Nikolaeva et al. 2015). Antibody levels are crucial for the efficacy of the RTS,S vaccine (White et al. 2015) and the same could be expected for a TBV; the efficacy of naturally induced sexual-stage antibodies is strongly influenced by antibody titer (Bousema et al. 2010).

In the absence of an efficacious TBV, transmission-reducing interventions now commonly rely on the deployment of antimalarial drugs to reduce the human infectious reservoir for malaria. Community-based chemotherapy studies have shown that only treating individuals positive by RDT had a very limited effect on transmission (Tiono et al. 2013; Cook et al. 2015). This limited effect is related to the proportion of infections that are capable of resulting in onward malaria transmission that is undetected and therefore not targeted (Tiono et al. 2013; Cook et al. 2015). In addition, the beneficial prophylactic effect of antimalarial drugs is withheld from a large proportion of the population if treatment is prompted by malaria diagnosis, which may further reduce the effect of screening-and-treatment approaches (Okell et al. 2011). At present, there is little data to indicate what density of parasites a diagnostic test needs to achieve for a screen-and-treat approach to become effective. On one hand, the proportion of populations that is diagnosed with malaria infections is increasing with the improvement of molecular diagnostics that examine larger blood volumes or use more sensitive molecular targets (Bousema et al. 2014; Hofmann et al. 2015). On the other hand, countries are eliminating malaria without a specific focus on these low-density carriers (Bousema et al. 2014; Lin et al. 2014). It appears likely, albeit formally unproven, that malaria elimination can be achieved sooner if field-deployable diagnostics become more sensitive and allow a larger proportion of the parasitemic and infectious human reservoir to be included in interventions.

It is important to note that infections are likely to cluster in a household and these households in turn may also be proximal. Studies in highland Kenya and low-endemic Tanzania found that individuals were 2–6 times more likely to be positive by molecular tests in the household of a person with a positive RDT (Cook et al. 2015; Stresman et al. 2015). This spatial heterogeneity in transmission has long been recognized at a macro scale but is only recently being described at micro scales (Bousema et al. 2012b; Bejon et al. 2014). The clustering of malaria infections in certain geographic areas (Bousema et al. 2012b; Bejon et al. 2014) or demographic populations (Wesolowski et al. 2012; Yangzom et al. 2012; Sturrock et al. 2013) has relevance for both the development of immunity to infection and long-term parasite carriage as well as for targeted control. In some instances in which malaria control nears elimination but isolated pockets of continued transmission persist, the value of targeted interventions is evident. In other settings in which malaria continues to be widespread but heterogeneous, the evidence that supports targeted interventions is less convincing. In these settings, individuals who are disproportionally exposed to (infected and uninfected) mosquitoes may spread malaria transmission to the larger population (Woolhouse et al. 1997). Targeting these areas or individuals theoretically forms a highly efficient approach to malaria control (Bousema et al. 2012b), but many uncertainties exist about the size, locality, detectability, and

stability of so-called malaria hot spots (Bejon et al. 2014). One cluster-randomized trial that quantified the effect of hot-spot-targeted interventions on surrounding malaria-endemic communities found very limited evidence for this community effect (Bousema et al. 2016) Uncertainties about the spatial and temporal dynamics of infected mosquitoes and human parasite carriers currently hinder the rational targeting of interventions in areas where malaria transmission is widespread but geographically heterogeneous.

CONCLUSIONS

Control and transmission reduction of malaria presents a uniquely complex challenge given its high transmissibility or R_0 (Smith et al. 2005). Notwithstanding this, there are encouraging reports of major reductions in malaria morbidity worldwide (Bhatt et al. 2015) and several countries have recently declared themselves malaria-free. However, lessons from history showed that the Global Malaria Eradication Program had little impact in Africa and, while this was attributed to decreasing efficacy of interventions, there was also major acknowledgment of our lack of fundamental understanding of basic biology. The currently available, field-deployable diagnostic approaches, such as microscopy and RDT, miss a substantial proportion of infectious individuals. This undiagnosed fraction of the human infectious reservoir may limit the impact of malaria interventions that depend on malaria diagnostics and extend the intervention phase that is required before elimination is achieved. TBV would be a highly desirable asset for malaria-elimination efforts and would avoid the challenges experienced by chemotherapy approaches that rely on malaria diagnosis. TBV are receiving significant investment, but their efficacy will depend on the longevity of the induced immune responses and the coverage of individuals transmitting infections to mosquitoes. A better understanding of the dynamics of the human infectious reservoir for malaria in the context of changing mosquito vector populations and other malaria-control interventions is urgently needed to support the implementation of TBV and other transmission-reducing interventions by setting evidence-based targets in terms of spatial and demographic coverage levels and the strength and longevity of the incurred protection.

ACKNOWLEDGMENTS

We thank Bronner Goncalves for discussion and advice and Sophie van Kempen for graphic design. T.B. is supported by the Bill and Melinda Gates Foundation (OPP1034789) and the European Research Council (ERC-2014-StG 639776). C.D. is supported by the Bill and Melinda Gates Foundation (OPP1034789) and the Wellcome Trust (091924).

REFERENCES

*Reference is also in this collection.

Ashley EA, White NJ. 2014. The duration of *Plasmodium falciparum* infections. *Malaria J* 13: 500.

Banoo S, Bell D, Bossuyt P, Herring A, Mabey D, Poole F, Smith PG, Sriram N, Wongsrichanalai C, Linke R, et al. 2006. Evaluation of diagnostic tests for infectious diseases: General principles. *Nat Rev Microbiol* 4: S20–S32.

Bastiaens GJ, Bousema T, Leslie T. 2014. Scale-up of malaria rapid diagnostic tests and artemisinin-based combination therapy: Challenges and perspectives in sub-Saharan Africa. *PLoS Med* 11: e1001590.

Baume CA, Marin MC. 2007. Intra-household mosquito net use in Ethiopia, Ghana, Mali, Nigeria, Senegal, and Zambia: Are nets being used? Who in the household uses them? *Am J Trop Med Hyg* 77: 963–971.

Bejon P, Williams TN, Nyundo C, Hay SI, Benz D, Gething PW, Otiende M, Peshu J, Bashraheil M, Greenhouse B, et al. 2014. A micro-epidemiological analysis of febrile malaria in Coastal Kenya showing hotspots within hotspots. *eLife* 3: e02130.

Bell D, Wongsrichanalai C, Barnwell JW. 2006. Ensuring quality and access for malaria diagnosis: How can it be achieved? *Nat Rev Microbiol* 4: 682–695.

Bernard J, Mtove G, Mandike R, Mtei F, Maxwell C, Reyburn H. 2009. Equity and coverage of insecticide-treated bed nets in an area of intense transmission of *Plasmodium falciparum* in Tanzania. *Malaria J* 8: 65.

Bhatt S, Weiss DJ, Cameron E, Bisanzio D, Mappin B, Dalrymple U, Battle KE, Moyes CL, Henry A, Eckhoff PA, et al. 2015. The effect of malaria control on *Plasmodium falciparum* in Africa between 2000 and 2015. *Nature* 526: 207–211.

Bonnet S, Gouagna LC, Paul RE, Safeukui I, Meunier JY, Boudin C. 2003. Estimation of malaria transmission from humans to mosquitoes in two neighbouring villages in south Cameroon: Evaluation and comparison of several indices. *Trans R Soc Trop Med Hyg* 97: 53–59.

Boudin C, Olivier M, Molez JF, Chiron JP, Ambroise-Thomas P. 1993a. High human malarial infectivity to laboratory-bred *Anopheles gambiae* in a village in Burkina Faso. *Am J Trop Med Hyg* 48: 700–706.

Boudin C, Olivier M, Molez JF, Chiron JP, Ambroise-Thomas P. 1993b. High human malarial infectivity to laboratory-bred *Anopheles gambiae* in a village in Burkina Faso. *Am J Trop Med Hyg* 48: 700–706.

Bousema T, Drakeley C. 2011. Epidemiology and infectivity of *Plasmodium falciparum* and *Plasmodium vivax* gametocytes in relation to malaria control and elimination. *Clin Microbiol Rev* 24: 377–410.

Bousema JT, Roeffen W, van der Kolk M, de Vlas SJ, van de Vegte-Bolmer M, Bangs MJ, Teelen K, Kurniawan L, Maguire JD, Baird JK, et al. 2006. Rapid onset of transmission-reducing antibodies in Javanese migrants exposed to malaria in Papua, Indonesia. *Am J Trop Med Hyg* 74: 425–431.

Bousema JT, Drakeley CJ, Kihonda J, Hendriks JC, Akim NI, Roeffen W, Sauerwein RW. 2007. A longitudinal study of immune responses to *Plasmodium falciparum* sexual stage antigens in Tanzanian adults. *Parasite Immunol* 29: 309–317.

Bousema T, Okell L, Shekalaghe S, Griffin J, Omar S, Sawa P, Sutherland C, Sauerwein R, Ghani A, Drakeley C. 2010. Revisiting the circulation time of *Plasmodium falciparum* gametocytes: Molecular detection methods to estimate the duration of gametocyte carriage and the effect of gametocytocidal drugs. *Malaria J* 9: 136.

Bousema T, Sutherland CJ, Churcher TS, Mulder B, Gouagna LC, Riley EM, Targett GA, Drakeley CJ. 2011. Human immune responses that reduce the transmission of *Plasmodium falciparum* in African populations. *Int J Parasitol* 41: 293–300.

Bousema T, Dinglasan RR, Morlais I, Gouagna LC, van Warmerdam T, Awono-Ambene PH, Bonnet S, Diallo M, Coulibaly M, Tchuinkam T, et al. 2012a. Mosquito feeding assays to determine the infectiousness of naturally infected *Plasmodium falciparum* gametocyte carriers. *PLoS ONE* 7: e42821.

Bousema T, Griffin JT, Sauerwein RW, Smith DL, Churcher TS, Takken W, Ghani A, Drakeley C, Gosling R. 2012b. Hitting hotspots: Spatial targeting of malaria for control and elimination. *PLoS Med* 9: e1001165.

Bousema T, Okell L, Felger I, Drakeley C. 2014. Asymptomatic malaria infections: Detectability, transmissibility and public health relevance. *Nat Rev Microbiol* 12: 833–840.

Bousema T, Stresman G, Baidjoe AY, Bradley J, Knight P, Stone W, Osoti V, Makori E, Owaga C, Odongo W, et al. 2016. The impact of hotspot-targeted interventions on malaria transmission in Rachuonyo South District in the Western Kenyan Highlands: A cluster-randomized controlled trial. *PLoS Med* 13: e1001993.

Braimah N, Drakeley C, Kweka E, Mosha F, Helinski M, Pates H, Maxwell C, Massawe T, Kenward MG, Curtis C. 2005. Tests of bednet traps (Mbita traps) for monitoring mosquito populations and time of biting in Tanzania and possible impact of prolonged insecticide treated net use. *Int J Trop Insect Sci* 25: 208–213.

Carnevale P, Frézil JL, Bosseno MF, Le Pont F, Lancien J. 1978. The aggressiveness of *Anopheles gambiae* A in relation to the age and sex of the human subjects. *Bull World Health Organ* **56:** 147–154.

Churcher TS, Bousema T, Walker M, Drakeley C, Schneider P, Ouedraogo AL, Basanez MG. 2013. Predicting mosquito infection from *Plasmodium falciparum* gametocyte density and estimating the reservoir of infection. *eLife* **2:** e00626.

Clyde DF, Shute GT. 1958. Selective feeding habits of Anophelines amongst Africans of different ages. *Am J Trop Med Hyg* **7:** 543–545.

Coleman RE, Kumpitak C, Ponlawat A, Maneechai N, Phunkitchar V, Rachapaew N, Zollner G, Sattabongkot J. 2004. Infectivity of asymptomatic *Plasmodium*-infected human populations to *Anopheles dirus* mosquitoes in western Thailand. *J Med Entomol* **41:** 201–208.

Cook J, Xu W, Msellem M, Vonk M, Bergstrom B, Gosling R, Al-Mafazy AW, McElroy P, Molteni F, Abass AK, et al. 2015. Mass screening and treatment on the basis of results of a *Plasmodium falciparum*–specific rapid diagnostic test did not reduce malaria incidence in Zanzibar. *J Infect Dis* **211:** 1476–1483.

Delrieu I, Leboulleux D, Ivinson K, Gessner BD; Malaria Transmission Blocking Vaccine Technical Consultation Group. 2015. Design of a phase III cluster randomized trial to assess the efficacy and safety of a malaria transmission blocking vaccine. *Vaccine* **33:** 1518–1526.

Drakeley CJ, Bousema JT, Akim NI, Teelen K, Roeffen W, Lensen AH, Bolmer M, Eling W, Sauerwein RW. 2006. Transmission-reducing immunity is inversely related to age in *Plasmodium falciparum* gametocyte carriers. *Parasite Immunol* **28:** 185–190.

Duffy PE, Kaslow DC. 1997. A novel malaria protein, Pfs28, and Pfs25 are genetically linked and synergistic as falciparum malaria transmission-blocking vaccines. *Infect Immun* **65:** 1109–1113.

Eksi S, Czesny B, van Gemert GJ, Sauerwein RW, Eling W, Williamson KC. 2006. Malaria transmission-blocking antigen, Pfs230, mediates human red blood cell binding to exflagellating male parasites and oocyst production. *Mol Microbiol* **61:** 991–998.

Eziefula AC, Bousema T, Yeung S, Kamya M, Owaraganise A, Gabagaya G, Bradley J, Grignard L, Lanke KHW, Wanzira H, et al. 2014. Single-dose primaquine for clearance of *P. falciparum* gametocytes in children with uncomplicated malaria in Uganda: A randomised controlled double-blinded dose-ranging trial. *Lancet Infect Dis* **14:** 130–139.

Gaye A, Bousema T, Libasse G, Ndiath MO, Konaté L, Jawara M, Faye O, Sokhna C. 2015. Infectiousness of the human population to *Anopheles arabiensis* by direct skin feeding in an area hypoendemic for malaria in Senegal. *Am J Trop Med Hyg* **92:** 648–652.

Githeko AK, Brandling-Bennett AD, Beier M, Atieli F, Owaga M, Collins FH. 1992. The reservoir of *Plasmodium falciparum* malaria in a holoendemic area of western Kenya. *Trans R Soc Trop Med Hyg* **86:** 355–358.

Graves PM, Burkot TR, Carter R, Cattani JA, Lagog M, Parker J, Brabin BJ, Gibson FD, Bradley DJ, Alpers MP. 1988. Measurement of malarial infectivity of human populations to mosquitoes in the Madang area, Papua New Guinea. *Parasitology* **96:** 251–263.

Grotendorst CA, Carter R, Rosenberg R, Koontz LC. 1986. Complement effects on the infectivity of *Plasmodium*

gallinaceum to *Aedes aegypti* mosquitoes. I: Resistance of zygotes to the alternative pathway of complement. *J Immunol* **136:** 4270–4274.

Hay SI, Guerra CA, Gething PW, Patil AP, Tatem AJ, Noor AM, Kabaria CW, Manh BH, Elyazar IR, Brooker S, et al. 2009. A world malaria map: *Plasmodium falciparum* endemicity in 2007. *PLoS Med* **6:** e1000048.

Hayward RE, Tiwari B, Piper KP, Baruch DI, Day KP. 1999. Virulence and transmission success of the malarial parasite *Plasmodium falciparum*. *Proc Natl Acad Sci* **96:** 4563–4568.

Healer J, McGuinness D, Carter R, Riley E. 1999. Transmission-blocking immunity to *Plasmodium falciparum* in malaria-immune individuals is associated with antibodies to the gamete surface protein Pfs230. *Parasitology* **119:** 425–433.

Hermsen CC, Telgt DS, Linders EH, van de Locht LA, Eling WM, Mensink EJ, Sauerwein RW. 2001. Detection of *Plasmodium falciparum* malaria parasites in vivo by real-time quantitative PCR. *Mol Biochem Parasitol* **118:** 247–251.

Hofmann N, Mwingira F, Shekalaghe S, Robinson LJ, Mueller I, Felger I. 2015. Ultra-sensitive detection of *Plasmodium falciparum* by amplification of multi-copy subtelomeric targets. *PLoS Med* **12:** e1001788.

Jeffery GM, Eyles DE. 1955. Infectivity to mosquitoes of *Plasmodium falciparum* as related to gametocyte density and duration of infection. *Am J Trop Med Hyg* **4:** 781–789.

Johnston GL, Smith DL, Fidock DA. 2013. Malaria's missing number: Calculating the human component of R_0 by a within-host mechanistic model of *Plasmodium falciparum* infection and transmission. *PLoS Comput Biol* **9:** e1003025.

Jones S, Grignard L, Nebie I, Chilongola J, Dodoo D, Sauerwein R, Theisen M, Roeffen W, Singh SK, Singh RK, et al. 2015. Naturally acquired antibody responses to recombinant Pfs230 and Pfs48/45 transmission blocking vaccine candidates. *J Infect* **71:** 117–127.

Kaslow DC, Bathurst IC, Barr PJ. 1992. Malaria transmission-blocking vaccines. *Trends Biotechnol* **10:** 388–391.

Killeen GF, Ross A, Smith T. 2006. Infectiousness of malaria-endemic human populations to vectors. *Am J Trop Med Hyg* **75:** 38–45.

Knols BGJ, de Jong R, Takken W. 1995. Differential attractiveness of isolated humans to mosquitoes in Tanzania. *Trans R Soc Trop Med Hyg* **89:** 604–606.

Kulkarni MA, Eng JV, Desrochers RE, Cotte AH, Goodson JL, Johnston A, Wolkon A, Erskine M, Berti P, Rakotoarisoa A, et al. 2010. Contribution of integrated campaign distribution of long-lasting insecticidal nets to coverage of target groups and total populations in malaria-endemic areas in Madagascar. *Am J Trop Med Hyg* **82:** 420–425.

Lasonder E, Ishihama Y, Andersen JS, Vermunt AM, Pain A, Sauerwein RW, Eling WM, Hall N, Waters AP, Stunnenberg HG, et al. 2002. Analysis of the *Plasmodium falciparum* proteome by high-accuracy mass spectrometry. *Nature* **419:** 537–542.

Lasonder E, Rijpma SR, van Schaijk BC, Hoeijmakers WA, Kensche PR, Gresnigt MS, Italiaander A, Vos MW, Woestenenk R, Bousema T, et al. 2016. Integrated transcriptomic and proteomic analyses of *P. falciparum* gametocytes: Molecular insight into sex-specific processes and translational repression. *Nucleic Acids Res* **44:** 6087–6101.

Le Roch KG, Johnson JR, Florens L, Zhou Y, Santrosyan A, Grainger M, Yan SF, Williamson KC, Holder AA, Carucci DJ, et al. 2004. Global analysis of transcript and protein levels across the *Plasmodium falciparum* life cycle. *Genome Res* **14:** 2308–2318.

Lin JT, Saunders DL, Meshnick SR. 2014. The role of submicroscopic parasitemia in malaria transmission: What is the evidence? *Trends Parasitol* **30:** 183–190.

Matovu F, Goodman C, Wiseman V, Mwengee W. 2009. How equitable is bed net ownership and utilisation in Tanzania? A practical application of the principles of horizontal and vertical equity. *Malaria J* **8:** 109.

* Meibalan E, Marti M. 2016. Biology of malaria transmission. *Cold Spring Harb Perspect Med* doi: 10.1101/cshperspect.a025452.

Miura K, Takashima E, Deng B, Tullo G, Diouf A, Moretz SE, Nikolaeva D, Diakite M, Fairhurst RM, Fay MP, et al. 2013. Functional comparison of *Plasmodium falciparum* transmission-blocking vaccine candidates by the standard membrane-feeding assay. *Infect Immun* **81:** 4377–4382.

Moiroux N, Gomez MB, Pennetier C, Elanga E, Djènontin A, Chandre F, Djègbé I, Guis H, Corbel V. 2012. Changes in *Anopheles funestus* biting behavior following universal coverage of long-lasting insecticidal nets in Benin. *J Infect Dis* **206:** 1622–1629.

Mosha JF, Sturrock HJ, Greenhouse B, Greenwood B, Sutherland CJ, Gadalla N, Atwal S, Drakeley C, Kibiki G, Bousema T, et al. 2013. Epidemiology of subpatent *Plasmodium falciparum* infection: Implications for detection of hotspots with imperfect diagnostics. *Malaria J* **12:** 221.

Muirhead-Thomson RC. 1951. Distribution of anopheline mosquito bites among different age groups. *BMJ* **1:** 1114–1117.

Muirhead-Thomson RC. 1957. The malarial infectivity of an African village population to mosquitoes (*Anopheles gambiae*); a random xenodiagnostic survey. *Am J Trop Med Hyg* **6:** 971–979.

Mukabana W, Takken W, Coe R, Knols B. 2002. Host-specific cues cause differential attractiveness of Kenyan men to the African malaria vector *Anopheles gambiae*. *Malaria J* **1:** 17.

Nassir E, Abdel-Muhsin AM, Suliaman S, Kenyon F, Kheir A, Geha H, Ferguson HM, Walliker D, Babiker HA. 2005. Impact of genetic complexity on longevity and gametocytogenesis of *Plasmodium falciparum* during the dry and transmission-free season of eastern Sudan. *Int J Parasitol* **35:** 49–55.

Nguyen HV, van den Eede P, van Overmeir C, Thang ND, Hung le X, D'Alessandro U, Erhart A. 2012. Marked age-dependent prevalence of symptomatic and patent infections and complexity of distribution of human *Plasmodium* species in central Vietnam. *Am J Trop Med Hyg* **87:** 989–995.

Nikolaeva D, Draper SJ, Biswas S. 2015. Toward the development of effective transmission-blocking vaccines for malaria. *Exp Rev Vaccines* **14:** 653–680.

Nwakanma D, Kheir A, Sowa M, Dunyo S, Jawara M, Pinder M, Milligan P, Walliker D, Babiker HA. 2008. High gametocyte complexity and mosquito infectivity of *Plasmodium falciparum* in the Gambia. *Int J Parasitol* **38:** 219–227.

Okell LC, Griffin JT, Kleinschmidt I, Hollingsworth TD, Churcher TS, White MJ, Bousema T, Drakeley CJ, Ghani AC. 2011. The potential contribution of mass treatment to the control of *Plasmodium falciparum* malaria. *PLoS ONE* **6:** e20179.

Okell LC, Bousema T, Griffin JT, Ouedraogo AL, Ghani AC, Drakeley CJ. 2012. Factors determining the occurrence of submicroscopic malaria infections and their relevance for control. *Nat Commun* **3:** 1237.

Ouédraogo AL, Schneider P, de Kruijf M, Nebie I, Verhave JP, Cuzin-Ouattara N, Sauerwein RW. 2007. Age-dependent distribution of *Plasmodium falciparum* gametocytes quantified by Pfs25 real-time QT-NASBA in a cross-sectional study in Burkina Faso. *Am J Trop Med Hyg* **76:** 626–630.

Ouédraogo AL, Bousema T, Schneider P, de Vlas SJ, Ilboudo-Sanogo E, Cuzin-Ouattara N, Nebie I, Roeffen W, Verhave JP, Luty AJ, et al. 2009. Substantial contribution of submicroscopical *Plasmodium falciparum* gametocyte carriage to the infectious reservoir in an area of seasonal transmission. *PLoS ONE* **4:** e8410.

Ouédraogo AL, Goncalves BP, Gneme A, Wenger EA, Guelbeogo MW, Ouedraogo A, Gerardin J, Bever CA, Lyons H, Pitroipa X, et al. 2015. Dynamics of the human infectious reservoir for malaria determined by mosquito feeding assays and ultrasensitive malaria diagnosis in Burkina Faso. *J Infect Dis* **213:** 90–99.

Ponnudurai T, Lensen AH, Van Gemert GJ, Bensink MP, Bolmer M, Meuwissen JH. 1989. Infectivity of cultured *Plasmodium falciparum* gametocytes to mosquitoes. *Parasitology* **98:** 165–173.

Port GR, Boreham PFL, Bryan JH. 1980. The relationship of host size to feeding by mosquitoes of the *Anopheles gambiae* Giles complex (Diptera: Culicidae). *Bull Entomol Res* **70:** 133–144.

Pradel G. 2007. Proteins of the malaria parasite sexual stages: Expression, function and potential for transmission blocking strategies. *Parasitology* **134:** 1911–1929.

Premawansa S, Gamage-Mendis A, Perera L, Begarnie S, Mendis K, Carter R. 1994. *Plasmodium falciparum* malaria transmission-blocking immunity under conditions of low endemicity as in Sri Lanka. *Parasite Immunol* **16:** 35–42.

Proietti C, Pettinato DD, Kanoi BN, Ntege E, Crisanti A, Riley EM, Egwang TG, Drakeley C, Bousema T. 2011. Continuing intense malaria transmission in northern Uganda. *Am J Trop Med Hyg* **84:** 830–837.

Qiu YT, Smallegange RC, Van Loon JJA, Ter Braak CJF, Takken W. 2006. Interindividual variation in the attractiveness of human odours to the malaria mosquito *Anopheles gambiae* s.s. *Med Vet Entomol* **20:** 280–287.

Ranawaka GR, Alejo-Blanco AR, Sinden RE. 1994. Characterization of the effector mechanisms of a transmission-blocking antibody upon differentiation of *Plasmodium berghei* gametocytes into ookinetes in vitro. *Parasitology* **109:** 11–17.

Reddy M, Overgaard H, Abaga S, Reddy V, Caccone A, Kiszewski A, Slotman M. 2011. Outdoor host seeking behaviour of *Anopheles gambiae* mosquitoes following initiation of malaria vector control on Bioko Island, Equatorial Guinea. *Malaria J* **10:** 184.

Rener J, Graves PM, Carter R, Williams JL, Burkot TR. 1983. Target antigens of transmission-blocking immunity on gametes of *Plasmodium falciparum*. *J Exp Med* **158:** 976–981.

Rogers NJ, Hall BS, Obiero J, Targett GA, Sutherland CJ. 2000. A model for sequestration of the transmission stages of *Plasmodium falciparum*: Adhesion of gametocyte-infected erythrocytes to human bone marrow cells. *Infect Immun* **68:** 3455–3462.

Ross A, Killeen G, Smith T. 2006. Relationships between host infectivity to mosquitoes and asexual parasite density in *Plasmodium falciparum*. *Am J Trop Med Hyg* **75:** 32–37.

Saeed M, Roeffen W, Alexander N, Drakeley CJ, Targett GA, Sutherland CJ. 2008. *Plasmodium falciparum* antigens on the surface of the gametocyte-infected erythrocyte. *PloS ONE* **3:** e2280.

Sawa P, Shekalaghe SA, Drakeley CJ, Sutherland CJ, Mweresa CK, Baidjoe AY, Manjurano A, Kavishe RA, Beshir KB, Yussuf RU, et al. 2013. Malaria transmission after artemether-lumefantrine and dihydroartemisinin-piperaquine: A randomized trial. *J Infect Dis* **207:** 1637–1645.

Schneider P, Bousema JT, Gouagna LC, Otieno S, van dV, Omar SA, Sauerwein RW. 2007. Submicroscopic *Plasmodium falciparum* gametocyte densities frequently result in mosquito infection. *Am J Trop Med Hyg* **76:** 470–474.

Shekalaghe SA, Bousema JT, Kunei KK, Lushino P, Masokoto A, Wolters LR, Mwakalinga S, Mosha FW, Sauerwein RW, Drakeley CJ. 2007. Submicroscopic *Plasmodium falciparum* gametocyte carriage is common in an area of low and seasonal transmission in Tanzania. *Trop Med Int Health* **12:** 547–553.

Silvestrini F, Lasonder E, Olivieri A, Camarda G, van Schaijk B, Sanchez M, Younis Younis S, Sauerwein R, Alano P. 2010. Protein export marks the early phase of gametocytogenesis of the human malaria parasite *Plasmodium falciparum*. *Mol Cell Proteomics* **9:** 1437–1448.

Sinden RE, Smalley ME. 1979. Gametocytogenesis of *Plasmodium falciparum* in vitro: The cell cycle. *Parasitology* **79:** 277–296.

Slater HC, Ross A, Ouedraogo AL, White LJ, Nguon C, Walker PG, Ngor P, Aguas R, Silal SP, Dondorp AM, et al. 2015. Assessing the impact of next-generation rapid diagnostic tests on *Plasmodium falciparum* malaria elimination strategies. *Nature* **528:** S94–101.

Smith DL, Dushoff J, Snow RW, Hay SI. 2005. The entomological inoculation rate and *Plasmodium falciparum* infection in African children. *Nature* **438:** 492–495.

Snounou G, Viriyakosol S, Jarra W, Thaithong S, Brown KN. 1993. Identification of the four human malaria parasite species in field samples by the polymerase chain reaction and detection of a high prevalence of mixed infections. *Mol Biochem Parasitol* **58:** 283–292.

Stone W, Goncalves BP, Bousema T, Drakeley C. 2015. Assessing the infectious reservoir of falciparum malaria: Past and future. *Trends Parasitol* **31:** 287–296.

Stresman GH, Baidjoe AY, Stevenson J, Grignard L, Odongo W, Owaga C, Osoti V, Makori E, Shagari S, Marube E, et al. 2015. Focal screening to identify the subpatent parasite reservoir in an area of low and heterogeneous transmission in the Kenya highlands. *J Infect Dis* **212:** 1768–1777.

Sturrock HJ, Hsiang MS, Cohen JM, Smith DL, Greenhouse B, Bousema T, Gosling RD. 2013. Targeting asymptomatic malaria infections: Active surveillance in control and elimination. *PLoS Med* **10:** e1001467.

Sutherland CJ. 2009. Surface antigens of *Plasmodium falciparum* gametocytes—A new class of transmission-blocking vaccine targets? *Mol Biochem Parasitol* **166:** 93–98.

Taylor LH, Read AF. 1997. Why so few transmission stages? Reproductive restraint by malaria parasites. *Parasitol Today* **13:** 135–140.

Thomas TCE. 1951. Biting activity of *Anopheles gambiae*. *BMJ* **2:** 1402–1402.

Tiono AB, Ouedraogo A, Ogutu B, Diarra A, Coulibaly S, Gansane A, Sirima SB, O'Neil G, Mukhopadhyay A, Hamed K. 2013. A controlled, parallel, cluster-randomized trial of community-wide screening and treatment of asymptomatic carriers of *Plasmodium falciparum* in Burkina Faso. *Malaria J* **12:** 79.

Tonwong N, Sattabongkot J, Tsuboi T, Iriko H, Takeo S, Sirichaisinthop J, Udomsangpetch R. 2012. Natural infection of *Plasmodium falciparum* induces inhibitory antibodies against gametocyte development in human hosts. *Jpn J Infect Dis* **65:** 152–156.

Tusting LS, Bousema T, Smith DL, Drakeley C. 2014. Measuring changes in *Plasmodium falciparum* transmission: Precision, accuracy and costs of metrics. *Adv Parasitol* **84:** 151–208.

van Dijk MR, Janse CJ, Thompson J, Waters AP, Braks JA, Dodemont HJ, Stunnenberg HG, van Gemert GJ, Sauerwein RW, Eling W. 2001. A central role for P48/45 in malaria parasite male gamete fertility. *Cell* **104:** 153–164.

Vermeulen AN, Ponnudurai T, Beckers PJ, Verhave JP, Smits MA, Meuwissen JH. 1985. Sequential expression of antigens on sexual stages of *Plasmodium falciparum* accessible to transmission-blocking antibodies in the mosquito. *J Exp Med* **162:** 1460–1476.

Wampfler R, Mwingira F, Javati S, Robinson L, Betuela I, Siba P, Beck HP, Mueller I, Felger I. 2013. Strategies for detection of *Plasmodium* species gametocytes. *PLoS ONE* **8:** e76316.

Wesolowski A, Eagle N, Tatem AJ, Smith DL, Noor AM, Snow RW, Buckee CO. 2012. Quantifying the impact of human mobility on malaria. *Science* **338:** 267–270.

White MT, Verity R, Griffin JT, Asante KP, Owusu-Agyei S, Greenwood B, Drakeley C, Gesase S, Lusingu J, Ansong D, et al. 2015. Immunogenicity of the RTS,S/AS01 malaria vaccine and implications for duration of vaccine efficacy: Secondary analysis of data from a phase 3 randomised controlled trial. *Lancet Infect Dis* **15:** 1450–1458.

Woolhouse ME, Dye C, Etard JF, Smith T, Charlwood JD, Garnett GP, Hagan P, Hii JL, Ndhlovu PD, Quinnell RJ, et al. 1997. Heterogeneities in the transmission of infectious agents: Implications for the design of control programs. *Proc Natl Acad Sci* **94:** 338–342.

Wu L, van den Hoogen LL, Slater H, Walker PGT, Ghani A, J DC, Okell LC. 2015. Detecting asymptomatic *Plasmodium falciparum* infections to inform control and elimination strategies—How do current diagnostics compare? *Nature* **528:** S86–93.

Yangzom T, Gueye CS, Namgay R, Galappaththy GN, Thimasarn K, Gosling R, Murugasampillay S, Dev V. 2012. Malaria control in Bhutan: Case study of a country embarking on elimination. *Malaria J* **11:** 9.

Biology of Malaria Transmission

Elamaran Meibalan and Matthias Marti

Harvard T.H. Chan School of Public Health, Department of Immunology and Infectious Diseases, Boston, Massachusetts 02115

Correspondence: mmarti@hsph.harvard.edu

Understanding transmission biology at an individual level is a key component of intervention strategies that target the spread of malaria parasites from human to mosquito. Gametocytes are specialized sexual stages of the malaria parasite life cycle developed during evolution to achieve crucial steps in transmission. As sexual differentiation and transmission are tightly linked, a deeper understanding of molecular and cellular events defining this relationship is essential to combat malaria. Recent advances in the field are gradually revealing mechanisms underlying sexual commitment, gametocyte sequestration, and dynamics of transmissible stages; however, key questions on fundamental gametocyte biology still remain. Moreover, species-specific variation between *Plasmodium falciparum* and *Plasmodium vivax* transmission dynamics pose another significant challenge for worldwide malaria elimination efforts. Here, we review the biology of transmission stages, highlighting numerous factors influencing development and dynamics of gametocytes within the host and determinants of human infectiousness.

Current measures for malaria elimination have been inspired by the Global Malaria Eradication Program (GMEP), which operated under the World Health Organization (WHO) between 1955 and 1969. The strategy of GMEP was largely based on dichlorodiphenyltrichloroethane (DDT)-based indoor residual spraying (DDT-IRS) complemented with mass drug administration (Pampana 1969). Although GMEP was able to eliminate malaria from many regions of the world, it was eventually abandoned because of technical challenges, increasing spread of both insecticide resistance and drug-resistant parasite strains, and lack of continuous political support (Najera et al. 2011). In 2007, the Bill and Melinda Gates Foundation, supported by WHO, called for a campaign to prioritize malaria eradication strategies with renewed focus on blocking transmission (Alonso et al. 2011; malERA Consultative Group on Drugs 2011). Indeed, malaria elimination can only be achieved by interrupting and reducing transmission in a defined area until no parasites remain (Cohen et al. 2010; Alonso et al. 2011). Tools currently used to reduce transmission focus on vector control efforts such as insecticide-treated nets (ITNs) and antimalarial combination therapy including a transmission-blocking drug. Artemisinin-based combination therapies (ACTs) are currently used as a first-line treatment worldwide (Global Partnership to Roll Back Malaria 2001). These efficiently clear asexual parasites and early transmission stages, whereas mature infectious transmission stages are unaffected. To block transmission, ACT is often combined with the only transmission-blocking drug on the market, Primaquine. However, recent emergence of artemisinin resistance in Southeast Asia asks for urgent evaluation of alternative treatment strategies (Noedl et al. 2008; Dondorp et al. 2009; Mbengue et al. 2015; Straimer et al. 2015).

Of the five *Plasmodium* species known to cause malaria in humans, *Plasmodium falciparum* is lethal and responsible for severe disease pathology and the majority of deaths due to malaria, especially in sub-Saharan Africa. *Plasmodium vivax* typically causes milder infections than *P. falciparum* but has a much greater geographical distribution (Gething et al. 2012). The clinical symptoms of malaria are largely a result of the replication of asexual stages in human blood, but transmission to mosquitoes is only achieved through the development of sexual stages, termed gametocytes. To abrogate transmission of *P. falciparum*, we must be able to clear asexual and sexual stages from the human host, eventually rendering an individual noninfectious to mosquitoes. However, in the case of *P. vivax*, elimination is highly challenging because of the relapse of dormant liver-stage hypnozoites that can persist as a transmission reservoir for several months after the initial infection (White 2011; Dembélé et al. 2014). Lack of sufficient knowledge on the infectivity of asymptomatic and symptomatic individuals harboring transmission parasite stages remains a major gap in understanding malaria transmission. Because of the complex and nonlinear relationship between parasite density in the human host and infectiousness to mosquitoes (Schneider et al. 2007; Bousema et al. 2012; Churcher et al. 2013), our knowledge of strategies used by the parasite for efficient transmission is still far from complete. Recent studies highlighting the bone marrow as the primary site of gametocyte development and sequestration (Farfour et al. 2012; Aguilar et al. 2014; Joice et al. 2014) raises questions on the timing of events from sequestration leading to reentry of mature gametocytes into the bloodstream

and potential migration to subdermal capillaries under the skin during an infection. As gametocytes represent a potential bottleneck in transmission, a deeper understanding of transmission biology is required to develop novel tools and strategies toward elimination and eradication of malaria. In this review, we discuss the current knowledge, recent advances, and open questions regarding key aspects of transmission biology, including mechanisms underlying gametocyte development, gametocyte sequestration, and assessment of the infectious reservoir in an individual. Targeted research on the highlighted knowledge gaps will be crucial to identify potential targets for intervention strategies. Although studies on the transmission biology of *P. vivax* are limited compared with *P. falciparum*, we have compared key features of sexual biology between both species.

DEVELOPMENT OF TRANSMISSION STAGES IN HUMAN MALARIA

The pathology of malaria infection and associated clinical manifestations are predominantly attributed to the asexual erythrocytic stages. During asexual blood stage development, the ring stages develop into replicative schizont forms that release multiple invasive daughter merozoites (Fig. 1A). Within each replication cycle, a small proportion ($\sim$0.1%–5%) of asexual parasites develop into male and female sexual stages called gametocytes (Sinden 1983), which are the only stages transmitted to the mosquito vector, albeit not directly contributing to disease pathology. The time required for gametocyte maturation differs strikingly between the different *Plasmodium* species. A *P. falciparum* gametocyte takes $\sim$8–10 days for maturation into five morphologically distinct phases (stages I–V) (Fig. 1B) (Hawking et al. 1971; Sinden et al. 1978). In the other *Plasmodium* species, asexual and sexual cycle are of similar length. *P. vivax* gametocytes require $\sim$48 h for development and disappear from circulation within 3 days of sexual maturation (Sinden and Gilles 2002). In the rodent malaria parasites, *Plasmodium berghei* (Mons et al. 1985) and *Plasmodium yoelii* (Gautret

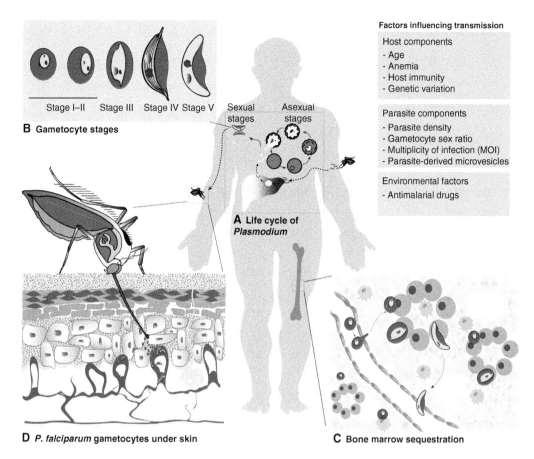

Figure 1. The *Plasmodium falciparum* life cycle in the human host. (*A*) Life cycle of *P. falciparum*. Human malaria infection is initiated when a female anopheline mosquito injects *Plasmodium* sporozoites into the skin during a blood meal. Sporozoites actively reach peripheral circulation and migrate to the liver in which they replicate within hepatocytes forming merozoites that are released into the bloodstream. Merozoites invade red blood cells (RBCs) and develop through ring, trophozoite, and schizont stages before forming new merozoites that are released at schizont egress and reinvade new RBCs. A small proportion of blood stage parasites develop into sexual stages called gametocytes that reach the dermis where they are taken up by another mosquito. After fertilization and sporogonic development in the mosquito midgut, infectious sporozoites are formed that reach the salivary glands for transmission into another host. (*B*) Schematic representation of *P. falciparum* gametocyte developmental stages. Gametocytes undergo five distinct morphological stages during development. Stage I and early stage II are morphologically similar to early stage asexual parasites, and late stage II is the first stage that can be distinguished from asexual trophozoites. Late stage III and stage IV are further elongated and characterized by their spindle shape, whereas in stage V gametocytes, the ends are more rounded forming a crescent shape with minimal visible host cell surface. (*C*) Model of bone marrow sequestration of *P. falciparum* gametocytes. Sexually committed parasitized RBCs home to the bone marrow by binding to endothelial wall of sinusoids followed by transmigration into the extravascular space and undergo development. Alternatively, early asexual parasite stages transmigrate into the extravascular space to produce sexually committed schizonts that release merozoites, which, on reinvasion, begins sexual developmental stages (models also reviewed in Nilsson et al. 2015). Increased rigidity of early gametocytes (Aingaran et al. 2012; Peatey et al. 2013) and the observed binding of immature gametocytes to erythroblastic islands (Joice et al. 2014) favor their maturation in the hematopoietic system. Mature gametocytes exit the microenvironment potentially because of restoration in their deformability (Tiburcio et al. 2012) and intravasate into circulation to be taken up by mosquitoes. (*D*) Model of *P. falciparum* gametocyte localization to the skin. Mature gametocytes preferentially sequester in the subdermal micro capillaries of skin where they are easily accessible to mosquito during a blood meal. (*Inset*) Factors influencing malaria transmission including host, parasite, and environmental conditions are listed.

et al. 1996a), gametocyte maturation requires only 24–27 h. The first recognizable gametocyte stages in *P. falciparum* are round compact forms containing hemozoin. These stages (stage I) and subsequent developmental forms (stage II–IV) are largely absent from blood circulation, but sequester in deep tissue in which they develop into mature sausage-shaped stage V gametocytes and reappear in the blood infective for mosquitoes (Thomson and Robertson 1935; Smalley et al. 1981). The density of mature *P. falciparum* gametocytes in peripheral circulation is typically <100 gametocytes/μL of blood (Drakeley et al. 2006), and in most cases they are present at submicroscopic levels. In contrast to *P. falciparum*, mature *P. vivax* gametocytes are large and round, filling up nearly the entire stippled red blood cell (RBC) with a prominent nucleus (Sinden and Gilles 2002). Because of their faster maturation period compared with *P. falciparum*, *P. vivax* gametocytes are present in blood circulation within a week after mosquito inoculation and before parasite detection by microscopy (Boyd and Stratman-Thomas 1934; Boyd et al. 1936; McKenzie et al. 2007). This poses a significant challenge to *P. vivax* elimination strategies, as infected people may be infectious before parasites are detectable by microscopy (see also below). On ingestion in the mosquito midgut, *P. falciparum* mature gametocytes egress from their host cell, differentiate into male and female gametes triggered by a drop in temperature, increase in pH and xanthurenic acid concentration, and, subsequently, undergo fertilization to form a diploid zygote (Billker et al. 1998, 2000). The zygote develops into motile ookinetes, which penetrate the mosquito midgut and develop into oocysts. *P. falciparum* oocysts mature over a period of 11–16 days (Meis et al. 1992) before releasing infectious sporozoites that migrate to the salivary glands for onward transmission. The likelihood of a mosquito acquiring an infection during a blood meal depends on a wide array of human, parasite, and mosquito factors. The development of gametocytes in humans is vital to the maintenance of malaria transmission and represents a potential bottleneck in the parasite's life cycle. Understanding the biology of

gametocyte development and the human infectious reservoir at both the individual and population level is therefore crucial to ablate disease transmission.

MECHANISMS OF SEXUAL COMMITMENT AND GAMETOCYTE SEQUESTRATION

Factors stimulating gametocytogenesis have been debated over the past decades. Early observational studies of infected individuals suggested that gametocyte production may be associated with clinical symptoms (Miller 1958), but the molecular mechanisms underlying this phenomenon remained unknown. The initiation of gametocytogenesis and modulation of gametocyte production in a natural infection is influenced by host environmental factors, including stress induced by host immunity (Bousema et al. 2006), antimalarial drug treatment (Dunyo et al. 2006), or anemia (Nacher et al. 2002), as well as host genetic factors such as human hemoglobin variants (Fig. 1, see inset, top) (Trager and Gill 1992; Gouagna et al. 2010). Similarly, under in vitro conditions, increased gametocyte production was seen at higher parasite densities (Bruce et al. 1990), in the presence of parasite-conditioned medium (Williams 1999; Dyer and Day 2003), and, on addition of human serum (Smalley and Brown 1981), erythroid progenitor cells (Peatey et al. 2013) or antimalarial drugs (Buckling et al. 1999). Total parasite density in an individual can influence gametocytogenesis as a relatively higher concentration of gametocytes was observed in individuals with low-density infections when compared with those with high-density infections (Drakeley et al. 2006). Evidence from clinical observations during human or experimental infections suggests an increased gametocyte production following drug treatment (Buckling et al. 1997; Price et al. 1999; Bousema et al. 2003; Sowunmi et al. 2011), indicating that inefficient treatment and/or parasite recrudescence are associated with higher gametocyte numbers (Price et al. 1999; Barnes et al. 2008). These studies suggest that selection of drug-resistant parasite clones may be associated with increased chances of transmission;

however, this hypothesis has yet to be systematically tested given the complex relationship between drug resistance and malaria transmission, which involves factors such as multiplicity of resistant clones, transmission intensity, and the genetic nature of resistance traits (Talisuna et al. 2003). Several other conditions have been associated with increased gametocyte production, including the time during transmission season (Ouédraogo et al. 2008), response to mosquito probing or bites from uninfected mosquitoes (Paul et al. 2004), and presence of vector-borne factors in the blood (Fischer et al. 2000).

Host Factors Associated with Gametocytogenesis

Naturally acquired immunity during a malaria infection limits the asexual parasite density, thereby affecting gametocyte production from the asexual precursors. However, there is also evidence for a direct influence of *Plasmodium*-induced host-immune response on gametocytogenesis. Increased gametocyte production in *P. falciparum* cultures was observed on addition of lymphocytes and sera from malaria-infected Gambian children (Smalley and Brown 1981) and after addition of anti−*P. falciparum* antibodies produced by hybridoma cell lines (Ono et al. 1986). Data from epidemiological studies suggest a role for anemia in triggering gametocytogenesis. A high proportion of gametocyte carriers were observed among anemic individuals in studies from Thailand and The Gambia (Price et al. 1999; von Seidlein et al. 2001; Nacher et al. 2002; Stepniewska et al. 2008), but the association may be a result of a longer duration of infection resulting in late gametocyte development in these individuals. More convincing data are from in vitro studies in which *P. falciparum* gametocytogenesis is promoted in the presence of young RBCs or reticulocytes (Trager et al. 1999; Trager 2005). On erythropoietin (EPO) treatment, which induces reticulocytosis, a marked increase in *Plasmodium chabaudi* (Gautret et al. 1996b) and *P. berghei* (Mons 1986) gametocyte production was observed in vivo. However, it is not clear which signal(s) associated with reticulocytosis stimulates gametocytogenesis.

Molecular Mechanism of Sexual Conversion

The rate of gametocyte production has historically been thought to be linked to the parasite's response to hostile growth conditions. Recent studies have started to unravel the molecular and cellular basis for the sexual developmental switch. Evidence from *P. falciparum* in vitro cultures indicates that sexual differentiation can be induced by depletion of nutrients in the parasite environment (culture media) (Williams 1999; Dyer and Day 2003). More recently, two studies have shown that extracellular vesicles (EVs) secreted by *P. falciparum* infected RBCs into the environment (or culture media) act as intercellular communicators to induce gametocytogenesis (Mantel et al. 2013; Regev-Rudzki et al. 2013). Purified EVs from the conditioned media of in vitro *P. falciparum* cultures can be internalized by infected RBCs and stimulate sexual stage development in a dose-dependent manner (Mantel et al. 2013). In addition, Regev-Rudzki et al. (2013) showed that drug treatment induces the release of EVs that can transfer nucleic acids to neighboring parasites promoting sexual conversion in the recipient cells as well as conferring drug resistance. The specific components of EVs that induce gametocytogenesis and the subsequent downstream mechanism in the sexual conversion pathway remain to be elucidated, which may open up new targets to ablate gametocyte development.

The genetic factors underlying sexual differentiation in *Plasmodium* parasites have remained elusive until recently. Early studies suggested that merozoites released from a schizont commit to either the asexual or sexual pathway (Inselburg 1983; Bruce et al. 1990) and that sexually committed parasites form exclusively male or female gametocytes (Silvestrini et al. 2000). These studies suggested a defined gene expression pathway responsible for commitment in malaria parasites. More recent work revealed that sexual commitment is regulated by a highly conserved apicomplexan-specific transcription factor, ApiAP2-G, both in *P. falciparum* (Kafsack et al. 2014) and in *P. berghei* (Sinha et al. 2014). In *P. berghei*, the disruption of another transcription factor from the AP2 family, AP-2G2, appears to inhibit male gametocyte development and may, therefore, be involved in maintenance of gametocyte sex ratio (Sinha et al. 2014). *P. falciparum* ApiAP2-G was found to be epigenetically regulated by at least two proteins, histone deacetylase 2 (PfHda2) and heterochromatin protein 1 (PfHP1), which causes repression of gametocytogenesis under nonpermissive conditions (Brancucci et al. 2014; Coleman et al. 2014). Conditional knockdown of PfHda1 or PfHP1 in asexual stage parasites in vitro leads to a cascade of gene activation, including *AP2-G*, and induction of gametocyte production (and decreased asexual replication) (Brancucci et al. 2014; Coleman et al. 2014). Together, these findings show epigenetic control of stage conversion; however, the upstream factors regulating these epigenetic control mechanisms remain unknown. In addition to ApiAP2-G-mediated epigenetic regulation, it is likely that additional factors are involved in the onset of gametocytogenesis. Moving forward, it will be important to understand how external stress factors are linked to the molecular mechanism(s) of sexual commitment and gametocyte development.

Sequestration of Transmission Stages

Tissue-specific sequestration of asexual parasite stages is associated with severe malaria pathology such as cerebral malaria and pregnancy-associated malaria (Miller et al. 2002). RBCs infected with the asexual stages of *P. falciparum* (mature trophozoites and schizonts) are sequestered away from peripheral circulation by adhering to endothelial receptors, such as CD36, ICAM-1, and CSA in the microvasculature (for reviews, see Miller et al. 2002; Sherman et al. 2003). Adherence to host receptors is mediated by expression of parasite-derived *P. falciparum* erythrocyte membrane protein-1 (PfEMP-1) on knob-like structures at the surface of infected RBCs (Kilejian 1979; Baruch et al. 1995). Although the transmission stages do not generally contribute to disease pathology, immature

stages of *P. falciparum* gametocytes sequester in tissues presumably to avoid clearance by the spleen. In contrast, all developmental stages of *P. vivax* gametocytes can be seen in the blood and no sequestration of *P. vivax* transmission stages has been reported so far. Because *P. vivax* develops exclusively in reticulocytes, RBCs infected with *P. vivax* have an increased surface area and are highly flexible (Suwanarusk et al. 2004; Handayani et al. 2009), which presumably helps them to pass through small capillaries or sinusoidal vessels and avoid clearance by the spleen.

Postmortem case studies from the early 1900s (Marchiafava and Bignami 1894; Thomson and Robertson 1935) and more recent field and clinical reports in the last two decades (Smalley et al. 1981; Farfour et al. 2012; Aguilar et al. 2014) have confirmed the presence of *P. falciparum* immature gametocytes in the spleen and bone marrow of malaria infected patients. Notably, a recent systematic histological and transcriptional analysis of autopsy tissues from children who died from cerebral malaria revealed gametocyte enrichment in the bone marrow parenchyma in which they are predominantly localized to the erythroblastic islands (Joice et al. 2014), suggesting that sexual stage development can occur in erythroid progenitor cells during infection. The underlying mechanism of gametocyte sequestration, including the parasite stages that home to bone marrow, is not yet well defined. However, the prevailing model suggests that sexually committed parasites or immature gametocytes traverse the endothelial barrier and home to the bone marrow parenchyma, in which they undergo development to produce mature gametocytes that eventually intravasate into the peripheral circulation (Fig. 1C) (Nilsson et al. 2015; Pelle et al. 2015). In contrast to asexual stages, early gametocytes do not significantly modify the RBC, as minimal levels of PfEMP-1 are expressed on the infected RBC surface and no significant knob structures were observed (Silvestrini et al. 2012; Tiburcio et al. 2013). This difference in surface protein expression is consistent with in vitro studies in which immature gametocytes showed significantly less, if any, binding to purified host ligands (CD36,

ICAM-1) (Day et al. 1998) and to bone marrow endothelium or other endothelial cell lines (Silvestrini et al. 2012). Altogether, these data suggest that gametocyte sequestration is PfEMP-1 independent, but may involve other exported parasite molecule(s) required for bone marrow homing and association with erythroblast islands in parenchyma. Based on *Plasmodium*-specific serum responses from malaria patients, the surface antigens of gametocytes seem to be distinct from those on the surface of asexual infected RBCs (Saeed et al. 2008), indicating that host–parasite interactions in tissues are likely gametocyte-specific. Products of multigene families involved in host cell modifications, such as STEVOR and RIFIN, are expressed during gametocyte development (McRobert et al. 2004; Petter et al. 2008), but their functional role in gametocytogenesis or cytoadherence has not been shown. Nevertheless, a switch in deformability of mature gametocytes (Aingaran et al. 2012; Dearnley et al. 2012; Tiburcio et al. 2012) is accompanied by reorganization of STEVOR in the RBC membrane of mature gametocytes (Tiburcio et al. 2012). Taken together, the sequestration and subsequent development of immature gametocytes in the bone marrow and spleen is likely to be maintained through mechanical retention and as-yet-uncharacterized binding properties, whereas the switch in deformability at the mature stage V gametocyte stage may facilitate their release from sequestration sites into the periphery.

Extravascular sequestration in the bone marrow may not only help young gametocytes to evade host immune responses and/or undergo development, but also provide a nutrient-rich and aerobic environment with abundant young RBCs for ideal gametocyte development. In agreement with this hypothesis, in vitro data indicates an enhanced invasion of erythroid progenitor cells with a concomitant increase in gametocyte formation within young RBCs (Tamez et al. 2009; Peatey et al. 2013). More focused studies are required to decipher the mechanism of gametocyte sequestration, including identification of parasite stages that home to the bone marrow, the receptor–ligand interactions involved, if any, and importantly,

whether sexual commitment occurs in the periphery or in the bone marrow microenvironment. Answers to these outstanding questions on gametocyte sequestration are crucial to understand transmission dynamics and to design novel transmission intervention strategies.

DETERMINANTS OF INFECTIOUSNESS

In the human host, a small subset of total parasite population differentiates into mature gametocytes, some of which may be ingested by a mosquito during a blood meal. Subsequent fertilization of gametes and development into sporozoites within the mosquito makes it infectious to another human. The human infectious reservoir is defined as the proportion of a population capable of successfully infecting mosquitoes (Drakeley et al. 2000). Gametocyte carriage and successful transmission from human to mosquito is influenced by several factors including age (Ouédraogo et al. 2010), gametocyte density (Robert et al. 2000; Schneider et al. 2007; Ouédraogo et al. 2009), gametocyte sex ratio (Robert et al. 1996b; Mitri et al. 2009), antimalarial drug treatment (Buckling et al. 1999; Robert et al. 2000; Sowunmi et al. 2004), and host immunity (Fig. 1, see inset, top) (Saeed et al. 2008; Sutherland 2009). Although mature gametocyte presence in the blood has long been thought to be crucial for an efficient transmission, these stages were rarely detected by microscopy (Dowling and Shute 1966; Bejon et al. 2006) and, therefore, it was previously assumed that only a small proportion of malaria-infected individuals carried gametocytes. With the use of sensitive molecular assays, it is now clear that gametocytes are present in most malaria infections and at highly variable densities (Schneider et al. 2007; Shekalaghe et al. 2007) that can successfully infect mosquitoes (Schneider et al. 2007; Bousema et al. 2012; Churcher et al. 2013). Given the highly variable and nonlinear relationship between gametocyte density and mosquito infection rate (Bousema et al. 2012; Churcher et al. 2013), quantifying the human component of the infectious reservoir is a challenging task. Mosquito-feeding assays have been routinely used to quantify the infectiousness of an individual and to evaluate the effects of transmission-blocking vaccines or gametocytocidal drugs. In direct skin-feeding assays, *Anopheles* mosquitoes are allowed to take a blood meal by direct contact with the skin of an individual recapitulating a natural infection (Bousema et al. 2012). In membrane-feeding assays, there are two types: (1) Direct membrane-feeding assay (DMFA) involves feeding uninfected *Anopheles* mosquitoes with a blood sample drawn from a naturally infected individual through an artificial membrane (parafilm) in the presence of autologous sera, and (2) standard membrane feeding assay (SMFA) involves feeding mosquitoes with in vitro cultured gametocytes mixed with RBCs and human serum through the membrane in a device (Bousema et al. 2012). Mosquito infectivity is measured in these assays by quantifying the number of oocysts present in the mosquito midgut (either as mean oocyst density or oocyst prevalence across mosquitoes) following a maturation period of 7 to 8 days. Although direct skin feeding assays may yield a more accurate estimate of human transmission potential, membrane-feeding assays are appropriate to compare infectiousness between individuals and to assess transmission-reducing interventions (Bousema et al. 2012; Miura et al. 2013). The SMFA, compared with DMFA, can be performed under standardized laboratory conditions and is considered the gold standard for measuring transmission-reducing activity. A more detailed review of the human infectious reservoir at the epidemiological level and tools to measure transmission is covered in Bousema and Drakely (2016).

Relationship between Gametocyte Density and Infectiousness to Mosquitoes

Human infectiousness is linked to asexual parasite density and gametocyte density in the blood. Although there is a positive correlation between gametocyte density and mosquito infection rate (Schneider et al. 2007; Ouédraogo et al. 2009), the association is highly variable and complex at low gametocyte densities (van der Kolk et al. 2005). High gametocyte densities

do not necessarily result in mosquito infection (Graves et al. 1988; Gamage-Mendis et al. 1991; Schneider et al. 2007), whereas individuals with low densities that carry no observable gametocytes have been found to be infectious (Jeffery and Eyles 1955; Muirhead-Thomson 1998; Coleman et al. 2004; Schneider et al. 2007). This heterogeneity in mosquito infection may result in part from sampling bias: Samples are generally collected via venipuncture but there may be a specified localization or clustering of gametocytes in the human vasculature during a blood meal (Pichon et al. 2000). Similarly, in *P. vivax* infections, the relationship between gametocyte density and mosquito infection is poorly defined which is attributed to limited sensitivity of microscopy to detect and differentiate gametocyte stages (Gamage-Mendis et al. 1991; Bharti et al. 2006). In one study, *P. vivax* infected patients were infectious to mosquitoes immediately after the appearance of asexual parasites detected by microscopy, but significantly before the emergence of gametocytes (Jeffery 1952). Similarly, several reports of infectivity at undetectable *P. vivax* gametocytemia have been published (Gamage-Mendis et al. 1991; Sattabongkot et al. 1991; McKenzie et al. 2002; Coleman et al. 2004; Pethleart et al. 2004; Bharti et al. 2006). Comparative studies of *P. falciparum* and *P. vivax* indicate that malaria transmission by *P. vivax* parasites is likely to be highly efficient, with lower gametocyte densities typically resulting in mosquito infection (Pukrittayakamee et al. 2008). The use of more sensitive tools, such as QT-NASBA to detect late gametocyte-specific mRNA markers, will help to evaluate the association between *P. vivax* gametocyte density and mosquito infection (Beurskens et al. 2009). Moreover, *P. vivax* transmission is much faster and more persistent than *P. falciparum* because of their ability to form gametocytes early and the relapse of blood stage infections caused by reactivation of hypnozoites (Galinski et al. 2013).

Dynamics of Parasite Genotypes (Complexity of Infection)

The evolutionary success of malaria transmission is attributed to the genetic complexity of

Cite this article as *Cold Spring Harb Perspect Med* doi: 10.1101/cshperspect.a025452

P. falciparum gametocytes in a natural infection and their infectivity to mosquitoes. A high degree of clonal multiplicity persists in malaria-endemic regions that varies with transmission intensity (Robert et al. 1996a), whereas cross-mating in mosquitoes produces new strains in the next generation. Multiple parasite clones in an individual were found to be equally transmissible to mosquitoes with a strong correlation between multiplicity of infection and frequency of cross-mating (Hill and Babiker 1995). However, in some cases, not all clones from the same infection were infectious resulting in less variable genotypes in the infected individual (Paul et al. 1995). In natural infections in The Gambia at the end of the dry season, a higher transmissibility of multiple clones was notably observed even if they existed as a minority parasite population in asymptomatic individuals (Nwakanma et al. 2008). Existing in vitro and population studies suggest that dynamics and degree of *P. falciparum* gametocyte production is associated with the parasite's genetic background (Graves et al. 1984; Teklehaimanot et al. 1987; Abdel-Wahab et al. 2002); however, factors favoring the production of different gametocyte clones within a mixed population are unknown.

Gametocyte Sex Ratio

Gametocyte sex ratio is one of the critical determinants of malaria transmission. Because one male gametocyte produces eight microgametes during final maturation, whereas the female gametocyte develops into one macrogamete, malaria parasites generally produce more female gametocytes than male, and they can also modulate the sex ratio during an infection. An optimal ratio of three or four females to one male gametocyte is commonly observed in *P. falciparum* infections (Robert et al. 1996b, 2003; Kar et al. 2009), but this varies considerably over the course of an infection and between malaria-endemic regions (Paul et al. 2002; Talman et al. 2004; Sowunmi et al. 2008). A higher production of male gametocytes relative to female gametocytes maximizes the success of transmission and this is especially important at lower gametocyte densities (Reece et al.

2008) where there is a need for male bias. The sex ratio is also influenced by stimulation of erythropoiesis (anemic state) and presence of competing parasite strains, which tends to favor a male-biased sex ratio in the infection (Paul et al. 2002; Reece et al. 2008). Differences in gametocyte sex ratio may be associated with the parasite's general response to host immunity during an infection (Paul et al. 2000) and/or stress factors affecting gametocytogenesis including parasite density (Reece et al. 2008).

Gametocyte Localization to the Skin Compartment

The availability of transmission stages ready to be picked up in a mosquito's blood meal is an essential component of human infectiousness and for efficient transmission, as mature gametocytes in circulation must traverse the microvasculature to reach the dermis. There is evidence for preferential parasite localization in the skin compartment. In a diagnostic study from the early 1950s conducted in the endemic regions of the Belgian Congo, skin scarification smears from acute and chronic malaria patients (children and adults) had a higher frequency of mature schizonts and gametocytes compared with thick peripheral blood films (van den and Chardome 1951; Chardome and Janssen 1952). Similarly, in the rodent *P. chabaudi* model, gametocyte numbers were higher in the mosquito's blood meal immediately after engorgement than in the venous tail blood (Gautret et al. 1996b), suggesting an enrichment of parasites in the skin microvasculature. A recent autopsy study of cerebral malaria patients from Malawi showed significant parasite sequestration in the skin microvasculature in a subset of patients by histological analysis (Milner et al. 2015); however, the stage composition of these parasites has not been determined. In another study, infection rates of mosquitoes that were fed directly on the skin were 2.4-fold higher than those observed after feeding on venous blood samples through an artificial membrane (Bousema et al. 2012). These studies suggest that infectious *P. falciparum* mature gametocytes may preferentially localize to subdermal capillaries beneath the skin (Fig. 1D). In addition, there is a distinct possibility that the parasite modulates gametocyte densities or sequestration according to the peak hours when mosquitoes take a blood meal (Hawking et al. 1971; Garnham 1974). Although conclusive evidence is still lacking, this scenario would likely enhance transmission success and maintain genetic diversity in the population by increasing the possibility of cotransmission of male and female gametocytes and of multiple genotypes in an infection. The increased deformability and subsequent interaction with specific receptors may aid in the localization of mature gametocytes to subdermal capillaries. This hypothesis needs to be rigorously tested using mosquito feeding assays and in vivo models.

CONCLUDING REMARKS AND FUTURE PERSPECTIVES

Understanding the biology of transmission stages in the human host leading to mosquito infectivity will be essential to successfully overcome current challenges in malaria elimination efforts. Despite their crucial role in transmission, many fundamental questions of gametocyte biology and development remain to be answered. In this review, we have discussed the sexual biology of malaria parasites and determinants of infectiousness emphasizing key factors influencing transmission in a human host. Transmission-blocking intervention strategies targeting sexual stages should take into account molecular targets including the genetic pathways of sexual conversion, sequestration mechanisms, intercellular parasite communication mechanisms, and gametocyte deformability. Increasing evidence in recent years point to the existence of a niche for gametocyte development in the extravascular environment of bone marrow (and presumably in the spleen) (Farfour et al. 2012; Aguilar et al. 2014; Joice et al. 2014) acting as the parasite's hideout. Identification of stage-specific markers and development of novel tools to study sequestration of immature gametocytes are warranted. Another important open question is how the developmental decision between asexual and sexual commitment is induced. The environmental cues influencing this decision are likely connected to precise signaling pathways leading to changes in gene expression. With the identification of genetic master regulators of sexual commitment (AP-2 and DOZI) (Mair et al. 2006; Kafsack et al. 2014; Sinha et al. 2014), the transcriptional and translational mechanisms regulating induction and maturation of gametocytes are becoming clearer. It remains to be answered if this regulation is conserved across *Plasmodium* species and whether a specific environment in the vertebrate host favors sexual differentiation. Finally, a major challenge for future research is to understand and define the infectious potential of malaria-infected individuals. Although highly sensitive molecular detection tools such as quantitative real-time PCR (qRT-PCR), RT-loop-mediated isothermal amplification (RT-LAMP), and quantitative nucleic acid-sequence-based amplification (QT-NASBA) indicate that a high proportion of asymptomatic individuals carry submicroscopic infections (Schneider et al. 2007; Shekalaghe et al. 2007; Bousema and Drakeley 2011), elimination of lingering parasite forms in these individuals is important. In conclusion, combined human, parasite, mosquito, and environmental factors play a key role in influencing transmission and the human infectious reservoir overall. To better understand the infectious reservoir in an individual and to develop transmission-blocking drugs and vaccines, further research on the basic biology of gametocytes and their dynamics within the host is essential. Building on exciting advances in the field discussed here, studies addressing the remaining knowledge gaps in transmission biology will open up new avenues for feasible targets to interrupt malaria transmission.

ACKNOWLEDGMENTS

The authors thank Kathleen Dantzler and Deepali Ravel for critical reading of the manuscript and helpful suggestions. Work in the Marti laboratory is funded by Grants 5R01AI077558 and 1R21AI105328 from the National Institutes of Health and a Career Development Award from the Burroughs Wellcome Fund to M.M.

REFERENCES

*Reference is also in this collection.

Abdel-Wahab A, Abdel-Muhsin AM, Ali E, Suleiman S, Ahmed S, Walliker D, Babiker HA. 2002. Dynamics of gametocytes among *Plasmodium falciparum* clones in natural infections in an area of highly seasonal transmission. *J Infect Dis* **185:** 1838–1842.

Aguilar R, Magallon-Tejada A, Achtman AH, Moraleda C, Joice R, Cistero P, Li Wai Suen CS, Nhabomba A, Macete E, Mueller I, et al. 2014. Molecular evidence for the localization of *Plasmodium falciparum* immature gametocytes in bone marrow. *Blood* **123:** 959–966.

Aingaran M, Zhang R, Law SK, Peng Z, Undisz A, Meyer E, Diez-Silva M, Burke TA, Spielmann T, Lim CT, et al. 2012. Host cell deformability is linked to transmission in the human malaria parasite *Plasmodium falciparum*. *Cell Microbiol* **14:** 983–993.

Alonso PL, Brown G, Arevalo-Herrera M, Binka F, Chitnis C, Collins F, Doumbo OK, Greenwood B, Hall BF, Levine MM, et al. 2011. A research agenda to underpin malaria eradication. *PLoS Med* **8:** e1000406.

Barnes KI, Little F, Mabuza A, Mngomezulu N, Govere J, Durrheim D, Roper C, Watkins B, White NJ. 2008. Increased gametocytemia after treatment: An early parasitological indicator of emerging sulfadoxine–pyrimethamine resistance in falciparum malaria. *J Infect Dis* **197:** 1605–1613.

Baruch DI, Pasloske BL, Singh HB, Bi X, Ma XC, Feldman M, Taraschi TF, Howard RJ. 1995. Cloning the *P. falciparum* gene encoding PfEMP1, a malarial variant antigen and adherence receptor on the surface of parasitized human erythrocytes. *Cell* **82:** 77–87.

Bejon P, Andrews L, Hunt-Cooke A, Sanderson F, Gilbert SC, Hill AV. 2006. Thick blood film examination for *Plasmodium falciparum* malaria has reduced sensitivity and underestimates parasite density. *Malaria J* **5:** 104.

Beurskens M, Mens P, Schallig H, Syafruddin D, Asih PB, Hermsen R, Sauerwein R. 2009. Quantitative determination of *Plasmodium vivax* gametocytes by real-time quantitative nucleic acid sequence-based amplification in clinical samples. *Am J Trop Med Hyg* **81:** 366–369.

Bharti AR, Chuquiyauri R, Brouwer KC, Stancil J, Lin J, Llanos-Cuentas A, Vinetz JM. 2006. Experimental infection of the neotropical malaria vector *Anopheles darlingi* by human patient-derived *Plasmodium vivax* in the Peruvian Amazon. *Am J Trop Med Hyg* **75:** 610–616.

Billker O, Lindo V, Panico M, Etienne AE, Paxton T, Dell A, Rogers M, Sinden RE, Morris HR. 1998. Identification of xanthurenic acid as the putative inducer of malaria development in the mosquito. *Nature* **392:** 289–292.

Billker O, Miller AJ, Sinden RE. 2000. Determination of mosquito bloodmeal pH in situ by ion-selective microelectrode measurement: Implications for the regulation of malarial gametogenesis. *Parasitology* **120:** 547–551.

Bousema T, Drakeley C. 2011. Epidemiology and infectivity of *Plasmodium falciparum* and *Plasmodium vivax* gametocytes in relation to malaria control and elimination. *Clin Microbiol Rev* **24:** 377–410.

* Bousema T, Drakely C. 2016. Determinants of malaria transmission at the population level. *Cold Spring Harb Perspect Med* doi: 10.1101/cshperspect.a025510.

Bousema JT, Gouagna LC, Meutstege AM, Okech BE, Akim NI, Githure JI, Beier JC, Sauerwein RW. 2003. Treatment failure of pyrimethamine-sulphadoxine and induction of *Plasmodium falciparum* gametocytaemia in children in western Kenya. *Trop Med Intl Health* **8:** 427–430.

Bousema JT, Drakeley CJ, Sauerwein RW. 2006. Sexual-stage antibody responses to *P. falciparum* in endemic populations. *Curr Mol Med* **6:** 223–229.

Bousema T, Dinglasan RR, Morlais I, Gouagna LC, van Warmerdam T, Awono-Ambene PH, Bonnet S, Diallo M, Coulibaly M, Tchuinkam T, et al. 2012. Mosquito feeding assays to determine the infectiousness of naturally infected *Plasmodium falciparum* gametocyte carriers. *PLoS ONE* **7:** e42821.

Boyd MF, Stratman-Thomas W. 1934. Studies on *Plasmodium vivax*. 7: Some observations on inoculation and onset. *Amer J Hyg* **20:** 488.

Boyd MF, Stratman-Thomas W, Muench H. 1936. The occurrence of gametocytes of *Plasmodium vivax* during the primary attack. *Am J Trop Med Hyg* **1:** 133–138.

Brancucci NM, Bertschi NL, Zhu L, Niederwieser I, Chin WH, Wampfler R, Freymond C, Rottmann M, Felger I, Bozdech Z, et al. 2014. Heterochromatin protein 1 secures survival and transmission of malaria parasites. *Cell Host Microbe* **16:** 165–176.

Bruce MC, Alano P, Duthie S, Carter R. 1990. Commitment of the malaria parasite *Plasmodium falciparum* to sexual and asexual development. *Parasitology* **100:** 191–200.

Buckling AG, Taylor LH, Carlton JM, Read AF. 1997. Adaptive changes in *Plasmodium* transmission strategies following chloroquine chemotherapy. *Proc Biol Sci* **264:** 553–559.

Buckling A, Ranford-Cartwright LC, Miles A, Read AF. 1999. Chloroquine increases *Plasmodium falciparum* gametocytogenesis in vitro. *Parasitology* **118:** 339–346.

Chardome M, Janssen P. 1952. Enquête sur l'incidence malarienne par la method dermique dans la region de Lubilash (Congo Belge) [Investigations on malaria incidence by skin scarification method in the Lubilash region (Belgian Congo)]. *Ann Soc Belge Med Trop* **32:** 209–211.

Churcher TS, Bousema T, Walker M, Drakeley C, Schneider P, Ouédraogo AL, Basanez MG. 2013. Predicting mosquito infection from *Plasmodium falciparum* gametocyte density and estimating the reservoir of infection. *eLife* **2:** e00626.

Cohen JM, Moonen B, Snow RW, Smith DL. 2010. How absolute is zero? An evaluation of historical and current definitions of malaria elimination. *Malaria J* **9:** 213.

Coleman RE, Kumpitak C, Ponlawat A, Maneechai N, Phunkitchar V, Rachapaew N, Zollner G, Sattabongkot J. 2004. Infectivity of asymptomatic *Plasmodium*-infected human populations to *Anopheles dirus* mosquitoes in western Thailand. *J Med Entomol* **41:** 201–208.

Coleman BI, Skillman KM, Jiang RH, Childs LM, Altenhofen LM, Ganter M, Leung Y, Goldowitz I, Kafsack BF, Marti M, et al. 2014. A *Plasmodium falciparum* histone deacetylase regulates antigenic variation and gametocyte conversion. *Cell Host Microbe* 16: 177–186.

Day KP, Hayward RE, Smith D, Culvenor JG. 1998. CD36-dependent adhesion and knob expression of the transmission stages of *Plasmodium falciparum* is stage specific. *Mol Biochem Parasitol* 93: 167–177.

Dearnley MK, Yeoman JA, Hanssen E, Kenny S, Turnbull L, Whitchurch CB, Tilley L, Dixon MW. 2012. Origin, composition, organization and function of the inner membrane complex of *Plasmodium falciparum* gametocytes. *J Cell Sci* 125: 2053–2063.

Dembélé L, Franetich JF, Lorthiois A, Gego A, Zeeman AM, Kocken CH, Le Grand R, Dereuddre-Bosquet N, van Gemert GJ, Sauerwein R. 2014. Persistence and activation of malaria hypnozoites in long-term primary hepatocyte cultures. *Nat Med* 20: 307–312.

Dondorp AM, Nosten F, Yi P, Das D, Phyo AP, Tarning J, Lwin KM, Ariey F, Hanpithakpong W, Lee SJ, et al. 2009. Artemisinin resistance in *Plasmodium falciparum* malaria. *N Engl J Med* 361: 455–467.

Dowling M, Shute G. 1966. A comparative study of thick and thin blood films in the diagnosis of scanty malaria parasitaemia. *Bull World Health Organ* 34: 249.

Drakeley CJ, Akim NI, Sauerwein RW, Greenwood BM, Targett GA. 2000. Estimates of the infectious reservoir of *Plasmodium falciparum* malaria in The Gambia and in Tanzania. *Trans R Soc Trop Med Hyg* 94: 472–476.

Drakeley C, Sutherland C, Bousema JT, Sauerwein RW, Targett GA. 2006. The epidemiology of *Plasmodium falciparum* gametocytes: Weapons of mass dispersion. *Trends Parasitol* 22: 424–430.

Dunyo S, Milligan P, Edwards T, Sutherland C, Targett G, Pinder M. 2006. Gametocytaemia after drug treatment of asymptomatic *Plasmodium falciparum*. *PLoS Clin Trials* 1: e20.

Dyer M, Day KP. 2003. Regulation of the rate of asexual growth and commitment to sexual development by diffusible factors from in vitro cultures of *Plasmodium falciparum*. *Am J Trop Med Hyg* 68: 403–409.

Farfour E, Charlotte F, Settegrana C, Miyara M, Buffet P. 2012. The extravascular compartment of the bone marrow: A niche for *Plasmodium falciparum* gametocyte maturation? *Malaria J* 11: 285.

Fischer P, Supali T, Wibowo H, Bonow I, Williams SA. 2000. Detection of DNA of nocturnally periodic *Brugia malayi* in night and day blood samples by a polymerase chain reaction-ELISA-based method using an internal control DNA. *Am J Trop Med Hyg* 62: 291–296.

Galinski MR, Meyer EV, Barnwell JW. 2013. *Plasmodium vivax*: Modern strategies to study a persistent parasite's life cycle. *Adv Parasitol* 81: 1–26.

Gamage-Mendis AC, Rajakaruna J, Carter R, Mendis KN. 1991. Infectious reservoir of *Plasmodium vivax* and *Plasmodium falciparum* malaria in an endemic region of Sri Lanka. *Am J Trop Med Hyg* 45: 479–487.

Garnham P. 1974. Periodicity of infectivity of plasmodial gametocytes: The "Hawking phenomenon." *Int J Parasitol* 4: 103–106.

Gautret P, Miltgen F, Chabaud AG, Landau I. 1996a. Synchronized *Plasmodium yoelii yoelii*: Pattern of gametocyte production, sequestration and infectivity. *Parassitologia* 38: 575–577.

Gautret P, Miltgen F, Gantier JC, Chabaud AG, Landau I. 1996b. Enhanced gametocyte formation by *Plasmodium chabaudi* in immature erythrocytes: Pattern of production, sequestration, and infectivity to mosquitoes. *J Parasitol* 82: 900–906.

Gething PW, Elyazar IR, Moyes CL, Smith DL, Battle KE, Guerra CA, Patil AP, Tatem AJ, Howes RE, Myers MF, et al. 2012. A long neglected world malaria map: *Plasmodium vivax* endemicity in 2010. *PLoS Negl Trop Dis* 6: e1814.

Global Partnership to Roll Back Malaria. 2001. *Antimalarial drug combination therapy: Report of a WHO technical consultation, 4–5 April 2001*. World Health Organization, Geneva.

Gouagna LC, Bancone G, Yao F, Yameogo B, Dabire KR, Costantini C, Simpore J, Ouédraogo JB, Modiano D. 2010. Genetic variation in human HBB is associated with *Plasmodium falciparum* transmission. *Nat Genet* 42: 328–331.

Graves PM, Carter R, McNeill KM. 1984. Gametocyte production in cloned lines of *Plasmodium falciparum*. *Am J Trop Med Hyg* 33: 1045–1050.

Graves PM, Burkot TR, Carter R, Cattani JA, Lagog M, Parker J, Brabin BJ, Gibson FD, Bradley DJ, Alpers MP. 1988. Measurement of malarial infectivity of human populations to mosquitoes in the Madang area, Papua, New Guinea. *Parasitology* 96: 251–263.

Handayani S, Chiu DT, Tjitra E, Kuo JS, Lampah D, Kenangalem E, Renia L, Snounou G, Price RN, Anstey NM, et al. 2009. High deformability of *Plasmodium vivax*–infected red blood cells under microfluidic conditions. *J Infect Dis* 199: 445–450.

Hawking F, Wilson ME, Gammage K. 1971. Evidence for cyclic development and short-lived maturity in the gametocytes of *Plasmodium falciparum*. *Trans R Soc Trop Med Hyg* 65: 549–559.

Hill WG, Babiker HA. 1995. Estimation of numbers of malaria clones in blood samples. *Proc Biol Sci* 262: 249–257.

Inselburg J. 1983. Gametocyte formation by the progeny of single *Plasmodium falciparum* schizonts. *J Parasitol* 69: 584–591.

Jeffery GM. 1952. The infection of mosquitoes by *Plasmodium vivax* (Chesson strain) during the early primary parasitemias. *Am J Trop Med Hyg* 1: 612–617.

Jeffery GM, Eyles DE. 1955. Infectivity to mosquitoes of *Plasmodium falciparum* as related to gametocyte density and duration of infection. *Am J Trop Med Hyg* 4: 781–789.

Joice R, Nilsson SK, Montgomery J, Dankwa S, Egan E, Morahan B, Seydel KB, Bertuccini L, Alano P, Williamson KC, et al. 2014. *Plasmodium falciparum* transmission stages accumulate in the human bone marrow. *Sci Transl Med* 6: 244re245.

Kafsack BF, Rovira-Graells N, Clark TG, Bancells C, Crowley VM, Campino SG, Williams AE, Drought LG, Kwiatkowski DP, Baker DA, et al. 2014. A transcriptional switch underlies commitment to sexual development in malaria parasites. *Nature* 507: 248–252.

Kar P, Dua V, Gupta N, Gupta A, Dash A. 2009. *Plasmodium falciparum* gametocytaemia with chloroquine chemotherapy in persistent malaria in an endemic area of India. *Indian J Med Res* **129**: 299–304.

Kilejian A. 1979. Characterization of a protein correlated with the production of knob-like protrusions on membranes of erythrocytes infected with *Plasmodium falciparum*. *Proc Natl Acad Sci* **76**: 4650–4653.

Mair GR, Braks JA, Garver LS, Wiegant JC, Hall N, Dirks RW, Khan SM, Dimopoulos G, Janse CJ, Waters AP. 2006. Regulation of sexual development of *Plasmodium* by translational repression. *Science* **313**: 667–669.

malERA Consultative Group on Drugs. 2011. A research agenda for malaria eradication: Drugs. *PLoS Med* **8**: e1000402.

Mantel PY, Hoang AN, Goldowitz I, Potashnikova D, Hamza B, Vorobjev I, Ghiran I, Toner M, Irimia D, Ivanov AR, et al. 2013. Malaria-infected erythrocyte-derived microvesicles mediate cellular communication within the parasite population and with the host immune system. *Cell Host Microbe* **13**: 521–534.

Marchiafava E, Bignami A. 1894. *On summer–autumn malarial fevers*. Book on Demand, Stoughton, WI.

Mbengue A, Bhattacharjee S, Pandharkar T, Liu H, Estiu G, Stahelin RV, Rizk SS, Njimoh DL, Ryan Y, Chotivanich K, et al. 2015. A molecular mechanism of artemisinin resistance in *Plasmodium falciparum* malaria. *Nature* **520**: 683–687.

McKenzie FE, Jeffery GM, Collins WE. 2002. *Plasmodium vivax* blood-stage dynamics. *J Parasitol* **88**: 521–535.

McKenzie FE, Jeffery GM, Collins WE. 2007. Gametocytemia and fever in human malaria infections. *J Parasitol* **93**: 627–633.

McRobert L, Preiser P, Sharp S, Jarra W, Kaviratne M, Taylor MC, Renia L, Sutherland CJ. 2004. Distinct trafficking and localization of STEVOR proteins in three stages of the *Plasmodium falciparum* life cycle. *Infect Immun* **72**: 6597–6602.

Meis JF, Wismans PG, Jap PH, Lensen AH, Ponnudurai T. 1992. A scanning electron microscopic study of the sporogonic development of *Plasmodium falciparum* in *Anopheles stephensi*. *Acta Tropica* **50**: 227–236.

Miller MJ. 1958. Observations on the natural history of malaria in the semi-resistant West African. *Trans R Soc Trop Med Hyg* **52**: 152–168.

Miller LH, Baruch DI, Marsh K, Doumbo OK. 2002. The pathogenic basis of malaria. *Nature* **415**: 673–679.

Milner DA Jr, Lee JJ, Frantzreb C, Whitten RO, Kamiza S, Carr RA, Pradham A, Factor RE, Playforth K, Liomba G, et al. 2015. Quantitative assessment of multiorgan sequestration of parasites in fatal pediatric cerebral malaria. *J Infect Dis* **212**: 1317–1321.

Mitri C, Thiery I, Bourgouin C, Paul RE. 2009. Density-dependent impact of the human malaria parasite *Plasmodium falciparum* gametocyte sex ratio on mosquito infection rates. *Proc Biol Sci* **276**: 3721–3726.

Miura K, Takashima E, Deng B, Tullo G, Diouf A, Moretz SE, Nikolaeva D, Diakite M, Fairhurst RM, Fay MP, et al. 2013. Functional comparison of *Plasmodium falciparum* transmission-blocking vaccine candidates by the standard membrane-feeding assay. *Infect Immun* **81**: 4377–4382.

Mons B. 1986. Intra erythrocytic differentiation of *Plasmodium berghei*. *Acta Leidensia* **54**: 1.

Mons B, Janse CJ, Boorsma EG, Van der Kaay HJ. 1985. Synchronized erythrocytic schizogony and gametocytogenesis of *Plasmodium berghei* in vivo and in vitro. *Parasitology* **91**: 423–430.

Muirhead-Thomson R. 1998. Where do most mosquitoes acquire their malarial (*Plasmodium falciparum*) infection? From adults or from children? *Ann Trop Med Parasitol* **92**: 891–893.

Nacher M, Singhasivanon P, Silachamroon U, Treeprasertsuk S, Tosukhowong T, Vannaphan S, Gay F, Mazier D, Looareesuwan S. 2002. Decreased hemoglobin concentrations, hyperparasitemia, and severe malaria are associated with increased *Plasmodium falciparum* gametocyte carriage. *J Parasitol* **88**: 97–101.

Najera JA, Gonzalez-Silva M, Alonso PL. 2011. Some lessons for the future from the Global Malaria Eradication Programme (1955–1969). *PLoS Med* **8**: e1000412.

Nilsson SK, Childs LM, Buckee C, Marti M. 2015. Targeting human transmission biology for malaria elimination. *PLoS Pathog* **11**: e1004871.

Noedl H, Se Y, Schaecher K, Smith BL, Socheat D, Fukuda MM; Artemisinin Resistance in Cambodia 1 Study C. 2008. Evidence of artemisinin-resistant malaria in western Cambodia. *N Engl J Med* **359**: 2619–2620.

Nwakanma D, Kheir A, Sowa M, Dunyo S, Jawara M, Pinder M, Milligan P, Walliker D, Babiker HA. 2008. High gametocyte complexity and mosquito infectivity of *Plasmodium falciparum* in The Gambia. *Int J Parasitol* **38**: 219–227.

Ono T, Nakai T, Nakabayashi T. 1986. Induction of gametocytogenesis in *Plasmodium falciparum* by the culture supernatant of hybridoma cells producing anti–*P. falciparum* antibody. *Biken J* **29**: 77–81.

Ouédraogo AL, de Vlas SJ, Nebie I, Ilboudo-Sanogo E, Bousema JT, Ouattara AS, Verhave JP, Cuzin-Ouattara N, Sauerwein RW. 2008. Seasonal patterns of *Plasmodium falciparum* gametocyte prevalence and density in a rural population of Burkina Faso. *Acta Tropica* **105**: 28–34.

Ouédraogo AL, Bousema T, Schneider P, de Vlas SJ, Ilboudo-Sanogo E, Cuzin-Ouattara N, Nebie I, Roeffen W, Verhave JP, Luty AJ, et al. 2009. Substantial contribution of submicroscopical *Plasmodium falciparum* gametocyte carriage to the infectious reservoir in an area of seasonal transmission. *PLoS ONE* **4**: e8410.

Ouédraogo AL, Bousema T, de Vlas SJ, Cuzin-Ouattara N, Verhave JP, Drakeley C, Luty A, Sauerwein R. 2010. The plasticity of *Plasmodium falciparum* gametocytaemia in relation to age in Burkina Faso. *Malaria J* **9**: 10.1186.

Pampana E. 1969. *A textbook of malaria eradication*. Oxford University Press, London.

Paul RE, Packer MJ, Walmsley M, Lagog M, Ranford-Cartwright LC, Paru R, Day KP. 1995. Mating patterns in malaria parasite populations of Papua New Guinea. *Science* **269**: 1709–1711.

Paul RE, Coulson TN, Raibaud A, Brey PT. 2000. Sex determination in malaria parasites. *Science* **287**: 128–131.

Paul RE, Brey PT, Robert V. 2002. *Plasmodium* sex determination and transmission to mosquitoes. *Trends Parasitol* **18:** 32–38.

Paul RE, Diallo M, Brey PT. 2004. Mosquitoes and transmission of malaria parasites—Not just vectors. *Malaria J* **3:** 39.

Peatey CL, Watson JA, Trenholme KR, Brown CL, Nielson L, Guenther M, Timmins N, Watson GS, Gardiner DL. 2013. Enhanced gametocyte formation in erythrocyte progenitor cells: A site-specific adaptation by *Plasmodium falciparum*. *J Infect Dis* **208:** 1170–1174.

Pelle KG, Oh K, Buchholz K, Narasimhan V, Joice R, Milner DA, Brancucci NM, Ma S, Voss TS, Ketman K, et al. 2015. Transcriptional profiling defines dynamics of parasite tissue sequestration during malaria infection. *Genome Med* **7:** 19.

Pethleart A, Prajakwong S, Suwonkerd W, Corthong B, Webber R, Curtis C. 2004. Infectious reservoir of *Plasmodium* infection in Mae Hong Son province, northwest Thailand. *Malaria J* **3:** 34.

Petter M, Bonow I, Klinkert MQ. 2008. Diverse expression patterns of subgroups of the *rif* multigene family during *Plasmodium falciparum* gametocytogenesis. *PLoS ONE* **3:** e3779.

Pichon G, Awono-Ambene HP, Robert V. 2000. High heterogeneity in the number of *Plasmodium falciparum* gametocytes in the bloodmeal of mosquitoes fed on the same host. *Parasitology* **121:** 115–120.

Price R, Nosten F, Simpson JA, Luxemburger C, Phaipun L, ter Kuile F, van Vugt M, Chongsuphajaisiddhi T, White NJ. 1999. Risk factors for gametocyte carriage in uncomplicated falciparum malaria. *Am J Trop Med Hyg* **60:** 1019–1023.

Pukrittayakamee S, Imwong M, Singhasivanon P, Stepniewska K, Day NJ, White NJ. 2008. Effects of different antimalarial drugs on gametocyte carriage in *P. vivax* malaria. *Am J Trop Med Hyg* **79:** 378–384.

Reece SE, Drew DR, Gardner A. 2008. Sex ratio adjustment and kin discrimination in malaria parasites. *Nature* **453:** 609–614.

Regev-Rudzki N, Wilson DW, Carvalho TG, Sisquella X, Coleman BM, Rug M, Bursac D, Angrisano F, Gee M, Hill AF, et al. 2013. Cell-cell communication between malaria-infected red blood cells via exosome-like vesicles. *Cell* **153:** 1120–1133.

Robert F, Ntoumi F, Angel G, Candito D, Rogier C, Fandeur T, Sarthou JL, Mercereau-Puijalon O. 1996a. Extensive genetic diversity of *Plasmodium falciparum* isolates collected from patients with severe malaria in Dakar, Senegal. *Trans R Soc Trop Med Hyg* **90:** 704–711.

Robert V, Read AF, Essong J, Tchuinkam T, Mulder B, Verhave JP, Carnevale P. 1996b. Effect of gametocyte sex ratio on infectivity of *Plasmodium falciparum* to *Anopheles gambiae*. *Trans R Soc Trop Med Hyg* **90:** 621–624.

Robert V, Awono-Ambene HP, Le Hesran JY, Trape JF. 2000. Gametocytemia and infectivity to mosquitoes of patients with uncomplicated *Plasmodium falciparum* malaria attacks treated with chloroquine or sulfadoxine plus pyrimethamine. *Am J Trop Med Hyg* **62:** 210–216.

Robert V, Sokhna CS, Rogier C, Ariey F, Trape JF. 2003. Sex ratio of *Plasmodium falciparum* gametocytes in inhabitants of Dielmo, Senegal. *Parasitology* **127:** 1–8.

Saeed M, Roeffen W, Alexander N, Drakeley CJ, Targett GA, Sutherland CJ. 2008. *Plasmodium falciparum* antigens on the surface of the gametocyte-infected erythrocyte. *PLoS ONE* **3:** e2280.

Sattabongkot J, Maneechai N, Rosenberg R. 1991. *Plasmodium vivax*: Gametocyte infectivity of naturally infected Thai adults. *Parasitology* **102:** 27–31.

Schneider P, Bousema JT, Gouagna LC, Otieno S, van de Vegte-Bolmer M, Omar SA, Sauerwein RW. 2007. Submicroscopic *Plasmodium falciparum* gametocyte densities frequently result in mosquito infection. *Am J Trop Med Hyg* **76:** 470–474.

Shekalaghe SA, Bousema JT, Kunei KK, Lushino P, Masokoto A, Wolters LR, Mwakalinga S, Mosha FW, Sauerwein RW, Drakeley CJ. 2007. Submicroscopic *Plasmodium falciparum* gametocyte carriage is common in an area of low and seasonal transmission in Tanzania. *Trop Med Intl Health* **12:** 547–553.

Sherman IW, Eda S, Winograd E. 2003. Cytoadherence and sequestration in *Plasmodium falciparum*: Defining the ties that bind. *Microbes Infect* **5:** 897–909.

Silvestrini F, Alano P, Williams JL. 2000. Commitment to the production of male and female gametocytes in the human malaria parasite *Plasmodium falciparum*. *Parasitology* **121:** 465–471.

Silvestrini F, Tiburcio M, Bertuccini L, Alano P. 2012. Differential adhesive properties of sequestered asexual and sexual stages of *Plasmodium falciparum* on human endothelial cells are tissue independent. *PLoS ONE* **7:** e31567.

Sinden RE. 1983. Sexual development of malarial parasites. *Adv Parasitol* **22:** 153–216.

Sinden R, Gilles H. 2002. The malaria parasites. In *Essential Malariology*, pp. 8–34. Hodder Arnold, London.

Sinden RE, Canning EU, Bray RS, Smalley ME. 1978. Gametocyte and gamete development in *Plasmodium falciparum*. *Proc R Soc Lond B Biol Sci* **201:** 375–399.

Sinha A, Hughes KR, Modrzynska KK, Otto TD, Pfander C, Dickens NJ, Religa AA, Bushell E, Graham AL, Cameron R, et al. 2014. A cascade of DNA-binding proteins for sexual commitment and development in *Plasmodium*. *Nature* **507:** 253–257.

Smalley ME, Brown J. 1981. *Plasmodium falciparum* gametocytogenesis stimulated by lymphocytes and serum from infected Gambian children. *Trans R Soc Trop Med Hyg* **75:** 316–317.

Smalley ME, Abdalla S, Brown J. 1981. The distribution of *Plasmodium falciparum* in the peripheral blood and bone marrow of Gambian children. *Trans R Soc Trop Med Hyg* **75:** 103–105.

Sowunmi A, Fateye BA, Adedeji AA, Fehintola FA, Happi TC. 2004. Risk factors for gametocyte carriage in uncomplicated falciparum malaria in children. *Parasitology* **129:** 255–262.

Sowunmi A, Balogun ST, Gbotosho GO, Happi CT. 2008. *Plasmodium falciparum* gametocyte sex ratios in children with acute, symptomatic, uncomplicated infections treated with amodiaquine. *Malaria J* **7:** 169.

Sowunmi A, Okuboyejo TM, Gbotosho GO, Happi CT. 2011. Risk factors for gametocyte carriage in uncomplicated falciparum malaria in children before and after

Cite this article as *Cold Spring Harb Perspect Med* doi: 10.1101/cshperspect.a025452

artemisinin-based combination treatments. *Chemotherapy* **57**: 497–504.

Stepniewska K, Price RN, Sutherland CJ, Drakeley CJ, von Seidlein L, Nosten F, White NJ. 2008. *Plasmodium falciparum* gametocyte dynamics in areas of different malaria endemicity. *Malaria J* **7**: 249.

Straimer J, Gnadig NF, Witkowski B, Amaratunga C, Duru V, Ramadani AP, Dacheux M, Khim N, Zhang L, Lam S, et al. 2015. Drug resistance. K13-propeller mutations confer artemisinin resistance in *Plasmodium falciparum* clinical isolates. *Science* **347**: 428–431.

Sutherland CJ. 2009. Surface antigens of *Plasmodium falciparum* gametocytes—A new class of transmission-blocking vaccine targets? *Mol Biochem Parasitol* **166**: 93–98.

Suwanarusk R, Cooke BM, Dondorp AM, Silamut K, Sattabongkot J, White NJ, Udomsangpetch R. 2004. The deformability of red blood cells parasitized by *Plasmodium falciparum* and *P. vivax*. *J Infect Dis* **189**: 190–194.

Talisuna AO, Langi P, Mutabingwa TK, Van Marck E, Speybroeck N, Egwang TG, Watkins WW, Hastings IM, D'Alessandro U. 2003. Intensity of transmission and spread of gene mutations linked to chloroquine and sulphadoxine-pyrimethamine resistance in falciparum malaria. *Int J Parasitol* **33**: 1051–1058.

Talman AM, Paul RE, Sokhna CS, Domarle O, Ariey F, Trape JF, Robert V. 2004. Influence of chemotherapy on the *Plasmodium* gametocyte sex ratio of mice and humans. *Am J Trop Med Hyg* **71**: 739–744.

Tamez PA, Liu H, Fernandez-Pol S, Haldar K, Wickrema A. 2009. Stage-specific susceptibility of human erythroblasts to *Plasmodium falciparum* malaria infection. *Blood* **114**: 3652–3655.

Teklehaimanot A, Collins WE, Nguyen-Dinh P, Campbell CC, Bhasin VK. 1987. Characterization of *Plasmodium falciparum* cloned lines with respect to gametocyte production in vitro, infectivity to *Anopheles* mosquitoes, and transmission to *Aotus* monkeys. *Trans R Soc Trop Med Hyg* **81**: 885–887.

Thomson JG, Robertson A. 1935. The structure and development of *Plasmodium falciparum* gametocytes in the internal organs and peripheral circulation. *Trans R Soc Trop Med Hyg* **29**: 31–40.

Tiburcio M, Niang M, Deplaine G, Perrot S, Bischoff E, Ndour PA, Silvestrini F, Khattab A, Milon G, David PH, et al. 2012. A switch in infected erythrocyte deformability at the maturation and blood circulation of *Plasmodium falciparum* transmission stages. *Blood* **119**: e172–e180.

Tiburcio M, Silvestrini F, Bertuccini L, Sander AF, Turner L, Lavstsen T, Alano P. 2013. Early gametocytes of the malaria parasite *Plasmodium falciparum* specifically remodel the adhesive properties of infected erythrocyte surface. *Cell Microbiol* **15**: 647–659.

Trager W. 2005. What triggers the gametocyte pathway in *Plasmodium falciparum*? *Trends Parasitol* **21**: 262–264.

Trager W, Gill GS. 1992. Enhanced gametocyte formation in young erythrocytes by *Plasmodium falciparum* in vitro. *J Protozool* **39**: 429–432.

Trager W, Gill GS, Lawrence C, Nagel RL. 1999. *Plasmodium falciparum*: Enhanced gametocyte formation in vitro in reticulocyte-rich blood. *Exp Parasitol* **91**: 115–118.

van den BL, Chardome M. 1951. An easier and more accurate diagnosis of malaria and filariasis through the use of the skin scarification smear. *Am J Trop Med Hyg* **31**: 411–413.

van der Kolk M, De Vlas SJ, Saul A, van de Vegte-Bolmer M, Eling WM, Sauerwein RW. 2005. Evaluation of the standard membrane feeding assay (SMFA) for the determination of malaria transmission-reducing activity using empirical data. *Parasitology* **130**: 13–22.

von Seidlein L, Drakeley C, Greenwood B, Walraven G, Targett G. 2001. Risk factors for gametocyte carriage in Gambian children. *Am J Trop Med Hyg* **65**: 523–527.

White NJ. 2011. Determinants of relapse periodicity in *Plasmodium vivax* malaria. *Malaria J* **10**: 297.

Williams JL. 1999. Stimulation of *Plasmodium falciparum* gametocytogenesis by conditioned medium from parasite cultures. *Am J Trop Med Hyg* **60**: 7–13.

The Biology of *Plasmodium vivax*

John H. Adams[1] and Ivo Mueller[2]

[1]Center for Global Health and Infectious Diseases, Department of Global Health, University of South Florida, Tampa, Florida 33612

[2]Population Health & Immunity Division, Walter & Eliza Hall Institute, Parkville, Victoria 3052, Australia

Correspondence: jadams3@health.usf.edu; ivomueller@fastmail.fm

Plasmodium vivax is the second most prevalent cause of malaria worldwide and the leading cause of malaria outside of Africa. Although infections are seldom fatal clinical disease can be debilitating and imposes significant health and economic impacts on affected populations. Estimates of transmission and prevalence intensity can be problematic because many episodes of vivax originate from hypnozoite stages in the liver that have remained dormant from previous infections by an unknown mechanism. Lack of treatment options to clear hypnozoites and the ability to infect mosquitoes before disease symptoms present represent major challenges for control and eradication of vivax malaria. Compounding these challenges is the unique biology of *P. vivax* and limited progress in development of experimental research tools, thereby hindering development of new drugs and vaccines. Renewed emphasis on vivax malaria research is beginning to make progress in overcoming some of these challenges.

Vivax malaria accounts for 14–80 million cases of clinical malaria each year with more than 70% of infections in Asia and the Americas (Mendis et al. 2001a; Price et al. 2007; WHO 2015). The last 10 years have seen a dramatic reduction in the burden of malaria, with many countries in the Asia-Pacific and the Americas with reductions of >90% in the number of clinical cases (WHO 2015). As a consequence, 34 countries are actively attempting to eliminate malaria and the leaders of Central American and East Asian countries have declared their intention to eliminate malaria from their regions by 2025 and 2030, respectively (PAHO 2013; APLMA 2014). In parallel to this reduction in overall incidence, a pronounced shift in species composition has been observed with *Plasmodium vivax*, now the predominant *Plasmodium* spp. in the vast majority of countries outside Africa, and is generally seen as the major obstacle to achieving malaria elimination in Asia and the Americas. The challenges in controlling and eliminating vivax malaria are likely to be related to the following aspects of *P. vivax* biology: (1) its ability to relapse from long-lasting, dormant liver stages (the hypnozoites) (White and Imwong 2012), and (2) its high transmission potential caused by early and continuous production of gametocytes, high infectivity to mosquitoes, and shorter development cycle in the vector host compared to other *Plasmodium* spp. (Mueller et al. 2009). These characteristics facilitate *P. vivax* transmission by seasonal mosquito vectors and at lower am-

Cite this article as *Cold Spring Harb Perspect Med* doi: 10.1101/cshperspect.a025585

bient environmental temperatures, thus extending the global distribution of *P. vivax* into temperate regions (Fig. 1) (Gething et al. 2011, 2012).

Although it has often been regarded as causing a benign self-limiting infection, there is increasing evidence that the overall burden, economic impact, and severity of disease from *P. vivax* have been underestimated (Price et al. 2007). Vivax malaria is known to incapacitate individuals of all ages resulting in repeated febrile episodes, severe anemia, respiratory distress, and, sometimes, poor outcomes in pregnancy. Increasing reports of clinical severity with complicated and lethal cases of vivax malaria, thus, challenge the perception of vivax malaria as benign (Anstey et al. 2012; Baird 2013). The increasingly widespread resistance to chloroquine, the primary frontline drug to treat vivax malaria (Baird et al. 1991; Ruebush et al. 2003; Teka et al. 2008; Ketema et al. 2009; Mohan and Maithani 2010; Rijken et al. 2011) represents an additional challenge to existing control and prevention programs for vivax malaria and highlights the critical need for more efforts toward development of new tools specifically targeting *P. vivax*.

Besides additional drugs targeting the dormant liver stages, the development of a vaccine against *vivax* malaria is especially important (Mueller et al. 2015). The rapid natural acquisition of immunity to *P. vivax* (Mueller et al. 2013) indicates that that the development of *P. vivax* vaccines should be feasible. Nevertheless, understanding correlates of protective immunity is as challenging for vivax malaria is it is for *Plasmodium falciparum*, because in most endemic areas, transmission is intermittent, with lack of sustained acquired immunity. Immune responses to the *P. vivax* vaccine candidate antigen, Duffy-binding protein (DBP), are often weak, short-lived, and biased toward strain-specific alleles (VanBuskirk et al. 2004; Ceravolo et al. 2009; Cole-Tobian et al. 2009; Chootong et al. 2010), which may be due, in part, to a high level degree of allelic diversity. Therefore, an effective vaccine against vivax malaria may face a greater challenge to have a substantial level of immunity against diverse strains.

In this article, we review the unique challenges associated with *P. vivax* experimental research, recent advances overcoming these obstacles, and breakthroughs needed to effectively deal with vivax malaria.

THE UNIQUE BIOLOGY OF *P. vivax*

Significant differences in the biology of *P. vivax* compared to *P. falciparum* are obvious by simple examination of a Giemsa-stained blood smear (Fig. 2) (Coatney et al. 1971). A typical parasitemia in vivax malaria is relatively low, which is attributed to restricted infection of only reticulocytes, often necessitating the use of thick smears to concentrate the blood for reliable diagnosis (Galinski and Barnwell 2008). Although not fixing the blood significantly increases sensitivity, it comes at the cost of retaining good morphology, which can present a challenge for parasite identification for nonexpert microscopists. Important for distinguishing different *Plasmodium* species is the observation of unique morphological features, such as the small dark granules in the reticulocyte cytoplasm, known as Schüffner's dots, representing caveola–vesicle complexes of parasite origin exported into the cytoplasm of the infected reticulocyte (Aikawa et al. 1975; Udagama et al. 1988), which increase in abundance as *P. vivax* develops. A second distinctive morphological feature for *P. vivax* is sexual-stage parasites have a round shape similar to the asexual stages. Finally, all *P. vivax* stages of blood-stage development can be observed in the peripheral blood.

The ability of *P. vivax* to remain in circulation is thought to be possible because of the increased plasticity of infected reticulocytes that is observed as the parasites develop, which is in contrast to the increased rigidity that occurs for *P. falciparum*–infected erythrocytes (Suwanarusk et al. 2004). Increased deformability is needed to periodically squeeze through the splenic chords and thereby evade removal from circulation (Handayani et al. 2009). Infected red blood cell (RBC) rigidity for *P. falciparum* is linked to cytoadherence and sequestration, but PfEMP1 knob proteins that are the key mediator of antigenic variant are absent in *P. vivax*.

Cite this article as *Cold Spring Harb Perspect Med* doi: 10.1101/cshperspect.a025585

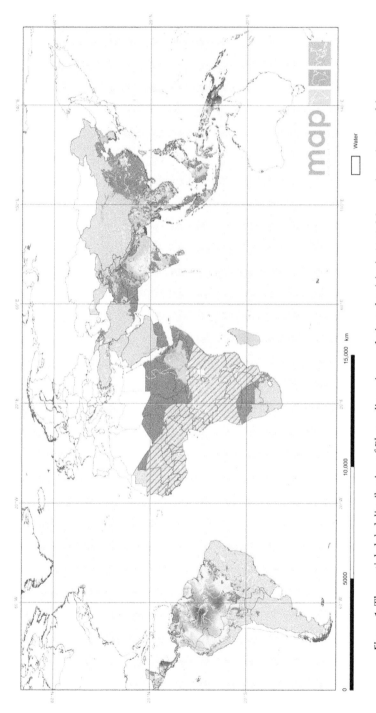

Figure 1. The spatial global distribution of *Plasmodium vivax* malaria endemicity in 2010. Mean point estimates of the age-standardized annual mean *P. vivax* parasite prevalence in 2- to 10-year olds within the spatial limits of stable transmission. Areas of no risk and unstable risk are also shown. Areas where Duffy negative prevalence was estimated as greater than or equal to 90% are hatched to provide additional context for the impact of *P. vivax* on the local population within these areas. Areas in light gray: *P. vivax* free; dark gray: unstable transmission; hatched marks: unstable transmission and high Duffy negative. Areas from red to light blue indicate $PvPR_{1-99} > 7\%$ to 0%, respectively. (From Gething et al. 2010; reprinted under the Creative Commons Attribution 3.0 Unported License.)

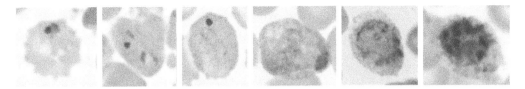

Figure 2. Light microscopic images of Giemsa-stained developmental stages of *Plasmodium vivax* during the blood-stage asexual cycle from early to late stages (*left* to *right*, respectively).

Antigenic variation originally described in the closely related vivax-like primate malaria *Plasmodium knowlesi* (Brown and Brown 1965) and is likely common to most, if not all, malaria parasites that are mediated by a large family of small surface variant antigens (Jemmely et al. 2010). In *P. vivax*, the VIR protein products of the *vir* multigene family are proposed to be the key molecule for antigenic variation in *P. vivax* (del Portillo et al. 2001). More recently, VIR proteins expressed on the reticulocyte surface are suggested to have a role mediating cytoadherence to endothelial cells and placenta, albeit much weaker than for *P. falciparum* (del Portillo et al. 2001; Fernandez-Becerra et al. 2005). Therefore, the lack of knobs and a strong sequestration mechanism does not mean that there is a lack of antigenic variation and sequestration, although cytoadherence to endothelium is less prevalent and possibly occurring only in more virulent infections (del Portillo et al. 2001; Fernandez-Becerra et al. 2005; Carvalho et al. 2010; Chotivanich et al. 2012). The lack of robust continuous culture methods have greatly hampered laboratory-based experimental studies of this and other unique biological properties of *P. vivax*.

In addition to their round morphology, *P. vivax* gametocytes are noteworthy for their very early appearance during the course of infection. In part, this may be caused by a rapid development time with gametocytes often detected within 3 days after the first asexual parasites are observed (Bousema and Drakeley 2011). In controlled experimental infections gametocytes appeared in the peripheral blood within 7 days of direct *P. vivax* sporozoite infection (Vallejo et al. 2016), indicating that in most natural infections mosquito transmission can occur before onset of clinical symptoms. Although early transmissibility can lead to rapid transmission with outbreaks spreading quickly, a side benefit attributed to this phenomenon is limiting the rapid spread of drug resistance for *P. vivax*. It is important to note that because transmission usually occurs before infections are treated, an effective transmission-blocking vaccine would help contain relapse infections that result from radical cure treatment failures (Douglas et al. 2013).

The key distinguishing feature of *P. vivax* biology is, however, its ability to form long-lasting liver stages, the hypnozoites (Krotoski et al. 1982). On entry into the liver, *P. vivax* sporozoites can take two distinct pathways. Some develop directly into liver-schizonts, which after 8 days, release merozoites to initiate the asexual cycle in the blood, although others, the hypnozoites, "arrest" their development beginning about the third day after infection (Coatney et al. 1971; Mikolajczak et al. 2015). Although hypnozoites are probably metabolically active, they do not divide and remain dormant for weeks if not months before reactivating. The frequency and timing of these relapses varies globally (White 2011), with the longest relapse periods present in temperate strains (Battle et al. 2014), indicating that relapse periodicity is under natural selection (White et al. 2016). The mechanisms underlying both commitment to dormancy and reactivation are poorly understood. However, it is increasingly clear that relapses from emerging such hypnozoites may contribute up to 80% of all *P. vivax* blood-stage infections (Betuela et al. 2012; Robinson et al. 2015). As there are no diagnostic tests that can diagnose dormant liver-stage infections, undetectable hypnozoite carriers are an important potential source of reintroduction of *P. vivax* and, if not treated appropriately, can cause new blood-stage infections months after the primary infection. Unfortunately, the only currently available drug to clear hypnozoites is primaquine, which can cause severe hemolysis in people with glucose 6-phosphate dehydrogenase (G6PD) deficiency (Baird et al. 2012). Given the lack of a cheap, reliable point-of-care G6PD test, many *P. vivax* patients do not currently receive adequate antihypnozoite treatment (Baird 2015).

GENETIC DIVERSITY/POPULATION OF *P. vivax*

Although its closest non-ape *Plasmodium* spp. are parasites of Southeast Asia monkeys, *P. vivax* is now thought to have originated in Africa with it closest relatives still circulating in African chimpanzee and gorilla populations (Liu et al. 2014). *P. vivax* shows a higher degree of genetic diversity and more global structure than *P. falciparum*. Comparative analyses revealed that *P. vivax* genomes show twice as much single-nucleotide polymorphism (SNP) diversity as *P. falciparum* and also have high microsatellite and gene family variability (Neafsey et al. 2012). Although *P. falciparum* microsatellite diversity is closely associated with regional levels of endemicity, *P. vivax* shows a high genetic diversity across all endemicities (Barry et al. 2015).

The global *P. vivax* population is nevertheless more strongly structured than that of *P. falciparum*. A comparative analyses of microsatellite diversity in a global panel of 841 *P. vivax* isolates showed very strong geographical structure with clearly distinct populations in South America, Africa and India, Southeast Asia, and the Southwest Pacific (Koepfli et al. 2015b). Similar global structure is also evident in sequences encoding for vaccine candidate antigens (Arnott et al. 2013) and has recently been confirmed using genome-wide SNPs (Hupalo et al. 2016; Pearson et al. 2016).

Contrary to the pronounced global structure, most studies found limited or no population structure at local or regional scale (Imwong et al. 2007; Getachew et al. 2015), even in areas where *P. falciparum* did show substantial population structure (Jennison et al. 2015; Noviyanti et al. 2015). This is likely to be caused by the generally higher genetic complexity of *P. vivax* infections (Barry et al. 2015), which increase the likelihood of genetic recombination and result in large effective population sizes. The exception to this pattern is found in the Americas, where pronounced local population structure is observed (Ferreira et al. 2007; Van den Eede et al. 2010; Delgado-Ratto et al. 2016), despite high continent-wide genetic diversity. This pattern is thought to be a reflection of both multiple introduction and more recent bottlenecks caused by intensified control.

Together, these patterns suggest a capacity for greater functional variation, a more distinct history of global colonization and a higher ability to maintain genetic diversity in the face of intensifying control efforts. More detailed studies of global and local *P. vivax* diversity are required to develop tools that will allow examination of the impact of control and elimination programs on the parasite gene pool. Of particular importance for local elimination would be to develop tools that allow for differentiation of locally acquired infections from imported *P. vivax* infections.

THE ROLE OF ASYMPTOMATIC INFECTIONS

Although *P. vivax* has a lower pyrogenic threshold than that of *P. falciparum* (Hemmer et al. 2006), asymptomatic *P. vivax* infections are very common at all levels of endemicity and often account for 90%–100% of all infections detected in cross-sectional surveys (Anstey et al. 2012). The vast majority of these *P. vivax* infections are of very low density, with submicroscopic infections accounting for 67% of all infections (Cheng et al. 2015). This is significantly higher than for *P. falciparum* in the same studies.

Several factors are thought to contribute to this very high rate of asymptomatic infections. Most importantly, clinical immunity to *P. vivax* infections is acquired rapidly. When malaria therapy patients were experimentally infected with *P. vivax*, effective clinical immunity, even against heterologous challenge, was often attained after as few as one to five *P. vivax* infections (Mueller et al. 2013; Snounou and Perignon 2013). Under natural exposure, clinical immunity to *P. vivax* is also acquired significantly more rapidly than to *P. falciparum*, both in high transmission settings such as Papua New Guinea, where the incidence of *P. vivax* malaria starts declining in the second year of life (Lin et al. 2010) and clinical disease is virtually absent in children >5 years, although *P. falciparum* episodes are common in primary school children (Michon et al. 2007), as well as in lower transmission settings such as Thailand (Phimpraphi et al. 2008), Sri Lanka (Mendis et al. 2001b), and Vanuatu (Maitland et al. 1996). With little evidence for naturally acquired immunity against (preerythrocytic) infections (Mueller et al. 2013), these patterns are indicative that, even in low transmission settings, semi-immune individuals develop effective blood-stage immunity characterized by a very good control of blood-stage parasitemia, which results in significant numbers of submicroscopic infections. The main driver for this rapid acquisition of immunity is the higher force of infections (Koepfli et al. 2013), caused largely by genetically distinct but related relapses (Bright et al. 2014) that account for up to 80% of all *P. vivax* blood-stage infections (Robinson et al. 2015).

The role of these asymptomatic infections in maintaining *P. vivax* transmission is not yet well understood. Most, if not all, of these asymptomatic infections produce gametocytes (Wampfler et al. 2013; Barbosa et al. 2014) with gametocyte densities closely correlated with overall parasitemia levels and thus at low levels (Koepfli et al. 2015a). Nevertheless, the asymptomatic cases are infectious to anopheline vectors, albeit at a substantially lower level than clinical cases (Pethleart et al. 2004; Alves et al. 2005), and may contribute substantially to maintaining *P. vivax* transmission given the high prevalence of the "silent" infections.

These asymptomatic infections may thus be a major impediment to the elimination of *P. vivax* malaria as they may not be efficiently cleared unless specifically targeted with active case detection and/or mass drug administration. Such a strategy is logistically challenging and would again require treating large numbers of individuals with asymptomatic infections, even those without detected blood-stage infections, with primaquine to clear the hypnozoite reservoir.

ADVANCES IN ENABLING TECHNOLOGIES TO SUPPORT *P. vivax* RESEARCH

The unique biology of *P. vivax* has presented major challenges for applying modern approaches in fundamental and translational research. In particular, the blood-stage requirement to infect reticulocytes and the hypnozoite liver stage have been difficult obstacles to overcome for laboratory-based research studies, thereby limiting most research efforts to using *P. vivax* from clinical isolates or nonhuman primate infections. In recent years, greater efforts from multiple laboratories have begun to provide new approaches to create more useful enabling technologies for research studies on the liver stages (Dembele et al. 2011; March et al. 2013; Mikolajczak et al. 2015). Unfortunately, similar success for developing a robust continuous culture system for blood-stage parasites has not been as successful with capabilities being limited primarily for short-term assays (Russell et al. 2011; Noulin et al. 2013; Roobsoong et al. 2015).

Because reticulocytes rapidly develop to mature erythrocytes at 37°C, a reticulocyte's half-life is shorter than the blood-stage asexual developmental cycle time. Therefore, reticulocytes must be replenished as each new generation matures or there is nothing for the parasites to infect. An important strategy to overcome the reticulocyte problem was exemplified in the Golenda study (Golenda et al. 1997). This 19-year-old study from the Walter Reed Army Institute of Research remains the gold standard for sustained growth of in vitro blood-stage culture of *P. vivax*. In the Golenda study, blood-stage parasites were grown for six to eight asexual cycles using an inventive, but complex labor-intensive culturing protocol not easily replicated. The success of the Golenda study was likely because

Cite this article as *Cold Spring Harb Perspect Med* doi: 10.1101/cshperspect.a025585

of a combination of variables that included use of the primate-adapted Chesson strain, obtaining reticulocytes from hemochromatosis patients undergoing traditional bloodletting treatments, which induces a reticulocytemia, and differential centrifugation methods for reticulocyte enrichment. Other important handling features of the protocol included exposure of the static cultures to intermittent agitation along with periodic addition of fresh reticulocytes. Of these variables, many subsequent studies identified the critical limiting factor for *P. vivax* blood-stage culture to be sustaining reticulocyte levels. Consequently, studies now include regular addition of relatively pure reticulocyte preparations so as to not dilute the culture with mature erythrocytes that cannot be invaded by *P. vivax*.

Traditional sources of reticulocytes to support *P. vivax* culture for most researchers have been placenta cord blood and adult peripheral blood, which are both readily available (Noulin et al. 2013). In both cases, reticulocytes constitute a subset of the total erythroid cell population and must be enriched (Udomsangpetch et al. 2007; Kumar et al. 2015). Over time, protocols have evolved to enable enrichment of nearly pure populations of reticulocytes from both of these traditional sources to overcome a historical limitation of attempts to establish *P. vivax* blood-stage cultures. Parallel to improvements in traditional approaches for enriching reticulocytes were the improvements and lowered costs in the hematopoietic stem cell (HSC) ex vivo production methods for creating reticulocytes (Douay and Giarratana 2005; Giarratana et al. 2005). These HSC reticulocytes have provided a third source, which also revealed the capacity of *P. vivax* to infected nucleated erythroid progenitor cells (Panichakul et al. 2007; Noulin et al. 2014). In addition, ex vivo reticulocytes produced from HSC can be experimentally manipulated to tease apart specific molecular interactions required for parasites infection (Crosnier et al. 2011; Egan et al. 2015). Despite being able to sustain abundant reticulocytes in vitro, a concomitant success in maintaining continuous long-term *P. vivax* culture has not been achieved yet, indicating factors beyond just reticulocytes are required to sustain parasites in vitro (Martin-Jaular et al. 2013; Roobsoong et al. 2015). Nonetheless, the value of studies reliant on traditional sources of *P. vivax* have improved considerably for support of fundamental and translational research (Price et al. 2010; Rijken et al. 2011; Marfurt et al. 2012; Lee et al. 2014; Malleret et al. 2015; Cho et al. 2016).

The basic capability to study complete in vitro development of *P. vivax*, *P. falciparum*, and other malaria parasites with primary hepatocytes and hepatocytoma cells has been established for many years (Mazier et al. 1984; Sattabongkot et al. 2006). With the increased awareness of the force of infection in *vivax* malaria caused by relapse (Betuela et al. 2012; Robinson et al. 2015), along with emergence of chloroquine resistance in many endemic regions (Baird et al. 1991; Ruebush et al. 2003; Teka et al. 2008; Ketema et al. 2009; Mohan and Maithani 2010; Rijken et al. 2011), there has been a renewed effort to develop higher throughput, more efficient, and longer duration systems for liver-stage studies, especially of hypnozoites (Wells et al. 2010; Campo et al. 2015). These efforts to improve capabilities for laboratory-based studies of the liver stages are yielding exciting results. Multiple new experimental platforms have emerged permitting researchers access to this least studied phase of *P. vivax* and human malaria parasites. Improvements in modified culture devices for in vitro enhancement of primary cell properties have progressed greatly to provide stability of viable primary human hepatocytes enhancing their potential use for malaria research (Dembele et al. 2011; March et al. 2013; Dembele et al. 2014; Maher et al. 2014; Ng et al. 2015). However, so far, the most significant innovations established are in vivo humanized mouse models (Shultz et al. 2007; Peltz 2013). These human liver-chimeric mice support complete liver-stage development, including persisting hypnozoites, of *P. vivax* and *Plasmodium ovale* (Mikolajczak et al. 2015; Soulard et al. 2015). These mouse models offer the potential to explore liver-stage biology and evaluate antimalarial candidates, in ways that were previously only possible through the use of primate models (Coatney et al. 1971).

CONCLUDING REMARKS

If the ambitious goals for the elimination of malaria are to be achieved, new tools specifically targeting *P. vivax* will be required. Accelerating the development of new drugs and vaccines will require both a better understanding of the unique *P. vivax* biology and the development of key research tools such as in vitro culture and in vivo models. Although significant progress has been made, many challenges remain.

Addressing these will require novel interdisciplinary research approaches that bridge from the field to the bedside and from the laboratory to the vivax research community backed by substantial investments in both basic and applied research.

ACKNOWLEDGMENTS

I.M. is supported by a National Health and Medical Research Council (NHMRC) Senior Research Fellowship (#1043345) and J.H.A. is supported by the National Institutes of Health (R01 AI064478). The authors thank Ashley Souza for assistance in preparation of this manuscript.

REFERENCES

Aikawa M, Miller LH, Rabbege J. 1975. Caveola–vesicle complexes in the plasmalemma of erythrocytes infected by *Plasmodium vivax* and *P. cynomolgi*. Unique structures related to Schuffner's dots. *Am J Pathol* **79:** 285–300.

Alves FP, Gil LH, Marrelli MT, Ribolla PE, Camargo EP, Da Silva LH. 2005. Asymptomatic carriers of *Plasmodium* spp. as infection source for malaria vector mosquitoes in the Brazilian Amazon. *J Med Entomol* **42:** 777–779.

Anstey NM, Douglas NM, Poespoprodjo JR, Price RN. 2012. *Plasmodium vivax*: Clinical spectrum, risk factors and pathogenesis. *Adv Parasitol* **80:** 151–201.

APLMA. 2014. East Asia Summit adopts unprecedented regional malaria goal. Asia Pacific Leaders Malaria Alliance Secretariat, Mandaluyong City, Philippines.

Arnott A, Mueller I, Ramsland PA, Siba PM, Reeder JC, Barry AE. 2013. Global population structure of the genes encoding the malaria vaccine candidate, *Plasmodium vivax* apical membrane antigen 1 (PvAMA1). *PLoS Negl Trop Dis* **7:** e2506.

Baird JK. 2013. Evidence and implications of mortality associated with acute *Plasmodium vivax* malaria. *Clin Microbiol Rev* **26:** 36–57.

Baird K. 2015. Origins and implications of neglect of G6PD deficiency and primaquine toxicity in *Plasmodium vivax* malaria. *Pathog Glob Health* **109:** 93–106.

Baird JK, Basri H, Purnomo, Bangs MJ, Subianto B, Patchen LC, Hoffman SL. 1991. Resistance to chloroquine by *Plasmodium vivax* in Irian Jaya, Indonesia. *Am J Trop Med Hyg* **44:** 547–552.

Baird KJ, Maguire JD, Price RN. 2012. Diagnosis and treatment of *Plasmodium vivax* malaria. *Adv Parasitol* **80:** 203–270.

Barbosa S, Gozze AB, Lima NF, Batista CL, Bastos Mda S, Nicolete VC, Fontoura PS, Goncalves RM, Viana SA, Menezes MJ, et al. 2014. Epidemiology of disappearing *Plasmodium vivax* malaria: A case study in rural Amazonia. *PLoS Negl Trop Dis* **8:** e3109.

Barry AE, Waltmann A, Koepfli C, Barnadas C, Mueller I. 2015. Uncovering the transmission dynamics of *Plasmodium vivax* using population genetics. *Pathog Glob Health* **109:** 142–152.

Battle KE, Karhunen MS, Bhatt S, Gething PW, Howes RE, Golding N, Van Boeckel TP, Messina JP, Shanks GD, Smith DL, et al. 2014. Geographical variation in *Plasmodium vivax* relapse. *Malaria J* **13:** 144.

Betuela I, Rosanas-Urgell A, Kiniboro B, Stanisic DI, Samol L, de Lazzari E, Del Portillo HA, Siba P, Alonso PL, Bassat Q, et al. 2012. Relapses contribute significantly to the risk of *Plasmodium vivax* infection and disease in Papua New Guinean children 1–5 years of age. *J Infect Dis* **206:** 1771–1780.

Bousema T, Drakeley C. 2011. Epidemiology and infectivity of *Plasmodium falciparum* and *Plasmodium vivax* gametocytes in relation to malaria control and elimination. *Clin Microbiol Rev* **24:** 377–410.

Bright AT, Manary MJ, Tewhey R, Arango EM, Wang T, Schork NJ, Yanow SK, Winzeler EA. 2014. A high resolution case study of a patient with recurrent *Plasmodium vivax* infections shows that relapses were caused by meiotic siblings. *PLoS Negl Trop Dis* **8:** e2882.

Brown KN, Brown IN. 1965. Immunity to malaria: Antigenic variation in chronic infections of *Plasmodium knowlesi*. *Nature* **208:** 1286–1288.

Campo B, Vandal O, Wesche DL, Burrows JN. 2015. Killing the hypnozoite—Drug discovery approaches to prevent relapse in *Plasmodium vivax*. *Pathog Glob Health* **109:** 107–122.

Carvalho BO, Lopes SC, Nogueira PA, Orlandi PP, Bargieri DY, Blanco YC, Mamoni R, Leite JA, Rodrigues MM, Soares IS, et al. 2010. On the cytoadhesion of *Plasmodium vivax*–infected erythrocytes. *J Infect Dis* **202:** 638–647.

Ceravolo IP, Sanchez BA, Sousa TN, Guerra BM, Soares IS, Braga EM, McHenry AM, Adams JH, Brito CF, Carvalho LH. 2009. Naturally acquired inhibitory antibodies to *Plasmodium vivax* Duffy binding protein are short-lived and allele-specific following a single malaria infection. *Clin Exp Immunol* **156:** 502–510.

Cheng Q, Cunningham J, Gatton ML. 2015. Systematic review of sub-microscopic *P. vivax* infections: Prevalence and determining factors. *PLoS Negl Trop Dis* **9:** e3413.

Cho JS, Russell B, Kosasaivee V, Zhang R, Colin Y, Bertrand O, Chandramohanadas R, Chu CS, Nosten F, Renia L, et al. 2016. Unambiguous determination of *Plasmodium vivax* reticulocyte invasion by flow cytometry. *Int J Parasitol* **46:** 31–39.

Chootong P, Ntumngia FB, VanBuskirk KM, Xainli J, Cole-Tobian JL, Campbell CO, Fraser TS, King CL, Adams JH. 2010. Mapping epitopes of the *Plasmodium vivax* Duffy binding protein with naturally acquired inhibitory antibodies. *Infect Immun* **78:** 1089–1095.

Chotivanich K, Udomsangpetch R, Suwanarusk R, Pukrittayakamee S, Wilairatana P, Beeson JG, Day NP, White NJ. 2012. *Plasmodium vivax* adherence to placental glycosaminoglycans. *PLoS ONE* **7:** e34509.

Coatney GR, Collins WE, Warren M, C PG. 1971. *The primate malarias*. U.S. Department of Health, Education and Welfare, Washington, DC.

Cole-Tobian JL, Michon P, Biasor M, Richards JS, Beeson JG, Mueller I, King CL. 2009. Strain-specific Duffy binding protein antibodies correlate with protection against infection with homologous compared to heterologous *Plasmodium vivax* strains in Papua New Guinean children. *Infect Immun* **77:** 4009–4017.

Crosnier C, Bustamante LY, Bartholdson SJ, Bei AK, Theron M, Uchikawa M, Mboup S, Ndir O, Kwiatkowski DP, Duraisingh MT, et al. 2011. Basigin is a receptor essential for erythrocyte invasion by *Plasmodium falciparum*. *Nature* **480:** 534–537.

Delgado-Ratto C, Gamboa D, Soto-Calle VE, Van den Eede P, Torres E, Sanchez-Martinez L, Contreras-Mancilla J, Rosanas-Urgell A, Rodriguez Ferrucci H, Llanos-Cuentas A, et al. 2016. Population genetics of *Plasmodium vivax* in the Peruvian Amazon. *PLoS Negl Trop Dis* **10:** e0004376.

del Portillo HA, Fernandez-Becerra C, Bowman S, Oliver K, Preuss M, Sanchez CP, Schneider NK, Villalobos JM, Rajandream MA, Harris D, et al. 2001. A superfamily of variant genes encoded in the subtelomeric region of *Plasmodium vivax*. *Nature* **410:** 839–842.

Dembele L, Gego A, Zeeman AM, Franetich JF, Silvie O, Rametti A, Le Grand R, Dereuddre-Bosquet N, Sauerwein R, van Gemert GJ, et al. 2011. Towards an in vitro model of *Plasmodium* hypnozoites suitable for drug discovery. *PLoS ONE* **6:** e18162.

Dembele L, Franetich JF, Lorthiois A, Gego A, Zeeman AM, Kocken CH, Le Grand R, Dereuddre-Bosquet N, van Gemert GJ, Sauerwein R, et al. 2014. Persistence and activation of malaria hypnozoites in long-term primary hepatocyte cultures. *Nat Med* **20:** 307–312.

Douay L, Giarratana MC. 2005. The cultured red blood cell: A study tool with therapeutic perspectives. *Cell Cycle* **4:** 999–1000.

Douglas NM, Simpson JA, Phyo AP, Siswantoro H, Hasugian AR, Kenangalem E, Poespoprodjo JR, Singhasivanon P, Anstey NM, White NJ, et al. 2013. Gametocyte dynamics and the role of drugs in reducing the transmission potential of *Plasmodium vivax*. *J Infect Dis* **208:** 801–812.

Egan ES, Jiang RH, Moechtar MA, Barteneva NS, Weekes MP, Nobre LV, Gygi SP, Paulo JA, Frantzreb C, Tani Y, et al. 2015. Malaria. A forward genetic screen identifies erythrocyte CD55 as essential for *Plasmodium falciparum* invasion. *Science* **348:** 711–714.

Fernandez-Becerra C, Pein O, de Oliveira TR, Yamamoto MM, Cassola AC, Rocha C, Soares IS, de Braganca Pereira CA, del Portillo HA. 2005. Variant proteins of *Plasmodium vivax* are not clonally expressed in natural infections. *Mol Microbiol* **58:** 648–658.

Ferreira MU, Karunaweera ND, da Silva-Nunes M, da Silva NS, Wirth DF, Hartl DL. 2007. Population structure and transmission dynamics of *Plasmodium vivax* in rural Amazonia. *J Infect Dis* **195:** 1218–1226.

Galinski MR, Barnwell JW. 2008. *Plasmodium vivax*: Who cares? *Malaria J* **7:** S9.

Getachew S, To S, Trimarsanto H, Thriemer K, Clark TG, Petros B, Aseffa A, Price RN, Auburn S. 2015. Variation in complexity of infection and transmission stability between neighbouring populations of *Plasmodium vivax* in Southern Ethiopia. *PLoS ONE* **10:** e0140780.

Gething PW, Van Boeckel TP, Smith DL, Guerra CA, Patil AP, Snow RW, Hay SI. 2011. Modelling the global constraints of temperature on transmission of *Plasmodium falciparum* and *P. vivax*. *Parasit Vectors* **4:** 92.

Gething PW, Elyazar IR, Moyes CL, Smith DL, Battle KE, Guerra CA, Patil AP, Tatem AJ, Howes RE, Myers MF, et al. 2012. A long neglected world malaria map: *Plasmodium vivax* endemicity in 2010. *PLoS Negl Trop Dis* **6:** e1814.

Giarratana MC, Kobari L, Lapillonne H, Chalmers D, Kiger L, Cynober T, Marden MC, Wajcman H, Douay L. 2005. Ex vivo generation of fully mature human red blood cells from hematopoietic stem cells. *Nat Biotechnol* **23:** 69–74.

Golenda CF, Li J, Rosenberg R. 1997. Continuous in vitro propagation of the malaria parasite *Plasmodium vivax*. *Proc Natl Acad Sci* **94:** 6786–6791.

Handayani S, Chiu DT, Tjitra E, Kuo JS, Lampah D, Kenangalem E, Renia L, Snounou G, Price RN, Anstey NM, et al. 2009. High deformability of *Plasmodium vivax*–infected red blood cells under microfluidic conditions. *J Infect Dis* **199:** 445–450.

Hemmer CJ, Holst FG, Kern P, Chiwakata CB, Dietrich M, Reisinger EC. 2006. Stronger host response per parasitized erythrocyte in *Plasmodium vivax* or *ovale* than in *Plasmodium falciparum* malaria. *Trop Med Int Health* **11:** 817–823.

Hupalo DN, Luo Z, Melnikov A, Sutton PL, Rogov P, Escalante A, Vallejo AF, Herrera S, Arévalo-Herrera M, Fan Q, et al. 2016. Population genomics reveals signatures of global dispersal and drug resistance in *Plasmodium vivax*. *Nat Genet* **48:** 953–958.

Imwong M, Nair S, Pukrittayakamee S, Sudimack D, Williams JT, Mayxay M, Newton PN, Kim JR, Nandy A, Osorio L, et al. 2007. Contrasting genetic structure in *Plasmodium vivax* populations from Asia and South America. *Int J Parasitol* **37:** 1013–1022.

Jemmely NY, Niang M, Preiser PR. 2010. Small variant surface antigens and *Plasmodium* evasion of immunity. *Future Microbiol* **5:** 663–682.

Jennison C, Arnott A, Tessier N, Tavul L, Koepfli C, Felger I, Siba PM, Reeder JC, Bahlo M, Mueller I, et al. 2015. *Plasmodium vivax* populations are more genetically diverse and less structured than sympatric *Plasmodium falciparum* populations. *PLoS Negl Trop Dis* **9**: e0003634.

Ketema T, Bacha K, Birhanu T, Petros B. 2009. Chloroquine-resistant *Plasmodium vivax* malaria in Serbo town, Jimma zone, south-west Ethiopia. *Malaria J* **8**: 177.

Koepfli C, Colborn KL, Kiniboro B, Lin E, Speed TP, Siba PM, Felger I, Mueller I. 2013. A high force of *Plasmodium vivax* blood-stage infection drives the rapid acquisition of immunity in Papua New Guinean children. *PLoS Negl Trop Dis* **7**: e2403.

Koepfli C, Robinson LJ, Rarau P, Salib M, Sambale N, Wampfler R, Betuela I, Nuitragool W, Barry AE, Siba P, et al. 2015a. Blood-stage parasitaemia and age determine *Plasmodium falciparum* and *P. vivax* gametocytaemia in Papua New Guinea. *PLoS ONE* **10**: e0126747.

Koepfli C, Rodrigues PT, Antao T, Orjuela-Sanchez P, Van den Eede P, Gamboa D, van Hong N, Bendezu J, Erhart A, Barnadas C, et al. 2015b. *Plasmodium vivax* diversity and population structure across four continents. *PLoS Negl Trop Dis* **9**: e0003872.

Krotoski WA, Collins WE, Bray RS, Garnham PC, Cogswell FB, Gwadz RW, Killick-Kendrick R, Wolf R, Sinden R, Koontz LC, et al. 1982. Demonstration of hypnozoites in sporozoite-transmitted *Plasmodium vivax* infection. *Am J Trop Med Hyg* **31**: 1291–1293.

Kumar AA, Lim C, Moreno Y, Mace CR, Syed A, Van Tyne D, Wirth DF, Duraisingh MT, Whitesides GM. 2015. Enrichment of reticulocytes from whole blood using aqueous multiphase systems of polymers. *Am J Hematol* **90**: 31–36.

Lee WC, Malleret B, Lau YL, Mauduit M, Fong MY, Cho JS, Suwanarusk R, Zhang R, Albrecht L, Costa FT, et al. 2014. Glycophorin C (CD236R) mediates vivax malaria parasite rosetting to normocytes. *Blood* **123**: e100–109.

Lin E, Kiniboro B, Gray L, Dobbie S, Robinson L, Laumea A, Schoepflin S, Lori L, Betuela I, Siba P, et al. 2010. Differential patterns of infection and disease with *P. falciparum* and *P. vivax* in young Papua New Guinean children. *PloS ONE* **5**: e9047.

Liu W, Li Y, Shaw KS, Learn GH, Plenderleith LJ, Malenke JA, Sundararaman SA, Ramirez MA, Crystal PA, Smith AG, et al. 2014. African origin of the malaria parasite *Plasmodium vivax*. *Nat Commun* **5**: 3346.

Maher SP, Crouse RB, Conway AJ, Bannister EC, Achyuta AK, Clark AY, Sinatra FL, Cuiffi JD, Adams JH, Kyle DE, et al. 2014. Microphysical space of a liver sinusoid device enables simplified long-term maintenance of chimeric mouse-expanded human hepatocytes. *Biomed Microdevices* **16**: 727–736.

Maitland K, Williams TN, Bennett S, Newbold CI, Peto TE, Viji J, Timothy R, Clegg JB, Weatherall DJ, Bowden DK. 1996. The interaction between *Plasmodium falciparum* and *P. vivax* in children on Espiritu Santo island, Vanuatu. *Trans R Soc Trop Med Hyg* **90**: 614–620.

Malleret B, Li A, Zhang R, Tan KS, Suwanarusk R, Claser C, Cho JS, Koh EG, Chu CS, Pukrittayakamee S, et al. 2015. *Plasmodium vivax*: Restricted tropism and rapid remodeling of CD71-positive reticulocytes. *Blood* **125**: 1314–1324.

March S, Ng S, Velmurugan S, Galstian A, Shan J, Logan DJ, Carpenter AE, Thomas D, Sim BK, Mota MM, et al. 2013. A microscale human liver platform that supports the hepatic stages of *Plasmodium falciparum* and *vivax*. *Cell Host Microbe* **14**: 104–115.

Marfurt J, Chalfein F, Prayoga P, Wabiser F, Wirjanata G, Sebayang B, Piera KA, Wittlin S, Haynes RK, Mohrle JJ, et al. 2012. Comparative ex vivo activity of novel endoperoxides in multidrug-resistant *Plasmodium falciparum* and *P. vivax*. *Antimicrob Agents Chemother* **56**: 5258–5263.

Martin-Jaular L, Elizalde-Torrent A, Thomson-Luque R, Ferrer M, Segovia JC, Herreros-Aviles E, Fernandez-Becerra C, Del Portillo HA. 2013. Reticulocyte-prone malaria parasites predominantly invade CD71hi immature cells: Implications for the development of an in vitro culture for *Plasmodium vivax*. *Malaria J* **12**: 434.

Mazier D, Landau I, Druilhe P, Miltgen F, Guguen-Guillouzo C, Baccam D, Baxter J, Chigot JP, Gentilini M. 1984. Cultivation of the liver forms of *Plasmodium vivax* in human hepatocytes. *Nature* **307**: 367–369.

Mendis K, Sina BJ, Marchesini P, Carter R. 2001a. The neglected burden of *Plasmodium vivax* malaria. *Am J Trop Med Hyg* **64**: 97–106.

Mendis K, Sina BJ, Mechesini P, Carter R. 2001b. The neglected burden of *Plasmodium vivax* malaria. *Am J Trop Med Hyg* **64**: 97–106.

Michon P, Cole-Tobian JL, Dabod E, Schoepflin S, Igu J, Susapu M, Tarongka N, Zimmerman PA, Reeder JC, Beeson JG, et al. 2007. The risk of malarial infections and disease in Papua New Guinean children. *Am J Trop Med Hyg* **76**: 997–1008.

Mikolajczak SA, Vaughan AM, Kangwanrangsan N, Roobsoong W, Fishbaugher M, Yimamnuaychok N, Rezakhani N, Lakshmanan V, Singh N, Kaushansky A, et al. 2015. *Plasmodium vivax* liver stage development and hypnozoite persistence in human liver-chimeric mice. *Cell Host Microbe* **17**: 526–535.

Mohan K, Maithani MM. 2010. Congenital malaria due to chloroquine-resistant *Plasmodium vivax*: A case report. *J Trop Pediatr* **56**: 454–455.

Mueller I, Galinski MR, Baird JK, Carlton JM, Kochar DK, Alonso PL, del Portillo HA. 2009. Key gaps in the knowledge of *Plasmodium vivax*, a neglected human malaria parasite. *Lancet Infect Dis* **9**: 555–566.

Mueller I, Galinski MR, Tsuboi T, Arevalo-Herrera M, Collins WE, King CL. 2013. Natural acquisition of immunity to *Plasmodium vivax*: Epidemiological observations and potential targets. *Adv Parasitol* **81**: 77–131.

Mueller I, Shakri AR, Chitnis CE. 2015. Development of vaccines for *Plasmodium vivax* malaria. *Vaccine* **33**: 7489–7495.

Neafsey DE, Galinsky K, Jiang RH, Young L, Sykes SM, Saif S, Gujja S, Goldberg JM, Young S, Zeng Q, et al. 2012. The malaria parasite *Plasmodium vivax* exhibits greater genetic diversity than *Plasmodium falciparum*. *Nat Genet* **44**: 1046–1050.

Ng S, Schwartz RE, March S, Galstian A, Gural N, Shan J, Prabhu M, Mota MM, Bhatia SN. 2015. Human iPSC-derived hepatocyte-like cells support *Plasmodium* liver-stage infection in vitro. *Stem Cell Rep* **4**: 348–359.

Cite this article as *Cold Spring Harb Perspect Med* doi: 10.1101/cshperspect.a025585

Noulin F, Borlon C, Van Den Abbeele J, D'Alessandro U, Erhart A. 2013. 1912–2012: A century of research on *Plasmodium vivax* in vitro culture. *Trends Parasitol* **29**: 286–294.

Noulin F, Manesia JK, Rosanas-Urgell A, Erhart A, Borlon C, Van Den Abbeele J, d'Alessandro U, Verfaillie CM. 2014. Hematopoietic stem/progenitor cell sources to generate reticulocytes for *Plasmodium vivax* culture. *PLoS ONE* **9**: e112496.

Noviyanti R, Coutrier F, Utami RA, Trimarsanto H, Tirta YK, Trianty L, Kusuma A, Sutanto I, Kosasih A, Kusriastuti R, et al. 2015. Contrasting transmission dynamics of co-endemic *Plasmodium vivax* and *P. falciparum*: Implications for malaria control and elimination. *PLoS Negl Trop Dis* **9**: e0003739.

PAHO. 2013. *Central America and Hispaniola seek to eliminate malaria by 2025.* Pan American Health Organization, Geneva.

Panichakul T, Sattabongkot J, Chotivanich K, Sirichaisinthop J, Cui L, Udomsangpetch R. 2007. Production of erythropoietic cells in vitro for continuous culture of *Plasmodium vivax*. *Int J Parasitol* **37**: 1551–1557.

Pearson RD, Amato R, Auburn S, Miotto O, Almagro-Garcia J, Amaratunga C, Seila S, Mao S, Noviyanti R, Trimarsanto H, et al. 2016. Genomic analysis of local variation and recent evolution in the *Plasmodium vivax* population. *Nat Genet* **48**: 959–964.

Peltz G. 2013. Can "humanized" mice improve drug development in the 21st century? *Trends Pharmacol Sci* **34**: 255–260.

Pethleart A, Prajakwong S, Suwonkerd W, Corthong B, Webber R, Curtis C. 2004. Infectious reservoir of *Plasmodium* infection in Mae Hong Son Province, north-west Thailand. *Malaria J* **3**: 34.

Phimpraphi W, Paul RE, Yimsamran S, Puangsa-art S, Thanyavanich N, Maneeboonyang W, Prommongkol S, Sornklom S, Chaimungkun W, Chavez IF, et al. 2008. Longitudinal study of *Plasmodium falciparum* and *Plasmodium vivax* in a Karen population in Thailand. *Malaria J* **7**: 99.

Price RN, Tjitra E, Guerra CA, Yeung S, White NJ, Anstey NM. 2007. Vivax malaria: Neglected and not benign. *Am J Trop Med Hyg* **77**: 79–87.

Price RN, Marfurt J, Chalfein F, Kenangalem E, Piera KA, Tjitra E, Anstey NM, Russell B. 2010. In vitro activity of pyronaridine against multidrug-resistant *Plasmodium falciparum* and *Plasmodium vivax*. *Antimicrob Agents Chemother* **54**: 5146–5150.

Rijken MJ, Boel ME, Russell B, Imwong M, Leimanis ML, Pyae Phyo A, Muehlenbachs A, Lindegardh N, McGready R, Renia L, et al. 2011. Chloroquine resistant vivax malaria in a pregnant woman on the western border of Thailand. *Malaria J* **10**: 113.

Robinson LJ, Wampfler R, Betuela I, Karl S, White MT, Li Wai Suen CS, Hofmann NE, Kinboro B, Waltmann A, Brewster J, et al. 2015. Strategies for understanding and reducing the *Plasmodium vivax* and *Plasmodium ovale* hypnozoite reservoir in Papua New Guinean children: A randomised placebo-controlled trial and mathematical model. *PLoS Med* **12**: e1001891.

Roobsoong W, Tharinjaroen CS, Rachaphaew N, Chobson P, Schofield L, Cui L, Adams JH, Sattabongkot J. 2015. Improvement of culture conditions for long-term in vitro culture of *Plasmodium vivax*. *Malaria J* **14**: 297.

Ruebush TK 2nd, Zegarra J, Cairo J, Andersen EM, Green M, Pillai DR, Marquino W, Huilca M, Arevalo E, Garcia C, et al. 2003. Chloroquine-resistant *Plasmodium vivax* malaria in Peru. *Am J Trop Med Hyg* **69**: 548–552.

Russell B, Suwanarusk R, Borlon C, Costa FT, Chu CS, Rijken MJ, Sriprawat K, Warter L, Koh EG, Malleret B, et al. 2011. A reliable ex vivo invasion assay of human reticulocytes by *Plasmodium vivax*. *Blood* **118**: e74–e81.

Sattabongkot J, Yimamnuaychoke N, Leelaudomlipi S, Rasameesoraj M, Jenwithisuk R, Coleman RE, Udomsangpetch R, Cui L, Brewer TG. 2006. Establishment of a human hepatocyte line that supports in vitro development of the exo-erythrocytic stages of the malaria parasites *Plasmodium falciparum* and *P. vivax*. *Am J Trop Med Hyg* **74**: 708–715.

Shultz LD, Ishikawa F, Greiner DL. 2007. Humanized mice in translational biomedical research. *Nat Rev Immunol* **7**: 118–130.

Snounou G, Perignon JL. 2013. Malariotherapy—Insanity at the service of malariology. *Adv Parasitol* **81**: 223–255.

Soulard V, Bosson-Vanga H, Lorthiois A, Roucher C, Franetich JF, Zanghi G, Bordessoulles M, Tefit M, Thellier M, Morosan S, et al. 2015. *Plasmodium falciparum* full life cycle and *Plasmodium ovale* liver stages in humanized mice. *Nat Commun* **6**: 7690.

Suwanarusk R, Cooke BM, Dondorp AM, Silamut K, Sattabongkot J, White NJ, Udomsangpetch R. 2004. The deformability of red blood cells parasitized by *Plasmodium falciparum* and *P. vivax*. *J Infect Dis* **189**: 190–194.

Teka H, Petros B, Yamuah L, Tesfaye G, Elhassan I, Muchohi S, Kokwaro G, Aseffa A, Engers H. 2008. Chloroquine-resistant *Plasmodium vivax* malaria in Debre Zeit, Ethiopia. *Malaria J* **7**: 220.

Udagama PV, Atkinson CT, Peiris JS, David PH, Mendis KN, Aikawa M. 1988. Immunoelectron microscopy of Schuffner's dots in *Plasmodium vivax*–infected human erythrocytes. *Am J Pathol* **131**: 48–52.

Udomsangpetch R, Somsri S, Panichakul T, Chotivanich K, Sirichaisinthop J, Yang Z, Cui L, Sattabongkot J. 2007. Short-term in vitro culture of field isolates of *Plasmodium vivax* using umbilical cord blood. *Parasitol Int* **56**: 65–69.

Vallejo AF, Garcia J, Amado-Garavito AB, Arevalo-Herrera M, Herrera S. 2016. *Plasmodium vivax* gametocyte infectivity in sub-microscopic infections. *Malaria J* **15**: 48.

VanBuskirk KM, Cole-Tobian JL, Baisor M, Sevova ES, Bockarie M, King CL, Adams JH. 2004. Antigenic drift in the ligand domain of *Plasmodium vivax* Duffy binding protein confers resistance to inhibitory antibodies. *J Infect Dis* **190**: 1556–1562.

Van den Eede P, Van der Auwera G, Delgado C, Huyse T, Soto-Calle VE, Gamboa D, Grande T, Rodriguez H, Llanos A, Anne J, et al. 2010. Multilocus genotyping reveals high heterogeneity and strong local population structure of the *Plasmodium vivax* population in the Peruvian Amazon. *Malaria J* **9**: 151.

Wampfler R, Mwingira F, Javati S, Robinson L, Betuela I, Siba P, Beck HP, Mueller I, Felger I. 2013. Strategies for detection of *Plasmodium* species gametocytes. *PLoS ONE* **8:** e76316.

Wells TN, Burrows JN, Baird JK. 2010. Targeting the hypnozoite reservoir of *Plasmodium vivax*: The hidden obstacle to malaria elimination. *Trends Parasitol* **26:** 145–151.

White NJ. 2011. Determinants of relapse periodicity in *Plasmodium vivax* malaria. *Malaria J* **10:** 297.

White NJ, Imwong M. 2012. Relapse. *Adv Parasitol* **80:** 113–150.

White M, Shirreff G, Karl S, Ghani A, Mueller I. 2016. Variation in relapse frequency and the transmission potential of *Plasmodium vivax* malaria. *Proc Biol Sci* **283:** 20160048.

WHO. 2015. World malaria report 2015. Global malaria programme. World Health Organization, Geneva.

Anopheline Reproductive Biology: Impacts on Vectorial Capacity and Potential Avenues for Malaria Control

Sara N. Mitchell and Flaminia Catteruccia

Harvard T.H. Chan School of Public Health, Department of Immunology and Infectious Diseases, Boston, Massachusetts 02115

Correspondence: fcatter@hsph.harvard.edu

Vectorial capacity is a mathematical approximation of the efficiency of vector-borne disease transmission, measured as the number of new infections disseminated per case per day by an insect vector. Multiple elements of mosquito biology govern their vectorial capacity, including survival, population densities, feeding preferences, and vector competence. Intriguingly, biological pathways essential to mosquito reproductive fitness directly or indirectly influence a number of these elements. Here, we explore this complex interaction, focusing on how the interplay between mating and blood feeding in female *Anopheles* not only shapes their reproductive success but also influences their ability to sustain *Plasmodium* parasite development. Central to malaria transmission, mosquito reproductive biology has recently become the focus of research strategies aimed at malaria control, and we discuss promising new methods based on the manipulation of key reproductive steps. In light of widespread resistance to all public health–approved insecticides targeting mosquito reproduction may prove crucial to the success of malaria-eradication campaigns.

PLASMODIUM SPOROGONIC DEVELOPMENT: A PROCESS INTIMATELY TIED TO MOSQUITO REPRODUCTION

Transmission of human *Plasmodium* parasites, the causative agents of malaria, relies on the infectious bite of female *Anopheles* mosquitoes. In the mosquito midgut, sporogonic development starts within minutes of a female taking a blood meal on an infected vertebrate host. At the same time, nutrients derived from the digestion of the blood meal accumulate in the ovaries during the process of oogenesis, which after 2–3 days will culminate in ovulation and oviposition. Sporogony and oogenesis are, therefore, temporally and physiologically coupled in the female mosquito (Fig. 1).

At the start of sporogonic development, male and female gametocytes—the sexual stage of the *Plasmodium* parasite—are ingested and enter the mosquito midgut where they immediately form gametes, triggered by a drop in surrounding temperature and by the presence of other mosquito-specific factors (Billker et al. 1997, 1998; McRobert et al. 2008; Kuehn and Pradel 2010). After escaping the enveloping

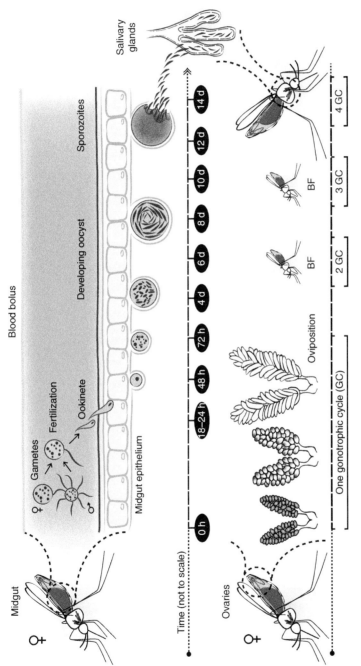

Figure 1. Plasmodium sporogony and anopheline oogenesis are temporally and physiologically tied in the mosquito. When a female *Anopheles* mosquito takes a blood meal from a malaria-infected host, two processes immediately begin within the midgut: *Plasmodium* gametogenesis, and digestion of the blood bolus for the production of nutrients vital for oogenesis. Within the first 3 days after feeding, a female will have completed her first gonotrophic cycle (GC) consisting of blood feeding, egg development, and oviposition. During this same 72-h period, the *Plasmodium* gametes will have fused to produce first a zygote and, subsequently, a motile ookinete form, which traverses the midgut epithelium before developing into an oocyst. Over the course of the next 10 days, the oocysts will produce transmission-stage sporozoites, whereas the female will undergo additional gonotrophic cycles, potentially becoming infectious on sporozoites reaching her salivary glands. BF, Blood feeding.

 Cite this article as *Cold Spring Harb Perspect Med* doi: 10.1101/cshperspect.a025593

erythrocyte, male gametocytes rapidly exflagellate to produce eight motile microgametes, which fuse with female macrogametes to form a diploid zygote. During the next 18–24 h, as the female digests the blood bolus in her midgut, the *Plasmodium* zygote will transform into a motile ookinete, which traverses the peritrophic matrix and midgut epithelium to reach the basal lamina. Here, the ookinete will encyst, differentiating into an oocyst. The initiation of oocyst development coincides with the completion of oogenesis in the mosquito ovaries, and if inseminated, the female will seek a suitable site to oviposit her eggs. Over the next 8–15 days (depending on *Plasmodium* species and extrinsic factors), the oocyst undergoes rapid growth and cellular division to produce thousands of infective sporozoites. After rupture of the oocyst wall, the mature sporozoites will migrate to and invade the salivary glands, ready to be injected into the host when the female takes her next blood meal. During this period, the female mosquito may undergo up to three additional gonotrophic cycles consisting of a blood meal, egg development, and oviposition (Fig. 1). This lengthy sporogonic cycle means that only a small proportion of female mosquitoes will actually survive long enough in nature to become infective with *Plasmodium* sporozoites and transmit disease (Charlwood et al. 1997; Killeen et al. 2000). Therefore, control interventions that target female mosquito life span are particularly successful in reducing malaria transmission in the field (Macdonald 1956; Smith et al. 2012).

Our understanding of the processes regulating egg development in the mosquito is largely derived from studies in the arboviral vector *Aedes aegypti* (reviewed in Attardo et al. 2005; Hansen et al. 2014). Oogenesis starts with the synthesis and secretion of yolk protein precursors (YPPs) and deposition into the developing oocytes. After a blood meal, the mosquito brain is triggered to release ovary ecdysteroidogenic hormone that stimulates the ovaries to produce the steroid hormone ecdysone (E). The latter, in turn, is hydroxylated to produce the active 20-hydroxyecdysone (20E) form in the fat body. A potent transcriptional regulator, 20E induces the expression of YPPs, including vitellogenin (Vg) and the lipid transporter lipophorin (Lp), which provision the developing oocytes with lipids. 20E and YPPs are integral to egg development in the malaria vector *Anopheles gambiae* (Atella et al. 2006; Bai et al. 2010), with 20E also fundamental to oogenesis in a number of insect species, including the fruit fly (*Drosophila melanogaster*) and the silk moth (*Bombyx mori*) (Swevers and Iatrou 2003; Belles and Piulachs 2015), suggesting conservation of this hormonally controlled process.

Interestingly, the YPPs that facilitate oogenesis also promote *Plasmodium* development via mechanisms that include protection from the mosquito's innate immune response (Vlachou et al. 2005; Mendes et al. 2008; Rono et al. 2010). RNAi-based knockdown of YPP *Lp* in *An. gambiae* infected with the rodent parasite *Plasmodium berghei* resulted in reduced oocyst numbers and abolished egg development (Vlachou et al. 2005). It was subsequently demonstrated that the expression and combined action of *Lp* and *Vg* after a blood meal blocks the parasite killing action of the complement-like factor thioester-containing protein 1 (TEP1) (Rono et al. 2010). TEP1 was previously shown to severely impair development of *Plasmodium* species (Levashina et al. 2001; Blandin et al. 2004), including the most deadly human malaria parasite *Plasmodium falciparum* (Dong et al. 2009; Garver et al. 2009; Eldering et al. 2016). In the absence of Vg, TEP1 binds more efficiently to the surface of *P. berghei* ookinetes, resulting in higher killing efficiency. Similarly, *Lp* knockdown resulted in reduced *P. falciparum* oocyst load, although the precise mechanism was not confirmed (Mendes et al. 2008). Others have shown incorporation of Lp loaded with lipids into the *Plasmodium* oocysts in *Aedes* mosquitoes (Atella et al. 2009) and, although the function of these lipids in the parasite is not known, silencing *Lp* reduces oocyst size in *An. gambiae* (Rono et al. 2010). Overall, it appears that malaria parasites have developed a system by which vitellogenic factors produced after a blood meal can be coopted to facilitate *Plasmodium* development within the mosquito.

THE COST OF INFECTION: POTENTIAL FOR TRADE-OFFS BETWEEN REPRODUCTION AND IMMUNITY DURING PARASITE DEVELOPMENT

Eliciting an immune response to infection is an energy-demanding process, as is the production of eggs. It has therefore been long postulated that *Plasmodium*-infected females may be faced with a trade-off of their resources in an effort to temper infection. A number of studies using the rodent malaria parasites *Plasmodium yoelii nigeriensis*, *P. chabaudi* and *P. berghei* have shown that infected females can experience decreased fecundity and fertility compared with noninfected counterparts (Hogg and Hurd 1997; Jahan and Hurd 1997; Ahmed et al. 2001; Ferguson et al. 2003; Olayemi and Ande 2013; reviewed in Hurd 2009). Oocyte resorption, initiated by apoptosis of epithelial cells surrounding the ovarian follicles, rather than a shortage of nutrients to provision-developing eggs, is believed to be the main driver of reduced fecundity in infected females (Hopwood et al. 2001; Hurd 2003; Ahmed and Hurd 2006). The timing of egg resorption coincides with ookinete traversal of the midgut epithelium (Hopwood et al. 2001), which is associated with epithelial cell pathology (Han and Barillas-Mury 2002) and strong immune induction (Dimopoulos 2003; Levashina 2004; Smith et al. 2014), which, in turn, may trigger apoptosis within the ovaries (Ahmed and Hurd 2006).

Yet, these studies suffer from the use of mosquito–parasite pairings that do not occur in nature. In natural pairings, we argue that the coevolution of parasite and vector over tens of thousands of years has led to a more "commensal" relationship in which immune induction is tempered and the potential cost of infection in the mosquito is minimized. Indeed, a number of studies using naturally occurring *Anopheles–Plasmodium* combinations have failed to show a negative impact of infection on mosquito fecundity (Ferguson et al. 2005; Yaro et al. 2012; Sangare et al. 2013, 2014). With only a modest negative effect on fecundity recorded in one field study in Tanzania, *An. gambiae* s.l. infected

with *P. falciparum* showed a ∼10% decrease in egg numbers (Hogg and Hurd 1997).

Although the potential trade-off between reproduction and *Plasmodium* infection remains somewhat unresolved, increasing evidence suggests that the parasite may have developed ways to circumvent damaging its invertebrate host. A recently proposed theory of malaria globalization suggests that *Plasmodium* parasites have evolved a mechanism to evade triggering the mosquito's midgut immune response in naturally occurring vector–parasite interactions (Molina-Cruz et al. 2015). This "lock-and-key theory" is based on parasite surface protein Pfs47 (the key), which suppresses the midgut nitration response (Molina-Cruz et al. 2013) through interaction with a yet-undetermined mosquito protein (the lock). It is therefore conceivable that in nonnatural infections the absence of the necessary coevolved "key" leads to immune triggering and, in turn, ovarian apoptosis and a reduction in reproductive fitness as reported in the aforementioned studies.

The mosquito may have also evolved mechanisms to overcome potential fitness costs incurred by *Plasmodium* infection. This fascinating topic warrants further exploration, although research must be based on *Anopheles–Plasmodium* combinations that naturally occur in malaria-endemic areas.

THE INTERPLAY BETWEEN MATING AND BLOOD FEEDING SHAPES VECTORIAL CAPACITY VIA THE STEROID HORMONE 20E

A number of studies point to an important role for the steroid hormone 20E during *Plasmodium* sporogony. 20E is the major ecdysteroid in insects where it regulates molting during juvenile stages (Yamanaka et al. 2013) and, as discussed, is also essential for egg development in many insect species including mosquitoes (Attardo et al. 2005; Belles and Piulachs 2015). Besides the induction of YPPs and their consequent modulation of the mosquito's complement-like system previously described (Rono et al. 2010), 20E regulates a number of additional genes that can either impair or facilitate parasite development within the female mosquito. In *An. gambiae* and *An. stephensi*, the 20E-induced immunomodulatory peroxidase HPX15 (also named IMPer)—alongside a role in ensuring mosquito fertility (Shaw et al. 2014)—protects *Plasmodium* parasites from the midgut epithelial immune response by catalyzing dityrosine network formation and decreasing epithelial permeability to immune elicitors (Kumar et al. 2010). On the other hand, 20E induces the expression of a number of immune genes with potential roles in curbing *Plasmodium* infections, including numerous prophenoloxidases (PPOs), which drive the *An. gambiae* melanization response to pathogens (Ahmed et al. 1999; Muller et al. 1999), and LRIM9 (leucine-rich repeat immune protein 9), an immunity factor that in *An. gambiae* reduces *P. berghei* infection intensity through as-yet-unknown mechanisms (Upton et al. 2015). The complex interaction between 20E and the innate immune response is therefore likely to influence the outcome of *Plasmodium* development in the mosquito.

Moreover, uniquely to anophelines, 20E is also produced by males and transferred to females during copulation. In most *Anopheles* species, mating occurs at dusk in large swarms formed by tens to hundreds of individuals. Females are attracted to swarms, most likely by a combination of olfactory, audial, and visual cues. On entering, females pair with a male before leaving to complete copulation. The female is inseminated only once in her lifetime (Tripet et al. 2003; Yuval 2006), and she uses sperm from this single copulation event to fertilize all egg batches produced during multiple gonotrophic cycles (Yaro et al. 2006). During this single mating event, females receive sperm into a specialized storage organ—the spermatheca—and seminal fluids secreted by the male accessory glands (MAGs), which in most anopheline species are coagulated to form a gelatinous mating plug deposited in the atrium (uterus) (Giglioli and Mason 1966; Rogers et al. 2009; Mitchell et al. 2015). Male 20E produced in the MAGs (Pondeville et al. 2008) is packaged into the mating plug during copulation and delivered to the

female atrium together with seminal proteins and lipids (Baldini et al. 2013; Mitchell et al. 2015). In *An. gambiae* and other *Anopheles* species, sexual transfer of male 20E triggers large behavioral and physiological responses paralleled by extensive transcriptional changes that result in a long-term refractoriness to further copulation, increased egg development following a blood meal, induction of oviposition in blood-fed females, and regulation of pathways that ensure fertility (Baldini et al. 2013; Gabrieli et al. 2014a; Shaw et al. 2014).

Sexual delivery of 20E modulates the expression of more than 800 *An. gambiae* genes in the female reproductive tract (Gabrieli et al. 2014a). Among these genes is the *Mating-Induced Stimulator of Oogenesis* (*MISO*), whose transcriptional level is strongly up-regulated by male 20E specifically in the female atrium (Rogers et al. 2008; Baldini et al. 2013). After expression, the interaction between MISO and male 20E activates downstream signaling cascades that ultimately promote oogenesis, via mechanisms that include elevated expression of the lipid transporter *Lp* and consequent increased lipid uptake into the ovaries (Baldini et al. 2013). The MISO-male 20E interaction therefore couples mating-induced pathways with blood feeding-activated processes, regulating the development of eggs in the ovaries and potentially affecting—based on the role of Lp in *Plasmodium* development (Vlachou et al. 2005; Mendes et al. 2008; Rono et al. 2010)— parasite survival in the midgut.

Significant divergence in the levels of 20E both produced by the MAGs and transferred to the female on mating is observed across *Anopheles* species worldwide (Mitchell et al. 2015). However, the function of this steroid hormone appears to be conserved in the genus, with the notable exception of the New World mosquito *Anopheles albimanus*, which in absence of 20E production in the MAGs must use alternative strategies to regulate oviposition and receptivity to mating (Mitchell et al. 2015). Given the effects of this steroid hormone on multiple pathways that also influence *Plasmodium* development, heterogeneity in levels of both female and male 20E across different anopheline vectors may result in variation in their ability to transmit malaria. Interestingly, phylogenetic and ancestral state analyses suggest that 20E synthesis in the MAGs and transfer via the mating plug are acquired traits that have evolved in the *Anopheles* lineage from a plugless and 20E-less ancestral species, inducing reciprocal adaptation in the 20E-interacting female protein MISO and likely other female reproductive factors (Mitchell et al. 2015). Although a direct link between male-transferred 20E and *Plasmodium* development in the female remains to be proven, these findings suggest the intriguing hypothesis that the evolution of a mating system based on sexual transfer of this steroid hormone may have affected vectorial capacity in anophelines. Consistent with this hypothesis, the *Anopheles* species that transfer the highest levels of 20E originate from areas with the largest malaria burden (see WHO 2015) and are among the most efficient vectors of the disease.

TARGETING MATING AND REPRODUCTION FOR MALARIA CONTROL

Current mosquito control methods based on long-lasting insecticide-treated nets (LLINs) and indoor residual spraying (IRS) are severely threatened by the rapid spread of resistance in natural mosquito populations and the lack of new insecticides coming to market (Toé et al. 2014; Hemingway et al. 2016). Of greatest concern are the reports of extensive high-level resistance to pyrethroid insecticides in sub-Saharan Africa (Ranson et al. 2011); pyrethroids are currently the only chemical class approved for use on LLINs, which are by far the most effective intervention against malaria transmission (Bhatt et al. 2015). A further challenge for the success of malaria control lies in those *Anopheles* populations that predominantly blood feed and rest outdoors, as these mosquitoes evade conventional indoor-based vector-control strategies and represent a significant barrier to malaria eradication (Alonso et al. 2011; Govella and Ferguson 2012).

Reproductive processes offer unexplored opportunities for the implementation of methods that may provide alternatives to, or enhance existing, insecticide interventions. In the mosquito life cycle, sex is a vulnerable step as females mate only once (Tripet et al. 2003; Yuval 2006). Interfering with mating is, therefore, a potential strategy for malaria control: If mating were disrupted or if virgin females were switched to a mated state without being successfully inseminated, the size of natural mosquito populations would be drastically reduced. Alternatively, manipulation of female reproductive physiology, whether in the form of preventing egg development, inhibiting egg laying, or inducing sterility in egg batches, would also provide a powerful means to reduce vectorial capacity.

SIT and Genetic Control Strategies

The idea of exploiting mating to control insect populations was first introduced by Raymond Bushland and Edward Knipling in the 1950s, who predicted that releasing mass numbers of sterile insects over a long period of time would collapse field populations (Fig. 2A). This concept, named sterile insect technique (SIT), has since been widely applied to the control of a number of economically important agricultural pests, including the New World screwworm fly (*Cochliomyia hominivorax*) in the Americas and North Africa (Lindquist et al. 1992; Wyss 2000), the melon fly (*Bactrocera cucurbitae*) in Japan (Koyama et al. 2004), and the medfly (*Ceratitis capitata*) in the United States and Central America (Hendrichs et al. 2002). As male mosquitoes do not feed on blood and are therefore not involved in the direct transmission of human disease, they are logical agents for campaigns based on release of sterile adults. However, SIT strategies have met limited success when used against *Anopheles* populations, with failures attributed to reduced male mating competitiveness resulting from sterilization and mass rearing-associated fitness costs (Dame et al. 2009; Howell and Knols 2009) and the lack of efficient mechanisms to separate females from males before a release (Benedict and Robinson 2003).

Major advances in the field of genetic engineering and the recent availability of genomic

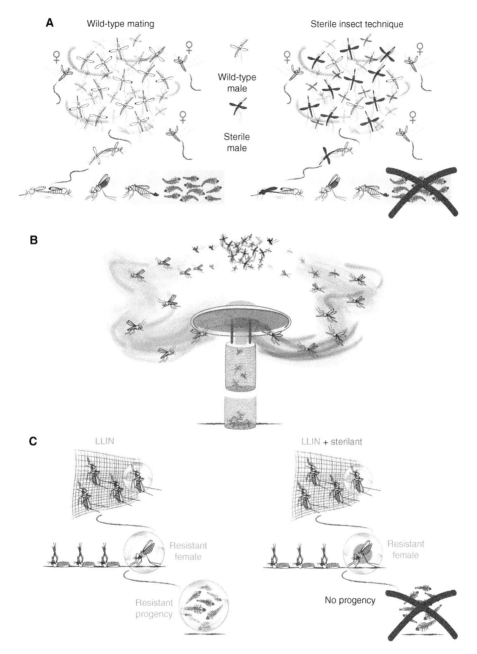

Figure 2. Exploiting anopheline reproductive biology for malaria control. (*A*) Sterile insect technique (SIT) involves the mass release of sterile males that, if released in high enough numbers, will outcompete normal wild-type males in the mating swarm (*right* panel) and mate with females. These females will then lay sterile egg batches and not produce any progeny, an effect that will eventually crash the population. (*B*) Chemical attractants such as aggregation or mating pheromones could be used in mating-disruption strategies to attract male and/or female mosquitoes to traps, diverting individuals from mating swarms. (*C*) The use of sterilants in combination with insecticides on long-lasting insecticide-treated nets (LLINs) could stop the spread of insecticide resistance. Females impervious to the effects of insecticides on nets (*left* panel) would not be able to pass genes conferring resistance on to subsequent generations if a sterilant is included on LLINs (*right* panel).

data for all major anopheline vectors (Neafsey et al. 2015) provide new opportunities for targeting reproductive processes via genetic manipulation of multiple natural vector populations. Since the generation of the first transgenic *Anopheles* strains more than a decade ago (Catteruccia et al. 2000), a wide array of gene editing tools with increased precision, flexibility, and level of sophistication have emerged (Urnov et al. 2010; Aryan et al. 2013; Mali et al. 2013). Our ability to introduce desired modifications in the genome while causing minimal perturbation to mosquito physiology has dramatically increased and can be exploited to effectively induce sterility while minimizing fitness costs to the insect. For instance, sterile, spermless males were generated by targeting a gene essential for germ cell development, "zero population growth" (ZPG), and although these males were able to mate successfully and induce refractoriness to further mating in females through the delivery of seminal secretions, mated blood-fed females laid only infertile eggs (Thailayil et al. 2011). Targeting sperm generation via genetic manipulation of *zpg* or similar genes offers promise as a SIT strategy, considering fertility can be specifically manipulated while minimizing any detrimental effects on male mating competitiveness. A similar strategy to SIT, "release of insects carrying a dominant lethal" (RIDL), eliminates the need for sterilization by producing fertile males whose progeny are killed during larval development (Phuc et al. 2007).

Gene Drives

Sterility or lethal transgenes can also be "driven" through populations using genetic selfish elements that can force their own spread in a non-Mendelian manner (reviewed in Gabrieli et al. 2014b). The most powerful example is CRISPR/Cas9, originally a bacterial-acquired immune defense system. It has been coopted to specifically recognize and cleave target sites in the genome through the action of Cas9 nuclease and small artificial guide RNAs (gRNAs) (Barrangou et al. 2007). When a transgene encoding Cas9 and gRNAs is inserted at the ho-

mologous chromosomal locus as their target sequence, DNA repair by homologous recombination results in the transgene being copied into the cleaved locus. When this occurs in the germline of heterozygous parents, the transgene can be inherited in >50% of the progeny, favoring the inheritance of the transgenic cassette (Esvelt et al. 2014). The ability to guarantee inheritance of transgenically encoded traits despite potential fitness defects would enable driving of otherwise highly costly sterility-causing cargoes through wild populations. Indeed, proof-of-principle examples of gene drives in mosquitoes have been generated by multiple laboratories (Gantz et al. 2015; Hammond et al. 2016), and improved "evolutionary stable" systems that prevent insurgence of deleterious mutations that block the drive are likely to emerge in the near future (Esvelt et al. 2014). By exploiting males and their need to find a mate, such genetic control strategies could play a significant role in the path to malaria eradication, contributing to the reduction of residual malaria transmission attributed to outdoor biting and resting mosquitoes that would evade even universal LLIN/IRS coverage.

Targeting Mating Behavior

Considering a female's lifetime reproductive output is centered on the quality of a single mate, the fitness of the preferred male has important implications for female mate choice decisions. A better understanding of male reproductive biology and the factors ensuring successful mating is therefore essential for SIT- or genetic-based strategies to succeed (Howell and Knols 2009; Lees et al. 2014; Diabate and Tripet 2015). Although the components of precopulatory sexual selection in *An. gambiae* remain unclear, chemical and acoustic signals appears to play a major role (Polerstock et al. 2002; Howard and Blomquist 2005; Cator et al. 2009, 2010). Before mating, the two sexes engage in a brief period of tarsal interaction, likely facilitating close-range chemical communication (Charlwood and Jones 1979). Longer-range chemical cues such as aggregation pheromones, on the other hand, may play a role in male lekking behavior, as suggested in *Aedes* mosquitoes (Cabrera and Jaffe 2007; Fawaz et al. 2014). Recent studies have also shown the importance of precopulatory acoustic signaling in the mating success of mosquito vectors including *An. gambiae* (Cator et al. 2009, 2010; Gibson et al. 2010; Pennetier et al. 2010). Once identified and characterized, these chemical and acoustic cues could be exploited to disrupt mating or be incorporated into traps to attract and kill mosquitoes looking for a mate, thus providing alternative tools to target insecticide-resistant mosquitoes and outdoor biting populations (Fig. 2B).

Recent advances in our understanding of the molecular determinants of female postmating and postblood feeding biology offer additional opportunities for the manipulation of reproductive success of mosquito populations (Rogers et al. 2008; Dottorini et al. 2013; Gabrieli et al. 2014a; Shaw et al. 2014; Mitchell et al. 2015). The steroid hormone 20E, produced by the male and transferred during copulation, has been identified as a major regulator for switching off female's receptivity to mating (Gabrieli et al. 2014a; Mitchell et al. 2015). If mating refractoriness could be triggered through application of 20E agonists, virgin females could be artificially switched to a mated state in the absence of insemination, dramatically reducing their reproductive output. Recent findings support the use of hormonal agonists as mosquito-control agents. Pyriproxyfen, an analog of the other major insect hormone juvenile hormone, produces both long-term sterility and life-shortening effects in *Anopheles* mosquitoes (Ohashi et al. 2012; Harris et al. 2013; Koama et al. 2015), with promising results when applied to resting surfaces and bednets in semifield trials (Kawada et al. 2014; Lwetoijera et al. 2014). By combining sterilizing compounds with insecticides, mosquitoes resistant to the killing action of the insecticide will be unable to propagate the resistance traits to the next generation, therefore preventing selection and spread of insecticide-resistant alleles in the population, an idea coined as "negative cross resistance" (Fig. 2C) (White et al. 2014).

FUTURE PERSPECTIVES

According to the World Health Organization, "mosquito control is the only intervention that can reduce malaria transmission from very high levels to close to zero" (see WHO 2014). This statement was recently validated by an extensive meta-analysis that established the effect of malaria control interventions on *P. falciparum* in Africa over the last decade; vector control accounted for 78% of the total 663 million cases averted (Bhatt et al. 2015).

The research community has begun to address the pressing need for new mosquito-control strategies that do not exclusively rely on current insecticides and can target exophilic *Anopheles* species. Genetic modification of mosquito vectors and, in particular, the use of gene drives that can spread rapidly through insect populations have been a major focus of research efforts (reviewed in Esvelt et al. 2014; Gabrieli et al. 2014b), but have also been met with criticism at both government and community levels (Macer 2006; Lavery et al. 2008; Brown et al. 2014). Given the potential for spread across borders and possible unanticipated ecological and environmental consequences, we believe that the release of gene drives for disease control should be the subject of wide and open debate between the scientific community, national and international funding and governmental agencies, and the general public (Esvelt et al. 2014; Oye and Esvelt 2014; Oye et al. 2014; Akbari et al. 2015). Moreover, two key research priorities are fundamental to the release of successful genetic drives: the generation of stable drives that can withstand the inevitable emergence of mutations; and the development of "counter-drive" mechanisms to reverse possible negative impacts following the release of the initial drive (Esvelt et al. 2014).

Additional strategies that can extend the efficacy of current insecticide-based control are urgently needed. We argue that the opportunities provided by targeting hormonal signaling essential to mosquito reproductive fitness, such as the juvenile hormone- and 20E-regulated pathways, need to be fully explored for the generation of control tools that target both mosquito survival and fertility. Moreover, the conservation of hormonal physiology across major malaria vector species will allow multiple disease vectors to be targeted with a single hormone analog, whereas the aforementioned ability to halt the reproductive output of females resistant to currently used insecticides will reduce the spread of this resistance in the wild.

Targeting outdoor biting mosquito populations and preventing residual malaria (defined as malaria transmission occurring despite universal LLINs or IRS) is proving particularly challenging. We believe that novel strategies, in addition to proposed genetic modification, are necessary to control these exophilic populations, and mating biology may prove key in the development of such tools. By bridging the knowledge gap between pre- and postcopulatory mating biology, we can harness essential chemical and acoustic signals for the development of traps that will target these mosquitoes outdoors.

Regardless of the strategies that will be developed, efforts to control malaria vectors must remain a top research and funding priority even in the face of emergencies such as the current Zika outbreak. Given the extraordinary success of mosquito-based interventions to date (Bhatt et al. 2015), "dropping the ball" now on *Anopheles* mosquito research and control would inevitably lead to disease resurgence, with disastrous consequences for millions worldwide.

CONCLUDING REMARKS

As *Plasmodium* transmission is contingent on the reproductive needs of its anopheline vector, with the processes of sporogony and oogenesis intimately tied within the female mosquito, it is unsurprising that reproductive pathways regulating oogenesis also impact *Plasmodium* development. Our increased power to explore the genomes of multiple *Anopheles* vectors, in combination with an exceptional ability to engineer them, provides unprecedented opportunity to target essential links in both parasite and mosquito reproductive cycles for malaria control. Whether by extending the duration of in-secticide effectiveness, enhancing the success of genetic control strategies, or providing novel strategies to disrupt mosquito mating, the study of reproductive biology is fundamental to this next generation of malaria-eradication efforts.

ACKNOWLEDGMENTS

We thank Manuela Bernardi for graphical contributions. We are grateful to members of the Catteruccia Laboratory for useful comments and discussion. We appreciate support from National Institutes of Health (NIH) grants R01-AI104956 and R21-AI117313 to F.C.

REFERENCES

Ahmed AM, Hurd H. 2006. Immune stimulation and malaria infection impose reproductive costs in *Anopheles gambiae* via follicular apoptosis. *Microbes Infect* **8:** 308–315.

Ahmed A, Martin D, Manetti AG, Han SJ, Lee WJ, Mathiopoulos KD, Muller HM, Kafatos FC, Raikhel A, Brey PT. 1999. Genomic structure and ecdysone regulation of the prophenoloxidase 1 gene in the malaria vector *Anopheles gambiae*. *Proc Natl Acad Sci* **96:** 14795–14800.

Ahmed AM, Maingon R, Romans P, Hurd H. 2001. Effects of malaria infection on vitellogenesis in *Anopheles gambiae* during two gonotrophic cycles. *Insect Mol Biol* **10:** 347–356.

Akbari OS, Bellen HJ, Bier E, Bullock SL, Burt A, Church GM, Cook KR, Duchek P, Edwards OR, Esvelt KM, et al. 2015. BIOSAFETY. Safeguarding gene drive experiments in the laboratory. *Science* **349:** 927–929.

Alonso PL, Brown G, Arevalo-Herrera M, Binka F, Chitnis C, Collins F, Doumbo OK, Greenwood B, Hall BF, Levine MM, et al. 2011. A research agenda to underpin malaria eradication. *PLoS Med* **8:** e1000406.

Aryan A, Anderson MA, Myles KM, Adelman ZN. 2013. TALEN-based gene disruption in the dengue vector *Aedes aegypti*. *PLoS ONE* **8:** e60082.

Atella GC, Silva-Neto MA, Golodne DM, Arefin S, Shahabuddin M. 2006. *Anopheles gambiae* lipophorin: Characterization and role in lipid transport to developing oocyte. *Insect Biochem Mol Biol* **36:** 375–386.

Atella GC, Bittencourt-Cunha PR, Nunes RD, Shahabuddin M, Silva-Neto MA. 2009. The major insect lipoprotein is a lipid source to mosquito stages of malaria parasite. *Acta Tropica* **109:** 159–162.

Attardo GM, Hansen IA, Raikhel AS. 2005. Nutritional regulation of vitellogenesis in mosquitoes: Implications for anautogeny. *Insect Biochem Mol Biol* **35:** 661–675.

Bai H, Gelman DB, Palli SR. 2010. Mode of action of methoprene in affecting female reproduction in the African malaria mosquito, *Anopheles gambiae*. *Pest Manag Sci* **66:** 936–943.

Cite this article as *Cold Spring Harb Perspect Med* doi: 10.1101/cshperspect.a025593

Baldini F, Gabrieli P, South A, Valim C, Mancini F, Catteruccia F. 2013. The interaction between a sexually transferred steroid hormone and a female protein regulates oogenesis in the malaria mosquito *Anopheles gambiae*. *PLoS Biol* **11**: e1001695.

Barrangou R, Fremaux C, Deveau H, Richards M, Boyaval P, Moineau S, Romero DA, Horvath P. 2007. CRISPR provides acquired resistance against viruses in prokaryotes. *Science* **315**: 1709–1712.

Belles X, Piulachs MD. 2015. Ecdysone signalling and ovarian development in insects: From stem cells to ovarian follicle formation. *Biochim Biophys Acta* **1849**: 181–186.

Benedict MQ, Robinson AS. 2003. The first releases of transgenic mosquitoes: An argument for the sterile insect technique. *Trends Parasitol* **19**: 349–355.

Bhatt S, Weiss DJ, Cameron E, Bisanzio D, Mappin B, Dalrymple U, Battle KE, Moyes CL, Henry A, Eckhoff PA, et al. 2015. The effect of malaria control on *Plasmodium falciparum* in Africa between 2000 and 2015. *Nature* **526**: 207–211.

Billker O, Shaw MK, Margos G, Sinden RE. 1997. The roles of temperature, pH and mosquito factors as triggers of male and female gametogenesis of *Plasmodium berghei* in vitro. *Parasitology* **115**: 1–7.

Billker O, Lindo V, Panico M, Etienne AE, Paxton T, Dell A, Rogers M, Sinden RE, Morris HR. 1998. Identification of xanthurenic acid as the putative inducer of malaria development in the mosquito. *Nature* **392**: 289–292.

Blandin S, Shiao SH, Moita LF, Janse CJ, Waters AP, Kafatos FC, Levashina EA. 2004. Complement-like protein TEP1 is a determinant of vectorial capacity in the malaria vector *Anopheles gambiae*. *Cell* **116**: 661–670.

Brown DM, Alphey LS, McKemey A, Beech C, James AA. 2014. Criteria for identifying and evaluating candidate sites for open-field trials of genetically engineered mosquitoes. *Vector Borne Zoonotic Dis* **14**: 291–299.

Cabrera M, Jaffe K. 2007. An aggregation pheromone modulates lekking behavior in the vector mosquito *Aedes aegypti* (Diptera: Culicidae). *J Am Mosq Control Assoc* **23**: 1–10.

Cator LJ, Arthur BJ, Harrington LC, Hoy RR. 2009. Harmonic convergence in the love songs of the dengue vector mosquito. *Science* **323**: 1077–1079.

Cator LJ, Ng'Habi KR, Hoy RR, Harrington LC. 2010. Sizing up a mate: Variation in production and response to acoustic signals in *Anopheles gambiae*. *Behav Ecol* **21**: 1033–1039.

Catteruccia F, Nolan T, Loukeris TG, Blass C, Savakis C, Kafatos FC, Crisanti A. 2000. Stable germline transformation of the malaria mosquito *Anopheles stephensi*. *Nature* **405**: 959–962.

Charlwood JD, Jones MDR. 1979. Mating behaviour in the mosquito, *Anopheles gambiae* s.l. *Physiol Entomol* **4**: 111–120.

Charlwood JD, Smith T, Billingsley PF, Takken W, Lyimo EOK, Meuwissen JHET. 1997. Survival and infection probabilities of anthropophagic anophelines from an area of high prevalence of *Plasmodium falciparum* in humans. *Bull Entomol Res* **87**: 445–453.

Dame DA, Curtis CF, Benedict MQ, Robinson AS, Knols BG. 2009. Historical applications of induced sterilisation in field populations of mosquitoes. *Malaria J* **8**: S2.

Diabate A, Tripet F. 2015. Targeting male mosquito mating behaviour for malaria control. *Parasit Vectors* **8**: 347.

Dimopoulos G. 2003. Insect immunity and its implication in mosquito–malaria interactions. *Cell Microbiol* **5**: 3–14.

Dong Y, Manfredini F, Dimopoulos G. 2009. Implication of the mosquito midgut microbiota in the defense against malaria parasites. *PLoS Pathog* **5**: e1000423.

Dottorini T, Persampieri T, Palladino P, Baker DA, Spaccapelo R, Senin N, Crisanti A. 2013. Regulation of *Anopheles gambiae* male accessory gland genes influences postmating response in female. *FASEB J* **27**: 86–97.

Eldering M, Morlais I, van Gemert GJ, van de Vegte-Bolmer M, Graumans W, Siebelink-Stoter R, Vos M, Abate L, Roeffen W, Bousema T, et al. 2016. Variation in susceptibility of African *Plasmodium falciparum* malaria parasites to TEP1 mediated killing in *Anopheles gambiae* mosquitoes. *Sci Rep* **6**: 20440.

Esvelt KM, Smidler AL, Catteruccia F, Church GM. 2014. Concerning RNA-guided gene drives for the alteration of wild populations. *eLife* doi: 10.7554/eLife.03401.

Fawaz EY, Allan SA, Bernier UR, Obenauer PJ, Diclaro JW II. 2014. Swarming mechanisms in the yellow fever mosquito: Aggregation pheromones are involved in the mating behavior of *Aedes aegypti*. *J Vector Ecol* **39**: 347–354.

Ferguson HM, Rivero A, Read AF. 2003. The influence of malaria parasite genetic diversity and anaemia on mosquito feeding and fecundity. *Parasitology* **127**: 9–19.

Ferguson HM, Gouagna LC, Obare P, Read AF, Babiker H, Githure J, Beier JC. 2005. The presence of *Plasmodium falciparum* gametocytes in human blood increases the gravidity of *Anopheles gambiae* mosquitoes. *Am J Trop Med Hyg* **73**: 312–320.

Gabrieli P, Kakani EG, Mitchell SN, Mameli E, Want EJ, Mariezcurrena Anton A, Serrao A, Baldini F, Catteruccia F. 2014a. Sexual transfer of the steroid hormone 20E induces the postmating switch in *Anopheles gambiae*. *Proc Natl Acad Sci* **111**: 16353–16358.

Gabrieli P, Smidler A, Catteruccia F. 2014b. Engineering the control of mosquito-borne infectious diseases. *Genome Biol* **15**: 535.

Gantz VM, Jasinskiene N, Tatarenkova O, Fazekas A, Macias VM, Bier E, James AA. 2015. Highly efficient Cas9-mediated gene drive for population modification of the malaria vector mosquito *Anopheles stephensi*. *Proc Natl Acad Sci* **112**: E6736–E6743.

Garver LS, Dong Y, Dimopoulos G. 2009. Caspar controls resistance to *Plasmodium falciparum* in diverse anopheline species. *PLoS Pathog* **5**: e1000335.

Gibson G, Warren B, Russell IJ. 2010. Humming in tune: Sex and species recognition by mosquitoes on the wing. *J Assoc Res Otolaryngol* **11**: 527–540.

Giglioli MEC, Mason GF. 1966. The mating plug in anopheline mosquitoes. *Proc R Entomol Soc Lond Ser A Gen Entomol* **41**: 123–129.

Govella NJ, Ferguson H. 2012. Why use of interventions targeting outdoor biting mosquitoes will be necessary to achieve malaria elimination. *Front Physiol* **3**: 199.

Hammond A, Galizi R, Kyrou K, Simoni A, Siniscalchi C, Katsanos D, Gribble M, Baker D, Marois E, Russell S, et al. 2016. A CRISPR-Cas9 gene drive system targeting female reproduction in the malaria mosquito vector *Anopheles gambiae*. *Nat Biotechnol* **34:** 78–83.

Han YS, Barillas-Mury C. 2002. Implications of Time Bomb model of ookinete invasion of midgut cells. *Insect Biochem Mol Biol* **32:** 1311–1316.

Hansen IA, Attardo GM, Rodriguez SD, Drake LL. 2014. Four-way regulation of mosquito yolk protein precursor genes by juvenile hormone-, ecdysone-, nutrient-, and insulin-like peptide signaling pathways. *Front Physiol* **5:** 103.

Harris C, Lwetoijera DW, Dongus S, Matowo NS, Lorenz LM, Devine GJ, Majambere S. 2013. Sterilising effects of pyriproxyfen on *Anopheles arabiensis* and its potential use in malaria control. *Parasites Vectors* **6:** 144.

Hemingway J, Ranson H, Magill A, Kolaczinski J, Fornadel C, Gimnig J, Coetzee M, Simard F, Roch DK, Hinzoumbe CK, et al. 2016. Averting a malaria disaster: Will insecticide resistance derail malaria control? *Lancet* **387:** 1785–1788.

Hendrichs J, Robinson A, Cayol J, Enkerlin W. 2002. Medfly area-wide sterile insect technique programmes for prevention, suppression or eradication: The importance of mating behavior studies. *Fla Entomol* **85:** 1–13.

Hogg JC, Hurd H. 1997. The effects of natural *Plasmodium falciparum* infection on the fecundity and mortality of *Anopheles gambiae* s.l. in north east Tanzania. *Parasitology* **114:** 325–331.

Hopwood JA, Ahmed AM, Polwart A, Williams GT, Hurd H. 2001. Malaria-induced apoptosis in mosquito ovaries: A mechanism to control vector egg production. *J Exp Biol* **204:** 2773–2780.

Howard RW, Blomquist GJ. 2005. Ecological, behavioral, and biochemical aspects of insect hydrocarbons. *Annu Rev Entomol* **50:** 371–393.

Howell PI, Knols BG. 2009. Male mating biology. *Malaria J* **8:** S8.

Hurd H. 2003. Manipulation of medically important insect vectors by their parasites. *Annu Rev Entomol* **48:** 141–161.

Hurd H. 2009. Evolutionary drivers of parasite-induced changes in insect life-history traits from theory to underlying mechanisms. *Adv Parasitol* **68:** 85–110.

Jahan N, Hurd H. 1997. The effects of infection with *Plasmodium yoelii* nigeriensis on the reproductive fitness of *Anopheles stephensi*. *Ann Trop Med Parasitol* **91:** 365–369.

Kawada H, Dida GO, Ohashi K, Kawashima E, Sonye G, Njenga SM, Mwandawiro C, Minakawa N. 2014. A small-scale field trial of pyriproxyfen-impregnated bed nets against pyrethroid-resistant *Anopheles gambiae* s.s. in western Kenya. *PLoS ONE* **9:** e111195.

Killeen GF, McKenzie FE, Foy BD, Schieffelin C, Billingsley PF, Beier JC. 2000. A simplified model for predicting malaria entomologic inoculation rates based on entomologic and parasitologic parameters relevant to control. *Am J Trop Med Hyg* **62:** 535–544.

Koama B, Namountougou M, Sanou R, Ndo S, Ouattara A, Dabire RK, Malone D, Diabate A. 2015. The sterilizing effect of pyriproxyfen on the malaria vector *Anopheles gambiae*: Physiological impact on ovaries development. *Malaria J* **14:** 101.

Koyama J, Kakinohana H, Miyatake T. 2004. Eradication of the melon fly, *Bactrocera cucurbitae*, in Japan: Importance of behavior, ecology, genetics, and evolution. *Annu Rev Entomol* **49:** 331–349.

Kuehn A, Pradel G. 2010. The coming-out of malaria gametocytes. *J Biomed Biotechnol* **2010:** 976827.

Kumar S, Molina-Cruz A, Gupta L, Rodrigues J, Barillas-Mury C. 2010. A peroxidase/dual oxidase system modulates midgut epithelial immunity in *Anopheles gambiae*. *Science* **327:** 1644–1648.

Lavery JV, Harrington LC, Scott TW. 2008. Ethical, social, and cultural considerations for site selection for research with genetically modified mosquitoes. *Am J Trop Med Hyg* **79:** 312–318.

Lees RS, Knols B, Bellini R, Benedict MQ, Bheecarry A, Bossin HC, Chadee DD, Charlwood J, Dabire RK, Djogbenou L, et al. 2014. Review: Improving our knowledge of male mosquito biology in relation to genetic control programmes. *Acta Tropica* **132:** S2–S11.

Levashina EA. 2004. Immune responses in *Anopheles gambiae*. *Insect Biochem Mol Biol* **34:** 673–678.

Levashina EA, Moita LF, Blandin S, Vriend G, Lagueux M, Kafatos FC. 2001. Conserved role of a complement-like protein in phagocytosis revealed by dsRNA knockout in cultured cells of the mosquito, *Anopheles gambiae*. *Cell* **104:** 709–718.

Lindquist DA, Abusowa M, Hall MJ. 1992. The New World screwworm fly in Libya: A review of its introduction and eradication. *Med Vet Entomol* **6:** 2–8.

Lwetoijera DW, Harris C, Kiware SS, Killeen GF, Dongus S, Devine GJ, Majambere S. 2014. Comprehensive sterilization of malaria vectors using pyriproxyfen: A step closer to malaria elimination. *Am J Trop Med Hyg* **90:** 852–855.

Macdonald G. 1956. Epidemiological basis of malaria control. *Bull World Health Organ* **15:** 613–626.

Macer DRJ. 2006. Ethics and community engagement for GM insect vector release. In *Genetically modified mosquitoes for malaria control* (ed. Boete C), pp. 152–165. Landes Bioscience, Austin, TX.

Mali P, Esvelt KM, Church GM. 2013. Cas9 as a versatile tool for engineering biology. *Nat Methods* **10:** 957–963.

McRobert L, Taylor CJ, Deng W, Fivelman QL, Cummings RM, Polley SD, Billker O, Baker DA. 2008. Gametogenesis in malaria parasites is mediated by the cGMP-dependent protein kinase. *PLoS Biol* **6:** e139.

Mendes AM, Schlegelmilch T, Cohuet A, Awono-Ambene P, De Iorio M, Fontenille D, Morlais I, Christophides GK, Kafatos FC, Vlachou D. 2008. Conserved mosquito/parasite interactions affect development of *Plasmodium falciparum* in Africa. *PLoS Pathog* **4:** e1000069.

Mitchell SN, Kakani EG, South A, Howell PI, Waterhouse RM, Catteruccia F. 2015. Mosquito biology. Evolution of sexual traits influencing vectorial capacity in anopheline mosquitoes. *Science* **347:** 985–988.

Molina-Cruz A, Garver LS, Alabaster A, Bangiolo L, Haile A, Winikor J, Ortega C, van Schaijk BC, Sauerwein RW, Taylor-Salmon E, et al. 2013. The human malaria parasite

Pfs47 gene mediates evasion of the mosquito immune system. *Science* **340:** 984–987.

Molina-Cruz A, Canepa GE, Kamath N, Pavlovic NV, Mu J, Ramphul UN, Ramirez JL, Barillas-Mury C. 2015. *Plasmodium* evasion of mosquito immunity and global malaria transmission: The lock-and-key theory. *Proc Natl Acad Sci* **112:** 15178–15183.

Muller HM, Dimopoulos G, Blass C, Kafatos FC. 1999. A hemocyte-like cell line established from the malaria vector *Anopheles gambiae* expresses six prophenoloxidase genes. *J Biol Chem* **274:** 11727–11735.

Neafsey DE, Waterhouse RM, Abai MR, Aganezov SS, Alekseyev MA, Allen JE, Amon J, Arca B, Arensburger P, Artemov G, et al. 2015. Mosquito genomics. Highly evolvable malaria vectors: The genomes of 16 *Anopheles* mosquitoes. *Science* **347:** 1258522.

Ohashi K, Nakada K, Ishiwatari T, Miyaguchi J, Shono Y, Lucas JR, Mito N. 2012. Efficacy of pyriproxyfen-treated nets in sterilizing and shortening the longevity of *Anopheles gambiae* (Diptera: Culicidae). *J Med Entomol* **49:** 1052–1058.

Olayemi IK, Ande AT. 2013. Plasmodium parasite-infection in the malaria vector mosquito, *Anopheles gambiae* (Diptera: Culicidae). *Eur J Biotechnol Biosci* **1:** 6–11.

Oye KA, Esvelt KM. 2014. Gene drives raise dual-use concerns—Response. *Science* **345:** 1010–1011.

Oye KA, Esvelt K, Appleton E, Catteruccia F, Church G, Kuiken T, Lightfoot SB, McNamara J, Smidler A, Collins JP. 2014. Biotechnology. Regulating gene drives. *Science* **345:** 626–628.

Pennetier C, Warren B, Dabire KR, Russell IJ, Gibson G. 2010. "Singing on the wing" as a mechanism for species recognition in the malarial mosquito *Anopheles gambiae*. *Curr Biol* **20:** 131–136.

Phuc HK, Andreasen MH, Burton RS, Vass C, Epton MJ, Pape G, Fu G, Condon KC, Scaife S, Donnelly CA, et al. 2007. Late-acting dominant lethal genetic systems and mosquito control. *BMC Biol* **5:** 11.

Polerstock AR, Eigenbrode SD, Klowden MJ. 2002. Mating alters the cuticular hydrocarbons of female *Anopheles gambiae* sensu stricto and *Aedes aegypti* (Diptera: Culicidae). *J Med Entomol* **39:** 545–552.

Pondeville E, Maria A, Jacques JC, Bourgouin C, Dauphin-Villemant C. 2008. *Anopheles gambiae* males produce and transfer the vitellogenic steroid hormone 20-hydroxyecdysone to females during mating. *Proc Natl Acad Sci* **105:** 19631–19636.

Ranson H, N'Guessan R, Lines J, Moiroux N, Nkuni Z, Corbel V. 2011. Pyrethroid resistance in African anopheline mosquitoes: What are the implications for malaria control? *Trends Parasitol* **27:** 91–98.

Rogers DW, Whitten MM, Thailayil J, Soichot J, Levashina EA, Catteruccia F. 2008. Molecular and cellular components of the mating machinery in *Anopheles gambiae* females. *Proc Natl Acad Sci* **105:** 19390–19395.

Rogers DW, Baldini F, Battaglia F, Panico M, Dell A, Morris HR, Catteruccia F. 2009. Transglutaminase-mediated semen coagulation controls sperm storage in the malaria mosquito. *PLoS Biol* **7:** e1000272.

Rono MK, Whitten MM, Oulad-Abdelghani M, Levashina EA, Marois E. 2010. The major yolk protein vitellogenin

interferes with the anti-*Plasmodium* response in the malaria mosquito *Anopheles gambiae*. *PLoS Biol* **8:** e1000434.

Sangare I, Michalakis Y, Yameogo B, Dabire R, Morlais I, Cohuet A. 2013. Studying fitness cost of *Plasmodium falciparum* infection in malaria vectors: Validation of an appropriate negative control. *Malaria J* **12:** 2.

Sangare I, Dabire R, Yameogo B, Da DF, Michalakis Y, Cohuet A. 2014. Stress dependent infection cost of the human malaria agent *Plasmodium falciparum* on its natural vector *Anopheles coluzzii*. *Infect Genet Evol* **25:** 57–65.

Shaw WR, Teodori E, Mitchell SN, Baldini F, Gabrieli P, Rogers DW, Catteruccia F. 2014. Mating activates the heme peroxidase HPX15 in the sperm storage organ to ensure fertility in *Anopheles gambiae*. *Proc Natl Acad Sci* **111:** 5854–5859.

Smith DL, Battle KE, Hay SI, Barker CM, Scott TW, McKenzie FE. 2012. Ross, Macdonald, and a theory for the dynamics and control of mosquito-transmitted pathogens. *PLoS Pathog* **8:** e1002588.

Smith RC, Vega-Rodriguez J, Jacobs-Lorena M. 2014. The *Plasmodium* bottleneck: Malaria parasite losses in the mosquito vector. *Mem Instit Oswaldo Cruz* **109:** 644–661.

Swevers L, Iatrou K. 2003. The ecdysone regulatory cascade and ovarian development in lepidopteran insects: Insights from the silkmoth paradigm. *Insect Biochem Mol Biol* **33:** 1285–1297.

Thailayil J, Magnusson K, Godfray HCJ, Crisanti A, Catteruccia F. 2011. Spermless males elicit large-scale female responses to mating in the malaria mosquito *Anopheles gambiae*. *Proc Natl Acad Sci* **108:** 13677–13681.

Toé KH, Jones CM, N'Fale S, Ismail HM, Dabiré RK, Ranson H. 2014. Increased pyrethroid resistance in malaria vectors and decreased bed net effectiveness, Burkina Faso. *Emerg Infect Dis* **20:** 1691–1696.

Tripet F, Toure YT, Dolo G, Lanzaro GC. 2003. Frequency of multiple inseminations in field-collected *Anopheles gambiae* females revealed by DNA analysis of transferred sperm. *Am J Trop Med Hyg* **68:** 1–5.

Upton LM, Povelones M, Christophides GK. 2015. *Anopheles gambiae* blood feeding initiates an anticipatory defense response to *Plasmodium berghei*. *J Innate Immun* **7:** 74–86.

Urnov FD, Rebar EJ, Holmes MC, Zhang HS, Gregory PD. 2010. Genome editing with engineered zinc finger nucleases. *Nat Rev Genet* **11:** 636–646.

Vlachou D, Schlegelmilch T, Christophides GK, Kafatos FC. 2005. Functional genomic analysis of midgut epithelial responses in *Anopheles* during *Plasmodium* invasion. *Curr Biol* **15:** 1185–1195.

White MT, Lwetoijera D, Marshall J, Caron-Lormier G, Bohan DA, Denholm I, Devine GJ. 2014. Negative cross resistance mediated by co-treated bed nets: A potential means of restoring pyrethroid-susceptibility to malaria vectors. *PLoS ONE* **9:** e95640.

WHO. 2014. World malaria report 2014. World Health Organization, Geneva.

WHO. 2015. World malaria report 2015. World Health Organization, Geneva.

Wyss JH. 2000. Screwworm eradication in the Americas. *Ann NY Acad Sci* **916:** 186–193.

Yamanaka N, Rewitz KF, O'Connor MB. 2013. Ecdysone control of developmental transitions: Lessons from *Drosophila* research. *Annu Rev Entomol* **58:** 497–516.

Yaro AS, Dao A, Adamou A, Crawford JE, Traore SF, Toure AM, Gwadz R, Lehmann T. 2006. Reproductive output of female *Anopheles gambiae* (Diptera: Culicidae): Comparison of molecular forms. *J Med Entomol* **43:** 833–839.

Yaro AS, Toure AM, Guindo A, Coulibaly MB, Dao A, Diallo M, Traore SF. 2012. Reproductive success in *Anopheles arabiensis* and the M and S molecular forms of *Anopheles gambiae*: Do natural sporozoite infection and body size matter? *Acta Tropica* **122:** 87–93.

Yuval B. 2006. Mating systems of blood-feeding flies. *Annu Rev Entomol* **51:** 413–440.

Cite this article as *Cold Spring Harb Perspect Med* doi: 10.1101/cshperspect.a025593

Modern Vector Control

Neil F. Lobo, Nicole L. Achee, John Greico, and Frank H. Collins

Department of Biological Sciences, University of Notre Dame, Notre Dame, Indiana 46556

Correspondence: frank@nd.edu

The rapid spread of mosquito resistance to currently available insecticides, and the current lack of an efficacious malaria vaccine are among many challenges that affect large-scale efforts for malaria control. As goals of malaria elimination and eradication are put forth, new vector-control paradigms and tools and/or further optimization of current vector-control products are required to meet public health demands. Vector control remains the most effective measure to prevent malaria transmission and present gains against malaria mortality and morbidity may be maintained as long as vector-intervention strategies are sustained and adapted to underlying vector-related transmission dynamics. The following provides a brief overview of vector-control strategies and tools either in use or under development and evaluation that are intended to exploit key entomological parameters toward driving down transmission.

Malaria, dengue, and other mosquito-borne diseases are public health problems in many parts of the world. There were an estimated 214 million cases and 438,000 deaths attributed to malaria in 2015 (WHO 2015a). Malaria-control strategies that have shown success include treatment of infected individuals with drugs, application of insecticide to reduce mosquito populations through indoor residual spray (IRS), and reduction of human contact with infected mosquitoes via insecticide-treated nets (ITNs) (D'Acremont et al. 2010; O'Meara et al. 2010). In 5 years (between 2000 and 2015), the global incidence of malaria fell 37% and malaria mortality decreased by 60% (WHO 2015a). However, ~3.2 billion people remain at risk of malaria, with continued associated morbidity and mortality.

Vector control remains the most effective measure to prevent malaria transmission. Vector-targeted interventions have been successful at reducing malaria mortality and morbidity worldwide—both historically and presently (WHO 2015a). The core goal of vector control is to reduce the vectorial capacity of a vector population below that required to maintain a malaria reproduction rate (R_0) of greater than 1—where R_0 is the number of human malaria cases that result from each human case in a population (malERA Consultative Group on Vector Control 2011). This has been shown from larval control in Brazil (Soper and Wilson 1943) and Egypt (Shousha 1948) in the 1940s, to the discovery of dichloro-diphenyl-trichloroethane (DDT) for use in IRS campaigns and present-day long-lasting insecticide-treated nets (LLINs). Vector control hence remains an integral part of the Global Malaria Control Strategy (GMSC) (WHO 1993). These remarkable effects and value to global health should be maintained as long as vector-related interventions are sustained and remain viable.

Effective vector control depends on the overlap between the specific intervention and susceptible vector behaviors (Elliott 1972; Bayoh et al. 2010; malERA Consultative Group on Vector Control 2011; Kiware et al. 2012; Killeen et al. 2013, 2014; Russell et al. 2013; Killeen 2014). Essentially, an intervention is more efficient if it functions on repeated vector behaviors such as ITNs killing susceptible mosquitoes when they look for a blood meal, which occurs once during a gonotrophic cycle and subsequently several times during the mosquito's life span (Killeen et al. 2014). Treated nets are, therefore, most efficient if the vector population host-seeks indoors while the local human population is asleep. In a similar manner, IRS is most effective against indoor resting vectors (Killeen et al. 2014). However, malaria transmission can be maintained by many vector species despite high coverage of ITNs and/or IRS as they may show behaviors that allow them to escape the effect of these interventions (Bugoro et al. 2011; Russell et al. 2013; Bayoh et al. 2014; Killeen 2014). With the case of ITNs, vector populations may avoid the intervention by feeding outside or early in the evening—at times when people are not sleeping under nets (Russell et al. 2013). Insecticide resistance will also impact the lethal effects of these interventions (Toe et al. 2014; Glunt et al. 2015).

Gains achieved by vector control in reducing malaria transmission cannot be relaxed without the expectation of a rebound in malaria incidence. Both a historical review and simulation modeling suggest that a scale-back of malaria vector control has a high probability of malaria resurgence for most scenarios, even where malaria transmission is very low or has been interrupted (WHO 2015b). In addition, residual transmission, that is, malaria transmission that happens outside the limits of the interventions in use (such as early-evening or outdoor biting in which ITNs are primary strategy) (Killeen 2014; WHO 2014), and insecticide resistance to pyrethroids—the most commonly used synthetic chemicals (Quinones et al. 2015; World Health Organization pesticide evaluation scheme [WHOPES], www.who.int/whopes/en), remain the biggest threats to control and elimination strategies. Indeed, studies suggest that current interventions strategies that rely primarily on ITNs and IRS are insufficient to eliminate or eradicate malaria (Shaukat et al. 2010) and a shift to the use of nonpyrethroids in Africa has occurred (N'Guessan et al. 2007; Mnzava et al. 2015). These points are the impetus for several novel intervention strategies being evaluated or developed. Such new tools are targeting transmission dynamics, vector species, and behaviors not susceptible to present interventions to include outdoor transmission, animal biting, sugar feeding, and the immature stage of the vector.

CORE WORLD HEALTH ORGANIZATION VECTOR-CONTROL STRATEGIES

Both ITNs and IRS remain core malaria-intervention strategies worldwide. These WHO-recommended interventions combined with chemoprevention in pregnant women and children, diagnostic testing, and access to treatment have largely contributed to the gains against malaria in the last few years (WHO 2015a). Typically, used independently, studies to determine impact from combination use have been conducted to help guide further gains. In Mozambique and Equatorial Guinea, protective effects of IRS with ITNs have been suggested to be additive (Kleinschmidt et al. 2009; Hamel et al. 2011; Fullman et al. 2013; West et al. 2014, 2015). Other studies found no evidence of an added benefit when combining ITS and ITNs (Nyarango et al. 2006; Corbel et al. 2012; Pinder et al. 2015; Protopopoff et al. 2015), whereas others remain unclear (Gimnig et al. 2016), pointing to the requirement of additional evidence (WHO 1993).

Insecticide-Treated Nets (ITNs)

ITNs, a form of personal protection, function by both providing a physical barrier to mosquitoes as well as the lethal effect of insecticides that are present on the bednet material. With high coverage, the size as well as the life span of the vector population is reduced—further protecting the community (Hawley et al. 2003). This intervention targets a permethrin (or insecticide-in-use) susceptible vector population that host-seeks indoors, whereas the local human population is asleep under a treated net and functions once per gonotrophic cycle. ITNs are consequently most effective against late-night and indoor-biting vectors. Historically, mosquito nets have been used against nuisance insects (Lindsay and Gibson 1988; Lengeler 2004). Studies in the 1980s showed that pyrethroids were safe for humans and both repelled and killed mosquitoes—showing that ITNs resulted in both individual and community-wide protection against malaria infection (Lengeler 2000, 2004). Driven by increasing access and distribution of ITNs, the proportion of the population sleeping under an ITN has increased dramatically in sub-Saharan Africa since 2000. However, the increasing number of ITNs have been insufficient to achieve universal coverage (WHO 2015a) and, this, along with the increasing spread of insecticide resistance (N'Guessan et al. 2007; Temu et al. 2012; Mulamba et al. 2014; Toe et al. 2014; Mnzava et al. 2015) and behavioral modification by the vector (Bayoh et al. 2010; Russell et al. 2013; Glunt et al. 2015), may point to the limits of the effectiveness of this intervention (Bayoh et al. 2014; WHO 2015a).

Indoor Residual Spraying (IRS)

IRS is the application of insecticide to the inside of human habitation, that is, walls and other surfaces that may serve as a resting place for malaria vectors. IRS effects result in knockdown and/or mortality of those vector populations that rest on these treated surfaces and are susceptible to the insecticide in use. IRS generally functions once per gonotrophic cycle when a mosquito rests on the sprayed surface before or after a blood meal. Historically, IRS with DDT has reduced malaria in many settings around the world. IRS contributed to the elimination of malaria from parts of Asia, Russia, Europe, and Latin America. Successful IRS programs were the primary mosquito intervention during the Global Malaria Eradication Campaign

(1955–1969) and have contributed to the elimination of malaria from parts of Asia, Russia, Europe, and Latin America, with successful IRS programs showed in parts of Africa. The successful use of IRS in Mozambique, South Africa, Swaziland, and Zimbabwe (Mabaso et al. 2004) prompted its present reintroduction as a primary tool in vector-control strategies with a shift to nonpyrethroids (N'Guessan et al. 2007; Mnzava et al. 2015) due to the increase in insecticide resistance of malaria vectors across Africa. Although IRS coverage has declined (primarily due to the cost of insecticides) in recent years, 2014 represents the largest proportion of the population being protected by IRS in Africa (WHO 2015a). Annual rotation of IRS insecticides is currently the best practice for resistance management in malaria vectors in most settings (Mnzava et al. 2015).

Both IRS and ITNs are effective tools for reducing disease. Studies in Mozambique and Equatorial Guinea have indicated that protective effects of IRS with ITNs may be (West et al. 2014, 2015) additive (Kleinschmidt et al. 2009; Hamel et al. 2011; Fullman et al. 2013). Other studies found no evidence of an added benefit when combining ITS and ITNs (Nyarango et al. 2006; Corbel et al. 2012; Pinder et al. 2015; Protopopoff et al. 2015), whereas others remained unclear (Gimnig et al. 2016), pointing to the requirement of additional evidence (WHO 1993).

Larval Source Management

Larval source management (LSM) is the management of bodies of water—potential larval habitats for mosquitoes, in an effort to prevent the completion of development of the immature stages (Tusting et al. 2013). Unlike IRS and LLINs, which target the adult stages, LSM targets the immature larval and pupal stages in the attempt to reduce the number of adult mosquitoes. LSM functions once in the lifetime of a mosquito during its larval stage. The four types of LSM—all directed toward limiting the adult population—include habitat modification, habitat manipulation, chemical larviciding, and biological control.

Habitat or environmental modification is meant to be permanent and includes drainage, filling, land leveling, and alteration of water reservoirs. Essentially, naturally occurring pools, pockets, and seepage ponds—suitable habitats for immature mosquitoes—are modified by the reinforcement of banks, deepening of channels, or diversion of flow (WHO 2013). Filling of holes, pits, and ponds in and around human habitation is a more simple method of habitat modification but requires more frequent management (WHO 2013). Habitat manipulation, on the other hand, is a recurrent activity more associated with agriculture, such as in rice cultivation (Mabaso et al. 2004; Temu et al. 2012). The manipulation temporarily reduces or removes mosquito habitat or kills immature stages. This includes changing the salinity of breeding sites (desalination or salination), flushing of streams and water bodies, regulation of the water level in reservoirs, as well as removal of vegetation for increased exposure to sunlight (WHO 2013). Larviciding is the regular application of insecticides, whether synthetic or natural, to water bodies (WHO 2013). These include a wide range of emulsifiable concentrates, suspension concentrates, water-dispersible granules, wettable powders, granules, pellets, and briquettes (WHO 2013). Bacterial, or biological, larvicides are highly effective with the added benefit of being selective, and having minimal nontarget effects. *Bacillus thuringiensis* subsp. *israelensis* (Bti) and *Bacillus sphaericus* (Bs) are the primary biologicals used for malaria vector control (WHO 2013). These bacteria produce a highly specific endotoxin, affecting only larvae of mosquitoes, black flies, and midges and are effective where target organisms are resistant to other larvicides (Fillinger et al. 2003; WHO 2013). Spinosad, another bacterial larvicide, is a combination of metabolites from the bacterium *Saccharopolyspora spinosa*. Insect growth regulators such as methoprene and pyriproxyfen, mimic mosquito juvenile hormone and prevent the development of larvae to the pupal stage subsequently killing the vector. Globally, trends indicate an increased use of insect growth regulators for the control of malaria vectors; however, this is minimal relative to oth-

er methods of vector control (WHOPES). Biological control is the introduction of natural aquatic predators into the breeding habitat (WHO 2013). These include fungi (e.g., *Laegenidium giganteum*) and mermithid nematodes (e.g., *Romanomermis culicivorax*), which parasitize and kill larval mosquitoes; however, these are not widely used because of inefficiency. Likewise, mosquito-eating fish (such as *Gambusia affinis* and *Poecilia reticulate*) have largely been ineffective except in a few studies. A recent Cochrane review (Tusting et al. 2013; Walshe et al. 2013) on the use of larvivorous fish as a malaria intervention concluded that there is a lack of evidence and insufficient research to show whether larvivorous fish consistently reduce the density of malaria vectors and malaria.

LSM has a long history of use in diverse settings with various levels of success in urban, low-transmission and elimination settings (Watson 1911, 1953; Hopkins 1940; Soper and Wilson 1943; Muirhead-Thomson 1945, 1951; Shousha 1948; Holstein 1954; Clyde 1967; Fillinger et al. 2009; Fillinger and Lindsay 2011). Its contributions to recent successes in reductions of malaria burden have not been considered substantial although there has been a significant amount of attention. A 2012 review by the WHO Malaria Policy Advisory Committee (WHO 2012b) combined with a 2013 Cochrane review on mosquito LSM for controlling malaria (Tusting et al. 2013), determined that larviciding should only have a limited role in malaria control in areas where mosquito breeding sites are few, fixed, and findable (Tusting et al. 2013; WHO 2012b). An additional term "fixable" (T Burkot, pers. comm.) has also been proposed to be required, with the concern that these may not be "fixable" with LSM (e.g., large lagoon breeding sites of *Anopheles farauti* in the Solomon Islands) (Bugoro 2011). An additional Cochrane review on larvivorous fish for preventing malaria transmission (Walshe et al. 2013) found no reliable studies that report that the introduction of larvivorous fish has an effect on malaria infection in nearby communities, on entomological inoculation rate, or on adult anopheline density.

A WHO operational manual (WHO 2013) provides guidance on the planning, implementation, management, and evaluation of LSM strategies. The combination of a lack of scientific studies showing effect as well as the need for better understanding of basic larval biology—habitats, abundance, behavior, and distribution of the larvae of malaria vectors (Fillinger et al. 2004) agree with the WHO emphasis that LSM programs need to be tailored to local environmental conditions and should be based on comprehensive and cost-effectiveness studies—that is, require evidence based decision making. LSM requires a comprehensive infrastructure composed of trained individuals, a monitoring system with appropriate logistical and analysis capabilities and a timely feedback and reaction system, with financial, community, and political commitment.

The success of LSM on malaria control depends, in part, on the basic reproductive number for malaria, R_0 and the EIR capacity (Garrett-Jones and Shidrawi 1969; Killeen et al. 2000; Smith et al. 2007). LSM, with the effect being on the larval and pupal stages, has a linear and not exponential effect on R_0 and is only as effective as its implementation. These interventions are affected by the heterogeneous distribution of adult emergence rates from larval habitats. If the removal of a few larval breeding sites drastically reduced adult mosquitoes populations, LSM may possibly produce a large effect on malaria transmission with little effort (Smith et al. 2007; WHO 2012b). Biological control may have a large impact in the steady state balance of an introduced insect but not necessarily on a naturally present vector.

Host-Mediated Control
Zooprophylaxis

In malaria-endemic settings where transmission is in part the result of zoophilic vectors, two routes of control have been suggested: diversion of vectors away from human hosts to alternative nonhuman blood meal sources (zooprophylaxis) and the use of nonhuman hosts as bait to attract vectors to a toxic host or blood meal source (insecticide-treated livestock/endectocides). This intervention targets a vector population that prefers feeding on animals and func-

tions once per gonotrophic cycle. The effect this intervention has on the vector population is directly proportional to the amount of zoophagy present.

Zooprophylaxis is considered to be controversial in its potential for both beneficial and detrimental outcomes. For example, despite diverting vectors to nonhuman host sources, the use of livestock may actually result in zoopotentiation (Saul 2003), suggesting that the larger numbers of animals and the ease of acquiring a blood meal could result in less time spent host-seeking. This would thereby correspond to reduced vector mortality overall and a potential increase in the number of blood meals taken on humans by infectious vectors. In situations where livestock are kept in close proximity to humans, animals may actually increase the risk of mosquito bites to individual persons by attracting vectors to the general proximity of human hosts (Schultz 1989; Hewitt et al. 1994; Bouma and Rowland 1995). Despite these scenarios, the use of insecticide-treated livestock and endectocides is gaining in popularity (Donnelly et al. 2015; Chaccour and Killeen 2016).

The expectation is that zooprophylaxis would have the greatest impact on malaria transmitted as a result of zoophilic vectors. The efficacy of zooprophylaxis may be enhanced by attracting vectors to insecticide-treated livestock. This approach has been attempted in both the United States (Nasci et al. 1990) and the Philippines (delas Llagas et al. 1996). Treatment of all domesticated animals with insecticides resulted in a decrease of malaria incidence and prevalence in Pakistan (Hewitt et al. 1994). Although there have been encouraging findings, the impact of insecticide-treated livestock on malaria transmission in Africa has yet to be assessed.

Endectocides

Endectocides are classified as systemic drugs with both endoparasitocidal and ectoparasitocidal activity (Foy et al. 2011). Drugs used against endoparasites such as Avermectin and Ivermectin have long been known to have a killing effect on a number of blood-sucking arthropods. Endectocides hold several advantages over traditional insecticides—these interventions travel with the host and do not rely on time or place to be effective. The primary advantage is that this strategy will be effective against endophagic, exophagic, and zoophilic vectors as well as crepuscular and night-biting vectors (Foy et al. 2011). In addition, the mode of action for endectocides ensures that there is a low probability of cross-resistance with current insecticidal strategies (Strycharz et al. 2008). This increases their usage where pyrethroid-based interventions are threatened by insecticide resistance. Last, these systemic drugs have the potential to inhibit the development of the malaria parasite, thus making them a viable target to combat drug resistance in the malaria parasite. Although endectocide use is an attractive option for malaria control, issues of cost (Burnham and Mebrahtu 2004; Goldman et al. 2007), long-term human use (Duke et al. 1990; Guzzo et al. 2002), and resistance build-up in both endo- and ectoparasites (Bourguinat et al. 2007) have been raised. Alternatives to this approach are to use treated livestock as the delivery medium for the endectocide to host-seeking vectors. Such approaches would again be focused on zoophagic vectors but would reduce health impacts associated with maintaining human populations on long-term drug therapy.

Focusing solely on these drugs ability to reduce vector abundance in intervention programs may be too simplistic (Wilson 1993), and these strategies need to be assessed for their ability to affect all variables associated with vectorial capacity.

Push–Pull Strategies

Personal protective measures have shown usage for preventing malaria (Hill et al. 2007, 2014; Syafruddin et al. 2014) and for reducing the overall intensity of outdoor biting (Goodyer et al. 2010). Using interventions focused on repelling mosquitoes from an individual, however, have prompted concerns that diverted vectors may result in higher attack rates on unprotected populations (Maia et al. 2013). Therefore, a strategy that relies on killing mos-

quitoes and reducing community-level risk is much more desirable (Howard et al. 2000).

One novel strategy currently being developed uses a push–pull approach that seeks to exploit the complementary effects of repellents and traps. Developed initially as a way to control agricultural and urban pests (Cook et al. 2007), push–pull interventions work by combining the repellency action of one component and the attractiveness of another to elicit movement away from a protected resource and toward a trap for subsequent removal from the environment (Pyke et al. 1987; Cook et al. 2007; Kitau et al. 2010; Reddy and Guerrero 2010; Paz-Soldan et al. 2011; Menger et al. 2014; Wagman et al. 2015). Accordingly, push–pull strategies for the control of mosquito vectors of human disease would use repellents to deter host-seeking mosquitoes from treated spaces toward a baited trap resulting in their capture and removal from the peridomestic environment thereby decreasing population densities for added community protection and/or personal protection of hosts in the outdoor environment (Cook et al. 2007; Kitau et al. 2010; Paz-Soldan et al. 2011). Although still in the proof-of-concept phase, preliminary studies have been encouraging (Kitau et al. 2010; Menger et al. 2014; Wagman et al. 2015), showing reduced biting rates and house entry.

Spatial Repellents

The term spatial repellent is used here as a general term to refer to chemical products designed to release volatile chemicals into the air and elicit a range of insect behaviors induced by airborne chemicals that result in a reduction in human–vector contact (Achee et al. 2012a; WHO 2012a). A large number of products are commercially available that use chemical actives registered as spatial repellents (U.S. Environmental Protection Agency [EPA]). These products range in cost and sophistication from expensive heat driven electrical outlet plugins used in the Europe to inexpensive mosquito coils that are widely used throughout Africa and Asia.

Spatial repellents can induce mosquitoes to move away from a chemical stimulus, interfere with their host detection (attraction–inhibition) and/or feeding response (WHO 2012a) and consequently can operate on all adult behaviors that incorporate movement. These effects have been measured in laboratory studies (Grieco et al. 2005; Suwannachote et al. 2009), in phase II testing under experimentally controlled conditions (Grieco et al. 2000, 2007; Ogoma et al. 2012), and in field settings (Pates et al. 2002; Kawada et al. 2004a,b; Lucas et al. 2007) against *Aedes* spp., *Anopheles* spp., and *Culex* spp. of varying insecticide resistance profiles. There is also evidence from a phase III study in Indonesia that spatial repellents can impact malaria incidence (Syafruddin et al. 2014).

The role for spatial repellents in modern vector control can best be conceptualized for transmission settings in which IRS and/or LLINs may not offer full protection or have reached their efficacy limits, especially in areas with residual transmission or areas where elimination is proposed. Control of malaria in these areas will require new approaches and this may be where spatial repellency would be most effective (Achee et al. 2012b; Ogoma et al. 2012, 2014). Spatial repellents may show effect against insecticide-resistant populations and have the potential to limit the spread of insecticide-resistant alleles because of reduced selection pressure when considering the nonlethality of effect (WHO 2012a). Spatial repellents could be offered as stand-alone tools where no other interventions are currently in use; or, most likely, combined with existing interventions to augment efficacy of these other tools.

Attractive Toxic Sugar Baits

Attractive toxic sugar baits (ATSBs) represent a new tool for the indoor and outdoor control of mosquito disease vectors. Mosquitoes are killed when they are attracted to and feed on toxic sugar meals that are either sprayed on plants or used in bait stations. This intervention targets a toxin susceptible vector population while sugar feeding. Because sugar feeding has been shown to occur repeatedly and often in the adult mosquito, the potential effects of this intervention on a vector population may be dramatic.

The use of sugar feeding to reduce mosquito populations was first reported in 1965 (Lea 1965) and then in several other studies (Schlein and Pener 1990; Robert et al. 1997; Muller and Schlein 2006; Xue et al. 2006; Schlein and Muller 2008; Muller et al. 2010b,c) in *Aedes* and other *Culicine* mosquitoes as well as sand flies. Effects on anopheline populations were shown in Israel and Mali (Muller et al. 2008, 2010b). This approach may be used in either of two ways, that is, direct mortality induced by feeding on the bait, and/or, the bait may be used to disseminate mosquito pathogens or toxins (Schlein and Pener 1990; Allan 2011).

Attractive toxic sugar bait solutions are composed of sugar, an attractant such as a flower scent, and an oral toxin. Toxins tested include malathion (Lea 1965), boric acid (Xue and Barnard 2003), spinosad (Muller and Schlein 2006), fipronil (Xue et al. 2008), as well as several other classes of insecticide (Muller and Schlein 2006). Toxins, such as boric acid, hold the added advantage of being safe for the environment. Attractants focus on locally acquired sugars, juices and fruit—as mosquitoes may be selective to carbohydrate choices originating from their geographic range (Grimstad and DeFoliart 1974; Muller and Schlein 2005; Muller et al. 2010a).

Sugars derived from plants are an integral component of mosquito nutrition and provide energy for survival, flight, and enhance fecundity and vectorial capacity (Nayar and Sauerman 1971, 1975a,b; Foster 1995; Briegel 2003; Gu et al. 2011). Both male and female mosquitoes may feed on sugar sources several times a day—primarily after emergence and then as required (Reisen et al. 1986; Foster 1995; Foster and Takken 2004; Gary and Foster 2006). Because sugar feeding occurs more often than blood feeding and continues throughout the life of the insect, this behavior represents an opportunity in a mosquito life cycle where a vector intervention may be placed. An accumulative effect of ATSBs on a mosquito population was shown for an area with readily available alternate sugar sources; however, the overall population level lethality was delayed relative to sugar poor areas (Beier et al. 2012). This suggests that ATSBs may be highly effective in arid, sugar-poor environments.

The recurrent nature of sugar feeding suggests a large ATSB effect on vectorial capacity (Garrett-Jones and Shidrawi 1969; Gu et al. 2011). A single application of ATSBs affected mosquito density, parity, survival, and hence vectorial capacity (Garrett-Jones and Shidrawi 1969; Beier et al. 2012). ATSBs in conjunction with other interventions like bednets might show an exponential effect as energy-deprived mosquitoes (e.g., those that are unable to acquire a blood meal because of bednets) seem to take more and larger sugar meals (Stone et al. 2012). A primary drawback of this strategy is the possibly effect on nontarget organisms—the killing of other sugar feeding insects (honey bees and pollinators in particular).

Altthough ATSB approaches are being developed and tested, they represent new powerful tools for the control of malaria vectors, especially because this method is simple, inexpensive, and environmentally friendly, and has been shown to be highly effective for mosquito control.

Genetic Control

Genetic control of malaria vector populations can be described as the dissemination of genetic or inheritable factors toward the decrease of disease and/or target vector populations. These control strategies rely on the dispersal of a modified organism for the purpose of mating with wild-type populations and are therefore species-specific. These strategies are expected to function synergistically with current and other proposed disease-intervention programs.

Curtis first presented the concept of genetic control in 1968 (Curtis 1968). Recent advances in molecular biology have resulted in the germline transformation of several anopheline species (Catteruccia et al. 2000; Grossman et al. 2001; Perera et al. 2002; Lobo et al. 2006). These systems have shown a reduction in vector competence (James et al. 1999; de Lara Capurro et al. 2000; Ito et al. 2002; Bian et al. 2013; Wilke and Marrelli 2015) and have further progressed to developing drivers that can disseminate these

systems into natural populations (Burt 2003; Deredec et al. 2008; Windbichler et al. 2011; Bian et al. 2013; Gantz et al. 2015; Hammond et al. 2016). Toward testing and wild release, large sets of molecular markers and genome sequences have been produced that can be used to study population structure and gene flow (Thomas et al. 2000; Black and Lanzaro 2001; Donnelly et al. 2001; Walton et al. 2001; Holt et al. 2002; Neafsey et al. 2015).

Genetic control can be broadly separated into germline transformation of mosquitoes, involving the germline manipulation of a genome and paratransgenesis—which works with transformation of obligate symbionts (Alphey et al. 2002). Paratransgenesis involves genetically modified organisms that can colonize vector species (Wilke and Marrelli 2015). Genetically modified symbiotic bacteria are reintroduced into the vector species where they express the genetic trait (Beard et al. 1993; Conte 1997; Favia et al. 2007; Coutinho-Abreu et al. 2010). These genetic traits may be a pathogenic effect in the host, interfering with reproduction, reducing vector competence (Bian et al. 2013) or the reproductive pathway (Yoshida et al. 2001; Chavshin et al. 2012; Bongio and Lampe 2015). *Wolbachia* have recently shown the ability to confer fitness costs on *Anopheles* vectors (Joshi et al. 2014) and inhibit *Plasmodium* infection (Jin et al. 2009; Kambris et al. 2010; Hughes et al. 2011). However, some studies have shown the opposite, where *Plasmodium* infections were enhanced in the presence of *Wolbachia* (Hughes et al. 2012). This finding necessitates a clearer understanding of underlying processes. Various other symbiotic bacteria species have been identified in anophelines and may be used for paratransgenesis, the choice of which is determined by the approach being used (Beard et al. 1993; Yoshida et al. 2001; Gonzalez-Ceron et al. 2003; Lindh et al. 2005; Favia et al. 2007; Wilke and Marrelli 2015). An advantage of paratransgenesis over that of genetic transformation is that a transgeneic strain is required for every species or reproductively isolated strain in the latter, while the same paratransgenic system may be used for multiple species as long as the bacteria being used can survive and the system function in the vector species used (Sayler and Ripp 2000; Riehle and Jacobs-Lorena 2005; Riehle et al. 2007; Wilke and Marrelli 2015).

Suppression and replacement strategies: Outcomes of genetic control strategies include (1) both population suppression, where the number of vectors in a target population is reduced, and (2) population replacement, where a trait is spread in the natural vector population toward the reduction of vectorial capacity at some point in the vector life cycle (Alphey et al. 2002; Wilke and Marrelli 2012). The "release of insects with dominant lethality" (RIDL) system uses a dominant lethal gene with a female-specific promoter (Heinrich and Scott 2000; Thomas et al. 2000; Atkinson et al. 2007). When genetically modified, males mate with wild females, sex-specific lethality results in inviable female progeny. Several genes and lethal mechanisms may be used with this system (Fortini et al. 1992; Alphey 2002). Population-replacement strategies have resulted in several anopheline species being genetically modified toward the disruption of *Plasmodium* transmission. *Anopheles stephensi* was transformed to express a peptide that blocked the majority of oocyte development (Ito et al. 2002). Other studies that have shown the ability of germline transformation to reduce or inhibit malaria transmission include the expression of venom phospholipase (Zieler et al. 2001; Moreira et al. 2002), single-chain antibodies (Isaacs et al. 2011) and other antimalaria genes (Meredith et al. 2011).

Self-limiting and self-sustaining strategies: Self-limiting as well as self-sustaining strategies may be used (Alphey et al. 2002). A strategy that incorporates a strong fitness penalty will result in the rapid reduction of the target population by natural selection. Sterile insect technique (SIT) (Alphey 2002) is a highly effective, area-wide method where periodic mass releases of irradiated and sterile males are required to maintain the selection pressure. Sterile-male methods incorporate the release of sterile males, which, because of infertile mating, results in population suppression (Helinski et al. 2008). Genetic sexing mechanisms that are self-sustained and stable offer a major benefit more than traditional SIT techniques that rely on ra-

diation-based sterilization (Heinrich and Scott 2000; Thomas et al. 2000; Alphey 2002). In general, population replacement strategies are self-sustaining, whereas population suppression strategies are self-limiting (Alphey et al. 2002; Jasinskiene et al. 2007; Wilke and Marrelli 2012). Self-sustaining paratransgenic systems such as *Wolbachia* invade and are maintained in the population once initially established in the target (Alphey et al. 2002; Wilke and Marrelli 2012). Genetic transforming self-sustaining strategies usually consist of two components—a genetic refractory mechanism that enable either population suppression or refractoriness to disease transmission, as well as a gene-drive system (Sinkins and Gould 2006) that disseminates the transgene cargo into the population toward the disruption of disease transmission (Zieler et al. 2001; Ito et al. 2002; Moreira et al. 2002; Isaacs et al. 2011; Meredith et al. 2011). There are several gene-drive systems that include the use of selfish genetic elements like transposons (Burt 2003; Chen et al. 2007; Sethuraman et al. 2007), meiotic drive genes (Lyttle 1991), and homing endonuclease genes (HEGs) (Burt 2003; Deredec et al. 2008).

Transposable elements are able to move within a genome and increase their number (Scott et al. 2002). The spread of the P element in *Drosophila melanogaster* is an example of the spread of a transposon in a population (Kidwell 1992; Engels 1997). Although common in malaria vectors (Holt et al. 2002) and having been used in germline transformation (Catteruccia et al. 2000; Grossman et al. 2001; Perera et al. 2002), there have not been any studies showing their use as a gene-drive system in *Anopheles* vectors (Sinkins and Gould 2006).

Meiotic drive, usually in males, occurs when a heterozygous locus segregates at a greater-than-expected frequency (Lyttle 1991; Sinkins and Gould 2006) through various mechanisms.

HEGs are selfish genetic elements naturally found in microbes (Burt and Koufopanou 2004; Stoddard 2005). They encode an endonuclease that recognizes and cleaves specific DNA sequences of ∼20–30 nucleotides that usually is present only once in the genome. This gene is inserted into the cleaved sequence. In a heterozygous genome, the chromosome without the endonuclease gets cleaved and the broken chromosome gets repaired using the homolog containing the HEG thereby propagating itself in the genome. In principle, an HEG with a transgene cargo is able to cleave a highly conserved target gene and should be capable of population invasion from a low starting frequency (Deredec et al. 2008) with germline incorporation of an HEG transgene. HEGs may be used in two ways (Burt and Koufopanou 2004; Deredec et al. 2008), that is, an HEG can be engineered to recognize a specific nuclear gene/sequence where, on insertion, it would knockout the gene. An HEG construct may be engineered to recognize and insert into a repeat sequence on the X chromosome, be linked to meiosis-specific control sequences, and inserted on the Y chromosome. The HEG bearing Y would propagate in the population biasing the sex ration toward males (Galizi et al. 2014).

Multiple genetic control strategies are presently being investigated and some have successfully been tested in the field with other field tests ongoing.

Integrated Vector Management (IVM)

IVM is a rational decision-making process for the optimal use of resources for vector control (WHO 2004, 2011; Beier et al. 2008). This encompassing approach to prevent disease transmission relies on evidence-based decision making and aims to maximize the efficiency, cost effectiveness, ecological soundness, and sustainability of a disease vector program based on all available tools. Central to IVM is an understanding of the vector, the disease transmission cycle, the environment, and how the intervention strategy reduces man–vector contact, vector survival, and the intensity of disease transmission. The acceptability and safety of the strategies, as well as flexibility of the program, is vital to its success. The global strategic framework for IVM and the WHO handbook (WHO 1982, 2004) establish broad principles and approaches to vector control. Distinguishing factors of IVM include advocacy, social mobilization and legislation, collaboration within and

outside the health sector, an integrated approach, evidence-based decision-making, and capacity building (WHO 2004; Beier et al. 2008). Success stories and various efforts in Africa include those in South Sudan (Chanda et al. 2013), Uganda (Mutero et al. 2012), Zambia (Chanda et al. 2008), among other countries (Alimi et al. 2015; Smith Gueye et al. 2016). Although, at present, the full extent of IVM on malaria transmission is unknown, historical implementations of IVM-like strategies have shown significant effects against disease transmission across a wide range of transmission settings (Beier et al. 2008). Evidence suggests that IVM can complement present malaria intervention programs such as ITN use, by avoiding the dependence on single intervention methods (Killeen et al. 2000; McKenzie et al. 2002; Caldas de Castro et al. 2004; Beier et al. 2008; Mutero et al. 2012, 2015).

Following on from evidence-based IVM strategies, central to the development and success of any intervention be it a combination or a single tool, is the understanding of the local vector species with their bionomic characteristics. The manner in which vector populations respond to these interventions and insecticide-associated selection pressures is required to evaluate effectiveness. Control measures may be profoundly impacted by the development of physiological insecticide resistance (Ranson et al. 2011; Gatton et al. 2013; Strode et al. 2014) and behavioral resistance—the ability of a vector population to change its bionomic characteristics in response to an intervention (Taylor 1975; Reddy et al. 2011; Russell et al. 2011, 2013; Bayoh et al. 2014). Epidemiology and entomology studies as well as vector-control programs require a strategic understanding of key local vector characteristics, such as feeding preferences and insecticide resistance, while also distinguishing vectors and nonvectors within anopheline cryptic species complexes, beyond the level of morphology. The wrong associations of local vector species with behavioral traits impact interpretations of species distributions, insecticide resistance, host preference studies, trap efficacy, and even screening for malaria parasites (Stevenson et al. 2012; Lobo

Cite this article as *Cold Spring Harb Perspect Med* doi: 10.1101/cshperspect.a025643

et al. 2015)—all of which influence the efficacy of an intervention.

CONCLUDING REMARKS AND FUTURE PERSPECTIVES

Present recommended vector-control strategies rely primarily on ITNs and IRS and have shown significant impact on malaria transmission. However, these alone may not be able to eliminate malaria and point to the requirement for additional tools, some of which are outlined in this review. Although, none of these tools present a "magic bullet," their combination with other strategies may enhance local vector control strategies toward the elimination of malaria. The greatest opportunity for impact on elimination/eradication is the better understanding of susceptible vector bionomic traits that may be used for the implementation, development, and use of effective vector control tools. The development and validation of novel vector control tools (such as ATSBs and genetic modification), as well as new insecticides, are required to fill in gaps in protection and provide additional weapons in residual transmission settings where our current tools are inadequate. Combinations of interventions that target different aspects of a vectors life cycle would be more efficacious and could enable the reduction of residual transmission. Other technologies—such as the use of satellite imagery—in combination with specific interventions can cater strategies to geographic requirements resulting in more efficacious interventions toward elimination.

The effectiveness of vector interventions toward elimination is dependent on local transmission dynamics that include nonvector factors such as access to health care, access to personal protective devices, and intervention distribution, human behavior, parasite species population dynamics, and drug resistance, among others. It is vital that a program aimed at geographic elimination or eradication incorporates both long-term feasibility and comprehensive primary stakeholder engagement (national, programmatic implementation, and research entities). Understanding and maximizing how various entities function in the inter-

vention and elimination sphere and using entomological intelligence to design policies will allow for a larger effect on transmission. A systems approach should collates and analyze existing data characterizing malaria transmission dynamics while also identifying data gaps. Vital data should include entomological endpoints such as vector bionomics, epidemiological incidence and prevalence, human components that contribute to transmission such as migratory and travel patterns, and an evaluation of all stakeholder malaria-control efforts to include implementation and surveillance. This will allow the evaluation of vector intervention strategies in place, with a focus on their optimization while also examining the gaps in protection based on entomological bionomic data. Molecular analysis of *Anopheles* specimens will allow for a temporal characterization and association of bionomics with specific species—enabling the direct association of intervention efficacy with *Anopheles* species. Insecticide resistance tests will enable an indication of insecticide efficacy at the sites based on local interventions in place. Epidemiological interventions, such as mass drug administration, and other parasites-related activity should also be evaluated. Risk factors associated with human behaviors that affect transmission as well as local knowledge and practices must be examined. This systems analysis with associated filling of data gaps will enable the characterization of residual transmission: the optimization of present strategies as well as outlining possible tools that will fill gaps based on local transmission dynamics. As countries strive for malaria elimination, they must adopt proactive versus reactive strategies that will delay the onset of insecticide and/or behavioral resistance. Improved and sustained access to appropriate vector-control tools and strategies will be essential for the elimination and eradication of malaria.

REFERENCES

Achee N, Masuoka P, Smith P, Martin N, Chareonviryiphap T, Polsomboon S, Hendarto J, Grieco J. 2012a. Identifying the effective concentration for spatial repellency of the dengue vector *Aedes aegypti*. *Parasit Vectors* **5:** 300.

Achee NL, Bangs MJ, Farlow R, Killeen GF, Lindsay S, Logan JG, Moore SJ, Rowland M, Sweeney K, Torr SJ, et al. 2012b. Spatial repellents: From discovery and development to evidence-based validation. *Malaria J* **11:** 164.

Alimi TO, Fuller DO, Quinones ML, Xue RD, Herrera SV, Arevalo-Herrera M, Ulrich JN, Qualls WA, Beier JC. 2015. Prospects and recommendations for risk mapping to improve strategies for effective malaria vector control interventions in Latin America. *Malaria J* **14:** 519.

Allan SA. 2011. Susceptibility of adult mosquitoes to insecticides in aqueous sucrose baits. *J Vector Ecol* **36:** 59–67.

Alphey L. 2002. Re-engineering the sterile insect technique. *Insect Biochem Mol Biol* **32:** 1243–1247.

Alphey L, Beard CB, Billingsley P, Coetzee M, Crisanti A, Curtis C, Eggleston P, Godfray C, Hemingway J, Jacobs-Lorena M, et al. 2002. Malaria control with genetically manipulated insect vectors. *Science* **298:** 119–121.

Atkinson MP, Su Z, Alphey N, Alphey LS, Coleman PG, Wein LM. 2007. Analyzing the control of mosquito-borne diseases by a dominant lethal genetic system. *Proc Natl Acad Sci* **104:** 9540–9545.

Bayoh MN, Mathias DK, Odiere MR, Mutuku FM, Kamau L, Gimnig JE, Vulule JM, Hawley WA, Hamel MJ, Walker ED. 2010. *Anopheles gambiae*: Historical population decline associated with regional distribution of insecticide-treated bed nets in western Nyanza Province, Kenya. *Malaria J* **9:** 62.

Bayoh MN, Walker ED, Kosgei J, Ombok M, Olang GB, Githeko AK, Killeen GF, Otieno P, Desai M, Lobo NF, et al. 2014. Persistently high estimates of late night, indoor exposure to malaria vectors despite high coverage of insecticide treated nets. *Parasit Vectors* **7:** 380.

Beard CB, O'Neill SL, Tesh RB, Richards FF, Aksoy S. 1993. Modification of arthropod vector competence via symbiotic bacteria. *Parasitol Today* **9:** 179–183.

Beier JC, Keating J, Githure JI, Macdonald MB, Impoinvil DE, Novak RJ. 2008. Integrated vector management for malaria control. *Malaria J* **7:** S4.

Beier JC, Muller GC, Gu W, Arheart KL, Schlein Y. 2012. Attractive toxic sugar bait (ATSB) methods decimate populations of *Anopheles* malaria vectors in arid environments regardless of the local availability of favoured sugar-source blossoms. *Malaria J* **11:** 31.

Bian G, Joshi D, Dong Y, Lu P, Zhou G, Pan X, Xu Y, Dimopoulos G, Xi Z. 2013. *Wolbachia* invades *Anopheles stephensi* populations and induces refractoriness to *Plasmodium* infection. *Science* **340:** 748–751.

Black WCt, Lanzaro GC. 2001. Distribution of genetic variation among chromosomal forms of *Anopheles gambiae* s.s.: Introgressive hybridization, adaptive inversions, or recent reproductive isolation? *Insect Mol Biol* **10:** 3–7.

Bongio NJ, Lampe DJ. 2015. Inhibition of *Plasmodium berghei* development in mosquitoes by effector proteins secreted from *Asaia* sp. bacteria using a novel native secretion signal. *PLoS ONE* **10:** e0143541.

Bouma M, Rowland M. 1995. Failure of passive zooprophylaxis: Cattle ownership in Pakistan is associated with a higher prevalence of malaria. *Trans R Soc Trop Med Hyg* **89:** 351–353.

Bourguinat C, Pion SD, Kamgno J, Gardon J, Duke BO, Boussinesq M, Prichard RK. 2007. Genetic selection of low fertile *Onchocerca volvulus* by ivermectin treatment. *PLoS Negl Trop Dis* **1:** e72.

Briegel H. 2003. Physiological bases of mosquito ecology. *J Vector Ecol* **28:** 1–11.

Bugoro H. 2011. "The bionomics of *Anopheles farauti* and prospects for malaria elimination in the Solomon Islands." PhD thesis, National Yang-Ming University, Institute of Clinical Medicine, Taipei, Taiwan.

Bugoro H, Iro'ofa C, Mackenzie DO, Apairamo A, Hevalao W, Corcoran S, Bobogare A, Beebe NW, Russell TL, Chen CC, et al. 2011. Changes in vector species composition and current vector biology and behaviour will favour malaria elimination in Santa Isabel Province, Solomon Islands. *Malaria J* **10:** 287.

Burnham G, Mebrahtu T. 2004. The delivery of ivermectin (Mectizan). *Trop Med Int Health* **9:** A26–44.

Burt A. 2003. Site-specific selfish genes as tools for the control and genetic engineering of natural populations. *Proc Biol Sci* **270:** 921–928.

Burt A, Koufopanou V. 2004. Homing endonuclease genes: The rise and fall and rise again of a selfish element. *Curr Opin Genet Dev* **14:** 609–615.

Caldas de Castro M, Yamagata Y, Mtasiwa D, Tanner M, Utzinger J, Keiser J, Singer BH. 2004. Integrated urban malaria control: A case study in Dar es Salaam, Tanzania. *Am J Trop Med Hyg* **71:** 103–117.

Catteruccia F, Nolan T, Loukeris TG, Blass C, Savakis C, Kafatos FC, Crisanti A. 2000. Stable germline transformation of the malaria mosquito *Anopheles stephensi*. *Nature* **405:** 959–962.

Chaccour C, Killeen GF. 2016. Mind the gap: Residual malaria transmission, veterinary endectocides and livestock as targets for malaria vector control. *Malaria J* **15:** 24.

Chanda E, Masaninga F, Coleman M, Sikaala C, Katebe C, Macdonald M, Baboo KS, Govere J, Manga L. 2008. Integrated vector management: The Zambian experience. *Malaria J* **7:** 164.

Chanda E, Govere JM, Macdonald MB, Lako RL, Haque U, Baba SP, Mnzava A. 2013. Integrated vector management: A critical strategy for combating vector-borne diseases in South Sudan. *Malaria J* **12:** 369.

Chavshin AR, Oshaghi MA, Vatandoost H, Pourmand MR, Raeisi A, Enayati AA, Mardani N, Ghoorchian S. 2012. Identification of bacterial microflora in the midgut of the larvae and adult of wild caught *Anopheles stephensi*: A step toward finding suitable paratransgenesis candidates. *Acta Trop* **121:** 129–134.

Chen CH, Huang H, Ward CM, Su JT, Schaeffer LV, Guo M, Hay BA. 2007. A synthetic maternal-effect selfish genetic element drives population replacement in *Drosophila*. *Science* **316:** 597–600.

Clyde DF. 1967. *Malaria in Tanzania*. Oxford University Press, London.

Conte JE Jr. 1997. A novel approach to preventing insect-borne diseases. *N Engl J Med* **337:** 785–786.

Cook SM, Khan ZR, Pickett JA. 2007. The use of push-pull strategies in integrated pest management. *Annu Rev Entomol* **52:** 375–400.

Corbel V, Akogbeto M, Damien GB, Djenontin A, Chandre F, Rogier C, Moiroux N, Chabi J, Banganna B, Padonou GG, et al. 2012. Combination of malaria vector control

Cite this article as *Cold Spring Harb Perspect Med* doi: 10.1101/cshperspect.a025643

interventions in pyrethroid resistance area in Benin: A cluster randomised controlled trial. *Lancet Infect Dis* **12:** 617–626.

Coutinho-Abreu IV, Zhu KY, Ramalho-Ortigao M. 2010. Transgenesis and paratransgenesis to control insect-borne diseases: Current status and future challenges. *Parasitol Int* **59:** 1–8.

Curtis CF. 1968. Possible use of translocations to fix desirable genes in insect pest populations. *Nature* **218:** 368–369.

D'Acremont V, Lengeler C, Genton B. 2010. Reduction in the proportion of fevers associated with *Plasmodium falciparum* parasitaemia in Africa: A systematic review. *Malaria J* **9:** 240.

De Lara Capurro M, Coleman J, Beerntsen BT, Myles KM, Olson KE, Rocha E, Krettli AU, James AA. 2000. Virus-expressed, recombinant single-chain antibody blocks sporozoite infection of salivary glands in *Plasmodium gallinaceum*–infected *Aedes aegypti*. *Am J Trop Med Hyg* **62:** 427–433.

delas Llagas L, Hernandez L, Samaniego J. 1996. Insecticidal zooprophylaxis. *ENHR Executive Brief (Philippines)* **2:** 3–7.

Deredec A, Burt A, Godfray HC. 2008. The population genetics of using homing endonuclease genes in vector and pest management. *Genetics* **179:** 2013–2026.

Donnelly MJ, Licht MC, Lehmann T. 2001. Evidence for recent population expansion in the evolutionary history of the malaria vectors *Anopheles arabiensis* and *Anopheles gambiae*. *Mol Biol Evol* **18:** 1353–1364.

Donnelly B, Berrang-Ford L, Ross NA, Michel P. 2015. A systematic, realist review of zooprophylaxis for malaria control. *Malaria J* **14:** 313.

Duke BO, Zea-Flores G, Castro J, Cupp EW, Munoz B. 1990. Effects of multiple monthly doses of ivermectin on adult *Onchocerca volvulus*. *Am J Trop Med Hyg* **43:** 657–664.

Elliott R. 1972. The influence of vector behavior on malaria transmission. *Am J Trop Med Hyg* **21:** 755–763.

Engels WR. 1997. Invasions of P elements. *Genetics* **145:** 11–15.

Favia G, Ricci I, Damiani C, Raddadi N, Crotti E, Marzorati M, Rizzi A, Urso R, Brusetti L, Borin S, et al. 2007. Bacteria of the genus *Asaia* stably associate with *Anopheles stephensi*, an Asian malarial mosquito vector. *Proc Natl Acad Sci* **104:** 9047–9051.

Fillinger U, Lindsay SW. 2011. Larval source management for malaria control in Africa: Myths and reality. *Malaria J* **10:** 353.

Fillinger U, Knols BG, Becker N. 2003. Efficacy and efficiency of new *Bacillus thuringiensis* var *israelensis* and *Bacillus sphaericus* formulations against Afrotropical anophelines in Western Kenya. *Trop Med Int Health* **8:** 37–47.

Fillinger U, Sonye G, Killeen GF, Knols BG, Becker N. 2004. The practical importance of permanent and semipermanent habitats for controlling aquatic stages of *Anopheles gambiae sensu lato* mosquitoes: Operational observations from a rural town in Western Kenya. *Trop Med Int Health* **9:** 1274–1289.

Fillinger U, Ndenga B, Githeko A, Lindsay SW. 2009. Integrated malaria vector control with microbial larvicides

and insecticide-treated nets in Western Kenya: A controlled trial. *Bull World Health Organ* **87:** 655–665.

Fortini ME, Simon MA, Rubin GM. 1992. Signalling by the sevenless protein tyrosine kinase is mimicked by Ras1 activation. *Nature* **355:** 559–561.

Foster WA. 1995. Mosquito sugar feeding and reproductive energetics. *Annu Rev Entomol* **40:** 443–474.

Foster WA, Takken W. 2004. Nectar-related vs. human-related volatiles: Behavioural response and choice by female and male *Anopheles gambiae* (Diptera: Culicidae) between emergence and first feeding. *Bull Entomol Res* **94:** 145–157.

Foy BD, Kobylinski KC, da Silva IM, Rasgon JL, Sylla M. 2011. Endectocides for malaria control. *Trends Parasitol* **27:** 423–428.

Fullman N, Burstein R, Lim SS, Medlin C, Gakidou E. 2013. Nets, spray or both? The effectiveness of insecticide-treated nets and indoor residual spraying in reducing malaria morbidity and child mortality in sub-Saharan Africa. *Malaria J* **12:** 62.

Galizi R, Doyle LA, Menichelli M, Bernardini F, Deredec A, Burt A, Stoddard BL, Windbichler N, Crisanti A. 2014. A synthetic sex ratio distortion system for the control of the human malaria mosquito. *Nat Commun* **5:** 3977.

Gantz VM, Jasinskiene N, Tatarenkova O, Fazekas A, Macias VM, Bier E, James AA. 2015. Highly efficient Cas9-mediated gene drive for population modification of the malaria vector mosquito *Anopheles stephensi*. *Proc Natl Acad Sci* **112:** E6736–E6743.

Garrett-Jones C, Shidrawi GR. 1969. Malaria vectorial capacity of a population of *Anopheles gambiae*: An exercise in epidemiological entomology. *Bull World Health Organ* **40:** 531–545.

Gary RE Jr, Foster WA. 2006. Diel timing and frequency of sugar feeding in the mosquito *Anopheles gambiae*, depending on sex, gonotrophic state and resource availability. *Med Vet Entomol* **20:** 308–316.

Gatton ML, Chitnis N, Churcher T, Donnelly MJ, Ghani AC, Godfray HC, Gould F, Hastings I, Marshall J, Ranson H, et al. 2013. The importance of mosquito behavioural adaptations to malaria control in Africa. *Evolution* **67:** 1218–1230.

Gimnig JE, Otieno P, Were V, Marwanga D, Abong'o D, Wiegand R, Williamson J, Wolkon A, Zhou Y, Bayoh MN, et al. 2016. The effect of indoor residual spraying on the prevalence of malaria parasite infection, clinical malaria and anemia in an area of perennial transmission and moderate coverage of insecticide treated nets in Western Kenya. *PLoS ONE* **11:** e0145282.

Glunt KD, Abilio AP, Bassat Q, Bulo H, Gilbert AE, Huijben S, Manaca MN, Macete E, Alonso P, Paaijmans KP. 2015. Long-lasting insecticidal nets no longer effectively kill the highly resistant *Anopheles funestus* of southern Mozambique. *Malaria J* **14:** 298.

Goldman AS, Guisinger VH, Aikins M, Amarillo ML, Belizario VY, Garshong B, Gyapong J, Kabali C, Kamal HA, Kanjilal S, et al. 2007. National mass drug administration costs for lymphatic filariasis elimination. *PLoS Negl Trop Dis* **1:** e67.

Gonzalez-Ceron L, Santillan F, Rodriguez MH, Mendez D, Hernandez-Avila JE. 2003. Bacteria in midguts of field-collected *Anopheles albimanus* block *Plasmodium vivax* sporogonic development. *J Med Entomol* **40**: 371–374.

Goodyer LI, Croft AM, Frances SP, Hill N, Moore SJ, Onyango SP, Debboun M. 2010. Expert review of the evidence base for arthropod bite avoidance. *J Travel Med* **17**: 182–192.

Grieco JP, Achee NL, Andre RG, Roberts DR. 2000. A comparison study of house entering and exiting behavior of *Anopheles vestitipennis* (Diptera: Culicidae) using experimental huts sprayed with DDT or deltamethrin in the southern district of Toledo, Belize, C.A. *J Vector Ecol* **25**: 62–73.

Grieco JP, Vogtsberger RC, Achee NL, Vanzie E, Andre RG, Roberts DR, Rejmankova E. 2005. Evaluation of habitat management strategies for the reduction of malaria vectors in northern Belize. *J Vector Ecol* **30**: 235–243.

Grieco JP, Achee NL, Chareonviriyaphap T, Suwonkerd W, Chauhan K, Sardelis MR, Roberts DR. 2007. A new classification system for the actions of IRS chemicals traditionally used for malaria control. *PLoS ONE* **2**: e716.

Grimstad PR, DeFoliart GR. 1974. Nectar sources of Wisconsin mosquitoes. *J Med Entomol* **11**: 331–341.

Grossman GL, Rafferty CS, Clayton JR, Stevens TK, Mukabayire O, Benedict MQ. 2001. Germline transformation of the malaria vector, *Anopheles gambiae*, with the *piggyBac* transposable element. *Insect Mol Biol* **10**: 597–604.

Gu W, Muller G, Schlein Y, Novak RJ, Beier JC. 2011. Natural plant sugar sources of *Anopheles* mosquitoes strongly impact malaria transmission potential. *PLoS ONE* **6**: e15996.

Guzzo CA, Furtek CI, Porras AG, Chen C, Tipping R, Clineschmidt CM, Sciberras DG, Hsieh JY, Lasseter KC. 2002. Safety, tolerability, and pharmacokinetics of escalating high doses of ivermectin in healthy adult subjects. *J Clin Pharmacol* **42**: 1122–1133.

Hamel MJ, Otieno P, Bayoh N, Kariuki S, Were V, Marwanga D, Laserson KF, Williamson J, Slutsker L, Gimnig J. 2011. The combination of indoor residual spraying and insecticide-treated nets provides added protection against malaria compared with insecticide-treated nets alone. *Am J Trop Med Hyg* **85**: 1080–1086.

Hammond A, Galizi R, Kyrou K, Simoni A, Siniscalchi C, Katsanos D, Gribble M, Baker D, Marois E, Russell S, et al. 2016. A CRISPR-Cas9 gene drive system targeting female reproduction in the malaria mosquito vector *Anopheles gambiae*. *Nat Biotechnol* **34**: 78–83.

Hawley WA, Phillips-Howard PA, ter Kuile FO, Terlouw DJ, Vulule JM, Ombok M, Nahlen BL, Gimnig JE, Kariuki SK, Kolczak MS, et al. 2003. Community-wide effects of permethrin-treated bed nets on child mortality and malaria morbidity in Western Kenya. *Am J Trop Med Hyg* **68**: 121–127.

Heinrich JC, Scott MJ. 2000. A repressible female-specific lethal genetic system for making transgenic insect strains suitable for a sterile-release program. *Proc Natl Acad Sci* **97**: 8229–8232.

Helinski ME, Hassan MM, El-Motasim WM, Malcolm CA, Knols BG, El-Sayed B. 2008. Towards a sterile insect technique field release of *Anopheles arabiensis* mosquitoes in Sudan: Irradiation, transportation, and field cage experimentation. *Malaria J* **7**: 65.

Hewitt S, Kamal M, Muhammad N, Rowland M. 1994. An entomological investigation of the likely impact of cattle ownership on malaria in an Afghan refugee camp in the North West Frontier Province of Pakistan. *Med Vet Entomol* **8**: 160–164.

Hill N, Lenglet A, Arnez AM, Carneiro I. 2007. Plant based insect repellent and insecticide treated bed nets to protect against malaria in areas of early evening biting vectors: Double blind randomised placebo controlled clinical trial in the Bolivian Amazon. *BMJ* **335**: 1023.

Hill N, Zhou HN, Wang P, Guo X, Carneiro I, Moore SJ. 2014. A household randomized, controlled trial of the efficacy of 0.03% transfluthrin coils alone and in combination with long-lasting insecticidal nets on the incidence of *Plasmodium falciparum* and *Plasmodium vivax* malaria in western Yunnan Province, China. *Malaria J* **13**: 208.

Holstein M. 1954. Biology of *Anopheles gambiae*: Research in French West Africa. Monograph series. World Health Organization, Geneva.

Holt RA, Subramanian GM, Halpern A, Sutton GG, Charlab R, Nusskern DR, Wincker P, Clark AG, Ribeiro JM, Wides R, et al. 2002. The genome sequence of the malaria mosquito *Anopheles gambiae*. *Science* **298**: 129–149.

Hopkins M. 1940. Afforestation as a method of drying up swamps. *East African Med J* **17**: 189–194.

Howard SC, Omumbo J, Nevill C, Some ES, Donnelly CA, Snow RW. 2000. Evidence for a mass community effect of insecticide-treated bednets on the incidence of malaria on the Kenyan coast. *Trans R Soc Trop Med Hyg* **94**: 357–360.

Hughes GL, Koga R, Xue P, Fukatsu T, Rasgon JL. 2011. *Wolbachia* infections are virulent and inhibit the human malaria parasite *Plasmodium falciparum* in *Anopheles gambiae*. *PLoS Pathog* **7**: e1002043.

Hughes GL, Vega-Rodriguez J, Xue P, Rasgon JL. 2012. *Wolbachia* strain wAlbB enhances infection by the rodent malaria parasite *Plasmodium berghei* in *Anopheles gambiae* mosquitoes. *Appl Environ Microbiol* **78**: 1491–1495.

Isaacs AT, Li F, Jasinskiene N, Chen X, Nirmala X, Marinotti O, Vinetz JM, James AA. 2011. Engineered resistance to *Plasmodium falciparum* development in transgenic *Anopheles stephensi*. *PLoS Pathog* **7**: e1002017.

Ito J, Ghosh A, Moreira LA, Wimmer EA, Jacobs-Lorena M. 2002. Transgenic anopheline mosquitoes impaired in transmission of a malaria parasite. *Nature* **417**: 452–455.

James AA, Beerntsen BT, Capurro Mde L, Coates CJ, Coleman J, Jasinskiene N, Krettli AU. 1999. Controlling malaria transmission with genetically engineered, *Plasmodium*-resistant mosquitoes: Milestones in a model system. *Parassitologia* **41**: 461–471.

Jasinskiene N, Coleman J, Ashikyan A, Salampessy M, Marinotti O, James AA. 2007. Genetic control of malaria parasite transmission: Threshold levels for infection in an avian model system. *Am J Trop Med Hyg* **76**: 1072–1078.

Jin C, Ren X, Rasgon JL. 2009. The virulent *Wolbachia* strain wMelPop efficiently establishes somatic infections in the malaria vector *Anopheles gambiae*. *Appl Environ Microbiol* **75**: 3373–3376.

Joshi D, McFadden MJ, Bevins D, Zhang F, Xi Z. 2014. *Wolbachia* strain wAlbB confers both fitness costs and benefit on *Anopheles stephensi. Parasit Vectors* 7: 336.

Kambris Z, Blagborough AM, Pinto SB, Blagrove MS, Godfray HC, Sinden RE, Sinkins SP. 2010. *Wolbachia* stimulates immune gene expression and inhibits *Plasmodium* development in *Anopheles gambiae. PLoS Pathog* 6: e1001143.

Kawada H, Maekawa Y, Tsuda Y, Takagi M. 2004a. Trial of spatial repellency of metofluthrin-impregnated paper strip against *Anopheles* and *Culex* in shelters without walls in Lombok, Indonesia. *J Am Mosq Control Assoc* 20: 434–437.

Kawada H, Maekawa Y, Tsuda Y, Takagi M. 2004b. Laboratory and field evaluation of spatial repellency with metofluthrin-impregnated paper strip against mosquitoes in Lombok Island, Indonesia. *J Am Mosq Control Assoc* 20: 292–298.

Kidwell MG. 1992. Horizontal transfer of P elements and other short inverted repeat transposons. *Genetica* 86: 275–286.

Killeen GF. 2014. Characterizing, controlling and eliminating residual malaria transmission. *Malaria J* 13: 330.

Killeen GF, McKenzie FE, Foy BD, Schieffelin C, Billingsley PF, Beier JC. 2000. The potential impact of integrated malaria transmission control on entomologic inoculation rate in highly endemic areas. *Am J Trop Med Hyg* 62: 545–551.

Killeen GF, Seyoum A, Sikaala C, Zomboko AS, Gimnig JE, Govella NJ, White MT. 2013. Eliminating malaria vectors. *Parasit Vectors* 6: 172.

Killeen GF, Seyoum A, Gimnig JE, Stevenson JC, Drakeley CJ, Chitnis N. 2014. Made-to-measure malaria vector control strategies: Rational design based on insecticide properties and coverage of blood resources for mosquitoes. *Malaria J* 13: 146.

Kitau J, Pates H, Rwegoshora TR, Rwegoshora D, Matowo J, Kweka EJ, Mosha FW, McKenzie K, Magesa SM. 2010. The effect of mosquito magnet liberty plus trap on the human mosquito biting rate under semi-field conditions. *J Am Mosq Control Assoc* 26: 287–294.

Kiware SS, Chitnis N, Devine GJ, Moore SJ, Majambere S, Killeen GF. 2012. Biologically meaningful coverage indicators for eliminating malaria transmission. *Biol Lett* 8: 874–877.

Kleinschmidt I, Schwabe C, Shiva M, Segura JL, Sima V, Mabunda SJ, Coleman M. 2009. Combining indoor residual spraying and insecticide-treated net interventions. *Am J Trop Med Hyg* 81: 519–524.

Lea AO. 1965. Sugar-baited insecticide residues against mosquitoes. *Mosq News* 25: 65–66.

Lengeler C. 2000. Insecticide-treated bednets and curtains for preventing malaria. *Cochrane Database Syst Rev* 2000: Cd000363.

Lengeler C. 2004. Insecticide-treated bed nets and curtains for preventing malaria. *Cochrane Database Syst Rev* 2004: Cd000363.

Lindh JM, Terenius O, Faye I. 2005. 16S rRNA gene-based identification of midgut bacteria from field-caught *Anopheles gambiae* sensu lato and *A. funestus* mosquitoes reveals new species related to known insect symbionts. *Appl Environ Microbiol* 71: 7217–7223.

Lindsay SW, Gibson ME. 1988. Bednets revisited—Old idea, new angle. *Parasitol Today* 4: 270–272.

Lobo NF, Clayton JR, Fraser MJ, Kafatos FC, Collins FH. 2006. High efficiency germ-line transformation of mosquitoes. *Nat Protoc* 1: 1312–1317.

Lobo NF, Laurent BS, Sikaala CH, Hamainza B, Chanda J, Chinula D, Krishnankutty SM, Mueller JD, Deason NA, Hoang QT, et al. 2015. Unexpected diversity of *Anopheles* species in Eastern Zambia: Implications for evaluating vector behavior and interventions using molecular tools. *Sci Rep* 5: 17952.

Lucas JR, Shono Y, Iwasaki T, Ishiwatari T, Spero N, Benzon G. 2007. U.S. laboratory and field trials of metofluthrin (SumiOne) emanators for reducing mosquito biting outdoors. *J Am Mosq Control Assoc* 23: 47–54.

Lyttle TW. 1991. Segregation distorters. *Annu Rev Genet* 25: 511–557.

Mabaso ML, Sharp B, Lengeler C. 2004. Historical review of malarial control in southern African with emphasis on the use of indoor residual house-spraying. *Trop Med Int Health* 9: 846–856.

Maia MF, Onyango SP, Thele M, Simfukwe ET, Turner EL, Moore SJ. 2013. Do topical repellents divert mosquitoes within a community? Health equity implications of topical repellents as a mosquito bite prevention tool. *PLoS ONE* 8: e84875.

malERA Consultative Group on Vector Control. 2011. A research agenda for malaria eradication: Vector control. *PLoS Med* 8: e1000401.

McKenzie FE, Baird JK, Beier JC, Lal AA, Bossert WH. 2002. A biologic basis for integrated malaria control. *Am J Trop Med Hyg* 67: 571–577.

Menger DJ, Otieno B, de Rijk M, Mukabana WR, van Loon JJ, Takken W. 2014. A push–pull system to reduce house entry of malaria mosquitoes. *Malaria J* 13: 119.

Meredith JM, Basu S, Nimmo DD, Larget-Thiery I, Warr EL, Underhill A, McArthur CC, Carter V, Hurd H, Bourgouin C, et al. 2011. Site-specific integration and expression of an anti-malarial gene in transgenic *Anopheles gambiae* significantly reduces *Plasmodium* infections. *PLoS ONE* 6: e14587.

Mnzava AP, Knox TB, Temu EA, Trett A, Fornadel C, Hemingway J, Renshaw M. 2015. Implementation of the global plan for insecticide resistance management in malaria vectors: Progress, challenges and the way forward. *Malaria J* 14: 173.

Moreira LA, Ito J, Ghosh A, Devenport M, Zieler H, Abraham EG, Crisanti A, Nolan T, Catteruccia F, Jacobs-Lorena M. 2002. Bee venom phospholipase inhibits malaria parasite development in transgenic mosquitoes. *J Biol Chem* 277: 40839–40843.

Muirhead-Thomson RC. 1945. Studies on the breeding places and control of *Anopheles gambiae* and *A. gambiae* var. melas in coastal districts of Sierra Leone. *Bull Entomol Res* 36: 185–252.

Muirhead-Thomson RC (ed.). 1951. *Behaviour in relation to malaria transmission and control in the tropics.* Edward Arnold & Co. London.

Mulamba C, Riveron JM, Ibrahim SS, Irving H, Barnes KG, Mukwaya LG, Birungi J, Wondji CS. 2014. Widespread pyrethroid and DDT resistance in the major malaria vector *Anopheles funestus* in East Africa is driven by metabolic resistance mechanisms. *PLoS ONE* **9:** e110058.

Muller G, Schlein Y. 2005. Plant tissues: The frugal diet of mosquitoes in adverse conditions. *Med Vet Entomol* **19:** 413–422.

Muller G, Schlein Y. 2006. Sugar questing mosquitoes in arid areas gather on scarce blossoms that can be used for control. *Int J Parasitol* **36:** 1077–1080.

Muller GC, Kravchenko VD, Schlein Y. 2008. Decline of *Anopheles sergentii* and *Aedes caspius* populations following presentation of attractive toxic (spinosad) sugar bait stations in an oasis. *J Am Mosq Control Assoc* **24:** 147–149.

Muller GC, Beier JC, Traore SF, Toure MB, Traore MM, Bah S, Doumbia S, Schlein Y. 2010a. Field experiments of *Anopheles gambiae* attraction to local fruits/seedpods and flowering plants in Mali to optimize strategies for malaria vector control in Africa using attractive toxic sugar bait methods. *Malaria J* **9:** 262.

Muller GC, Junnila A, Schlein Y. 2010b. Effective control of adult *Culex pipiens* by spraying an attractive toxic sugar bait solution in the vegetation near larval habitats. *J Med Entomol* **47:** 63–66.

Muller GC, Beier JC, Traore SF, Toure MB, Traore MM, Bah S, Doumbia S, Schlein Y. 2010c. Successful field trial of attractive toxic sugar bait (ATSB) plant-spraying methods against malaria vectors in the *Anopheles gambiae* complex in Mali, West Africa. *Malaria J* **9:** 210.

Mutero CM, Schlodder D, Kabatereine N, Kramer R. 2012. Integrated vector management for malaria control in Uganda: Knowledge, perceptions and policy development. *Malaria J* **11:** 21.

Mutero CM, Mbogo C, Mwangangi J, Imbahale S, Kibe L, Orindi B, Girma M, Njui A, Lwande W, Affognon H, et al. 2015. An assessment of participatory integrated vector management for malaria control in Kenya. *Environ Health Perspect* **123:** 1145–1151.

Nasci RS, McLaughlin RE, Focks D, Billodeaux JS. 1990. Effect of topically treating cattle with permethrin on blood feeding of *Psorophora columbiae* (Diptera: Culicidae) in a southwestern Louisiana rice-pasture ecosystem. *J Med Entomol* **27:** 1031–1034.

Nayar JK, Sauerman DM Jr. 1971. The effects of diet on lifespan, fecundity and flight potential of *Aedes taeniorhynchus* adults. *J Med Entomol* **8:** 506–513.

Nayar JK, Sauerman DM Jr. 1975a. The effects of nutrition on survival and fecundity in Florida mosquitoes. Part 1: Utilization of sugar for survival. *J Med Entomol* **12:** 92–98.

Nayar JK, Sauerman DM Jr. 1975b. The effects of nutrition on survival and fecundity in Florida mosquitoes. Part 3: Utilization of blood and sugar for fecundity. *J Med Entomol* **12:** 220–225.

Neafsey DE, Waterhouse RM, Abai MR, Aganezov SS, Alekseyev MA, Allen JE, Amon J, Arca B, Arensburger P, Artemov G, et al. 2015. Mosquito genomics. Highly evolvable malaria vectors: The genomes of 16 *Anopheles* mosquitoes. *Science* **347:** 1258522.

N'Guessan R, Corbel V, Akogbeto M, Rowland M. 2007. Reduced efficacy of insecticide-treated nets and indoor residual spraying for malaria control in pyrethroid resistance area, Benin. *Emerg Infect Dis* **13:** 199–206.

Nyarango PM, Gebremeskel T, Mebrahtu G, Mufunda J, Abdulmumini U, Ogbamariam A, Kosia A, Gebremichael A, Gunawardena D, Ghebrat Y, et al. 2006. A steep decline of malaria morbidity and mortality trends in Eritrea between 2000 and 2004: The effect of combination of control methods. *Malaria J* **5:** 33.

Ogoma SB, Ngonyani H, Simfukwe ET, Mseka A, Moore J, Killeen GF. 2012. Spatial repellency of transfluthrin-treated hessian strips against laboratory-reared *Anopheles arabiensis* mosquitoes in a semi-field tunnel cage. *Parasit Vectors* **5:** 54.

Ogoma SB, Ngonyani H, Simfukwe ET, Mseka A, Moore J, Maia MF, Moore SJ, Lorenz LM. 2014. The mode of action of spatial repellents and their impact on vectorial capacity of *Anopheles gambiae* sensu stricto. *PLoS ONE* **9:** e110433.

O'Meara WP, Mangeni JN, Steketee R, Greenwood B. 2010. Changes in the burden of malaria in sub-Saharan Africa. *Lancet Infect Dis* **10:** 545–555.

Pates HV, Line JD, Keto AJ, Miller JE. 2002. Personal protection against mosquitoes in Dar es Salaam, Tanzania, by using a kerosene oil lamp to vaporize transfluthrin. *Med Vet Entomol* **16:** 277–284.

Paz-Soldan VA, Plasai V, Morrison AC, Rios-Lopez EJ, Guedez-Gonzales S, Grieco JP, Mundal K, Chareonviriyaphap T, Achee NL. 2011. Initial assessment of the acceptability of a push–pull *Aedes aegypti* control strategy in Iquitos, Peru and Kanchanaburi, Thailand. *Am J Trop Med Hyg* **84:** 208–217.

Perera OP, Harrell IR, Handler AM. 2002. Germ-line transformation of the South American malaria vector, *Anopheles albimanus*, with a *piggyBac/EGFP* transposon vector is routine and highly efficient. *Insect Mol Biol* **11:** 291–297.

Pinder M, Jawara M, Jarju LB, Salami K, Jeffries D, Adiamoh M, Bojang K, Correa S, Kandeh B, Kaur H, et al. 2015. Efficacy of indoor residual spraying with dichlorodiphenyltrichloroethane against malaria in Gambian communities with high usage of long-lasting insecticidal mosquito nets: A cluster-randomised controlled trial. *Lancet* **385:** 1436–1446.

Protopopoff N, Wright A, West PA, Tigererwa R, Mosha FW, Kisinza W, Kleinschmidt I, Rowland M. 2015. Combination of insecticide treated nets and indoor residual spraying in Northern Tanzania provides additional reduction in vector population density and malaria transmission rates compared to insecticide treated nets alone: A randomised control trial. *PLoS ONE* **10:** e0142671.

Pyke B, Rice M, Sabine B, Zalucki M. 1987. The push-pull strategy—Behavioural control of *Heliothis*. *Austr Cotton Grow* **8:** 7–9.

Quinones ML, Norris DE, Conn JE, Moreno M, Burkot TR, Bugoro H, Keven JB, Cooper R, Yan G, Rosas A, et al. 2015. Insecticide resistance in areas under investigation by the international centers of excellence for malaria research: A challenge for malaria control and elimination. *Am J Trop Med Hyg* **93:** 69–78.

Cite this article as *Cold Spring Harb Perspect Med* doi: 10.1101/cshperspect.a025643

Ranson H, N'Guessan R, Lines J, Moiroux N, Nkuni Z, Corbel V. 2011. Pyrethroid resistance in African anopheline mosquitoes: What are the implications for malaria control? *Trends Parasitol* **27**: 91–98.

Reddy GV, Guerrero A. 2010. New pheromones and insect control strategies. *Vitam Horm* **83**: 493–519.

Reddy MR, Overgaard HJ, Abaga S, Reddy VP, Caccone A, Kiszewski AE, Slotman MA. 2011. Outdoor host seeking behaviour of *Anopheles gambiae* mosquitoes following initiation of malaria vector control on Bioko Island, Equatorial Guinea. *Malaria J* **10**: 184.

Reisen WK, Meyer RP, Milby MM. 1986. Patterns of fructose feeding by *Culex tarsalis* (Diptera: Culicidae). *J Med Entomol* **23**: 366–373.

Riehle MA, Jacobs-Lorena M. 2005. Using bacteria to express and display anti-parasite molecules in mosquitoes: Current and future strategies. *Insect Biochem Mol Biol* **35**: 699–707.

Riehle MA, Moreira CK, Lampe D, Lauzon C, Jacobs-Lorena M. 2007. Using bacteria to express and display anti-*Plasmodium* molecules in the mosquito midgut. *Int J Parasitol* **37**: 595–603.

Robert LL, Perich MJ, Schlein Y, Jacobson RL, Wirtz RA, Lawyer PG, Githure JI. 1997. Phlebotomine sand fly control using bait-fed adults to carry the larvicide *Bacillus sphaericus* to the larval habitat. *J Am Mosq Control Assoc* **13**: 140–144.

Russell TL, Govella NJ, Azizi S, Drakeley CJ, Kachur SP, Killeen GF. 2011. Increased proportions of outdoor feeding among residual malaria vector populations following increased use of insecticide-treated nets in rural Tanzania. *Malaria J* **10**: 80.

Russell TL, Beebe NW, Cooper RD, Lobo NF, Burkot TR. 2013. Successful malaria elimination strategies require interventions that target changing vector behaviours. *Malaria J* **12**: 56.

Saul A. 2003. Zooprophylaxis or zoopotentiation: The outcome of introducing animals on vector transmission is highly dependent on the mosquito mortality while searching. *Malaria J* **2**: 32.

Sayler GS, Ripp S. 2000. Field applications of genetically engineered microorganisms for bioremediation processes. *Curr Opin Biotechnol* **11**: 286–289.

Schlein Y, Muller GC. 2008. An approach to mosquito control: Using the dominant attraction of flowering *Tamarix jordanis* trees against *Culex pipiens*. *J Med Entomol* **45**: 384–390.

Schlein Y, Pener H. 1990. Bait-fed adult *Culex pipiens* carry the larvicide *Bacillus sphaericus* to the larval habitat. *Med Vet Entomol* **4**: 283–288.

Schultz GW. 1989. Animal influence on man-biting rates at a malarious site in Palawan, Philippines. *Southeast Asian J Trop Med Public Health* **20**: 49–53.

Scott TW, Takken W, Knols BG, Boete C. 2002. The ecology of genetically modified mosquitoes. *Science* **298**: 117–119.

Sethuraman N, Fraser MJ Jr, Eggleston P, O'Brochta DA. 2007. Post-integration stability of *piggyBac* in *Aedes aegypti*. *Insect Biochem Mol Biol* **37**: 941–951.

Shaukat AM, Breman JG, McKenzie FE. 2010. Using the entomological inoculation rate to assess the impact of vector control on malaria parasite transmission and elimination. *Malaria J* **9**: 122.

Shousha AT. 1948. Species-eradication: The eradication of *Anopheles gambiae* from Upper Egypt, 1942–1945. *Bull World Health Organ* **1**: 309–352.

Sinkins SP, Gould F. 2006. Gene drive systems for insect disease vectors. *Nat Rev Genet* **7**: 427–435.

Smith DL, McKenzie FE, Snow RW, Hay SI. 2007. Revisiting the basic reproductive number for malaria and its implications for malaria control. *PLoS Biol* **5**: e42.

Smith Gueye C, Newby G, Gosling RD, Whittaker MA, Chandramohan D, Slutsker L, Tanner M. 2016. Strategies and approaches to vector control in nine malaria-eliminating countries: A cross-case study analysis. *Malaria J* **15**: 2.

Soper FL, Wilson DB. 1943. *Anopheles gambiae in Brazil.* The Rockefeller Foundation, New York.

Stevenson J, St Laurent B, Lobo NF, Cooke MK, Kahindi SC, Oriango RM, Harbach RE, Cox J, Drakeley C. 2012. Novel vectors of malaria parasites in the western highlands of Kenya. *Emerg Infect Dis* **18**: 1547–1549.

Stoddard BL. 2005. Homing endonuclease structure and function. *Q Rev Biophys* **38**: 49–95.

Stone CM, Jackson BT, Foster WA. 2012. Effects of bed net use, female size, and plant abundance on the first meal choice (blood vs sugar) of the malaria mosquito *Anopheles gambiae*. *Malaria J* **11**: 3.

Strode C, Donegan S, Garner P, Enayati AA, Hemingway J. 2014. The impact of pyrethroid resistance on the efficacy of insecticide-treated bed nets against African anopheline mosquitoes: Systematic review and meta-analysis. *PLoS Med* **11**: e1001619.

Strycharz JP, Yoon KS, Clark JM. 2008. A new ivermectin formulation topically kills permethrin-resistant human head lice (Anoplura: Pediculidae). *J Med Entomol* **45**: 75–81.

Suwannachote N, Grieco JP, Achee NL, Suwonkerd W, Wongtong S, Chareonviriyaphap T. 2009. Effects of environmental conditions on the movement patterns of *Aedes aegypti* (Diptera: Culicidae) into and out of experimental huts in Thailand. *J Vector Ecol* **34**: 267–275.

Syafruddin D, Bangs MJ, Sidik D, Elyazar I, Asih PB, Chan K, Nurleila S, Nixon C, Hendarto J, Wahid I, et al. 2014. Impact of a spatial repellent on malaria incidence in two villages in Sumba, Indonesia. *Am J Trop Med Hyg* **91**: 1079–1087.

Taylor B. 1975. Changes in the feeding behaviour of a malaria vector, *Anopheles farauti* Lav., following the use of DDT as a residual spray in houses in the British Solomon Islands Protectorate. *Trans R Entomol Soc London* **127**: 277–292.

Temu EA, Maxwell C, Munyekenye G, Howard AF, Munga S, Avicor SW, Poupardin R, Jones JJ, Allan R, Kleinschmidt I, et al. 2012. Pyrethroid resistance in *Anopheles gambiae*, in Bomi County, Liberia, compromises malaria vector control. *PLoS ONE* **7**: e44986.

Thomas DD, Donnelly CA, Wood RJ, Alphey LS. 2000. Insect population control using a dominant, repressible, lethal genetic system. *Science* **287**: 2474–2476.

Toe KH, Jones CM, N'Fale S, Ismail HM, Dabire RK, Ranson H. 2014. Increased pyrethroid resistance in malaria vectors and decreased bed net effectiveness, Burkina Faso. *Emerg Infect Dis* **20**: 1691–1696.

Tusting LS, Thwing J, Sinclair D, Fillinger U, Gimnig J, Bonner KE, Bottomley C, Lindsay SW. 2013. Mosquito larval source management for controlling malaria. *Cochrane Database Syst Rev* **8**: CD008923.

Wagman JM, Grieco JP, Bautista K, Polanco J, Briceno I, King R, Achee NL. 2015. The field evaluation of a push-pull system to control malaria vectors in northern Belize, Central America. *Malaria J* **14**: 184.

Walshe DP, Garner P, Abdel-Hameed Adeel AA, Pyke GH, Burkot T. 2013. Larvivorous fish for preventing malaria transmission. *Cochrane Database Syst Rev* **12**: CD008090.

Walton C, Handley JM, Collins FH, Baimai V, Harbach RE, Deesin V, Butlin RK. 2001. Genetic population structure and introgression in *Anopheles dirus* mosquitoes in South-east Asia. *Mol Ecol* **10**: 569–580.

Watson M. 1911. *The prevention of malaria in the Federated Malay States*. Liverpool School of Tropical Medicine, Liverpool, UK.

Watson M (ed.). 1953. *African highway: The battle for health in central Africa*. John Murray, London.

West PA, Protopopoff N, Wright A, Kivaju Z, Tigererwa R, Mosha FW, Kisinza W, Rowland M, Kleinschmidt I. 2014. Indoor residual spraying in combination with insecticide-treated nets compared to insecticide-treated nets alone for protection against malaria: A cluster randomised trial in Tanzania. *PLoS Med* **11**: e1001630.

West PA, Protopopoff N, Wright A, Kivaju Z, Tigererwa R, Mosha FW, Kisinza W, Rowland M, Kleinschmidt I. 2015. Enhanced protection against malaria by indoor residual spraying in addition to insecticide treated nets: Is it dependent on transmission intensity or net usage? *PLoS ONE* **10**: e0115661.

WHO. 1982. Manual on environmental management for mosquito control with special emphasis on malaria vectors. WHO offset publication No. 66. World Health Organization, Geneva.

WHO. 1993. A global strategy for malaria control. World Health Organization, Geneva.

WHO. 2004. Global strategic framework for integrated vector management. World Health Organization, Geneva.

WHO. 2011. Position statement on integrated vector management to control malaria and lymphatic filariasis. *Wkly Epidemiol Rec* **86**: 121–127.

WHO. 2012a. Global plan for insecticide resistance management in malaria vectors. World Health Organization, Geneva.

WHO. 2012b. Interim position statement: The role of larviciding for malaria control in sub-Saharan Africa. World Health Organization, Geneva.

WHO. 2013. Larval source management. A supplementary measure for malaria vector control. An operational manual. World Health Organization, Geneva.

WHO. 2014. Guidance note: Control of residual malaria parasite transmission. World Health Organization, Geneva.

WHO. 2015a. World malaria report 2015. World Health Organization, Geneva.

WHO. 2015b. Information note on the risks associated with the scale back of vector control in areas where transmission has been reduced. World Health Organization, Geneva.

Wilke AB, Marrelli MT. 2012. Genetic control of mosquitoes: Population suppression strategies. *Rev Inst Med Trop Sao Paulo* **54**: 287–292.

Wilke AB, Marrelli MT. 2015. Paratransgenesis: A promising new strategy for mosquito vector control. *Parasit Vectors* **8**: 342.

Wilson ML. 1993. Avermectins in arthropod vector management—Prospects and pitfalls. *Parasitol Today* **9**: 83–87.

Windbichler N, Menichelli M, Papathanos PA, Thyme SB, Li H, Ulge UY, Hovde BT, Baker D, Monnat RJ Jr, Burt A, et al. 2011. A synthetic homing endonuclease-based gene drive system in the human malaria mosquito. *Nature* **473**: 212–215.

Xue RD, Barnard DR. 2003. Boric acid bait kills adult mosquitoes (Diptera: Culicidae). *J Econ Entomol* **96**: 1559–1562.

Xue RD, Kline DL, Ali A, Barnard DR. 2006. Application of boric acid baits to plant foliage for adult mosquito control. *J Am Mosq Control Assoc* **22**: 497–500.

Xue RD, Ali A, Kline DL, Barnard DR. 2008. Field evaluation of boric acid- and fipronil-based bait stations against adult mosquitoes. *J Am Mosq Control Assoc* **24**: 415–418.

Yoshida S, Ioka D, Matsuoka H, Endo H, Ishii A. 2001. Bacteria expressing single-chain immunotoxin inhibit malaria parasite development in mosquitoes. *Mol Biochem Parasitol* **113**: 89–96.

Zieler H, Keister DB, Dvorak JA, Ribeiro JM. 2001. A snake venom phospholipase A$_2$ blocks malaria parasite development in the mosquito midgut by inhibiting ookinete association with the midgut surface. *J Exp Biol* **204**: 4157–4167.

Cite this article as *Cold Spring Harb Perspect Med* doi: 10.1101/cshperspect.a025643

Current and Future Prospects for Preventing Malaria Transmission via the Use of Insecticides

Hilary Ranson

Department of Vector Biology, Liverpool School of Tropical Medicine, Liverpool L3 5QA, United Kingdom

Correspondence: hilary.ranson@lstmed.ac.uk

Malaria vectors have developed resistance to all classes of insecticides that are used to target the adult mosquito to prevent parasite transmission. The number of resistant mosquito populations has increased dramatically in recent years, most likely as a result of the scale-up of vector control activities, and the intensity of this resistance is increasing rapidly and compromising the performance of vector control tools. Bednets and indoor residual spray formulations containing alternative active ingredients have shown promise in field trials but are still several years away from implementation. As existing insecticides become less effective at killing mosquitoes in the countries with the highest burden of malaria, there is growing concern that the advances made in reducing malaria transmission will be eroded by insecticide resistance. The likelihood of this scenario, and strategies that may help mitigate against this, are reviewed below.

USE OF INSECTICIDES IN MALARIA CONTROL

Wide-scale implementation of tools to prevent malaria transmission by the mosquito vectors has achieved dramatic results across Africa. It is estimated that nearly half of the population at risk of malaria in Africa are protected by insecticide-treated nets (ITNs) and approximately 7% live in houses that have received indoor residual spraying (IRS). The scale-up in coverage with these preventative measures has contributed to an approximate halving of malaria mortality in Africa between 2000 and 2013 (WHO 2014a). Outside of Africa, the feeding patterns of malaria vectors mean that ITNs are generally less effective and, hence, us-age patterns are lower. IRS is reportedly used in over half of the countries in the Americas and Asia that have ongoing malaria transmission (WHO 2014a).

Only pyrethroid insecticides are approved for bednet treatment and with hundreds of millions of ITNs in use today, this imposes a major selection pressure on mosquitoes. Until recently, the majority of IRS programs were also reliant on this insecticide class although an increasing number of countries are switching to organophosphates (principally primiphos-methyl) or, in some cases, carbamates (bendiocarb) in response to emerging pyrethroid resistance. The organochlorine, DDT, is also still used in some IRS programs in Africa and in India.

Cite this article as *Cold Spring Harb Perspect Med* doi: 10.1101/cshperspect.a026823

THE EMERGENCE AND SPREAD OF RESISTANCE

Pyrethroid resistance was first detected in African malaria vectors in Sudan in the 1970s and later in West Africa in the early 1990s (Brown 1986; Elissa et al. 1993). These early instances of resistance were likely selected for by exposure of mosquitoes to pyrethroids used to protect agricultural crops against insect damage and pyrethroid resistance remained relatively rare until the end of the 20th century (Ranson and Lissenden 2016). But in recent years, reports of pyrethroid resistance in the major African malaria vectors have increased markedly and it is now becoming increasingly difficult to find a population of *Anopheles gambiae* s.l. that is fully susceptible to this insecticide class (Fig. 1). Pyrethroid resistance is also widespread in *Anopheles funestus* in southern Africa and resistance has been detected in West and East African populations of this vector species (Riveron et al. 2013; Mulamba et al. 2014).

DDT resistance is also prevalent across Africa. In *An. gambiae* s.s. and *An. coluzzi* cross resistance between DDT and pyrethroids, caused by alterations in the common target site of both insecticide classes, the voltage-gated sodium channel (known as *kdr* mutations or alleles), is common (Donnelly et al. 2009). Kdr is less common in *An. arabiensis* and absent in *An. funestus* but metabolic resistance can confer DDT resistance in both these species (see below).

Resistance to carbamates and organophosphates is also on the increase (Ranson and Lissenden 2016). Cross resistance between these insecticide classes can be caused by mutations in their shared target site. Of increasing concern is the emergence of mosquito populations that are resistant to all four classes of insecticide. This can arise when multiple resistance mechanisms are selected for in the same population (e.g., *An. gambiae* and *An. coluzzi* in West Africa containing multiple target site resistance alleles have been reported [Dabire et al. 2008; Edi et al. 2012; Essandoh et al. 2013]) or when a single

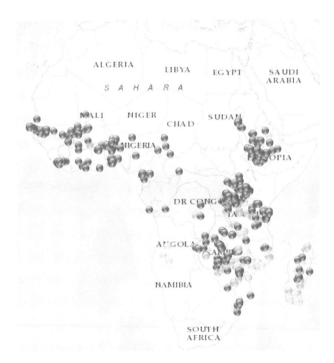

Figure 1. Pyrethroid resistance in malaria vectors. Flags indicate mortality in WHO bioassays (red <90% mortality, orange 90%–97% mortality, green >97% mortality). Data shown are from 2011 to 2016 (Source: IR Mapper [www.irmapper.com], September 2016).

 Cite this article as *Cold Spring Harb Perspect Med* doi: 10.1101/cshperspect.a026823

resistance mechanism can cause resistance to multiple insecticide classes (e.g., elevated activity of enzymes that detoxify pyrethroids, DDT, organophosphates, and/or carbamates [Mitchell et al. 2012; Edi et al. 2014]).

RESISTANCE MECHANISMS

Understanding the genetic basis of insecticide resistance can help elucidate patterns of cross resistance, as described above, and also lead to field-based diagnostics to track and manage resistance (Donnelly et al. 2015).

Target Site Resistance

The best-characterized resistance mechanisms are mutations in the insecticide target sites that reduce the binding of the toxicant. In *An. gambiae*, two alternative substitutions in the same codon of the voltage-gated sodium channel, the 1014F and 1014S *kdr* alleles, are now widely distributed across the continent (Donnelly et al. 2009; Djegbe et al. 2011). An additional mutation (N1575Y) in the same target site gene is present in West Africa but is only found in mosquitoes that contain the 1014F *kdr* mutation (Jones et al. 2012a). In vitro binding studies have shown that the 1575Y allele alone does not confer pyrethroid resistance but it acts synergistically with 1014F to confer a stronger level of resistance in mosquitoes with this double mutation (Wang et al. 2015). This example highlights a common pattern in the emergence of resistance—the overlayering of multiple resistance mutations, each of which serves to further increase the level of resistance of the individual to the toxicant.

Carbamates and organophosphates both target the acetylcholine esterase (AchE) enzyme, which is responsible for degrading the neurotransmitter acetylcholine in the nerve synapses. By inhibiting this enzyme, the insecticides cause a toxic level of acetylcholine to accumulate. A glycine to serine substitution in codon 119 of AchE is strongly associated with resistance to carbamates and/or organophosphates in some West African countries (Essandoh et al. 2013; Edi et al. 2014). The frequency of this mutation

is increasing, which is of great concern, particularly in areas where these insecticide classes are replacing pyrethroids for IRS.

Metabolic Resistance

Metabolic resistance refers to the ability of the mosquito to detoxify the insecticide before it reaches the target site. Several enzyme families have been implicated in insecticide detoxification (Li et al. 2007), but the two families most strongly associated with resistance in malaria vectors are the glutathione transferases (GSTs) and the cytochrome P450s. Overexpression of, or amino acids substitutions in, the GSTE2 enzyme can confer DDT resistance in *An. gambiae* and *An. funestus* and molecular diagnostics have been used to demonstrate the association between genotype and phenotype at this locus (Ranson et al. 2001; Mitchell et al. 2014; Riveron et al. 2014).

Increased expression of multiple cytochrome P450s have been associated with pyrethroid resistance. Several *Anopheles* P450 enzymes have been expressed in vitro and their ability to metabolize pyrethroids demonstrated, with some also metabolizing other insecticide classes (Muller et al. 2008; Edi et al. 2014; Mitchell et al. 2014). Nevertheless, the genetic mechanism responsible for elevated P450 gene expression in mosquitoes has proved elusive so far. In *An. funestus*, there is strong genetic evidence to implicate a mutation in a regulatory element in the vicinity of the CYP9P9 genes (Riveron et al. 2013) and, thus, it is hopeful that a molecular diagnostic for this resistance mechanism will be available soon. The situation is less clear in *An. gambiae* s.l. Although genetic mapping, transcriptomic studies, and whole-genome sequencing have identified several strong candidates for P450-mediated resistance, they have so far failed to coalesce on a single major locus controlling the overexpression of P450s. This may indicate that P450-based resistance has emerged independently in multiple *An. gambiae* populations with different enzymes responsible for resistance in separate populations. Although the search for DNA markers for resistance continues (Donnelly et al. 2015), robust qPCR diagnostic tools to detect the major pyrethroid-resistance-associated P450s are now available.

Reduced Penetration

Until recently, reduced penetration, sometimes referred to as cuticular resistance, was considered a minor, secondary resistance mechanism in mosquitoes. However, several indirect lines of evidence suggest this mechanism may be evolving in African malaria vectors. Measurements of the cuticle in *An. funestus* and *An. gambiae* have found a significant thickening in pyrethroid-resistant mosquitoes (Wood et al. 2010; Balabanidou et al. 2016) and a reduced uptake of pyrethroids has been demonstrated in a resistant *An. gambiae* strain (Balabanidou et al. 2016). Multiple genes implicated in cuticular hydrocarbon synthesis have been found elevated in pyrethroid-resistant strains of *Anopheles arabiensis* in Zanzibar (Jones et al. 2013) and *An. coluzzi* in Burkina Faso (Toe et al. 2015). Both of these populations have very high pyrethroid-resistance phenotypes, which cannot be attributed to other known resistance mechanisms alone. Two cytochrome P450s genes (CYP4G16 and CYP4G17) are elevated in these populations but these P450s do not metabolize insecticides. Instead CYP4G16, and its ortholog in *Drosophila melanogaster* CYP4G1, catalyzes a critical step in the production of CHCs (Qiu et al. 2012; Balabanidou et al. 2016). Finally, several members of the ABC transporter family belonging to a subfamily that, in other insects, has been implicated in transport of lipids to the cuticle are elevated in insecticide-resistant populations of *An. gambiae* (Broehan et al. 2013; Jones et al. 2013). Ongoing work measuring insecticide uptake rates and cuticle composition will hopefully clarify the importance of reduced penetration in insecticide resistance in malaria vectors.

Behavioral Resistance

Increased use of insecticides in the domestic environment may be selecting for genetic changes in the behavior of malaria vectors that increase the rates of outdoor feeding and/or resting, making them less amenable to control by ITNs or IRS. Outdoor transmission is a major obstacle to effective vector control in South East Asia and South America (Santos et al. 2009; Gryseels et al. 2015). In Africa, outdoor transmission has previously been thought to account for only a very small percentage of malaria cases and it is clear that, even in countries that have had sustained coverage with ITNs over many years, the majority of malaria transmission still occurs indoors (Bayoh et al. 2014). However, if African malaria vectors do change their behavior as a result of intensive indoor use of insecticide the implications for malaria control could be catastrophic (Gatton et al. 2013; WHO 2014b). This is clearly something that needs careful monitoring.

LIMITATIONS IN INSECTICIDE-RESISTANCE MONITORING

Understanding the extent and magnitude of resistance in the local vector population is an essential requirement for the design and implementation of effective resistance management strategies. Yet, less than half the 96 countries reporting the use of ITNs and IRS for malaria control, were able to produce any data on resistance for the previous year (WHO 2014a), suggesting monitoring is intermittent at best. However, before criticizing programs for the lack of data on resistance, it is worth reflecting on the utility of the data routinely collected for evidence-based decision making in malaria control.

The vast majority of insecticide resistance monitoring, including the data in the map in Figure 1, relies entirely on the use of discriminating dose bioassays using World Health Organization tube assays or, in a small number of cases, CDC bottle bioassays. Data are reported as percentage mortality and a threshold of less than 90% mortality is used to define resistance (WHO 2013). This standardized methodology is useful for tracking the spread of resistance but does not provide information on the strength of this resistance or its impact. It is not uncommon to find close to zero mortality after exposure of the main African malaria vectors, *An. gambiae*

Cite this article as *Cold Spring Harb Perspect Med* doi: 10.1101/cshperspect.a026823

or *An. funestus*, to the discriminating dose of pyrethroids but simply collating data on the prevalence of resistance may mask important changes in the strength of this resistance. For example, 3 years of monitoring insecticide resistance in *An. gambiae* from Vallé de Kou in Southwest Burkina Faso using discriminating dose assays showed no significant difference in percentage mortality between the years, but when a more quantitative measure was used to assess the strength of this resistance, resistance was found to have increased $10\times$ in a single year (Toe et al. 2014).

Several bioassays that measure the strength of resistance have been described and are compared in a recent publication (Bagi et al. 2015). A consensus on the most suitable methodology would facilitate geographic comparisons and also aid evaluations of the efficacy of resistance-management strategies. However, measuring the intensity of resistance is only the first step. As discussed below, agreement is also needed on what level of resistance has an operational impact. In the agricultural sector, definitions of operationally significant resistance are often related to the field dose of insecticide by dividing the insecticide concentration required to achieve 50% mortality (LC_{50}) by the field dose (Zimmer and Nauen 2011). This is not so straightforward in vector control as formulation issues can have a major impact on the bioavailability of insecticide making the field dose difficult to determine. Furthermore, as discussed below, to assess the public health impact of resistance, we are not only interested in whether or not a mosquito survives exposure to insecticide, but also how this exposure impacts the vectorial capacity. The disconnect between the data generated by resistance monitoring and the data needed to assess the impact of this resistance on malaria control activities must be addressed if this information is going to be used to drive decision making.

IMPACT OF RESISTANCE ON VECTOR CONTROL

The data shown in Figure 1 provide a snapshot of the location of known pyrethroid-resistant ma-

laria vectors in Africa. From the limited number of studies assessing the strength of resistance it is clear that pyrethroid-resistance levels have reached extremely high levels in some sites, with LC_{50}s 100- or even 1000-fold higher than standard laboratory susceptible strains being reported (Edi et al. 2012; Mawejje et al. 2013; Toe et al. 2014). However, the evidence for the impact of this resistance on current control activities is less clear. Part of the reasons for this uncertainty is methodological. As discussed above, the use of discriminating dose assays, which bear no resemblance to the application rates and measure resistance prevalence rather than intensity makes correlations between bioassays and control failure difficult to infer. Inclusion of cone bioassays, in which mosquitoes are exposed directly to a sprayed surface or an ITN can partially help fill these gaps and several studies have now shown that the level of resistance in the field is sufficient to compromise the performance of currently available ITNs (Ochomo et al. 2013; Toe et al. 2014). It is important that these cone bioassays are not just performed on freshly sprayed surfaces or new ITNs as the public health impact of resistance is most likely to manifest itself as insecticide rates decay (Churcher et al. 2016). Studies in Burkina Faso and Kenya both found ITNs that had been in use for a year or more in the field were much less effective at killing resistant mosquitoes than new nets. (Toe et al. 2014; Wanjala et al. 2015).

Experimental Hut Studies Have Been Used to Demonstrate Reduced Personal Protection from ITNs in Areas of Resistance

One of the first such studies was conducted in Benin, in an era when the malaria vectors in the North of the country were still fully susceptible to insecticides but in the South the majority of the vectors were resistant to pyrethroids. Using experimental huts containing volunteers sleeping under holed nets, the study found that ITNs reduced blood-feeding by 96% at the Northern site with susceptible vectors, but had almost no impact in the Southern site with high levels of pyrethroid resistance (N'Guessan et al. 2007). Furthermore the mortality of mosquitoes entering huts at the susceptible site was nearly three times as high as that at the site with high levels of pyrethroid resistance. This was followed up with household studies in 2007, which showed that sleeping under an ITN was no more protective than sleeping under an untreated net in areas with high pyrethroid resistance (Asidi et al. 2012).

It is important to remember that ITNs work by providing both personal protection to users and community protection to non-ITN users and, assuming the ITNs are of good physical quality, it is the latter effect that is most likely to be reduced as resistance increases (Thomas and Read, 2016). Experimental hut studies can measure how personal protection is impacted by resistance (see, for example, Strode et al. 2014) but modeling approaches are needed to extrapolate from this to assess the public health impact of resistance on the entire community. Using a meta-analysis of experimental hut data and a mathematical model of malaria transmission Churcher found that personal protection remained substantial until pyrethroid resistance reached high levels in the population however, the community protection dissipated much more rapidly as resistance increased (Churcher et al. 2016). Although ITN use has increased greatly in recent years, most countries are still a long way from universal coverage and use of ITNs. It is, therefore, critical that the impact of resistance on both ITN used and nonusers is considered when measuring the public health impact of resistance.

In addition, it is important that models of malaria transmission also consider other possible impacts of the resistance phenotype, the majority of which are woefully under studied. Most assays record mortality 24-h post-exposure as the end point; there is very little data on the long-term impact on the mosquito after surviving exposure to insecticides. Yet to quantify the public health impact of insecticide resistance, it is necessary to measure the impact of resistance on all traits that impact the ability of the mosquito to transmit the parasite. As an example, a recent laboratory study found that exposure to ITNs reduced the mean lifespan of adult mosquitoes. Including this delayed mortality in models of malaria transmission suggested that

ITNs would still dramatically reduce the malaria transmission potential even in areas where the mosquito population was largely resistant to the immediate killing effect of the pyrethroids (Viana et al. 2016). Furthermore, it is already established that older mosquitoes are less resistant then their younger counterparts (on which bioassays are routinely conducted). If resistance declines with mosquito age, to the extent that mosquitoes old enough to transmit malaria are still killed by field doses of insecticide, the impact of resistance will again be diminished (Lines and Nassor 1991; Jones et al. 2012b). Other studies have found that exposure of insecticide-resistant mosquitoes to ITNs reduces the likelihood of parasite development (Kristan et al. 2016). These are all important parameters that must be investigated and quantified. However, it is already abundantly clear that, although these factors may possibly reduce the impact of resistance, they will not remove the threat altogether. In Kenya (Ochomo et al. 2013) and Benin (Gnanguenon et al. 2013), mosquitoes with fully developed sporozoites have been found resting inside ITNs, clearly unperturbed by the presence of the insecticide.

The epidemiological impact of resistance will be influenced by a large number of non-vector factors (e.g., efficacy of case management approaches, drug resistance, etc.). Thus, it is complex to attribute an effect directly to insecticide resistance, and even harder to extrapolate between different ecological settings. Longitudinal studies, with accurate records of malaria transmission and resistance levels, afford one of the best chances of demonstrating the impact of resistance. The most widely cited evidence for the impact of resistance comes from such a study in KwaZulu Natal, which demonstrated a correlation between the emergence of pyrethroid resistance and a spike in malaria cases, which was later contained by the reintroduction of DDT (Barnes et al. 2005). More recently, a similar conclusion was reached in Senegal, where reduction in ITN efficacy was attributed to resistance, although the absence of longitudinal resistance data makes this conclusion difficult to validate (Trape et al. 2011). Unfortunately, the opportunity for initiating new

Cite this article as *Cold Spring Harb Perspect Med* doi: 10.1101/cshperspect.a026823

studies of this nature, at least for pyrethroid resistance in Africa, may have passed, unless good historical data sets already exist.

Indirect evidence that insecticide resistance is impacting on malaria transmission can be obtained from retrospective analysis in countries that have changed insecticide class in IRS programs (usually either in response to reports of resistance or increases in malaria cases) and seen an improvement in control. As an example, DDT and pyrethroids were being used for IRS in Uganda, despite the known presence of resistance. When these insecticides were replaced with bendiocarb, a marked improvement in slide positivity rates was observed (Kigozi et al. 2012). Similarly, in Ghana, pyrethroid resistance triggered a switch to use of the organophosphate insecticide Actellic (primiphos-methyl) for IRS, which was associated with a noticeable

impact on key indicators (Fig. 2) (President's Malaria Initiative 2015).

RESISTANCE-MANAGEMENT STRATEGIES

Although there are many challenges to definitively linking insecticide resistance with increased malaria transmission most stakeholders remain in no doubt that if the selection pressure on malaria mosquitoes is allowed to continue unchecked, resistance will eventually result in the failure of existing tools. In 2012, WHO published the Global Plan for Insecticide Resistance Management (GPIRM) (WHO 2012). This document outlined a number of strategies designed to prevent this scenario becoming a reality and provided guidelines to vector control programs on how best to respond to the presence of resistance.

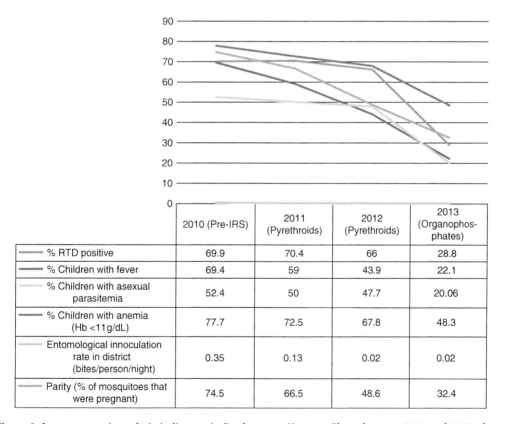

	2010 (Pre-IRS)	2011 (Pyrethroids)	2012 (Pyrethroids)	2013 (Organophosphates)
% RTD positive	69.9	70.4	66	28.8
% Children with fever	69.4	59	43.9	22.1
% Children with asexual parasitemia	52.4	50	47.7	20.06
% Children with anemia (Hb <11g/dL)	77.7	72.5	67.8	48.3
Entomological innoculation rate in district (bites/person/night)	0.35	0.13	0.02	0.02
Parity (% of mosquitoes that were pregnant)	74.5	66.5	48.6	32.4

Figure 2. Improvement in malaria indicators in Bunkpurugu-Yunyoo, Ghana between 2010 and 2013 after a switch in insecticide class from pyrethroids to carbamates for indoor residual spraying. (Source: President's Malaria Initiative 2015.) RTD, Rapid diagnostic test; IRS, indoor residual spraying.

Resistance-management strategies for programs reliant on ITNs are clearly very limited given that WHO recommends universal coverage with bednets (WHO 2014c) and yet there are currently no alternative insecticides to pyrethroids for net impregnation. Some net manufacturers have introduced new nets to the market that contain pyrethroids, plus the synergist piperonyl butoxide (PBO): PermaNet 3.0, is a mosaic long-lasting insecticide treated net with PBO on the roof of the net and deltamethrin on the sides, while Olyset Plus has PBO and permethrin combined throughout the net. Both of these ITNs have interim approval from the WHO pesticide evaluation scheme (WHOPES) as conventional LLINs and the Vector Control Advisory Group (VCAG) have supported the PermaNet 3.0 manufacturers' claim that this net has increased bioefficacy against mosquitoes that have developed metabolic resistance to insecticides (WHO 2014d). Despite this, these LLINs are not in widespread use against resistant populations and instead WHO recommends pilot implementations only (WHO 2015a).

Bednets containing alternative insecticides with new modes of action that differ to the currently available adulticides are under evaluation in the field. Interceptor G$_2$, from BASF, contains the slow acting insecticide chlorfenapyr and the pyrethroid alphacypermethrin and is currently being reviewed by WHOPES (WHO 2015b). Olyset Duo, from Sumitomo Chemicals, contains permethrin and an insect growth regulator, pyriproxyfen. This is also undergoing WHOPES evaluation and, as the idea of sterilizing the resistant mosquitoes that survive contact with the bi-treated net is a novel paradigm, this net is being evaluated in a clinical trial in Burkina Faso (Tiono et al. 2015). It is anticipated that one or both of these new nets with novel modes of action will be on the market by 2017–2018.

For malaria control programs using IRS, it should theoretically be possible to manage insecticide resistance by careful preplanned rotation of insecticide classes with different modes of action (i.e., alternating between DDT or pyrethroids and carbamates or organophosphates). This can be effective if implemented in a proactive manner to prevent the emergence of resistance. However, in reality, rotation of insecticide class is usually triggered by reports of resistance or perceived failures of the current product (e.g., increases in malaria cases, increased reports of mosquitoes inside homes). If resistance to one or more classes of insecticide to be used in rotation has already developed, effective resistance management will only be achieved if resistance has a fitness cost. In the worst-case scenario, the end result may be a more rapid selection of resistance to both chemicals. Little is known about the fitness costs of different resistance mechanisms in mosquitoes and this raises questions over the long-term efficacy of current IRM strategies. Furthermore, simply changing insecticide class may not be sufficient to relieve the selection pressure on the mosquito. Three of the four insecticide classes used in public health are widely used in agriculture and hence mosquitoes may be continually exposed to low doses of these chemicals even if their use in vector control is suspended. For programs including pyrethroids in their IRS rotations, the reality of continued selection pressure from ITNs and the use of coils and pyrethroid-based repellents and aerosols must be factored in. Finally, the possibility that increased expression of a single enzyme could render three or more insecticide classes obsolete is obviously a major impediment to even the best-planned IRM strategies (Edi et al. 2014).

As with ITNs, new products for IRS are under development. However, for these to be implemented in the timeframe necessary to prevent resistance from derailing malaria control, a more coordinated approach to their evaluation, regulation, and to the production of guidelines on when and where they should be deployed is essential (Hemingway et al. 2016).

FUTURE PERSPECTIVES

It is vital that the lessons learned from the current resistance crisis are used to inform future insecticide development and deployment. This will be dependent on the coordinated action of a wide range of stakeholders (Hemingway et al.

2016) and will also require brave decisions to be made to ensure the stewardship of these new products. The introduction of a single new insecticide into the market place would provide a very short-term solution and inevitably lead to the same issues now being faced with pyrethroid resistance. Selection pressure might be reduced if this product was not widely used in agriculture but, if this new insecticide met the desired criteria (reviewed in Vontas et al. 2014), it would likely be used at scale very rapidly, exerting intense selection pressure on mosquito populations. Resistance-management strategies, including plans for monitoring, recording, and sharing data on resistance evolution, must be planned from the outset and should be evidence-based.

CONCLUDING REMARKS

With resistance to one or more insecticides in African malaria vectors now becoming the norm, rather than the exception, it is time to switch the emphasis from simply describing the problem to providing effective, practical solutions. This includes revisiting the way we monitor for resistance to provide information that is of more direct value to implementers and funders, providing a more robust set of evidence on the current and projected impact of resistance to aid in planning and budgeting malaria control activities, evaluating current options to tackle resistance, and, finally, synthesizing lessons learned to develop guidelines for the effective stewardship of new insecticide products as they are introduced into the market. It may be too late to preserve the pyrethroids for future generations but now is the time to start planning evidence-based insecticide-resistance-management strategies for new public health insecticides.

REFERENCES

Asidi A, N'Guessan R, Akogbeto M, Curtis C, Rowland M. 2012. Loss of household protection from use of insecticide-treated nets against pyrethroid-resistant mosquitoes, benin. *Emerg Infect Dis* **18**: 1101–1106.

Bagi J, Grisales N, Corkill R, Morgan JC, N'Fale S, Brogdon WG, Ranson H. 2015. When a discriminating dose assay is not enough: Measuring the intensity of insecticide resistance in malaria vectors. *Malaria J* **14**: 210.

Balabanidou V, Kampouraki A, MacLean M, Blomquist GJ, Tittiger C, Mijailovsky SJ, Chalepakis G Anthousi A, Lynd A, Sanou A, Hemingway J, et al. 2016. Cytochrome P450 associated with insecticide resistance catalyses cuticular hydrocarbon production in *An. gambiae*. *Proc Natl Acad Sci* **113**: 9268–9273.

Barnes KI, Durrheim DN, Little F, Jackson A, Mehta U, Allen E, Dlamini SS, Tsoka J, Bredenkamp B, Mthembu DJ, et al. 2005. Effect of artemether–lumefantrine policy and improved vector control on malaria burden in KwaZulu-Natal, South Africa. *PLoS Med* **2**: e330.

Bayoh MN, Walker ED, Kosgei J, Ombok M, Olang GB, Githeko AK, Killeen GF, Otieno P, Desai M, Lobo NF, et al. 2014. Persistently high estimates of late night, indoor exposure to malaria vectors despite high coverage of insecticide treated nets. *Parasit Vectors* **7**: 380.

Broehan G, Kroeger T, Lorenzen M, Merzendorfer H. 2013. Functional analysis of the ATP-binding cassette transporter family in *Tribolium castaneum*. *BMC Genomics* **14**: 6.

Brown AW. 1986. Insecticide resistance in mosquitoes: A pragmatic review. *J Am Mosq Control Assoc* **2**: 123–140.

Churcher TS, Lissenden N, Griffin JT, Worrall E, Ranson H. 2016. The impact of pyrethroid resistance on the efficacy and effectiveness of bednets for malaria control in Africa. *eLife* **5**: e16090.

Dabire KR, Diabate A, Djogbenou L, Ouari A, N'Guessan R, Ouedraogo JB, Hougard JM, Chandre F, Baldet T. 2008. Dynamics of multiple insecticide resistance in the malaria vector *Anopheles gambiae* in a rice growing area in South-Western Burkina Faso. *Malaria J* **7**: 188.

Djegbe I, Boussari O, Sidick A, Martin T, Ranson H, Chandre F, Akogbeto M, Corbel V. 2011. Dynamics of insecticide resistance in malaria vectors in Benin: First evidence of the presence of L1014S *kdr* mutation in *Anopheles gambiae* from West Africa. *Malaria J* **10**: 261.

Donnelly MJ, Corbel V, Weetman D, Wilding CS, Williamson MS, Black WCt. 2009. Does *kdr* genotype predict insecticide-resistance phenotype in mosquitoes? *Trends Parasitol* **25**: 213–219.

Donnelly MJ, Issacs AT, Weetman D. 2015. Identification, validation and application of molecular diagnostics for insecticide resistance in malaria vectors. *Trends Parasitol* **32**: 197–206.

Edi CV, Koudou BG, Jones CM, Weetman D, Ranson H. 2012. Multiple-insecticide resistance in *Anopheles gambiae* mosquitoes, Southern Cote d'Ivoire. *Emerg Infect Dis* **18**: 1508–1511.

Edi CV, Djogbenou L, Jenkins AM, Regna K, Muskavitch MA, Poupardin R, Jones CM, Essandoh J, Ketoh GK, Paine MJ, et al. 2014. CYP6 P450 enzymes and ACE-1 duplication produce extreme and multiple insecticide resistance in the malaria mosquito *Anopheles gambiae*. *PLoS Genet* **10**: e1004236.

Elissa N, Mouchet J, Riviere F, Meunier JY, Yao K. 1993. Resistance of *Anopheles gambiae* s.s. to pyrethroids in Cote d'Ivoire. *Ann Soc Belg Med Trop* **73**: 291–294.

Essandoh J, Yawson AE, Weetman D. 2013. Acetylcholinesterase (Ace-1) target site mutation 119S is strongly diagnostic of carbamate and organophosphate resistance in

Anopheles gambiae s.s. and *Anopheles coluzzii* across southern Ghana. *Malaria J* **12**: 404.

Gatton ML, Chitnis N, Churcher T, Donnelly MJ, Ghani AC, Godfray HC, Gould F, Hastings I, Marshall J, Ranson H, et al. 2013. The importance of mosquito behavioural adaptations to malaria control in Africa. *Evolution: Int J Organ Evol* **67**: 1218–1230.

Gnanguenon V, Azondekon R, Oke-Agbo F, Sovi A, Osse R, Padonou G, Aikpon R, Akogbeto MC. 2013. Evidence of man-vector contact in torn long-lasting insecticide-treated nets. *BMC Public Health* **13**: 751.

Gryseels C, Durnez L, Gerrets R, Uk S, Suon S, Set S, Phoeuk P, Sluydts V, Heng S, Sochantha T, et al. 2015. Re-imagining malaria: Heterogeneity of human and mosquito behaviour in relation to residual malaria transmission in Cambodia. *Malaria J* **14**: 165.

Hemingway J, Ranson H, Magill A, Kolaczinski J, Fornadel C, Gimnig J, Coetzee M, Simard F, Roch DK, Hinzoumbe CK, et al. 2016. Averting a malaria disaster: Will insecticide resistance derail malaria control? *Lancet* **387**: 1785–1788.

Jones CM, Liyanapathirana M, Agossa FR, Weetman D, Ranson H, Donnelly MJ, Wilding CS. 2012a. Footprints of positive selection associated with a mutation (N1575Y) in the voltage-gated sodium channel of *Anopheles gambiae*. *Proc Natl Acad Sci* **109**: 6614–6619.

Jones CM, Sanou A, Guelbeogo WM, Sagnon N, Johnson PC, Ranson H. 2012b. Aging partially restores the efficacy of malaria vector control in insecticide-resistant populations of *Anopheles gambiae* s.l. from Burkina Faso. *Malaria J* **11**: 24.

Jones CM, Toe HK, Sanou A, Namountougou M, Hughes A, Diabate A, Dabire R, Simard F, Ranson H. 2012c. Additional selection for insecticide resistance in urban malaria vectors: DDT resistance in *Anopheles arabiensis* from Bobo-Dioulasso, Burkina Faso. *PLoS ONE* **7**: e45995.

Jones CM, Haji KA, Khatib BO, Bagi J, Mcha J, Devine GJ, Daley M, Kabula B, Ali AS, Majambere S, et al. 2013. The dynamics of pyrethroid resistance in *Anopheles arabiensis* from Zanzibar and an assessment of the underlying genetic basis. *Parasit Vectors* **6**: 343.

Kigozi R, Baxi SM, Gasasira A, Sserwanga A, Kakeeto S, Nasr S, Rubahika D, Dissanayake G, Kamya MR, Filler S, et al. 2012. Indoor residual spraying of insecticide and malaria morbidity in a high transmission intensity area of Uganda. *PLoS ONE* **7**: e42857.

Kristan M, Lines J, Nuwa A, Ntege C, Meek SR, Abeku TA. 2016. Exposure to deltamethrin affects development of *Plasmodium falciparum* inside wild pyrethroid resistant *Anopheles gambiae* s.s. mosquitoes in Uganda. *Parasites Vectors* **9**: 100.

Li X, Schuler MA, Berenbaum MR. 2007. Molecular mechanisms of metabolic resistance to synthetic and natural xenobiotics. *Annu Rev Entomol* **52**: 231–253.

Lines JD, Nasssor N.S. 1991. DDT resistance in *Anopheles gambiae* declines with mosquito age. *Med Vet Entomol* **5**: 261–265.

Mawejje HD, Wilding CS, Rippon EJ, Hughes A, Weetman D, Donnelly MJ. 2013. Insecticide resistance monitoring of field-collected *Anopheles gambiae* s.l. populations from Jinja, eastern Uganda, identifies high levels of pyrethroid resistance. *Med Vet Entomol* **27**: 276–283.

Mitchell SN, Stevenson BJ, Muller P, Wilding CS, Egyir-Yawson A, Field SG, Hemingway J, Paine MJ, Ranson H, Donnelly MJ. 2012. Identification and validation of a gene causing cross-resistance between insecticide classes in *Anopheles gambiae* from Ghana. *Proc Natl Acad Sci* **109**: 6147–6152.

Mitchell SN, Rigden DJ, Dowd AJ, Lu F, Wilding CS, Weetman D, Dadzie S, Jenkins AM, Regna K, Boko P, et al. 2014. Metabolic and target-site mechanisms combine to confer strong DDT resistance in *Anopheles gambiae*. *PLoS ONE* **9**: e92662.

Mulamba C, Riveron JM, Ibrahim SS, Irving H, Barnes KG, Mukwaya LG, Birungi J, Wondji CS. 2014. Widespread pyrethroid and DDT resistance in the major malaria vector *Anopheles funestus* in East Africa is driven by metabolic resistance mechanisms. *PLoS ONE* **9**: e110058.

Muller P, Warr E, Stevenson BJ, Pignatelli PM, Morgan JC, Steven A, Yawson AE, Mitchell SN, Ranson H, Hemingway J, et al. 2008. Field-caught permethrin-resistant *Anopheles gambiae* overexpress CYP6P3, a P450 that metabolises pyrethroids. *PLoS Genet* **4**: e1000286.

N'Guessan R, Corbel V, Akogbeto M, Rowland M. 2007. Reduced efficacy of insecticide-treated nets and indoor residual spraying for malaria control in pyrethroid resistance area, Benin. *Emerg Infect Dis* **13**: 199–206.

Ochomo EO, Bayoh NM, Walker ED, Abongo BO, Ombok MO, Ouma C, Githeko AK, Vulule J, Yan G, Gimnig JE. 2013. The efficacy of long-lasting nets with declining physical integrity may be compromised in areas with high levels of pyrethroid resistance. *Malaria J* **12**: 368.

President's Malaria Initiative. 2015. Ghana: Malaria operational plan FY 2015. USAID, Washington, DC.

Qiu Y, Tittiger C, Wicker-Thomas C, Le Goff G, Young S, Wajnberg E, Fricaux T, Taquet N, Blomquist GJ, Feyereisen R. 2012. An insect-specific P450 oxidative decarbonylase for cuticular hydrocarbon biosynthesis. *Proc Natl Acad Sci* **109**: 14858–14863.

Ranson H, Lissenden N. 2016. Insecticide resistance in African *Anopheles* mosquitoes: A worsening situation that needs urgent action to maintain malaria control. *Trends Parasitol* **32**: 187–196.

Ranson H, Rossiter L, Ortelli F, Jensen B, Wang X, Roth CW, Collins FH, Hemingway J. 2001. Identification of a novel class of insect glutathione S−transferases involved in resistance to DDT in the malaria vector *Anopheles gambiae*. *Biochem J* **359**: 295–304.

Riveron JM, Irving H, Ndula M, Barnes KG, Ibrahim SS, Paine MJ, Wondji CS. 2013. Directionally selected cytochrome P450 alleles are driving the spread of pyrethroid resistance in the major malaria vector *Anopheles funestus*. *Proc Natl Acad Sci* **110**: 252–257.

Riveron JM, Yunta C, Ibrahim SS, Djouaka R, Irving H, Menze BD, Ismail HM, Hemingway J, Ranson H, Albert A, et al. 2014. A single mutation in the GSTe2 gene allows tracking of metabolically based insecticide resistance in a major malaria vector. *Genome Biol* **15**: R27.

Santos RL, Padilha A, Costa MD, Costa EM, Dantas-Filho Hde C, Povoa MM. 2009. Malaria vectors in two indigenous reserves of the Brazilian Amazon. *Rev Saude Publica* **43**: 859–868.

 Cite this article as *Cold Spring Harb Perspect Med* doi: 10.1101/cshperspect.a026823

Strode C, Donegan S, Garner P, Enayati AA, Hemingway J. 2014. The impact of pyrethroid resistance on the efficacy of insecticide treated bednets against African anopheline mosquitoes: Systematic review and meta analysis. *Plos Med* **18:** 11.

Thomas MB, Read AF. 2016. The threat (or not) of insecticide resistance for malaria control. *Proc Natl Acad Sci* **113:** 8900–8902.

Tiono AB, Pinder M, N'Fale S, Faragher B, Smith T, Silkey M, Ranson H, Lindsay SW. 2015. The AvecNet Trial to assess whether addition of pyriproxyfen, an insect juvenile hormone mimic, to long-lasting insecticidal mosquito nets provides additional protection against clinical malaria over current best practice in an area with pyrethroid-resistant vectors in rural Burkina Faso: Study protocol for a randomised controlled trial. *Trials* **16:** 113.

Toe KH, Jones CM, N'Fale S, Ismail HM, Dabire RK, Ranson H. 2014. Increased pyrethroid resistance in malaria vectors and decreased bed net effectiveness, Burkina Faso. *Emerg Infect Dis* **20:** 1691–1696.

Toe KH, N'Fale S, Dabire RK, Ranson H, Jones CM. 2015. The recent escalation in strength of pyrethroid resistance in *Anopheles coluzzi* in West Africa is linked to increased expression of multiple gene families. *BMC Genomics* **16:** 146.

Trape JF, Tall A, Diagne N, Ndiath O, Ly AB, Faye J, Dieye-Ba F, Roucher C, Bouganali C, Badiane A, et al. 2011. Malaria morbidity and pyrethroid resistance after the introduction of insecticide-treated bednets and artemisinin-based combination therapies: A longitudinal study. *Lancet Infect Dis* **11:** 925–932.

Viana M, Hughes A, Matthiopoulos J, Ranson H, Ferguson HM. 2016. Delayed mortality effects cut the malaria transmission potential of insecticide-resistant mosquitoes. *Proc Natl Acad Sci* **113:** 8975–8980

Vontas J, Moore S, Kleinschmidt I, Ranson H, Lindsay S, Lengeler C, Hamon N, McLean T, Hemingway J. 2014. Framework for rapid assessment and adoption of new vector control tools. *Trends Parasitol* **30:** 191–204.

Wang L, Nomura Y, Du Y, Liu N, Zhorov BS, Dong K. 2015. A mutation in the intracellular loop III/IV of mosquito sodium channel synergizes the effect of mutations in helix IIS6 on pyrethroid resistance. *Molec Pharmacol* **87:** 421–429.

Wanjala CL, Zhou G, Mbugi J, Simbauni J, Afrane YA, Ototo E, et al. 2015. Insecticidal decay effects of long-lasting insecticide nets and indoor residual spraying on *Anopheles gambiae* and *Anopheles arabiensis* in Western Kenya. *Parasit Vectors* **8:** 588

Wood O, Hanrahan S, Coetzee M, Koekemoer L, Brooke B. 2010. Cuticle thickening associated with pyrethroid resistance in the major malaria vector *Anopheles funestus*. *Parasit Vectors* **3:** 67.

WHO. 2012. Global plan for insecticide resistance management in malaria vectors. Global Malaria Programme, World Health Organization, Geneva.

WHO. 2013. Test procedures for insecticide resistance monitoring in malaria vector mosquitoes. World Health Organization, Geneva.

WHO. 2014a. World malaria report. World Health Organization, Geneva.

WHO. 2014b. Control of residual malaria parasite transmission. WHO/HTM/GMP/MPAC/2014.5. World Health Organization, Geneva.

WHO. 2014c. WHO recommendations for achieving universal coverage with long-lasting insecticidal nets in malaria control September 2013 (revised March 2014). World Health Organization, Geneva.

WHO. 2014d. Second meeting of the vector control advisory group. World Health Organization, Geneva.

WHO. 2015a. Conditions for use of long-lasting insecticidal nets treated with a pyrethroid and piperonyl butoxide. World Health Organization, Geneva.

WHO. 2015b. Pesticide products under WHOPES laboratory and or field testing and evaluation. World Health Organization, Geneva.

Zimmer C, Nauen R. 2011. Pyrethroid resistance and thiacloprid baseline susceptibility of European populations of *Meligethes aeneus* (Coleoptera: Nitidulidae collected in winter oilseed rape. *Pest Manag Sci* **67:** 599–608.

Plasmodium Sporozoite Biology

Friedrich Frischknecht[1] and Kai Matuschewski[2]

[1]Integrative Parasitology, Center for Infectious Diseases, University of Heidelberg Medical School, 69120 Heidelberg, Germany

[2]Department of Molecular Parasitology, Institute of Biology, Humboldt University Berlin, 10115 Berlin, Germany

Correspondence: freddy.frischknecht@med.uni-heidelberg.de; kai.matuschewski@hu-berlin.de

Plasmodium sporozoite transmission is a critical population bottleneck in parasite life-cycle progression and, hence, a target for prophylactic drugs and vaccines. The recent progress of a candidate antisporozoite subunit vaccine formulation to licensure highlights the importance of sporozoite transmission intervention in the malaria control portfolio. Sporozoites colonize mosquito salivary glands, migrate through the skin, penetrate blood vessels, breach the liver sinusoid, and invade hepatocytes. Understanding the molecular and cellular mechanisms that mediate the remarkable sporozoite journey in the invertebrate vector and the vertebrate host can inform evidence-based next-generation drug development programs and immune intervention strategies.

Malaria-related pathology is exclusively caused by asexual parasite propagation inside vertebrate erythrocytes, rendering the life-cycle phases preceding blood infection a prime window of opportunity for targeted prophylactic interventions. The time from an infectious *Anopheles* bite to the occurrence of the first parasites in the peripheral blood, the so-called prepatent period, reflects the obligate preerythrocytic tissue phase that leads to a dramatic expansion of the *Plasmodium* population from a tiny sporozoite inoculum. This phase is clinically silent and remains diagnostically inaccessible. Intriguingly, phylogenetic placement of mammalian *Plasmodium* parasites suggests that asexual blood replication is the exception rather than the rule (Perkins 2014). Closely related taxa, including *Hepato-*cystis and *Nycteria*, are nonpathogenic, and first-generation tissue merozoites do not replicate asexually inside erythrocytes. Instead, these parasites differentiate straight into microgametes and macrogametes. In any case, successful completion of the obligate preerythrocytic development is most critical for host colonization, propagation of parasite populations, and onward transmission. Despite the recent awareness of the central importance of sporozoite-based interventions for malaria control many fundamental knowledge gaps remain and a broader molecular, cellular, and immunological understanding of sporozoite–host cross talk is urgently needed. Here, we present an overview of the foundation, recent discoveries, and challenges in *Plasmodium* sporozoite biology.

THE NATURAL HISTORY OF SPOROZOITES

Plasmodium sporogony, an extracellular phase of asexual replication, occurs in *Anopheles* mosquitoes, although some species of lizard plasmodia, for instance *Plasmodium mexicanum*, can also be transmitted by sand flies (Ayala 1971). The onset of sporogony is marked when ookinetes settle after their journey from the blood meal across the midgut epithelium. They transform and develop into oocysts underneath the basal lamina surrounding the digestive organ of *Anopheles* mosquitoes (Beier 1998). Curiously, the distribution of oocysts can differ in mosquitoes depending on the insect's ability to agglutinate blood. In mosquitoes that agglutinate blood, parasites settle at the bottom of the digestive organ following the force of gravity, whereas in those who do not, for example, in *Anopheles stephensi*, they distribute randomly (Shortt 1948; Kan et al. 2014). Within the oocysts, sporozoites develop over the course of 10 days to 4 weeks depending on the *Plasmodium* species and ambient temperature before they emerge into the circulatory fluid of the insect, the hemolymph (Figs. 1 and 2). They are crescent-shaped, 8- to 14-μm long, and display substrate-dependent locomotion known as gliding motility (Figs. 3 and 4). Within the hemolymph, sporozoites are transported throughout the body cavity but seem to specifically interact with and enter into salivary glands, crossing the basal lamina surrounding this organ and passing through the saliva-producing acinar cells (Sterling et al. 1973; Pimenta et al. 1994; Douglas et al. 2015). Sporozoites accumulate in the salivary cavities from where they can also move into the narrow salivary ducts that connect to the proboscis. Sporozoites are considered mature once they reach the salivary cavities, but experimental infections with sporozoites liberated from oocysts or collected from the hemolymph can initiate a malaria episode (Shute 1943; Vanderberg 1975; Sato et al. 2014). During an infectious bite, the mosquito ejects saliva and with it a small fraction of the sporozoites in the gland. Most sporozoites are deposited in the dermis of the host during the probing phase when the mosquito searches for a blood vessel to puncture (Sidjanski and Vanderberg 1997; Matsuoka et al. 2002; Vanderberg and Frevert 2004; Amino et al. 2006). Once the mosquito sucks up blood, sporozoites that continue to be ejected with the saliva appear to be largely reingested into the mosquito midgut by the stronger flow and, thus, are lost for transmission (Kebaier and Vanderberg 2006). Sporozoites in the dermis can actively migrate at high-speed passing through several skin cells and

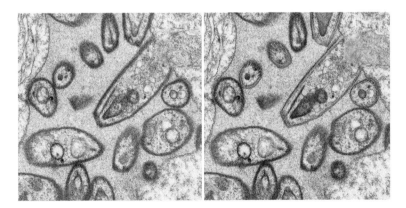

Figure 1. Sporozoite formation within the oocyst. Transmission electron micrograph showing *Plasmodium berghei* sporozoites budding from sporoblasts 10 days after the uptake of parasites by the mosquito. On the *right* image, some selected structures are highlighted. Blue, plasma membrane; yellow, inner membrane complex; green, microtubules; magenta, nascent rhoptries; cyan, nascent micronemes; brown, rootlet fiber; light blue, nucleus. The image is 4 μm wide. (Image courtesy of Mirko Singer and Stefan Hillmer.)

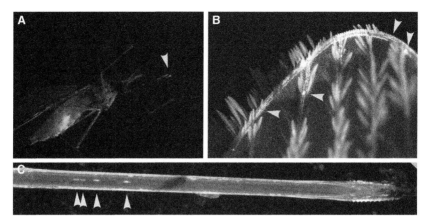

Figure 2. Sporozoites in the *Anopheles* vector. (*A*) A mosquito infected with green fluorescent parasites. Note the green fluorescence of sporozoites secreted with saliva at the front of the proboscis (arrowhead). (*B*) Sporozoites in the veins of a mosquito wing. Arrowheads point to two sporozoites stuck in the veins and two that are streaked out because of the fast movement of the hemolymph. (*C*) Sporozoites (arrowheads) within the salivary canal of the proboscis as they are ejected from the mosquito. (Courtesy of Biology of Parasitism course 2015 at the Marine Biological Laboratory, Woods Hole.)

enter blood or lymphatic vessels (Amino et al. 2006, 2008). Sporozoites of plasmodia that infect birds and lizards can enter into and differentiate within phagocytic cells of the reticulo-endothelial system, including within the skin. Sporozoites of plasmodia that infect mammals need to enter the bloodstream to be transported to the liver, in which they specifically differentiate in hepatocytes. To access this niche sporozoites arrest in the sinusoids of the liver and pass through endothelial cells or Kupffer cells, liver resident macrophages, to gain access to the underlying hepatocytes (Baer et al. 2007; Tavares et al. 2013). Here again, they usually migrate through a few hepatocytes before settling in one for differentiation into thousands of red blood cell–invading merozoites (Mota et al. 2001; Prudêncio et al. 2006). Hence, sporozoites are the most versatile of *Plasmodium* stages because they are formed in the invertebrate host to eventually differentiate in the vertebrate host. On their journey, sporozoites undergo massive changes in their proteomic makeup, migrate actively through different cells in different tissues, and use the circulatory fluid of vector and host for reaching their intermediate (salivary gland) and final (hepatocyte) destination. It is no surprise then that the sporozoite is

as exciting and enigmatic a parasite stage to study with still plenty of scope for fundamental discovery.

THE IMMUNE-DOMINANT SPOROZOITE ANTIGEN: CSP

The circumsporozoite precipitation test was the first antigen assay that permitted a correlation of antisporozoite antibody titers with sterile protection in a volunteer that was immunized with high doses of *Plasmodium falciparum*–infected irradiated mosquitoes (Clyde et al. 1973). In this test, sporozoite surface antigens were broadly precipitated and the major protein was termed circumsporozoite protein (CSP). CSP is thought to be secreted at the anterior sporozoite tip, translocated backward to the anterior end, and abundantly shed into the microenvironment (Stewart and Vanderberg 1991). CSP was among the first cloned and sequenced *Plasmodium* antigens (Dame et al. 1984; Enea et al. 1984) and is structurally similar in different *Plasmodium* species (Sinnis and Nardin 2002). CSP is a glycosylphosphatidylinositol (GPI)-anchored membrane protein and contains two conserved regions flanking a central repeat region of various lengths.

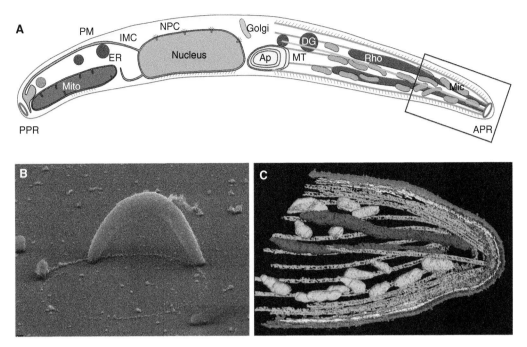

Figure 3. Shape and subcellular structure of the *Plasmodium* sporozoite. (*A*) Schematic showing the cellular organelles and their position and relative size in the *Plasmodium* sporozoite. PPR, proximal polar ring; Mito, mitochondrion; PM, plasma membrane (blue); ER, endoplasmic reticulum; IMC, inner membrane complex (yellow); NPC, nuclear pore complex; Ap, apicoplast (yellow); MT, microtubules (green); DG, dense granules (brown); Rho, rhoptries (magenta); Mic, micronemes (cyan); APR, apical polar ring (red). Note the single stack Golgi apparatus and the nucleus being associated to the IMC. (*B*) Scanning electron micrograph of a *Plasmodium berghei* sporozoite. Sporozoites are an elongated crescent shape and tailored for lasting continuous locomotion and host cell invasion. When deposited on a substrate sporozoites alternate gliding periods with nongliding phases. Sporozoite material that is shed during gliding locomotion marks the trails. (Image from Montagna et al. 2012c; adapted, with permission, from the authors.) (*C*) Computer tomogram of the apical end of a sporozoite. Highlighted are plasma membrane (blue), inner membrane complex (yellow), microtubules (green), rhoptries (magenta), and micronemes (cyan).

A formulation that contains a fusion protein of the *P. falciparum* CSP carboxyl terminus, including 19 repeats, the hepatitis B surface (S) antigen, and the very strong, investigational adjuvant AS01, termed RTS,S/AS01, is the first advanced candidate antimalaria vaccine (Cohen et al. 2010). The recent completion of the first multicenter phase III antimalaria vaccine trial in sub-Saharan Africa (RTS,S Clinical Trials Partnership 2015) highlighted the reputation of targeting sporozoite transmission on a population level. Among the aims of the RTS,S/AS01 vaccine and improved formulations was to elicit a strong, nonnatural immune response against sporozoites, which is typically not ac-

quired during natural transmission in endemic areas (Offeddu et al. 2012).

As predicted for a stage-specific major surface protein, targeted deletion of *Plasmodium berghei* CSP did not affect blood infection but aborted sporozoite formation, yielding vacuolated oocysts (Ménard et al. 1997). This was further confirmed by down-regulation of *CSP*, which resulted in aberrant development of oocyst membranes and stumpy, noninfectious sporozoites (Thathy et al. 2002). The amino-terminal region I apparently mediates sporozoite invasion of invertebrate and mammalian host cells (Sidjanski et al. 1997; Aldrich et al. 2012). Region I and a carboxy-terminal region II bind

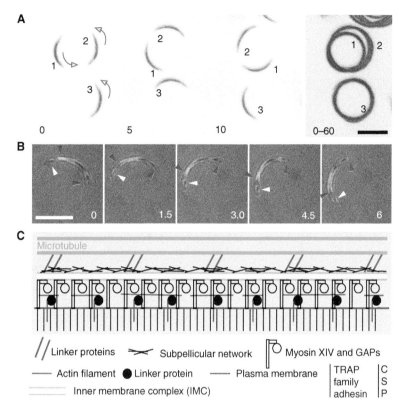

Figure 4. Sporozoite motility in vitro. (*A*) Three sporozoites move in a circular fashion with their apical end leading (red arrowheads) at speeds above 1 μm/sec. Their near-perfect circular trajectory is revealed by the maximum intensity projection (0–60). Time between images is indicated in seconds. Scale bar, 10 μm. (*B*) Reflection interference contrast microscopy reveals the contact points between sporozoites and substrate (dark areas). Arrowheads point to the same positions of a migrating sporozoite. Note that at these positions the dark and bright areas appear and disappear highlighting the dynamic adhesion to the substrate. Time between images is indicated in seconds. Scale bar, 10 μm. (*C*) Schematic of the sporozoite pellicle with a focus on the core gliding motility machinery.

heparin-sulfate proteoglycans on the surface of liver cells (Cerami et al. 1992; Frevert et al. 1993). On the developmental switch from cell traversal to invasion CSP is proteolytically cleaved thereby exposing region II, indicating that this region is important for liver colonization and covered throughout most of the sporozoite journey to prevent premature cell invasion (Coppi et al. 2011). Proteolytic processing of CSP can be targeted by protective antibodies (Espinosa et al. 2015), indicating that RTS,S/AS01 might be considerably improved by replacing the truncated antigen with full length CSP.

An attractive path for in vivo testing of CSP-based vaccines was the generation of transgenic *P. berghei* parasites that harbor a CSP from human-infecting parasites. This proved difficult for *Pf*CSP, because complemented *P. berghei* parasites are severely impaired in salivary gland colonization and yield only very few and impaired sporozoites for transmission experiments (Tewari et al. 2002). However, *P. berghei* parasites harboring a chimeric CSP containing the repeat region from *P. falciparum* or *Plasmodium vivax* CSP (Persson et al. 2002; Espinosa et al. 2013) and, more recently, complemented *Plasmodium yoelii* sporozoites (Zhang et al. 2016) can be used in robust infection models. Naturally acquired antisporozoite antibody responses are almost exclusively directed against CSP repeats but a potential association with immunity against malaria in children and adults remains elusive (Offeddu et al. 2012). This remarkable immunodominance could well be a mechanism of immune evasion (Schofield 1990) and could explain the modest efficacy of the RTS,S/AS01 vaccine (RTS,S Clinical Trials Partnership 2015). Hence, deciphering the cellular and immunological functions of CSP in parasite–host interactions and discovering additional protective sporozoite antigens remain research priorities (Hafalla et al. 2011, 2013).

SPOROZOITE GLIDING MOTILITY, TRAP FAMILY ADHESINS, AND ACTIN FILAMENTS

Sporozoites need to be motile to succeed in their arduous journey. Evidence suggests that sporozoites actively exit the oocysts, but the requirement of motility has not been formally shown. Several proteins, including CSP and egress cysteine protease 1 (ECP1) (Aly and Matuschewski 2005; Wang et al. 2005), function in sporozoite egress indicating an active participation by the sporozoites, but liberation might be further aided by oocyst rupture. Subsequently, sporozoites need to actively migrate to enter salivary glands. Inside the salivary glands, most sporozoites stop moving and aggregate within the salivary cavities, whereas a few move slowly down the salivary ducts (Frischknecht et al. 2004). Once in the dermis, sporozoites move at average speeds between 1 and 2 μm/sec, about 10 times as fast as neutrophils migrate (Amino et al. 2006). Without this motility, sporozoites are stuck in the skin and hosts remain largely uninfected after mosquito bites (Montagna et al. 2012a). After entering blood vessels, sporozoites use their motility to infect the liver, although they can efficiently accomplish this with much diminished migration capacity (Montagna et al. 2012a).

To move, sporozoites need to attach to a substrate and generate a force against this substrate. Furthermore, they must continuously generate new substrate attachment sites and

turn them over (Fig. 4B). How this is all achieved is not yet understood completely but a complex picture emerges; plasma-membrane-spanning proteins of the thrombosponin-related anonymous protein (TRAP) family, actin filaments, and actin-binding proteins including the motor protein myosin and a complex of myosin anchoring proteins form a transient motor complex that integrates signaling proteins and molecules, such as calcium and possibly cAMP and cGMP (Ono et al. 2008; Montagna et al. 2012b; Carey et al. 2014; Lakshmanan et al. 2015).

The gene coding for TRAP was the first gene to be deleted from the parasite genome that revealed an effect in parasite motility (Sultan et al. 1997). TRAP is specifically expressed in sporozoites and $trap^-$ sporozoites can neither move continuously nor enter into salivary glands, resulting in a complete life-cycle arrest just before sporozoite transmission. Curiously, $trap^-$ sporozoites still attach to substrates and move back and forth over single adhesion sites (Münter et al. 2009). It thus appears that TRAP plays a role in generating directional migration, although precisely how it does this is currently not understood. Parasites expressing TRAP with point mutations in conserved residues of the cytoplasmic tail also show aberrant motility suggesting that TRAP links extracellular interactions with the interior to modulate motility (Kappe et al. 1999). Subtle mutations in the extracellular domains of TRAP that mediate adhesion to the substrate lead to no effect on gliding motility of sporozoites but abrogate sporozoite invasion into salivary glands and liver cells (Matuschewski et al. 2002a). Notably, replacement of *P. berghei* TRAP with the *P. falciparum* ortholog affects gliding motility and partly reproduces the defects observed in $trap^-$ sporozoites (Wengelnik et al. 1999). This finding is in agreement with species-specific signaling roles during motility, as suggested by structural studies of the adhesive domains (Song et al. 2012).

TRAP is the founding member of a larger family of TRAP-like adhesins, and sporozoites express two additional members, TRAP-like protein (TLP) and TREP/S6/UOS3. Ablation of these genes revealed a major function for

TREP during sporozoite invasion of salivary glands (Combe et al. 2009; Steinbüchel and Matuschewski 2009) and a role for TLP during migration in the skin (Moreira et al. 2008; Hegge et al. 2010a; Hellmann et al. 2011). Replacing the cytoplasmic tail of TRAP with that of TLP showed that sporozoites expressing this hybrid protein could still move, albeit not as efficiently as wild-type sporozoites (Heiss et al. 2008). This result suggests that the cytoplasmic tails of TRAP and TLP bind to the same protein(s) but possibly with different affinities. TRAP family proteins are trafficked to and stored within micronemes and released to the surface on activation of sporozoites (Gantt et al. 2000; Carey et al. 2014). Sporozoites can be activated by serum albumin (Vanderberg 1974) or small ligands (Perschmann et al. 2011), which leads to an increase in intracellular calcium followed by exocytosis of TRAP (Carey et al. 2014). Strikingly, only a small percentage of the total amount of TRAP family proteins is on the surface of activated sporozoites (Gantt et al. 2000), and it appears that their number is limited for efficient migration (Perschmann et al. 2011). This scarceness of TRAP family proteins makes investigation of their role in motility using classic GFP tagging and microscopy localization approaches a formidable challenge.

Actin filaments are moved by myosin motors in most examined cells and such is the case also in *Plasmodium*. Myosin is anchored to the inner membrane complex (IMC), a flattened organelle that subtends the plasma membrane of apicomplexan parasites at a close distance of ~30 nm in sporozoites (Fig. 4C). Myosin is likely also connected across the IMC to the subpellicular network, which gives the sporozoite its shape (Khater et al. 2004; Kudryashev et al. 2012). The subpellicular network can be considered to be a rigid structure that provides a counterforce for the moving myosin. Thus, myosin can push actin filaments toward the back of a sporozoite, and when TRAP family adhesins are connected to the filaments the adhesins are pushed back simultaneously. This retrograde flow can be indirectly seen by the motion of tissue debris or small microspheres attached to

activated sporozoites (Münter et al. 2009; Quadt et al. 2016). When sporozoites are attached to a rigid substrate they move forward by the same mechanism of force and counterforce.

Yet, actin filaments are elusive structures in sporozoites. Unlike actin in metazoan cells, which forms long filaments, *Plasmodium* actin filaments are short and feature a highly dynamic turnover (Schmitz et al. 2005; Schüler et al. 2005). This dynamic turnover is mediated by a number of actin-binding proteins (Sattler et al. 2011) and is also built into the structure of *Plasmodium* actin itself (Skillman et al. 2011; Vahokoski et al. 2014). Again, reverse genetic analysis has revealed some insight into which proteins are important in regulating actin dynamics in sporozoites. For example, sporozoites lacking a subunit of the heterodimeric actin filament capping protein (CP) moved in a similar fashion as *trap*⁻ sporozoites and also failed to enter salivary glands (Ganter et al. 2009). The resulting life-cycle arrest could only be rescued by both orthologous *P. falciparum* CP subunits, indicating distinct species-specific adaptations of microfilament regulation in sporozoites (Ganter et al. 2015). One basic open question is how actin filaments are oriented in the sporozoite. For directed forward motility, it is generally envisaged that actin filaments are aligned along the parasite long axis so that myosin motors can move them backward. The phenotypic back-and-forth movements of *trap*⁻ and *cp*⁻ sporozoites suggest that in these parasites the actin filaments might not be properly oriented thus leading to aberrant movement, but without direct visualization of the filaments this hypothesis remains conjecture.

Even if we were to understand the interplay between TRAP family adhesins and actin, the process of movement likely involves more players. TRAP itself is likely cleaved by an intramembrane protease of the rhomboid family and this cleavage is important to achieve continuous migration (Ejigiri et al. 2012). Moreover, an inhibitor of cysteine proteases is necessary for sporozoite motility, and *icp*⁻ sporozoites reproduce the life-cycle arrest observed in *trap*⁻-infected mosquitoes (Boysen and Matuschewski 2013; Lehmann et al. 2014).

Several *Plasmodium*-specific membrane proteins that do not belong to the TRAP family of adhesins, including SIAP-1/ag17/S5, S23/SSP3, PCRMP3, and PCRMP4, play critical roles in sporozoite transmission (Engelmann et al. 2009; Douradinha et al. 2011; Harupa et al. 2014), indicative of a complex and nonredundant protein network that mediates sporozoite–host interactions. Deletion of the small heat shock protein HSP20 also slowed motility, which showed the essential role of sporozoite migration in the skin, as *hsp20⁻* parasites still entered the salivary gland but moved at very low speed and could not migrate efficiently through the dermis (Montagna et al. 2012a,c). Considering the numbers of unexplored proteins present in sporozoites (Matuschewski et al. 2002b; Kaiser et al. 2004; Lasonder et al. 2008; Lindner et al. 2013a), it is likely that many of these will be important for migration, moving a complete understanding of this crucial and fascinating process a few decades into the future.

IN AND OUT OF CELLS: FROM GLIDING TO INVASION

During sporozoite migration the parasites need to pass through cells of the hosts to cross the barriers constituted by the salivary gland, the skin, and the liver (Fig. 5) (see online Movie 1 at perspectivesinmedicine.cshlp.org). To do so, the sporozoite uses CSP, TRAP, and other proteins that recognize target cells and allow sporozoites to pass them (Ishino et al. 2004, 2005).

The salivary gland surface is likely initially recognized by MAEBL (Kariu et al. 2002; Saenz et al. 2008). Thereafter, TRAP interacts specifically with the mosquito protein saglin to allow entry into the glands (Ghosh et al. 2009), a process so far only observed by electron microscopy (Sterling et al. 1973; Pimenta et al. 1994). These studies suggest that sporozoites form a tight junction with the acinar cells of the salivary gland on their way in and curiously "bud" out from the cells at the apical end facing the salivary cavities such that they are initially surrounded by a host cell membrane (Pimenta et al. 1994). How they shed this membrane and arrange in large nonmotile aggregates is not clear. Once in the skin, sporozoites pass through dermal cells by breaching their membranes as revealed by in vivo imaging of migrating sporozoites injected into mice along with a cell-wounding marker (Formaglio et al. 2014). This wounding phenomenon is clearly associated with the capacity of the sporozoite to migrate over long distances in the dermis because ablation of genes preventing cell wounding inhibits intradermal motility (Bhanot et al. 2005; Amino et al. 2008; Risco-Castillo et al. 2015).

It is currently not clear whether sporozoites also need to breach endothelial cells to enter the bloodstream but they clearly can do so when they move from the bloodstream toward the hepatocytes (Tavares et al. 2013). They can also enter through the liver resident macrophages called Kupffer cells (Baer et al. 2007). In both cases, sporozoites need their capacity to wound

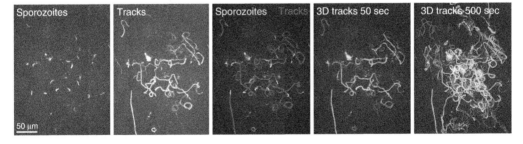

Figure 5. Sporozoite migration in vivo. Sporozoite migration after transmission into the dermis. Shown are sporozoites (white) (*far left*), the tracks of sporozoites migrating for 50 sec (*left*), sporozoites (yellow) at the start of the movie overlaid by the tracks (red) (*center*), and tracks over 50 sec (*right*) and 500 sec (*far right*) spatially color-coded such that red, green, and blue colors represent different confocal planes 10 μm apart. (Shots taken from movie courtesy of Rogerio Amino, Institut Pasteur, Paris.)

Cite this article as *Cold Spring Harb Perspect Med* doi: 10.1101/cshperspect.a025478

the cells to progress toward hepatocytes. Even when they reach hepatocytes they continue to wound several cells before settling in a last hepatocyte (Mota et al. 2001; Frevert et al. 2005).

Two competing models aim at explaining how a sporozoite finally productively infects a hepatocyte. The first model suggests that specific signaling occurs to "prepare" the sporozoite for entry (Mota et al. 2002), whereas the second one suggests a switch of the sporozoite from a generic "wounding and transmigration" mode to an invasion mode (Amino et al. 2008). In the first model, the host cells play a role in providing a signal to the sporozoite. The second model suggests a stochastic process that stipulates that the number of proteins needed for transmigration is limited and that once they have been used up the sporozoite will settle in whichever cell is the next on its path. Experiments suggest that both mechanisms might play a role. The lack of one of the major proteins needed for transmigration, termed SPECT, causes sporozoites to invade and develop within fibroblasts in the dermis (Amino et al. 2008; Gueirard et al. 2010). Hence, it is clear that in the absence of SPECT no further signal is required to a full invasion mode, which apparently is the default activity of sporozoites. However, this does not rule out that in the presence of SPECT additional regulatory processes also play a role. One such process could be the sensing by the sporozoite of the higher potassium concentration within cells than in the extracellular medium (Kumar et al. 2007; Ono et al. 2008). High potassium buffers have been shown to increase the intracellular cAMP concentration, which causes increased intracellular Ca^{2+} concentrations followed by exocytosis of micronemes. This brings more TRAP onto the surface of sporozoites, arrests their motility, and leads to more invasion (Ono et al. 2008). Also, as described above, the processing of CSP on contact to highly sulfated proteoglycans was shown to switch the sporozoite toward an invasive mode (Coppi et al. 2011). Thus, a stepwise process involving first CSP processing followed by potassium signaling might, among others, contribute to sporozoite invasion.

Intriguingly, we still do not know the receptor–ligand pairs involved in the formation of a tight junction that appears to be essential for host cell invasion in *Plasmodium* and related parasites and thus possibly also in sporozoite invasion of hepatocytes. TRAP and AMA-1 on the sporozoite appear to be involved (Matuschewski et al. 2002a; Silvie et al. 2004). On the host cell side, several proteins have been suggested to be important for invasion including fetuin (Jethwaney et al. 2005), CD81 (Silvie et al. 2003; Risco-Castillo et al. 2014), and CD68 (Cha et al. 2015). Although fetuin might directly interact with TRAP, the roles of CD81 and CD68 are likely more complex as no direct interaction with a sporozoite protein could be shown yet.

Once in the host cells, the sporozoite rapidly dedifferentiates, not undetected by the host. During this dedifferentiation, the IMC and the subpellicular network disassemble leading to a round parasite. Curiously, a similar rounding up of sporozoites can be detected in vitro in the absence of host cells (Kaiser et al. 2003; Hegge et al. 2010b). This transformation program is initiated prematurely in salivary gland sporozoites that lack *UIS1/IK2*, a sporozoite-specific protein kinase (Zhang et al. 2010), or *PUF2*, which encodes an RNA-binding protein (Gomes-Santos et al. 2011; Müller et al. 2011; Lindner et al. 2013b). Sporozoites transcribe and store mRNAs that encode proteins required for liver-stage development. For instance, translational repression of *UIS4*, encoding an essential component of the liver-stage parasitophorous vacuolar membrane, is important for sporozoite infectivity and subsequent stage conversion (Silvie et al. 2014). Deciphering the entire signaling network that controls translational repression and sporozoite latency is central to a better understanding of the host switch between the insect and mammalian hosts.

PERSPECTIVES

Considering the potential medical application of whole sporozoite vaccination, it would be a fundamental progress if initial results of axenic sporozoite cultures (Warburg and Miller 1992;

Warburg and Schneider 1993; Al-Olayan et al. 2002; Porter-Kelley et al. 2006) could be substantially improved to allow mass production of sporozoites without the need for mosquito colonies. Especially, if this could be applied to the different human infective parasite species research on the sporozoite would be boosted to new heights, as the parasite would become workable without the need of running an insectary, which for the case of human parasites needs to be in a costly biosafety environment. Furthermore, one of the black boxes of sporozoite biology concerns its interaction with the salivary gland. Also, this would be pushed forward if it were possible to culture salivary glands in vitro for extended periods or generate stable cell lines from the terminally differentiated salivary gland cells, which clearly is no minor task. Furthermore, most in vitro assays currently used to investigate the sporozoite are not considering the flow of the blood, so incorporating microfluidic devices into sporozoite research also promises a molecular and biophysical understanding of the key interactions that arrest the sporozoite at the liver.

Last, the field would benefit from standardized in vitro liver culture systems that would allow higher throughput research on the fascinating sporozoite liver cell interaction, which could lead to the discovery of the molecular mechanism of sporozoite liver cell entry. Ideally, such a culture system would also include other liver cells with which the sporozoite interacts such as endothelial and immune cells to retrace and dissect its journey into the liver. Such functional assays would then also require a higher computerized image data throughput, which should not be the bottleneck considering the progress in imaging techniques in other fields. Such a set of new assay systems would be valuable for investigating innovative approaches to stop the sporozoite, which might ultimately contribute to control malaria.

CONCLUDING REMARKS

The *Plasmodium* sporozoite constitutes the first form of the malaria parasite entering the human body and, hence, provides the first and leading targets to control an infection. Only few ($\sim$10–100) sporozoites are injected by infected mosquitoes, suggesting that they form excellent intervention targets. Nonetheless, it might be particularly challenging to eliminate every one of these few individuals, because a single sporozoite breakthrough will initiate a fulminant blood infection. Sporozoites could be targeted by small molecules and/or antibodies by either stopping the rapid migration and liver entry of sporozoites or direct killing. Yet, intervention programs focusing on sporozoites remain scarce and underexplored. Antibodies against the major surface protein CSP have been shown to prevent a detectable blood infection under experimental conditions. However, the clinical trials results of RTS,S/AS01 were unsatisfactory and failed to prevent the occurrence of natural infections. The search for new sporozoite antigens and a better understanding of the molecular mechanisms that drive sporozoite motility and liver cell entry are expected to yield previously unrecognized targets that could turn into urgently needed control measures.

ACKNOWLEDGMENTS

We thank Ross Douglas and Alyssa Ingmundson for comments on the manuscript.

REFERENCES

Aldrich C, Magini A, Emiliani C, Dottorini T, Bistoni F, Crisanti A, Spaccapelo R. 2012. Roles of the amino terminal region and repeat region of the *Plasmodium berghei* circumsporozoite protein in parasite infectivity. *PLoS ONE* 7: e32524.

Al-Olayan AM, Beetsma AL, Butcher GA, Sinden RE, Hurd H. 2002. Complete development of mosquito phases of malaria parasite in vitro. *Science* 295: 677–679.

Aly AS, Matuschewski K. 2005. A malarial cysteine protease is necessary for *Plasmodium* sporozoite egress from oocysts. *J Exp Med* 202: 225–230.

Amino R, Thiberge S, Martin B, Celli S, Shorte S, Frischknecht F, Ménard R. 2006. Quantitative imaging of *Plasmodium* transmission from mosquito to mammal. *Nat Med* 12: 220–224.

Amino R, Giovannini D, Thiberge S, Gueirard P, Boisson B, Dubremetz JF, Prévost MC, Ishino T, Yuda M, Ménard R. 2008. Host cell traversal is important for progression of the malaria parasite through the dermis to the liver. *Cell Host Microbe* 3: 88–96.

Cite this article as *Cold Spring Harb Perspect Med* doi: 10.1101/cshperspect.a025478

Ayala SC. 1971. Sporogony and experimental transmission of *Plasmodium mexicanum*. *J Parasitol* **57:** 598–602.

Baer K, Roosevelt M, Clarkson AB Jr, Van Rooijen N, Schnieder T, Frevert U. 2007. Kupffer cells are obligatory for *Plasmodium yoelii* sporozoite infection of the liver. *Cell Microbiol* **9:** 397–412.

Beier JC. 1998. Malaria parasite development in mosquitoes. *Annu Rev Entomol* **43:** 519–543.

Bhanot P, Schauer K, Coppens I, Nussenzweig V. 2005. A surface phospholipase is involved in the migration of *Plasmodium* sporozoites through cells. *J Biol Chem* **280:** 6752–6760.

Boysen K, Matuschewski K. 2013. Inhibitor of cysteine proteases is critical for motility and infectivity of *Plasmodium* sporozoites. *mBio* **4:** e00874–13

Carey AF, Singer M, Bargieri D, Thiberge S, Frischknecht F, Ménard R, Amino R. 2014. Calcium dynamics of *Plasmodium berghei* sporozoite motility. *Cell Microbiol* **16:** 768–783.

Cerami C, Frevert U, Sinnis U, Takacs B, Clavijo P, Santos MJ, Nussenzweig V. 1992. The basolateral domain of the hepatocyte plasma membrane bears receptors for the circumsporozoite protein of *Plasmodium falciparum* sporozoites. *Cell* **70:** 1021–1033.

Cha SJ, Park K, Srinivasan P, Schindler CW, van Rooijen N, Stins M, Jacobs-Lorena M. 2015. CD68 acts as a major gateway for malaria sporozoite liver infection. *J Exp Med* **212:** 1391–1403.

Clyde DF, Most H, McCarthy VC, Vanderberg JP. 1973. Immunization of man against sporozoite-induced falciparum malaria. *Am J Med Sci* **266:** 169–177.

Cohen J, Nussenzweig V, Vekemans J, Leach A. 2010. From the circumsporozoite protein to the RTS,S/AS candidate vaccine. *Hum Vacc* **6:** 90–96.

Combe A, Moreira C, Ackerman S, Thiberge S, Templeton TJ, Ménard R. 2009. TREP, a novel protein necessary for gliding motility of the malaria sporozoite. *Int J Parasitol* **39:** 489–496.

Coppi A, Natarajan R, Pradel G, Bennett BL, James ER, Roggero MA, Corradin G, Persson C, Tewari R, Sinnis P. 2011. The malaria circumsporozoite protein has two functional domains, each with distinct roles as sporozoites journey from mosquito to mammalian host. *J Exp Med* **208:** 341–356.

Dame JB, Williams JL, McCutchan TF, Weber JL, Wirtz RA, Hockmeyer WT, Maloy L, Heynes JD, Scheider I, Roberts D, et al. 1984. Structure of the gene encoding the immunodominant surface antigen on the sporozoite of the human malaria parasite *Plasmodium falciparum*. *Science* **225:** 593–599.

Douglas RG, Amino R, Sinnis P, Frischknecht F. 2015. Active migration and passive transport of malaria parasites. *Trends Parasitol* **31:** 357–362.

Douradinha B, Augustijn KD, Moore SG, Ramesar J, Mota MM, Waters AP, Janse CJ, Thompson J. 2011. *Plasmodium* cysteine repeat modular proteins 3 and 4 are essential for malaria parasite transmission from the mosquito to the host. *Malar J* **10:** 71.

Ejigiri I, Ragheb DR, Pino P, Coppi A, Bennett BL, Soldati-Favre D, Sinnis P. 2012. Shedding of TRAP by a rhomboid protease from the malaria sporozoite surface is essential for gliding motility and sporozoite infectivity. *PLoS Pathog* **8:** e1002725.

Enea V, Ellis J, Zavala F, Arnot DE, Asavanich A, Masuda A, Quakyi I, Nussenzweig RS. 1984. DNA cloning of *Plasmodium falciparum* circumsporozoite gene: Amino acid sequence of repetitive epitope. *Science* **225:** 628–630.

Engelmann S, Silvie O, Matuschewski K. 2009. Disruption of *Plasmodium* sporozoite transmission by depletion of sporozoite invasion-associated protein 1. *Eukaryot Cell* **8:** 640–648.

Espinosa DA, Yadava A, Angov E, Maurizio PL, Ockenhouse CF, Zavala F. 2013. Development of a chimeric *Plasmodium berghei* strain expressing the repeat region of *P. vivax* circumsporozoite protein for in vivo evaluation of vaccine efficacy. *Infect Immun* **81:** 2882–2887.

Espinosa DA, Gutierrez GM, Rojas-López M, Noe AR, Shi L, Tse SW, Sinnis P, Zavala F. 2015. Proteolytic cleavage of the *Plasmodium falciparum* circumsporozoite protein is a target of protective antibodies. *J Infect Dis* **212:** 1111–1119.

Formaglio P, Tavares J, Ménard R, Amino R. 2014. Loss of host cell plasma membrane integrity following cell traversal by *Plasmodium* sporozoites in the skin. *Parasitol Int* **63:** 237–244.

Frevert U, Sinnis P, Cerami C, Shreffler W, Takacs B, Nussenzweig V. 1993. Malaria circumsporozoite protein binds to heparin sulfate proteoglycans associated with the surface membrane of hepatocytes. *J Exp Med* **177:** 1287–1298.

Frevert U, Engelmann S, Zougbédé S, Stange J, Ng B, Matuschewski K, Liebes L, Yee H. 2005. Intravital observation of *Plasmodium berghei* sporozoite infection of the liver. *PLoS Biol* **3:** e192.

Frischknecht F, Baldacci P, Martin B, Zimmer C, Thiberge S, Olivo-Marin JC, Shorte SL, Ménard R. 2004. Imaging movement of malaria parasites during transmission by *Anopheles* mosquitoes. *Cell Microbiol* **6:** 687–694.

Ganter M, Schüler H, Matuschewski K. 2009. Vital role for the *Plasmodium* actin capping protein (CP) β-subunit in motility of malaria sporozoites. *Mol Microbiol* **74:** 1356–1367.

Ganter M, Rizopoulos Z, Schüler H, Matuschewski K. 2015. Pivotal and distinct role for *Plasmodium* capping protein α during blood infection of the malaria parasite. *Mol Microbiol* **96:** 84–94.

Gantt S, Persson C, Rose K, Birkett AJ, Abagyan R, Nussenzweig V. 2000. Antibodies to TRAP do not inhibit *Plasmodium* sporozoite infectivity in vivo. *Infect Immun* **68:** 3667–3673.

Ghosh AK, Devenport M, Jethwaney D, Kalume DE, Pandey A, Anderson VE, Sultan AA, Kumar N, Jacobs-Lorena M. 2009. Malaria parasite invasion of the mosquito salivary gland requires interaction between the *Plasmodium* TRAP and the *Anopheles* saglin proteins. *PLoS Pathog* **5:** e1000265.

Gomes-Santos CS, Braks J, Prudêncio M, Carret C, Gomes AR, Pain A, Feltwell T, Khan S, Waters A, Janse C, et al. 2011. Transition of *Plasmodium* sporozoites into liver stage-like forms is regulated by the RNA binding protein Pumilio. *PLoS Pathog* **7:** e1002046.

Gueirard P, Tavares J, Thiberge S, Bernex F, Ishino T, Milon G, Franke-Fayard B, Janse CJ, Ménard R, Amino R. 2010.

Development of the malaria parasite in the skin of the mammalian host. *Proc Natl Acad Sci* **107:** 18640–18645.

Hafalla JC, Silvie O, Matuschewski K. 2011. Cell biology and immunology of malaria. *Immun Rev* **240:** 297–316.

Hafalla JCR, Bauza K, Friesen J, Gonzalez-Aseguinolaza G, Hill AVS, Matuschewski K. 2013. Identification of targets of CD8+ T cell responses to malaria liver stages by genome-wide epitope profiling. *PLoS Pathog* **9:** e1003303.

Harupa A, Sack BK, Lakshmanan V, Arang N, Douglass AN, Oliver BG, Stuart AB, Sather DN, Lindner SE, Hybiske K, et al. 2014. SSP3 is a novel *Plasmodium yoelii* sporozoite surface protein with a role in gliding motility. *Infect Immun* **82:** 4643–4653.

Hegge S, Münter S, Steinbüchel M, Heiss K, Engel U, Matuschewski K, Frischknecht F. 2010a. Multistep adhesion of *Plasmodium* sporozoites. *FASEB J* **24:** 2222–2234.

Hegge S, Kudryashev M, Barniol L, Frischknecht F. 2010b. Key factors regulating *Plasmodium berghei* sporozoite survival and transformation revealed by an automated visual assay. *FASEB J* **24:** 5003–5012.

Heiss K, Nie H, Kumar S, Daly TM, Bergman LW, Matuschewski K. 2008. Functional characterization of a redundant *Plasmodium* TRAP family invasin, TRAP-like protein, by aldolase binding and a genetic complementation test. *Eukaryot Cell* **7:** 1062–1070.

Hellmann JK, Münter S, Kudryashev M, Schulz S, Heiss K, Müller AK, Matuschewski K, Spatz JP, Schwarz US, Frischknecht F. 2011. Environmental constrains guide migration of malaria parasites during transmission. *PLoS Pathog* **7:** e1002080.

Ishino T, Yano K, Chinzei Y, Yuda M. 2004. Cell-passage activity is required for the malaria parasite to cross the liver sinusoidal cell layer. *PLoS Biol* **2:** e4.

Ishino T, Chinzei Y, Yuda M. 2005. A *Plasmodium* sporozoite protein with a membrane attack complex domain is required for breaching the liver sinusoidal cell layer prior to hepatocyte infection. *Cell Microbiol* **7:** 199–208.

Jethwaney D, Lepore T, Hassan S, Mello K, Rangarajan R, Jahnen-Dechent W, Wirth D, Sultan AA. 2005. Fetuin-A, a hepatocyte-specific protein that binds *Plasmodium berghei* thrombospondin-related adhesive protein: A potential role in infectivity. *Infect Immun* **73:** 5883–5891.

Kaiser K, Camargo N, Kappe SH. 2003. Transformation of sporozoites into early exoerythrocytic malaria parasites does not require host cells. *J Exp Med* **197:** 1045–1050.

Kaiser K, Matuschewski K, Camargo N, Ross J, Kappe SHI. 2004. Differential transcriptome profiling identifies *Plasmodium* genes encoding pre-erythrocytic stage-specific proteins. *Mol Microbiol* **51:** 1221–1232.

Kan A, Tan YH, Angrisano F, Hanssen E, Rogers KL, Whitehead L, Mollard VP, Cozijnsen S, Sinden RE, McFadden GI, et al. 2014. Quantitative analysis of *Plasmodium* ookinete motion in three dimensions suggests a critical role for cell shape in the biomechanics of malaria parasite gliding locomotion. *Cell Microbiol* **16:** 734–750.

Kappe S, Bruderer T, Gantt S, Fujioka H, Nussenzweig V, Ménard R. 1999. Conservation of a gliding motility and cell invasion machinery in Apicomplexan parasites. *J Cell Biol* **147:** 937–944.

Kariu T, Yuda M, Yano K, Chnizei Y. 2002. MAEBL is essential for malaria sporozoite infection of the mosquito salivary gland. *J Exp Med* **195:** 1317–1323.

Kebaier C, Vanderberg JP. 2006. Re-ingestion of *Plasmodium berghei* sporozoites after delivery into the host by mosquitoes. *Am J Trop Med Hyg* **75:** 1200–1204.

Khater EI, Sinden RE, Dessens JT. 2004. A malaria membrane skeletal protein is essential for normal morphogenesis, motility, and infectivity of sporozoites. *J Cell Biol* **167:** 425–432.

Kudryashev M, Münter S, Lemgruber L, Montagna G, Stahlberg H, Matuschewski K, Meissner M, Cyrklaff M, Frischknecht F. 2012. Structural basis for chirality and directional motility of *Plasmodium* sporozoites. *Cell Microbiol* **14:** 1757–1768.

Kumar KA, Garcia CR, Chandran VR, van Roojen N, Zhou Y, Winzeler E, Nusssenzweig V. 2007. Exposure of *Plasmodium* sporozoites to the intracellular concentration of potassium enhances infectivity and reduces cell passage activity. *Mol Biochem Parasitol* **156:** 32–40.

Lakshmanan V, Fishbaugher ME, Morrison B, Baldwin M, Macarulay M, Vaughan AM, Mikolajczak SA, Kappe SH. 2015. Cyclic GMP balance is critical for malaria parasite transmission from the mosquito to the mammalian host. *mBio* **17:** e02330.

Lasonder E, Janse CJ, van Gemert GJ, Mair GR, Vermunt AM, Douradinha BG, van Noort V, Huynen MA, Luty AJ, Kroeze H, et al. 2008. Proteomic profiling of *Plasmodium* sporozoite maturation identifies new proteins essential for parasite development and infectivity. *PLoS Pathog* **4:** e1000195.

Lehmann C, Heitmann A, Mishra S, Burda PC, Singer M, Prado M, Niklaus L, Lacroix C, Ménard R, Frischknecht F, et al. 2014. A cysteine protease inhibitor of *Plasmodium berghei* is essential for exo-erythrocytic development. *PLoS Pathog* **10:** e1004336.

Lindner SE, Swearingen KE, Harupa A, Vaughan AM, Sinnis P, Moritz RL, Kappe SH. 2013a. Total and putative surface proteomics of malaria parasite salivary gland sporozoites. *Mol Cell Proteomics* **12:** 1127–1143.

Lindner SE, Mikolajczak SA, Vaughan AM, Moon W, Joyce BR, Sullivan WJ Jr, Kappe SH. 2013b. Perturbations of *Plasmodium* Puf2 expression and RNA-seq of Puf2-deficient sporozoites reveal a critical role in maintaining RNA homeostasis and parasite transmissibility. *Cell Microbiol* **15:** 1266–1283.

Matsuoka H, Yoshida S, Hirai M, Ishii A. 2002. A rodent malaria, *Plasmodium berghei*, is experimentally transmitted to mice by merely probing of infective mosquito, *Anopheles stephensi*. *Parasitol Int* **51:** 17–23.

Matuschewski K, Nunes AC, Nussenzweig V, Ménard R. 2002a. *Plasmodium* sporozoite invasion of insect and mammalian cells is directed by the same dual binding system. *EMBO J.* **21:** 1597–1606.

Matuschewski K, Ross J, Brown S, Kaiser K, Nussenzweig V, Kappe SHI. 2002b. Infectivity-associated changes in the transcriptional repertoire of the malaria parasite sporozoite stage. *J Biol Chem* **277:** 41948–41953.

Ménard R, Sultan AA, Cortes C, Altszuler R, van Dijk MR, Janse CJ, Waters AP, Nussenzweig RS, Nussenzweig V. 1997. Circumsporozoite protein is required for development of malaria sporozoites in mosquitoes. *Nature* **385**: 336–340.

Montagna GN, Buscaglia CA, Münter S, Goosmann C, Frischknecht F, Brinkmann V, Matuschewski K. 2012a. Critical role for heat shock protein 20 (HSP20) in migration of malarial sporozoites. *J Biol Chem* **287**: 2410–2422.

Montagna GN, Matuschewski K, Buscaglia CA. 2012b. *Plasmodium* sporozoite motility: An update. *Front Biosci* **17**: 726–744.

Montagna GN, Matuschewski K, Buscaglia CA. 2012c. Small heat shock proteins in cellular adhesion and migration. *Cell Adh Migr* **6**: 78–84.

Moreira CK, Templeton TJ, Lazavec C, Haward RE, Hobbs CV, Kroeze H, Janse CJ, Waters AP, Sinnis P, Coppi A. 2008. The *Plasmodium* TRAP/MIC2 family member, TRAP-like protein (TLP), is involved in tissue traversal by sporozoites. *Cell Microbiol* **10**: 1505–1516.

Mota MM, Pradel G, Vanderberg JP, Hafalla JC, Frevert U, Nussenzweig RS, Nussenzweig V, Rodriguez A. 2001. Migration of *Plasmodium* sporozoites through cells before infection. *Science* **291**: 141–144.

Mota MM, Hafalla JC, Rodriguez A. 2002. Migration through host cells activates *Plasmodium* sporozoites for infection. *Nat Med* **8**: 1318–1322.

Müller K, Matuschewski K, Silvie O. 2011. The Puf-family RNA-binding protein Puf2 controls sporozoite conversion to liver stages in the malaria parasite. *PLoS ONE* **6**: e19860.

Münter S, Sabass B, Selhuber-Unkel C, Kudryashev M, Hegge S, Engel U, Spatz JP, Matuschewski K, Schwarz US, Frischknecht F. 2009. Malaria parasite motility is limited by turnover of discrete adhesion sites. *Cell Host Microbe* **6**: 551–562.

Offeddu V, Thathy V, Marsh K, Matuschewski K. 2012. Naturally acquired immune responses against *Plasmodium falciparum* sporozoites and liver infection. *Int J Parasitol* **42**: 535–548.

Ono T, Cabrita-Santos L, Leitao R, Bettiol E, Purcell LA, Diaz-Pulido O, Andrews LB, Tadakuma T, Bhanot P, Mota MM, et al. 2008. Adenyl cyclase α and cAMP signaling mediate *Plasmodium* sporozoite apical regulated exocytosis and hepatocyte infection. *PLoS Pathog* **4**: e1000008.

Perkins SL. 2014. Malaria's many mates: Past, present, and future of the systematics of the order Haemosporida. *J Parasitol* **100**: 11–25.

Perschmann N, Hellmann JK, Frischknecht F, Spatz JP. 2011. Induction of malaria parasite migration by synthetically tunable microenvironments. *Nano Lett* **11**: 4468–4474.

Persson C, Oliveira GA, Sultan AA, Bhanot P, Nussenzweig V, Nardin E. 2002. Cutting edge: A new tool to evaluate human pre-erythrocytic malaria vaccines: Rodent parasites bearing a hybrid *Plasmodium falciparum* circumsporozoite protein. *J Immunol* **169**: 6681–6685.

Pimenta PF, Touray M, Miller L. 1994. The journey of malaria sporozoites in the mosquito salivary gland. *J Euk Microbiol* **41**: 608–624.

Porter-Kelley JM, Dinglasan RR, Alam U, Ndeta GA, Sacci JB Jr, Azad AF. 2006. *Plasmodium yoelii*: Axenic develop-ment of the parasite mosquito stages. *Exp Parasitol* **112**: 99–108.

Prudêncio M, Rodriguez A, Mota MM. 2006. The silent path to thousands of merozoites: The *Plasmodium* liver stage. *Nat Rev Microbiol* **4**: 849–856.

Quadt KA, Streichfuss M, Moreau CA, Spatz JP, Frischknecht F. 2016. Coupling of retrograde flow to force production during malaria parasite migration. *ACS Nano* **10**: 2091–2102.

Risco-Castillo V, Topçu S, Son O, Briquet S, Manzoni G, Silvie O. 2014. CD81 is required for rhoptry discharge during host cell invasion by *Plasmodium yoelii* sporozoites. *Cell Microbiol* **16**: 1533–1548.

Risco-Castillo V, Topçu S, Marinach C, Manzoni G, Bigorgne AE, Briquet S, Baudin X, Lebrun M, Dubremetz JF, Silvie O. 2015. Malaria sporozoite traverse host cells with transient vacuoles. *Cell Host Microbe* **18**: 593–603.

RTS,S Clinical Trials Partnership. 2015. Efficacy and safety of RTS,S/AS01 malaria vaccine with or without final booster in infants and children in Africa: Final results of a phase 3, individually randomised, controlled trial. *Lancet* **386**: 31–45.

Saenz FE, Balu B, Smith J, Mendonca SR, Adams JH. 2008. The transmembrane isoform of *Plasmodium falciparum* MAEBL is essential for the invasion of *Anopheles* salivary glands. *PLoS ONE* **3**: e2287.

Sato Y, Montagna GN, Matuschewski K. 2014. *Plasmodium berghei* sporozoites acquire virulence and immunogenicity during mosquito hemocoel transit. *Infect Immun* **82**: 1164–1172.

Sattler JM, Ganter M, Hliscs M, Matuschewski K, Schüler H. 2011. Actin regulation in the malaria parasite. *Eur J Cell Biol* **90**: 966–971.

Schmitz S, Grainger M, Howell S, Calder LJ, Gaeb M, Pinder JC, Holder AA, Veigel C. 2005. Malaria parasite actin filaments are very short. *J Mol Biol* **349**: 113–125.

Schofield L. 1990. The circumsporozoite protein of *Plasmodium*: A mechanism of immune evasion by the malaria parasite? *Bull WHO* **68**: 66–73.

Schüler H, Mueller AK, Matuschewski K. 2005. Unusual properties of *Plasmodium falciparum* actin: New insights into microfilament dynamics of apicomplexan parasites. *FEBS Lett* **579**: 655–660.

Shortt HE. 1948. The life cycle of *Plasmodium cynomolgi* in its insect and mammalian hosts. *Trans R Soc Med Hyg* **42**: 227–230.

Shute PG. 1943. Successful transmission of human malaria with sporozoites which have not come into contact with the salivary glands of the insect host. *J Trop Med Hyg* **46**: 57–58.

Sidjanski S, Vanderberg JP. 1997. Delayed migration of *Plasmodium* sporozoites from the mosquito bite site to the blood. *Am J Trop Med Hyg* **57**: 426–429.

Sidjanski S, Vanderberg JP, Sinnis P. 1997. *Anopheles stephensi* salivary glands bear receptors for region I of circumsporozoite protein of *Plasmodium falciparum*. *Mol Biochem Parasitol* **90**: 33–41.

Silvie O, Rubinstein E, Franetich JF, Prenant M, Belnoue E, Rénia L, Hannoun L, Eling W, Levy S, Boucheix C, et al. 2003. Hepatocyte CD81 is required for *Plasmodium fal*-

ciparum and *Plasmodium yoelii* sporozoite infectivity. *Nat Med* **9**: 93–96.

Silvie O, Franetich JF, Charrin S, Mueller MS, Siau A, Bodescout M, Rubinstein E, Hannoun L, Charoenvit Y, Kocken CH, et al. 2004. A role for apical membrane antigen 1 during invasion of hepatocytes by *Plasmodium falciparum* sporozoites. *J Biol Chem* **279**: 9490–9496.

Silvie O, Briquet S, Müller K, Manzoni G, Matuschewski K. 2014. Post-transcriptional silencing of *UIS4* in *Plasmodium berghei* sporozoites is important for host switch. *Mol Microbiol* **91**: 1200–1213.

Sinnis P, Nardin E. 2002. Sporozoite antigens: Biology and immunology of the circumsporozoite protein and thrombospondin-related anonymous protein. *Chem Immunol* **80**: 70–96.

Skillman KM, Diraviyam K, Khan A, Tang K, Sept D, Sibley LD. 2011. Evolutionary divergent, unstable filamentous actin is essential for gliding motility in apicomplexan parasites. *PLoS Pathog* **7**: e1002280.

Song G, Koksal AC, Lu C, Springer TA. 2012. Shape change in the receptor for gliding motility in *Plasmodium* sporozoites. *Proc Natl Acad Sci* **109**: 21420–21425.

Steinbüchel M, Matuschewski K. 2009. Role for the *Plasmodium* sporozoite-specific transmembrane protein S6 in parasite motility and efficient malaria transmission. *Cell Microbiol* **11**: 279–288.

Sterling CR, Aikawa M, Vanderberg JP. 1973. The passage of *Plasmodium berghei* sporozoites through the salivary glands of *Anopheles stephensi*: An electronmicroscopic study. *J Parasitol* **59**: 593–605.

Stewart MJ, Vanderberg JP. 1991. Malaria sporozoites release circumsporozoite protein from their apical end and translocate it along their surface. *J Protozool* **38**: 411–421.

Sultan AA, Thathy V, Frevert U, Robson KJ, Crisanti A, Nussenzweig V. 1997. TRAP is necessary for gliding motility and infectivity of *Plasmodium* sporozoites. *Cell* **90**: 511–522.

Tavares J, Formaglio P, Thiberge S, Mordelet E, Van Rooijen N, Medvinsky A, Ménard R, Amino R. 2013. Role of host cell traversal by the malaria sporozoite during liver infection. *J Exp Med* **210**: 905–915.

Tewari R, Spaccapelo R, Bistoni F, Holder AA, Crisanti A. 2002. Function of region I and II adhesive motifs of *Plasmodium falciparum* circumsporozoite protein in sporo-

zoite motility and infectivity. *J Biol Chem* **277**: 47613–47618.

Thathy V, Fujioka H, Gantt S, Nussenzweig R, Nussenzweig V, Ménard R. 2002. Levels of circumsporozoite protein in the *Plasmodium* oocyst determine sporozoite morphology. *EMBO J* **21**: 1586–1596.

Vahokoski J, Bhargav SP, Desfosses A, Andreadaki M, Kumpula EP, Martinez SM, Ignatev A, Lepper S, Frischknecht F, Sidén-Kiamos, et al. 2014. Structural differences explain diverse functions of *Plasmodium* actins. *PLoS Pathog* **10**: e1004091.

Vanderberg JP. 1974. Studies on the motility of *Plasmodium* sporozoites. *J Protozool* **21**: 527–537.

Vanderberg JP. 1975. Development of infectivity by the *Plasmodium berghei* sporozoite. *J Parasitol* **61**: 43–50.

Vanderberg JP, Frevert U. 2004. Intravital microscopy demonstrating antibody-mediated immobilisation of *Plasmodium berghei* sporozoites injected into skin by mosquitoes. *Int J Parasitol* **34**: 991–996.

Wang Q, Fujioka H, Nussenzweig V. 2005. Exit of *Plasmodium* sporozoites from oocysts is an active process that involves the circumsporozoite protein. *PLoS Pathog* **1**: e9.

Warburg A, Miller LH. 1992. Sporogonic development of a malaria parasite in vitro. *Science* **255**: 448–450.

Warburg A, Schneider I. 1993. In vitro culture of the mosquito stages of *Plasmodium falciparum*. *Exp Parasitol* **76**:121–126.

Wengelnik K, Spaccapelo R, Naitza S, Robson KJ, Janse CJ, Bistoni F, Waters AP, Crisanti A. 1999. The A-domain and thrombospondin-related motif of *Plasmodium falciparum* TRAP are implicated in the invasion process of mosquito salivary glands. *EMBO J* **18**: 5195–5204.

Zhang M, Fennell C, Ranford-Cartwright L, Sakthivel R, Gueirard P, Meister S, Caspi A, Doerig C, Nussenzweig RS, Tuteja N, et al. 2010. The *Plasmodium* eukaryotic initiation factor-2alpha kinase IK2 controls the latency of sporozoites in the mosquito salivary glands. *J Exp Med* **207**: 1465–1474.

Zhang M, Kaneko I, Tsao T, Mitchell R, Nardin EH, Iwanaga S, Yuda M, Tsuji M. 2016. A highly infectious *Plasmodium yoelii* parasite, bearing *Plasmodium falciparum* circumsporozoite protein. *Malaria J* **15**: 201.

Cite this article as *Cold Spring Harb Perspect Med* doi: 10.1101/cshperspect.a025478

Malaria Parasite Liver Infection and Exoerythrocytic Biology

Ashley M. Vaughan[1] and Stefan H.I. Kappe[1,2]

[1]Center for Infectious Disease Research, formerly Seattle Biomedical Research Institute, Seattle, Washington 98109

[2]Department of Global Health, University of Washington, Seattle, Washington 98195

Correspondence: stefan.kappe@cidresearch.org

In their infection cycle, malaria parasites undergo replication and population expansions within the vertebrate host and the mosquito vector. Host infection initiates with sporozoite invasion of hepatocytes, followed by a dramatic parasite amplification event during liver stage parasite growth and replication within hepatocytes. Each liver stage forms up to 90,000 exoerythrocytic merozoites, which are in turn capable of initiating a blood stage infection. Liver stages not only exploit host hepatocyte resources for nutritional needs but also endeavor to prevent hepatocyte cell death and detection by the host's immune system. Research over the past decade has identified numerous parasite factors that play a critical role during liver infection and has started to delineate a complex web of parasite–host interactions that sustain successful parasite colonization of the mammalian host. Targeting the parasites' obligatory infection of the liver as a gateway to the blood, with drugs and vaccines, constitutes the most effective strategy for malaria eradication, as it would prevent clinical disease and onward transmission of the parasite.

The genus *Plasmodium* consists of many different parasite species, each with a narrow host range and the causative agent of the disease malaria in its respective host. *Plasmodium* parasites have evolved exceedingly complex life cycles, using mosquitoes as the vehicle of transmission to infect reptiles, birds, and mammals, including humans. Human malaria parasite infection inflicts tremendous morbidity and significant mortality, mainly caused by two parasite species, *Plasmodium falciparum* and *Plasmodium vivax*. When the parasites' sporozoite stages are transmitted by a mosquito bite, these preerythrocytic forms establish the gateway to host infection by invading host cells and initiating the first round of intracellular replication. Preerythrocytic infection precedes blood stage infection and, for all *Plasmodium* species that infect mammals, takes place in hepatocytes within the liver. Hence, the intrahepatocytic replication stages are called liver stages or exoerythrocytic forms (EEFs). Liver infection is completely asymptomatic; thus, it cannot be detected in humans and, in consequence, cannot be directly studied during natural infection. Fritz Schaudinn's infamous blunder at the turn of the 19th century, the alleged observation that sporozoites could directly infect red blood cells, held back research on preerythrocytic infection for decades, and it was only in the late 1940s that the liver stages of the parasite were discovered. This breakthrough was made possible by the discovery of rodent malaria parasites such as *Plasmodium yoelii* and *Plasmodium berghei*, and their introduction into laboratory research, which provided exceptionally powerful experimental tools for the direct analysis of liver infection. Indeed, most of the data concerning preerythrocytic infection have been generated with these models. Preerythrocytic stages of human malaria parasites remain exceedingly difficult to study. However, the development of in vitro platforms for the culture of human hepatocytes and the development of liver-humanized mice provide, for the first time, powerful preerythrocytic infection models, which are revolutionizing research on the initial stages of human malaria parasite infection. Here, we review the biology of liver infection by sporozoites and liver stage development, raise outstanding questions regarding the field, highlight opportunities for future research, and argue for the liver stages as the essential target for malaria eradication efforts.

HEPATOCYTE INVASION AND TRANSITION TO LIVER STAGE

After an infectious mosquito bite, sporozoites must leave the bite site and find their way to hepatocytes, where liver stage development occurs. The dermis-to-hepatocyte journey (reviewed in Ejigiri and Sinnis 2009) is complex and perilous for the sporozoites and their numbers are modest, yet a single infectious mosquito bite leads to liver infection, thereby setting the stage for successful host colonization. The sporozoite (Fig. 1A) is a unique invasive stage—unlike the parasite's ookinete stage that only traverses across the basal lamina of the mosquito midgut (Vinetz 2005) and the merozoites that only invade red blood cells (Cowman et al. 2012)—sporozoites are highly motile and must *traverse* and *invade* cells. They enter the bloodstream by traversing a dermal capillary, are transported to the hepatic capillary network (the sinusoids), and then traverse across

the endothelial barrier to enter the hepatic parenchyma. Here, sporozoites traverse multiple hepatocytes and then finally undergo a functional switch that allows them to invade a hepatocyte to take up residence. During and after invasion, the sporozoite releases the contents of a unique set of invasive organelles, the micronemes and rhoptries, whose constituent proteins mediate molecular interactions with the host cell (Fig. 1A–C). The molecular mechanisms and sequence of events in cell invasion have been extremely well dissected with regard to merozoite invasion of red blood cells, but much less is known about hepatocyte infection by sporozoites. Merozoite and sporozoite host cell invasion share commonalities, such as the parasite actin–myosin motor that powers active entry into the host cell (Fowler et al. 2004) and the host cell plasma membrane invagination during invasion that ensconces the intracellular parasite within a host membrane, known as the parasitophorous vacuole membrane (PVM) (Fig. 1D) (Meis et al. 1983). The PVM is extensively modified by the developing liver stage parasite and acts not only as a barrier to the host cell cytoplasm but also as a conduit for communication and nutrient acquisition (Figs. 1E and 2A,B). Research has revealed some of the key molecular players, both parasite and host, in the hepatocyte invasion process, many of which are unique to sporozoites.

The major sporozoite surface protein, circumsporozoite protein (CSP), is a key mediator of the sporozoites' interaction with the host during its journey to the liver and the infection of hepatocytes. CSP is composed of a central repeat region, diverse across *Plasmodium* species, flanked by two conserved domains—the amino-terminal region I and a cell-adhesive carboxy-terminal motif known as the type I thrombospondin repeat (TSR). Region I masks the adhesive TSR until the sporozoite reaches the liver at which time it is cleaved, allowing the TSR to mediate hepatocyte adhesion (Coppi et al. 2011). This begs the question, how does the sporozoite know it has reached the liver? Localized within the liver sinusoid are highly sulfated heparin sulfate proteoglycans (HSPGs), produced by stellate cells within the space of

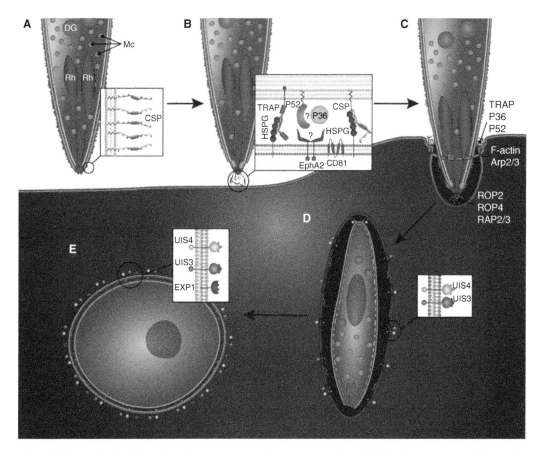

Figure 1. Sporozoite invasion of host hepatocytes. Graphic representation of the invasion steps that culminate in the productive infection of the hepatocyte host cell. (*A*) The surface of the motile sporozoite is coated with circumsporozoite protein (CSP) (shown in *inset*), which engages heparin sulfate proteoglycans (HSPGs) on the hepatocyte surface. The apical end of the sporozoite contains organelles whose contents are essential for hepatocyte invasion: rhoptries (Rh, pink), micronemes (Mc, orange), and likely dense granules (DG, blue), although the latter have not been unequivocally identified. (*B,C*) Contact with an invasion-permissive hepatocyte (brown) triggers CSP processing, which, via an unknown mechanism, triggers the release of invasion-essential proteins from the micronemes (*inset*). These proteins include thrombospondin-related adhesive protein (TRAP), which binds to HSPGs on the hepatocyte cell surface and to the sporozoite internal glideosome complex (not shown) via its cytoplasmic domain to provide traction for the invading sporozoite at the moving junction (also known as the tight junction, shown as a gray ring). The microneme proteins P52 and P36 are also involved in the invasion process and may interact with each other as well as interacting with the hepatocyte Ephrin A2 receptor (EphA2). The P52/P36/EphA2 axis appears to be critical for the formation of the parasitophorous vacuole (PV). The hepatocyte receptor CD81 is also important for the invasion process and PV formation, but it is not clear whether the sporozoite directly interacts with it. The inner membrane complex (IMC) (in yellow) anchors the internal glideosome complex, allowing for sporozoite movement into the hepatocyte. Hepatocyte invasion occurs through the moving junction at the point of entry and is accompanied by the polymerization of host F-actin in association with Arp2/3. Invasion results in the invagination of the hepatocyte plasma membrane and the release of rhoptry proteins, including ROP2, ROP4, and RAP2/3. (*D*) Successful invasion results in the sporozoite residing within a PV surrounded by a parasitophorous vacuole membrane (PVM) of hepatocyte origin. The PVM is extensively modified by the parasite and the putative dense granule proteins UIS3 and UIS4 are released and trafficked to the PVM, as is EXP-1 (*inset*). During sporozoite dedifferentiation, the IMC (dashed yellow line) and the apical organelles are broken down. (*E*) The nascent liver stage trophozoite resides within a PV, has its own parasite plasma membrane still coated by CSP (green), and is surrounded by a PVM (blue).

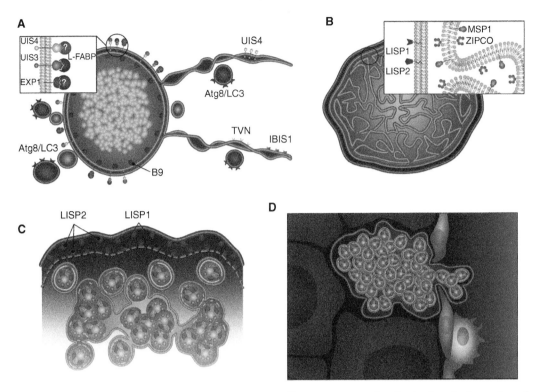

Figure 2. Liver stage development. Graphic representation of liver stage maturation that leads to the formation of exoerythrocytic merozoites. (*A*) The tubulovesicular network (TVN) (blue)—membrane-bound extensions and whorls that emanate from the parasitophorous vacuole membrane (PVM)—interacts with the hepatocyte's autophagosomes (which express Atg8/LC3) likely for nutrient uptake. Parasite proteins expressed on the PVM/TVN include IBIS1, EXP1, UIS4, and UIS3, which has been shown to interact with host L-FABP. The parasite plasma membrane (PPM)-associated protein B9 is known to be important for liver stage development. (*B*) As the liver stage parasite matures, multiple invaginations of the PPM occur (cytomere formation), and this is accompanied by the expression of MSP1 and ZIPCO. Additionally, LISP1 and LISP2 expression occur on the PVM. (*C*) Toward the end of liver stage development, individual exoerythrocytic merozoites begin to form, the PVM breaks down (a process that relies on LISP1), and LISP2 is released into the host hepatocyte. (*D*) Merosomes, merozoites surrounded by hepatocyte plasma membrane, are released into the bloodstream through the liver sinusoid, which is demarcated by epithelial cells (red) and liver resident macrophages, the Kupffer cells (yellow).

Disse, and these HSPGs are recognized by the sporozoite via CSP (Fig. 1B) (Frevert et al. 1993). This might lead to a signaling event that switches the sporozoite to an invasive phenotype (Coppi et al. 2007), resulting in the aforementioned cleavage of region I, a process that is catalyzed by a sporozoite protease (Coppi et al. 2005).

CSP cleavage appears to be a prerequisite for productive infection, but what other molecules are involved in the process? A number of sporozoite micronemal proteins are known to be crucial and they include thrombospondin-

related anonymous protein (TRAP) and the 6-cys domain proteins P52 and P36 (Fig. 1B). TRAP is a type 1 transmembrane protein, and like CSP, it contains a TSR domain but also an integrin-like domain. TRAP is released onto the sporozoite surface from the micronemes during invasion and, during this process, TRAP binds to the sporozoite actin–myosin motor through its carboxy-terminal cytoplasmic domain and binds to HSPGs through its extracellular domain (Kappe et al. 1999). During invasion, TRAP is translocated from the anterior to the posterior of the sporozoite and is subsequently shed from the sporozoite by cleavage within its transmembrane domain, likely by the rhomboid protease ROM4, which allows for hepatocyte invasion, because the cleavage releases the TRAP–HSPG bond (Baker et al. 2006; Ejigiri et al. 2012) (Fig. 1B). The micronemal proteins P52, a predicted GPI-anchored protein, and P36, a predicted secreted protein, are members of the 6-cys protein family (Templeton and Kaslow 1999), and they are critical for hepatocyte infection (Fig. 1B,C). Other members of the 6-cys family that are expressed in different parasite stages also have roles in parasite–parasite or host–parasite interactions (Pradel 2007; van Dijk et al. 2010; Molina-Cruz et al. 2013; Sala et al. 2015). The 6-cys domains are likely involved in protein–protein interaction, but evidence for this has been scarce. P52 is released from the micronemes to the sporozoite surface before invasion and disruption of either *P52* or *P36* in *P. berghei* (Ishino et al. 2005; van Schaijk et al. 2008), and *P52* in *P. falciparum* (van Schaijk et al. 2008) results in sporozoites that are defective in hepatocyte invasion. In *P. yoelii*, the simultaneous deletion of *P36* and *P52* renders sporozoites unable to form or maintain a PVM, resulting in early abortion of liver stage development (Labaied et al. 2007). Similarly, *P. falciparum* sporozoites lacking *P36* and *P52* cannot develop after hepatocyte entry (VanBuskirk et al. 2009). Recent work revealed the hepatocyte receptor that directly interacts with these proteins: the transmembrane receptor Ephrin A2 (EphA2) (Fig. 1B). EphA2 is essential for sporozoite invasion and concomitant PVM formation in rodent and human malaria parasites and antibodies to EphA2 block sporozoite infection (Kaushansky et al. 2015). Intriguingly, its natural ligand EphrinA1 shares structural similarity with the 6-cys fold and there is strong evidence that EphA2 directly interacts with P36, thus constituting the first bona fide host receptor–parasite ligand pair with a critical role in hepatocyte infection (Fig. 1B).

In addition to EphA2, other hepatocyte surface proteins are critical for successful sporozoite infection. The tetraspanin membrane protein "cluster of differentiation 81" (CD81) (Fig. 1B) is required on hepatocytes for *P. yoelii* and *P. falciparum* sporozoite invasion with PVM formation but interestingly not for *P. berghei*. *P. yoelii* sporozoites are unable to infect CD81-deficient mouse hepatocytes, and antibodies against mouse and human CD81 inhibit the in vitro hepatocyte infection by *P. yoelii* and *P. falciparum* sporozoites (Silvie et al. 2003). Yet, a sporozoite ligand for CD81 has not been identified. Cholesterol is involved in the assembly of CD81-rich microdomains on the cell surface, and this assembly is necessary for sporozoite infection (Silvie et al. 2006), indicating that it is the organization and composition of microdomains, rather than a direct interaction with CD81, that enable successful sporozoite infection of hepatocytes. A further hepatocyte membrane receptor, scavenger receptor BI (SR-BI), which mediates the selective uptake of cholesteryl esters from both high- and low-density lipoproteins, plays a role in hepatocyte infection. This role appears rather indirect because SR-BI deficiency causes a decreased expression of CD81 on the hepatocyte surface (Yalaoui et al. 2008). Antibodies to SR-BI do not block sporozoite invasion (Foquet et al. 2015), adding credence to the idea that SR-BI expression is necessary for CD81 microdomain formation but not a receptor for the sporozoite. Recently, an important link between the initial interaction of the sporozoite with the hepatocyte surface and the signaling to trigger processes within sporozoites has been revealed—the presence of CD81 on hepatocytes appears to be critical for the subsequent discharge of the rhoptries (Risco-Castillo et al. 2014). Research thus indicates an orchestrated sequence of events whereby sporozoite interaction with the hepatocyte promotes downstream signaling that triggers the secretion of proteins necessary for the formation and modification of the PVM.

Once the sporozoite lies completely ensconced in the PVM (Fig. 1D), it must metamorphose into a highly metabolically active intracellular replication machine, a process that requires jettisoning or disassembling its invasive organelles and inner membrane complex (IMC) (Fig. 1D). IMC breakdown is accompanied by spherical plasma membrane expansion in the center of the still elongated parasite and the contraction of its distal ends (Jayabalasing-ham et al. 2010). This shape conversion is accompanied by the clearance of the IMC and invasion-associated organelles, which are discharged as large exocytic vesicles or possibly undergo autophagy. However, the presence of autophagy in *Plasmodium* is controversial because the key autophagy marker protein Atg8/LC3 localizes to the parasite apicoplast and does not relocalize to autophagosome-like vesicles or vacuoles (Eickel et al. 2013; Jayabalasingham et al. 2014). The nascent liver stage preferentially develops in the host juxtanuclear region and the PVM appears to form an association with the host endoplasmic reticulum (ER) (Bano et al. 2007). Parasite modification of the PVM allows the passage of molecules of up to 855 Da from the host cytosol to the PV through open channels, and it is possible that host-derived cholesterol that accumulates at the PVM may modulate channel activity (Bano et al. 2007). These channels ensure that molecules from the nutrient-rich hepatocyte can feed the growing liver stage, although a tubulovesicular network, described below, likely allows for the uptake of larger molecules. Although the PVM is vital for successful liver stage development, the initial metamorphosis from sporozoite to trophozoite can occur outside a host cell. This indicates that the intracellular environment does not provide specific signals to trigger this process but rather that more general changes that occur with the sporozoites transition into a mammalian host, such as an elevation in temperature and the presence of serum components (Kaiser et al. 2003).

As described above, the initiation of liver stage development is a complex process that is initiated when the sporozoite detects a suitable hepatocyte for infection. Once the sporozoite has invaded its host cell, it must then dedifferentiate from an invasive extracellular parasite into an intracellular trophozoite contained within a PVM. During this process, signaling events prevent the parasites' destruction by the host cell. Finally, the trophozoite transitions into a highly replicative schizont that relies on nutrient uptake from its host as well as its own metabolic processes to ensure its

eventual goal of exoerythrocytic merozoite release.

It must be noted that the transition to schizogony, which always occurs in *P. falciparum* liver stage development, does not always occur in *P. vivax*. The *P. vivax* sporozoite, once it has entered a host hepatocyte, dedifferentiates and can then become a dormant trophozoite, known as the hypnozoite. The hypnozoite can lie dormant for months and even years and then reactivate and fully develop, leading to *P. vivax* malaria relapses. The processes that lead to hypnozoite formation and reactivation are very poorly understood, and malaria elimination must address the radical cure of the dormant hypnozoite.

LIVER STAGE DEVELOPMENT

The liver stage undergoes schizogony—nuclear division without cell division—during its maturation and only in the final phase of this process do invasive exoerythrocytic merozoites form. Liver stage schizogony constitutes one of the most rapid eukaryotic replication events—in a little >2 d, rodent malaria sporozoites can transform into a mature ellipsoid liver stage containing up to 29,000 exoerythrocytic merozoites (Baer et al. 2007). Liver stage development in *P. falciparum* takes longer, ~6.5 d, with estimates of up to 90,000 exoerythrocytic merozoites packaged in the fully mature parasite (Vaughan et al. 2012). Liver stage schizogony is characterized by the rapid branching and growth of the parasite's organelles such as the mitochondria and the relict plastid organelle, the apicoplast (Stanway et al. 2009), as well as massive DNA replication. Studies utilizing parasite and host transgenesis have shed light on the important pathways that allow for parasite growth, and, not surprisingly, a number of parasite proteins involved in PVM formation and modification are essential for liver stage formation and development.

The liver stage PVM proteins UIS3 and UIS4 are encoded by genes belonging to the up-regulated in infective sporozoites (UIS) group (Figs. 1D–E, 2A, 3A–C,F). These genes are highly transcribed in sporozoites when they

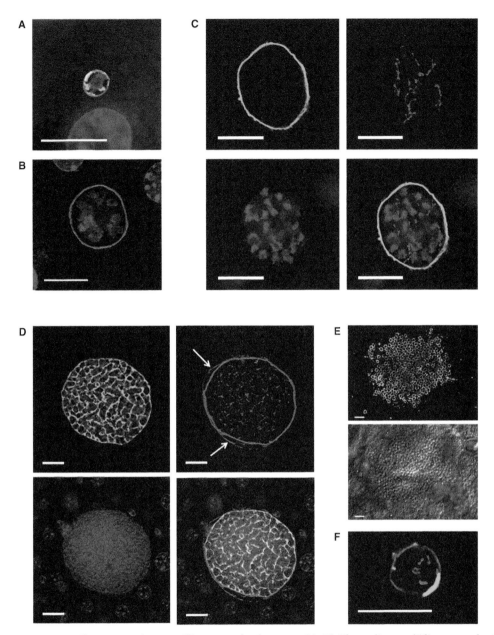

Figure 3. Immunofluorescence images of liver stage development. (*A–E*) *Plasmodium yoelii* liver stage development in a mouse liver. (*A*) The spherical, early liver stage parasite, 12 h after sporozoite invasion, is significantly smaller than the host hepatocyte nucleus (blue). The liver stage parasitophorous vacuole (PVM) is shown in red (UIS4 expression), the endoplasmic reticulum (ER) is shown in green (BiP expression), and the parasite contains a single nuclear center (blue). (*B*) By 24 h, the *P. yoelii* liver stage parasite (the UIS4-positive PVM is shown in red) has entered schizogony (multiple centers of nuclear replication [blue]). (*C*) At 30 h of development, the *P. yoelii* liver stage (the UIS4 PVM is shown in green) has undergone multiple rounds of nuclear replication (blue) and contains a highly branched apicoplast (acyl carrier protein expression, shown in red). (*D*) Late in *P. yoelii* liver stage development (48 h), the parasite plasma membrane (PPM) undergoes extensive invagination resulting in cytomere formation (MSP1, green). LISP2 (red) is expressed on the PVM as well as the hepatocyte membrane (white arrows). The nuclei (blue) of the individual parasites can be seen within the liver stage parasite. (*E*) At the end of liver stage development (52 h), individual exoerythrocytic merozoites (MSP1 expression in green, *upper* panel, delineates the merozoite membrane) can be seen within the mature liver stage parasite (differential interference contrast, *lower* panel). (*F*) Image of a *P. vivax* hypnozoite in a humanized mouse liver. The hypnozoite remains latent, is small, and does not replicate its DNA, and its PVM has a unique UIS4-positive prominence (green). The hypnozoite mitochondrion (HSP60 expression) is shown in red and is branched. Scale bars, 10 μm.

still reside in the mosquito salivary glands but some are translationally repressed with protein production peaking only after hepatocyte invasion. This "just in time" protein expression from stored mRNAs exemplifies one of the approaches the sporozoite has evolved to ready itself for the rapid transition to liver stage replication and indicates that proteins such as UIS3 and UIS4 must be playing an important role starting very early in liver stage development. Indeed, deletion of either *UIS3* or *UIS4* gene causes arrest of early liver stage development (Mueller et al. 2005a,b; Jobe et al. 2007). The carboxyl termini of both UIS3 and UIS4 face the hepatocyte cytoplasm and the amino termini the PV lumen, suggestive of roles in parasite– hepatocyte interactions. Indeed, UIS3 interacts with liver fatty acid protein (L-FABP) (Fig. 2A) (Mikolajczak et al. 2007), suggesting an interaction that could serve as a conduit for the transport of lipid into the liver stage to support growth. Lipid transport within and between eukaryotic cells can occur through membrane-bound ATP-binding cassette (ABC) transporters, and the ABCC class of transporters is expressed by both *P. berghei* and *P. falciparum* liver stages. Interestingly, the deletion of *ABCC2* (also known as *MRP2*) in both *P. berghei* and *P. falciparum* leads to liver stage arrest, demonstrating the importance of parasite ABC transporters in liver stage development and hinting to their role in lipid transport (Rijpma et al. 2016). To date, UIS4 function has remained elusive, as has the function of a second PVM-resident protein exported protein 1 (EXP1, also known as Hep17 in rodent malaria parasites) (Fig. 2A). Later in liver stage development, two further PVM-associated proteins are expressed, LISP1 and LISP2 (Figs. 2B,C and 3D) (Ishino et al. 2009; Orito et al. 2013). LISP1 is involved in PVM breakdown and subsequent merozoite release, whereas LISP2 (which contains a modified 6-cys domain) is localized to the PV and PVM and is also transported to the cytoplasm and plasma membrane of infected hepatocytes (Figs. 2B,C and 3D). Although the functions of these two proteins are not fully understood, gene deletion studies in *P. berghei* have indicated their importance in late liver

stage growth because parasites that lack LISP1 or LISP2 do not mature effectively. Further critical proteins expressed by liver stage parasites include the 6-cys-like protein, B9, expressed on the parasite plasma membrane (PPM) (Fig. 2A) (Annoura et al. 2014) and ZIPCO, an iron transporter expressed on the late liver stage PPM (Fig. 2B) (Sahu et al. 2014). Although an increasing number of PV and PVM proteins have been identified that play important roles in liver stage development, an important future goal is the comprehensive identification of all liver stage PVM, PV, and PPM proteins that will supersede the current identification of important players using candidate approaches. Importantly, research needs to go beyond the assembly of "parts lists" and ought to delineate the relationship and interaction among liver stage PVM and PV proteins and their interaction with host proteins to establish a network of important liver stage–hepatocyte interactions.

Although the liver stage clearly parasitizes the extremely metabolically active host hepatocyte, the massive increase in parasite biomass during liver stage development likely requires the participation of parasite anabolic pathways. Indeed, combined transcriptome and proteome analysis of liver stage development showed that the parasite de novo type II fatty acid synthesis pathway (FAS II) is highly active (Tarun et al. 2008). To assess the importance of FAS II, which is localized to the parasite apicoplast, gene knockouts in rodent malarias have been performed and showed that FAS II is critical for late liver stage development (Yu et al. 2008; Vaughan et al. 2009; Pei et al. 2010; Falkard et al. 2013; Lindner et al. 2014). These reports show that the liver stage requires its own fatty acid synthesis, but it is not currently understood why the fatty acids are synthesized—they might be incorporated into exoerythrocytic merozoite membranes, but they could also be incorporated into the growing hepatocyte plasma membrane or the PVM. As mentioned above, the UIS3/L-FABP interaction likely allows for lipid acquisition from the hepatocyte. The cholesterol component of this lipid can be derived from low-density lipoprotein internalization by the hepatocyte as well as de novo synthesized hepa-

Cite this article as *Cold Spring Harb Perspect Med* doi: 10.1101/cshperspect.a025486

tocyte cholesterol (Labaied et al. 2011). Further research has shown that hepatocyte phosphatidylcholine, the major membrane phospholipid, is taken up by liver stages, and preventing the rate-limiting steps in the synthesis of hepatocyte phosphatidylcholine affects liver stage development (Itoe et al. 2014). All of these studies show that liver stage parasites critically depend on both lipid uptake from the host hepatocyte and endogenous lipid synthesis to support their dramatic growth and differentiation.

During growth, liver stage mass increases so much that the infected hepatocyte must significantly expand to accommodate the replicating parasite. However, the liver stage parasites remain relatively undifferentiated until shortly before completion of liver stage maturation. Late in development, the PPM undergoes rapid expansion and extensive invagination (called cytomere formation) (Figs. 2B and 3D), which dramatically increases parasite surface area and enables rapid formation of individual exoerythrocytic merozoites (Figs. 2C and 3E). This process also requires coordinated nuclear and organellar fission to ensure partitioning of nuclei and organelles into nascent merozoites (Stanway et al. 2011). This coordinated fission likely relies on both DNA- and RNA-binding proteins, and a liver stage–specific RNA-binding protein, PlasMei2, appears to be essential for the partitioning of nuclear DNA. The deletion of *PlasMei2* in *P. yoelii*, without affecting liver stage growth, prevents the partitioning of nuclear DNA, and this in turn prevents the formation of exoerythrocytic merozoites (Dankwa et al. 2016). Once merozoites have fully formed, the PVM must break down (Fig. 2C) before they can be released, and this process is a result of changes in PVM permeability (Sturm et al. 2009) and relies on a parasite phospholipase, which localizes to the PVM (Burda et al. 2015).

Intravital microscopic observations of live-fluorescent *P. yoelii* and *P. berghei* mature liver stages in mice have shown that they induce the detachment of their host hepatocyte, leading to the budding of merosomes (merozoite-filled vesicles) into the sinusoidal lumen (Fig. 2D) (Sturm et al. 2006; Tarun et al. 2006). The mer-

osome membrane derives from the host hepatocyte plasma membrane (Graewe et al. 2011), allowing the merosome to hide from the immune system and thereby avoid uptake and destruction by the numerous liver-resident macrophages (the Kupffer cells), on its way to the bloodstream. Merosomes have also been observed in mature *P. falciparum* liver stages (Vaughan et al. 2012), confirming their existence in human malaria parasite liver stages. Most *P. yoelii* merosomes exit the liver intact and adapt to a relatively uniform size, within which 100 to 200 merozoites reside (Baer et al. 2007). Merosomes eventually break up inside pulmonary capillaries, resulting in merozoite liberation and red blood cell infection.

PARASITE PERTURBATIONS OF HOST HEPATOCYTES

So far, we have discussed parasite proteins and some host molecules that are necessary for sporozoite invasion and liver stage development, but to acquire nutrients and grow, the parasite must not simply reside in the hepatocyte and exploit it but actively manipulate and subvert it to avoid its demise. How does this happen? Already at the point of invasion, the parasite subverts its host. As the sporozoite invades, it induces the formation of a ring-shaped structure in the hepatocyte composed of de novo polymerized host F-actin (Fig. 1C) (Gonzalez et al. 2009). The hepatocyte Arp2/3 complex, an actin-nucleating factor, is recruited to this ring structure and is necessary for parasite invasion (Fig. 1C). The PVM is essential for liver stage development, and the formation of a productive PVM is a prerequisite for the parasite's ability to render its host hepatocyte resistant to apoptosis (van de Sand et al. 2005; van Dijk et al. 2005; Kaushansky et al. 2013a). Although the sensitivity to apoptosis is dependent on the Bcl-2 family of mitochondrial proteins that the parasite subverts (Kaushansky et al. 2013a), the parasite molecules that interfere with hepatocyte apoptosis are not known. A line of defense used by many host cells against pathogen infection is the synthesis of stress granules, thereby shutting down protein synthesis. However, there is no evidence that hepatocyte infection causes stress granule formation, which implies that the parasite has evolved to prevent this response from occurring in the hepatocyte (Hanson and Mair 2014). In a surprising twist on parasite–host manipulation, liver stage survival actually benefits from the host ER stress response pathway (Inacio et al. 2015), which typically shuts down cellular activity. Proteins and transcripts that act in the unfolded protein response leading to ER stress were found to be elevated in hepatocytes in response to infection, but why the parasite perturbs its host in this way is not clear. It is possible that ER stress supports parasite growth by regulating lipid metabolism, vital for parasite growth (Itoe et al. 2014), or diminishing antigen presentation so the liver stage can remain hidden from the immune system—a trick used by hepatitis C (Tardif and Siddiqui 2003).

The perturbations of the host hepatocyte have been explored by analyzing changes in hepatocyte transcription and protein expression early during liver stage infection (Albuquerque et al. 2009; Kaushansky et al. 2013b). Transcriptome data showed that parasite infection initially causes a global stress response, which then morphs into an engagement of host metabolic processes and the maintenance of cell viability to ensure parasite and host cell survival (Albuquerque et al. 2009). Using cell lysate arrays to simultaneously monitor many protein perturbations, a subset of hepatocyte protein levels and accompanying posttranslational modifications were measured 24 h postinfection with rodent malaria parasites and compared with uninfected hepatocytes (Kaushansky et al. 2013b). This revealed a signaling network aimed at preventing host cell death but also determined that the tumor suppressor P53 is substantially dampened in infected hepatocytes. This is of functional significance because increasing P53 levels whether chemically or genetically nearly eliminates liver stage infection and development and mice lacking P53 are hypersusceptible to infection (Kaushansky et al. 2013b).

During liver stage development, a tubulovesicular network (TVN) forms, which includes membranous extensions of the PVM as well

as the creation of autonomous vesicular structures within the infected hepatocyte (Fig. 2A) (Mueller et al. 2005a). The TVN likely functions in hepatocyte interactions and in accessing nutrients from the hepatocyte, but these functions need to be experimentally verified. Fluorescent tagging of two *P. berghei* PVM proteins, UIS4 and IBIS1, and the use of correlative light-electron microscopy have shown that the TVN membranes extend throughout the host cell and include dynamic vesicles as well as long tubules that extend and contract from the PVM (Fig. 2A) (Grutzke et al. 2014). Additionally, labeling of host hepatocyte compartments revealed an association of late endosomes and lysosomes with the TVN-associated elongated membrane clusters. Furthermore, the host autophagosome protein Atg8/LC3 colocalizes with UIS4 at the PVM and TVN (Fig. 2A). These data suggest that the intimate association between the TVN and host endosomes/lysosomes allows for parasite–hepatocyte signaling as well as nutrient uptake. Further studies have shown that complete parasite development actually correlates with the gradual loss of autophagy marker proteins and associated lysosomes from the PVM even though other autophagic events such as nonselective canonical autophagy continue in the host cell (Prado et al. 2015). Thus, it is possible that the parasite continues to benefit from nonselective canonical autophagy for its growth.

Supporting the hypothesis that the endosomal system supports liver stage growth, the growth of the parasite is dependent on phosphoinositide 5-kinase (PIKfyve), which converts phosphatidylinositol 3-phosphate into phosphatidylinositol 3,5-bisphosphate (PI (3,5) P2) within the endosomal system—an enzymatic reaction essential for late endocytic membrane fusion (Thieleke-Matos et al. 2014). Indeed, the PI (3,5) P2 effector protein TRPML1, involved in late endocytic membrane fusion, was shown to be present in vesicles in close contact with the PVM and PIKfyve inhibition delayed parasite growth. Additionally, contents of late endocytic vesicles have been found within the parasite cytoplasm (Lopes da Silva et al. 2012). We are only just beginning to un-

Cite this article as *Cold Spring Harb Perspect Med* doi: 10.1101/cshperspect.a025486

derstand how the parasite manipulates its host, and many questions remain unanswered. Most notably, there is a complete lack of understanding of how the liver stage, during its own massive growth, also enables the growth of the PVM and expansion of the host hepatocyte to accommodate its heft—cells do not normally dramatically increase in size, but the mature liver stage–infected hepatocyte can expand to 200 times its normal volume.

The developing liver stage parasite, as well as interacting with its host hepatocyte to ensure its survival, must also evade the host's immune system to ensure merozoite maturation and release. As noted above, the autophagy marker Atg8/LC3 colocalizes with UIS4 at the PVM and TVN, and aids in liver stage growth. Conversely, autophagy has been identified as a downstream pathway that is activated in response to interferon γ (IFN-γ) in the control of intracellular infections (Deretic et al. 2013). Indeed, IFN-γ, a master regulator of immune functions, has been known for many years to induce the elimination of liver stage parasites in vivo (Ferreira et al. 1986). Thus, the parasite needs to precisely coordinate autophagy for its benefit. Research on *P. vivax* liver stages has shown that IFN-γ-mediated restriction of liver stage *P. vivax* depends on autophagy-related proteins including Beclin-1, PI3K, and Atg5 and enhanced the recruitment of LC3 to the PVM. In this case, the LC3 decoration of the PVM led to a noncanonical autophagy pathway resembling that of LC3-associated phagocytosis, promoting the fusion of *P. vivax* compartments with lysosomes and subsequent killing of the pathogen (Boonhok et al. 2016). Thus, research has uncovered positive and negative aspects of autophagy on parasite survival, and it is clear that although the parasite can take advantage of host cell autophagy, it can also be killed by the pathway and thus must carefully control this intracellular process for its own gain.

IFN-γ production in response to liver stage parasite detection is part of a programmed innate immune response to liver stage infection (Liehl and Mota 2012). This innate immune response to infection is pronounced and can actually lead to the effective killing of a second-

ary liver stage infection (Miller et al. 2014). This response is in part initiated by liver-resident cells and driven by *Plasmodium* RNA, which acts as a pathogen-associated molecular pattern capable of activating the type I IFN response via the cytosolic pattern recognition receptor Mda5 (Liehl et al. 2014). Furthermore, the response is abrogated in mice deficient in IFN-γ, as well as the type I IFN-α/β receptor (IFNAR), demonstrating the important role of IFNAR in driving the innate immune response (Liehl et al. 2014; Miller et al. 2014). The cell type linked to the secretion of IFN-γ was shown to be $CD49b^+CD3^+$ natural killer T (NKT) cells and an increase in CD1d-restricted NKT cells was critical in reducing liver stage burden of a secondary infection (Miller et al. 2014). In turn, the lack of IFNAR signaling abrogated the increase in NKT cell numbers in the liver, showing a link between type I IFN signaling, cell recruitment, and parasite elimination (Miller et al. 2014).

The above highlights the extent of our current knowledge on how the liver stage parasite influences both the host hepatocyte and the host innate immune system. Far more research is necessary and will help in the design and implementation of drugs to target the liver stage parasite and effective vaccines that engender appropriate immune responses to liver stage parasites. For these advances to take place, we need better models for liver stage development and liver stage isolation.

ADVANCES IN MODEL DEVELOPMENT FOR HUMAN MALARIA PARASITE LIVER INFECTION

A natural sporozoite infection typically results in the productive invasion of only a small number of hepatocytes. Because of this bottleneck, the liver stage parasite has been extremely difficult to study. However, such studies are essential to uncover pathways that are necessary for parasite survival and replication. These pathways can then be perturbed to prevent development and ultimately to thwart life cycle progression to blood stage disease. To this end, parasite transgenesis has enabled the creation of fluorescent parasites and this led to the sorting of murine hepatocytes infected with *P. yoelii* fluorescent liver stages, resulting in the first extensive liver stage transcriptomes and proteomes (Tarun et al. 2008; Albuquerque et al. 2009). However, extensive -omic analysis of human malaria liver stages has still not been completed and needs to be performed. Such analysis is important for the reason that numerous studies have shown significant biological differences between rodent and human malaria parasites. Nevertheless, platforms for the growth of human malaria parasite liver stages are not easily established, because of the limitation that *P. falciparum* and *P. vivax* preerythrocytic stages only infect human and some nonhuman primate hepatocytes and do not grow well in hepatoma cells. Additionally, the *P. vivax* sporozoite, unlike the model rodent malaria sporozoite, can develop into either a liver stage schizont *or* a liver stage hypnozoite (Krotoski et al. 1982)—a dormant liver stage form (Fig. 3F) that can activate and cause malaria relapse infections in affected individuals.

In vitro development of *P. vivax* liver stages in primary human hepatocytes was first documented in 1984 (Mazier et al. 1984) and for *P. falciparum* in 1985 (Mazier et al. 1985), and both parasites were later shown to mature in the human hepatocyte cell line HC-04 (Sattabongkot et al. 2006), albeit poorly. Rapid advances in cryopreservation methods for primary human hepatocytes make this cell type more easily available, and investigators no longer depend on cells fresh from liver surgery. Recently, an improved in vitro system using primary human hepatocytes in a microscale human liver platform was shown to support *P. falciparum* and *P. vivax* liver stages development including *P. vivax* hypnozoite formation (March et al. 2013). An additional promising platform uses induced pluripotent stem cell-derived hepatocyte-like cells and liver stage development of both *P. falciparum* and *P. vivax* appears to mirror that observed in primary human hepatocytes (Ng et al. 2015). Thus, this platform is an attractive alternative because it enables a potential unlimited production of hepatocytes.

Although in vitro models for infection have greatly improved over the past years, robust in vivo infection models for preerythrocytic stages of human malaria parasites are highly desirable. Fortunately, human-liver chimeric mouse models that were originally developed for drug metabolism studies and hepatitis research are promising as animal models for human malaria liver infection. These models are all built around some form of immunocompromised background plus genetically encoded liver injury that selectively ablates mouse hepatocytes, thereby creating niches in the liver that can then be repopulated with primary human hepatocytes. An initial study using the SCID Alb-uPA mouse transplanted with human hepatocytes showed that *P. falciparum* liver stages developed after intravenous sporozoite injection (Sacci et al. 2006).

A second liver-chimeric mouse model, the FRG huHep mouse (Azuma et al. 2007), can yield up to 95% human hepatocyte chimerism. After intravenous injection of *P. falciparum* sporozoites into FRG huHep mice, complete liver stage development occurred, resulting in the creation of schizonts packed with tens of thousands of exoerythrocytic merozoites that were able to transition in vivo to red blood cell infection, which was then continuously maintained in vitro (Vaughan et al. 2012). This enabled the creation of *P. falciparum* genetic crosses, which were previously possible only in splenectomized chimpanzees (Vaughan et al. 2015). The FRG huHep mouse has, in addition, been used to show the efficacy of antibodies against sporozoite proteins to reduce or prevent *P. falciparum* liver infection (Sack et al. 2014). This has also been achieved in SCID Alb-uPA mice (Behet et al. 2014; Foquet et al. 2014). Together, the work establishes liver-chimeric mice as an important preclinical tool to assess interventions against human malaria parasite preerythrocytic stages and further refinement could ascertain their use as a new stepping-stone toward clinical testing of interventions in controlled human malaria infection trials.

Intriguingly, the FRG huHep mouse was also recently used for infections with *P. vivax* (Mikolajczak et al. 2015). In this study, robust liver infection with *P. vivax* sporozoites was observed that culminated in complete liver stage development and exoerythrocytic merozoite release 9.5 d after infection and infectious merozoites could be captured by the injection of human reticulocytes. Alongside liver stage development, the establishment and persistence of hypnozoites was observed, enabling, for the first time, a detailed characterization of this unique latent EEF. Although DNA replication did indeed not occur in hypnozoites as previously thought, in contrast to previously held assumptions, latent hypnozoites were not "dormant" but metabolically active, showing limited organelle replication and modest growth over time. Hypnozoites also exhibited a unique thickening of the PVM, called a "prominence," that appears to distinguish them from replicating liver stages (Fig. 3F). The study also showed that the FRG huHep mouse will be useful to model hypnozoite activation, which leads to the production of second- and third-generation exoerythrocytic merozoites and relapsing blood stage infection, which is a distinguishing clinical feature of *P. vivax* infection. Thus, the FRG huHep model might prove useful to test the effectiveness of drugs that can eliminate hypnozoites and thus prevent relapsing infection with *P. vivax*.

VACCINATION WITH ATTENUATED PREERYTHROCYTIC PARASITES

Following earlier research on bird malaria (which do not have a liver stage), a study in 1967 showed that mice inoculated with irradiation-attenuated *P. berghei* sporozoites induced protection from a subsequent infection with wild-type sporozoites (Nussenzweig et al. 1967) and with this, the concept of an attenuated, whole sporozoite malaria vaccine was born. Similar studies in humans with irradiated *P. falciparum* sporozoites showed equal promise (Clyde et al. 1973; Rieckmann et al. 1974). Subsequent work showed that attenuated sporozoites have to be infectious and invade hepatocytes to unfold their protective potential likely by virtue of expressing new antigens before the cessation of liver stage development. Live sporozoite immunization elicits both protective humoral responses and cellular responses (Doll and

Harty 2014). In the 1970s, irradiation-attenuated sporozoites were not considered a practical vaccine because of the issues with irradiation, mass production, preservation, and delivery. However, increasing success in producing and storing *P. falciparum* sporozoites, irradiated sporozoites gained a resurgent interest in the 2000s and intravenous inoculation of humans with cryopreserved, irradiated *P. falciparum* sporozoites recently showed complete protection from infectious sporozoite challenge (Seder et al. 2013).

The discovery of genes that are essential for liver stage development, discussed earlier, gave rise to the idea that attenuation of the parasite could be accomplished through engineered gene deletion within the parasite's complex genome, thus rendering irradiation obsolete. In this effort, vaccine development meets parasite biology and synergizes effectively to create a biologically informed malaria vaccine strategy. Today, numerous genes essential for liver stage development have been identified, mostly in rodent malaria models (Table 1). Gene deletions arrest the parasite at distinct points during liver stage development, and studies have shown that late liver stage–arresting parasites afford superior immunity when compared with both an early arresting, genetically engineered parasite and irradiation-attenuated sporozoites. This is due to the significant increase in antigen load and breadth, which engenders a broader and diversified immune response (Butler et al. 2011; Sack et al. 2015). Engineering of *P. falciparum* liver stage–attenuated parasites has been undertaken (VanBuskirk et al. 2009); the parasites have undergone initial human clinical trial testing and are now undergoing improvements in attenuation (Table 1) (Mikolajczak et al. 2014; van Schaijk et al. 2014b). Ultimately, this will likely yield an engineered parasite that can replace irradiated sporozoites and such a vaccine will play a crucial role in malaria elimination.

FUTURE PERSPECTIVES

A call for malaria eradication by 2040 is perceived to be an achievable goal (endmalaria

Table 1. *Plasmodium* gene knockouts that lead to liver stage arrest

Gene knockout	Function	Temporal/spatial expression	Knockout phenotype			References
			Pb	Py	Pf	
B9	Unknown	PPM	Late arrest/partial attenuation	Late arrest/partial attenuation	—	Annoura et al. 2014
β-Ketoacyl-acyl-carrier protein synthase I/II (Fab B/F)	Fatty acid synthesis	Apicoplast throughout development	—	Late arrest/complete attenuation	No sporozoites	Vaughan et al. 2009; van Schaijk et al. 2014a
cGMP-dependent protein kinase (PKG) (conditional knockout)	Protein phosphorylation	Throughout development	Late arrest/complete attenuation	—	—	Falae et al. 2010
Glycerol 3-phosphate acyltransferase (G3PAT)	Phosphatidic acid synthesis	Apicoplast throughout development	—	Late arrest/complete attenuation	—	Lindner et al. 2014
Glycerol 3-phosphate dehydrogenase (G3PDH)	Phosphatidic acid synthesis	Apicoplast throughout development	—	Late arrest/complete attenuation	—	Lindner et al. 2014
Lipoic acid protein ligase B (LipB)	Fatty acid synthesis	Apicoplast throughout development	Late arrest/partial attenuation	—	—	Falkard et al. 2013
Liver stage antigen 1 (LSA1)	Unknown	PV late in development	—	—	Aberrant maturation	Mikolajczak et al. 2011
Liver-specific protein 1 (LISP1)	Unknown	PVM late in development	Late arrest/partial attenuation	—	—	Ishino et al. 2009
Liver-specific protein 1 (LISP2)	Unknown	PVM late in development/host hepatocyte	Late arrest/partial attenuation	—	—	Orito et al. 2013; Annoura et al. 2014

Cite this article as *Cold Spring Harb Perspect Med* doi: 10.1101/cshperspect.a025486

	Function	Localization		Decreased size/ partial attenuation		References
Macrophage migration inhibitory factor (MIF)	Unknown	Cytoplasm	—	—	—	Miller et al. 2012
MSP1 (conditional knockout)	Invasion	PPM late in development	Late arrest/ complete attenuation	—	—	Combe et al. 2009
MRP2 (ABCC2)	Unknown	Liver stage	Mid arrest/ complete attenuation	—	Mid-arrest	Rijpma et al. 2016
P52	Invasion	Sporozoite microneme/PPM during hepatocyte invasion	Early arrest/ partial attenuation	—	Early arrest	van Dijk et al. 2005; Douradinha et al. 2007; van Schaijk et al. 2008
Plasmodium-specific apicoplast protein for liver merozoite formation (PALM)	Unknown	Apicoplast late in development	Late arrest/ partial attenuation	—	—	Haussig et al. 2011
Pyruvate dehydrogenase subunit E1α (PDH E1α)	Acetyl COA synthesis	Apicoplast throughout development	Late arrest/ partial attenuation	Late arrest/ complete attenuation	No sporozoites	Pei et al. 2010; Cobbold et al. 2013; Nagel et al. 2013
Plasmei2	RNA binding	Mid-to-late liver stage cytoplasm	—	Late arrest/ complete attenuation	—	Dankwa et al. 2016
Pyruvate dehydrogenase subunit E3 (PDH E3)	Acetyl CoA synthesis	Apicoplast throughout development	—	Late arrest/ complete attenuation	—	Pei et al. 2010
Sporozoite asparagine-rich protein 1 (SAP1)/sporozoite and liver stage asparagine-rich protein (SLARP)	mRNA stability	Sporozoite cytoplasm	Early arrest/ complete attenuation	Early arrest/ complete attenuation	—	Aly et al. 2008; Silvie et al. 2008
trans-2-Enoyl-acyl carrier protein reductase (Fab I)	Fatty acid synthesis	Apicoplast throughout development	Late arrest/ partial attenuation	—	No sporozoites	Yu et al. 2008; van Schaijk et al. 2014a

Continued

Table 1. *Continued*

Gene knockout	Function	Temporal/spatial expression	Knockout phenotype				References
			Pb	Py	Pf		
Up-regulated in infective sporozoites gene 3 (UIS3)	Lipid uptake	Sporozoite microneme then PVM throughout development	Early arrest/ complete attenuation	Early arrest/ complete attenuation	Gene deletion unsuccessful		Mueller et al. 2005b; Tarun et al. 2007
Up-regulated in infective sporozoites gene 4 (UIS4)	Unknown	Sporozoite microneme then PVM throughout development	Early arrest/ partial attenuation	Early arrest/ complete attenuation	Gene deletion unsuccessful		Mueller et al. 2005a; Tarun et al. 2007
Zrt-, Irt-like protein domain-containing protein (ZIPCO)	Iron uptake	PPM late in development	Late arrest/ partial attenuation	–	–		Sahu et al. 2014
B9/SAP1 (SLARP)	–	–	Early arrest/ complete attenuation	–	Early arrest		van Schaijk et al. 2014b
P52/P36	–	–	Early arrest/ partial attenuation	Early arrest/ partial attenuation	Early arrest/ partial attenuation		Labaied et al. 2007; VanBuskirk et al. 2009; Ploemen et al. 2012; Spring et al. 2013
P52/P36/SAP1 (SLARP)	–	–	–	–	Early arrest		Mikolajczak et al. 2014
UIS3/UIS4	–	–	Early arrest/ complete attenuation	–	–		Jobe et al. 2007

Cite this article as *Cold Spring Harb Perspect Med* doi: 10.1101/cshperspect.a025486

2040.org). However, *P. falciparum* malaria will not be eradicated globally without an effective preerythrocytic vaccine that will prevent the onset of disease-causing blood stage infection and onward transmission through the mosquito vector. In addition, the elusive *P. vivax* preerythrocytic hypnozoite forms must be targeted by radical cure drugs to ensure full malaria eradication, and thus drug development ought to place more emphasis on finding compounds with activity against liver stages. A robust understanding of hypnozoite biology might well be a prerequisite to develop new drugs that afford radical cure. A further critical research question in this context is whether preerythrocytic vaccination can be used to provide an "immunological radical cure" and as such should be a major aspect of *P. vivax* vaccine research. Overall, we must be continuously guided by the principle that novel and innovative intervention strategies will emerge only from critical research of parasite biology and the immunology of infection and vaccination.

CONCLUDING REMARKS

The past decade has seen an unprecedented progress in research on liver stage malaria. This has brought forth the identification of numerous parasite and host factors that are of critical importance to hepatocyte infection and intra-hepatocytic parasite development. Without doubt, research in the coming years will identify additional important factors. However, the study of parasite–hepatocyte interaction must now enter the next phase, by not only identifying critical host–pathogen interactions but also assembling these interactions into a temporal and spatial cascading network that fully delineates parasite infection of and development within hepatocytes at the molecular level, from the point of invasion to the release of merozoites. These studies will be likely performed with rodent malaria models, but the increased maturity of in vitro and in vivo hepatocyte infection models of human malaria parasites gives hope that at least some of this work can be achieved with medically relevant parasite species. This is particularly important for the study of *P. vivax* hypnozoites in gaining insights into the molecular mechanisms of their latency, their activation, and their interaction with hepatocytes during long periods of persistence.

Finally, identification of parasite molecules that are critical for liver stage development has transcended basic biology in that it enabled the development and use of genetically engineered, attenuated parasite strains for vaccination. It is hoped that the continued biological interrogation of liver stage malaria will carry on to bear fruit for parasite immunology and vaccine development, thereby potentiating its role in helping to develop new tools for the eradication of human malaria infection.

ACKNOWLEDGMENTS

Research being performed in the Kappe Laboratory is partly funded by the U.S. National Institutes of Health and the Bill and Melinda Gates Foundation. We thank laboratory members past and present for their scientific contributions as well as our dedicated insectary and vivarium staff.

REFERENCES

Albuquerque SS, Carret C, Grosso AR, Tarun AS, Peng X, Kappe SH, Prudencio M, Mota MM. 2009. Host cell transcriptional profiling during malaria liver stage infection reveals a coordinated and sequential set of biological events. *BMC Genomics* **10:** 270.

Aly AS, Mikolajczak SA, Rivera HS, Camargo N, Jacobs-Lorena V, Labaied M, Coppens I, Kappe SH. 2008. Targeted deletion of SAP1 abolishes the expression of infectivity factors necessary for successful malaria parasite liver infection. *Mol Microbiol* **69:** 152–163.

Annoura T, van Schaijk BC, Ploemen IH, Sajid M, Lin JW, Vos MW, Dinmohamed AG, Inaoka DK, Rijpma SR, van Gemert GJ, et al. 2014. Two *Plasmodium* 6-Cys family-related proteins have distinct and critical roles in liver-stage development. *FASEB J* **28:** 2158–2170.

Azuma H, Paulk N, Ranade A, Dorrell C, Al-Dhalimy M, Ellis E, Strom S, Kay MA, Finegold M, Grompe M. 2007. Robust expansion of human hepatocytes in Fah$^{-/-}$/Rag2$^{-/-}$/Il2rg$^{-/-}$ mice. *Nat Biotechnol* **25:** 903–910.

Baer K, Klotz C, Kappe SH, Schnieder T, Frevert U. 2007. Release of hepatic *Plasmodium yoelii* merozoites into the pulmonary microvasculature. *PLoS Pathog* **3:** e171.

Baker RP, Wijetilaka R, Urban S. 2006. Two *Plasmodium* rhomboid proteases preferentially cleave different adhesins implicated in all invasive stages of malaria. *PLoS Pathog* **2:** e113.

Bano N, Romano JD, Jayabalasingham B, Coppens I. 2007. Cellular interactions of *Plasmodium* liver stage with its host mammalian cell. *Int J Parasitol* **37:** 1329–1341.

Behet MC, Foquet L, van Gemert GJ, Bijker EM, Meuleman P, Leroux-Roels G, Hermsen CC, Scholzen A, Sauerwein RW. 2014. Sporozoite immunization of human volunteers under chemoprophylaxis induces functional antibodies against pre-erythrocytic stages of *Plasmodium falciparum*. *Malar J* **13:** 136.

Boonhok R, Rachaphaew N, Duangmanee A, Chobson P, Pattaradilokrat S, Utaisincharoen P, Sattabongkot J, Ponpuak M. 2016. LAP-like process as an immune mechanism downstream of IFN-γ in control of the human malaria *Plasmodium vivax* liver stage. *Proc Natl Acad Sci* **113:** E3519–E3528.

Burda PC, Roelli MA, Schaffner M, Khan SM, Janse CJ, Heussler VT. 2015. A *Plasmodium* phospholipase is involved in disruption of the liver stage parasitophorous vacuole membrane. *PLoS Pathog* **11:** e1004760.

Butler NS, Schmidt NW, Vaughan AM, Aly AS, Kappe SH, Harty JT. 2011. Superior antimalarial immunity after vaccination with late liver stage-arresting genetically attenuated parasites. *Cell Host Microbe* **9:** 451–462.

Clyde DF, Most H, McCarthy VC, Vanderberg JP. 1973. Immunization of man against sporozite-induced falciparum malaria. *Am J Med Sci* **266:** 169–177.

Cobbold SA, Vaughan AM, Lewis IA, Painter HJ, Camargo N, Perlman DH, Fishbaugher M, Healer J, Cowman AF, Kappe SH, et al. 2013. Kinetic flux profiling elucidates two independent acetyl-CoA biosynthetic pathways in *Plasmodium falciparum*. *J Biol Chem* **288:** 36338–36350.

Combe A, Giovannini D, Carvalho TG, Spath S, Boisson B, Loussert C, Thiberge S, Lacroix C, Gueirard P, Menard R. 2009. Clonal conditional mutagenesis in malaria parasites. *Cell Host Microbe* **5:** 386–396.

Coppi A, Natarajan R, Pradel G, Bennett BL, James ER, Roggero MA, Corradin G, Persson C, Tewari R, Sinnis P. 2011. The malaria circumsporozoite protein has two functional domains, each with distinct roles as sporozoites journey from mosquito to mammalian host. *J Exp Med* **208:** 341–356.

Coppi A, Pinzon-Ortiz C, Hutter C, Sinnis P. 2005. The *Plasmodium* circumsporozoite protein is proteolytically processed during cell invasion. *J Exp Med* **201:** 27–33.

Coppi A, Tewari R, Bishop JR, Bennett BL, Lawrence R, Esko JD, Billker O, Sinnis P. 2007. Heparan sulfate proteoglycans provide a signal to *Plasmodium* sporozoites to stop migrating and productively invade host cells. *Cell Host Microbe* **2:** 316–327.

Cowman AF, Berry D, Baum J. 2012. The cellular and molecular basis for malaria parasite invasion of the human red blood cell. *J Cell Biol* **198:** 961–971.

Dankwa DA, Davis MJ, Kappe SH, Vaughan AM. 2016. A *Plasmodium yoelii* Mei2-like RNA binding protein is essential for completion of liver stage schizogony. *Infect Immun* **84:** 1336–1345.

Deretic V, Saitoh T, Akira S. 2013. Autophagy in infection, inflammation and immunity. *Nat Rev Immunol* **13:** 722–737.

Doll KL, Harty JT. 2014. Correlates of protective immunity following whole sporozoite vaccination against malaria. *Immunol Res* **59:** 166–176.

Douradinha B, van Dijk MR, Ataide R, van Gemert GJ, Thompson J, Franetich JF, Mazier D, Luty AJ, Sauerwein R, Janse CJ, et al. 2007. Genetically attenuated P36p-deficient *Plasmodium* berghei sporozoites confer long-lasting and partial cross-species protection. *Int J Parasitol* **37:** 1511–1519.

Eickel N, Kaiser G, Prado M, Burda PC, Roelli M, Stanway RR, Heussler VT. 2013. Features of autophagic cell death in *Plasmodium* liver-stage parasites. *Autophagy* **9:** 568–580.

Ejigiri I, Sinnis P. 2009. *Plasmodium* sporozoite-host interactions from the dermis to the hepatocyte. *Curr Opin Microbiol* **12:** 401–407.

Ejigiri I, Ragheb DR, Pino P, Coppi A, Bennett BL, Soldati-Favre D, Sinnis P. 2012. Shedding of TRAP by a rhomboid protease from the malaria sporozoite surface is essential for gliding motility and sporozoite infectivity. *PLoS Pathog* **8:** e1002725.

Falae A, Combe A, Anburaj A, Carvalho TG, Menard R, Bhanot P. 2010. The role of *Plasmodium berghei* cGMP dependent protein kinase in late liver stage development. *J Biol Chem* **285:** 3282–3288.

Falkard B, Kumar TR, Hecht LS, Matthews KA, Henrich PP, Gulati S, Lewis RE, Manary MJ, Winzeler EA, Sinnis P, et al. 2013. A key role for lipoic acid synthesis during *Plasmodium* liver stage development. *Cell Microbiol* **15:** 1585–1604.

Ferreira A, Schofield L, Enea V, Schellekens H, van der Meide P, Collins WE, Nussenzweig RS, Nussenzweig V. 1986. Inhibition of development of exo-erythrocytic forms of malaria parasites by γ-interferon. *Science* **232:** 881–884.

Foquet L, Hermsen CC, van Gemert GJ, Van Braeckel E, Weening KE, Sauerwein R, Meuleman P, Leroux-Roels G. 2014. Vaccine-induced monoclonal antibodies targeting circumsporozoite protein prevent *Plasmodium falciparum* infection. *J Clin Invest* **124:** 140–144.

Foquet L, Hermsen CC, Verhoye L, van Gemert GJ, Cortese R, Nicosia A, Sauerwein RW, Leroux-Roels G, Meuleman P. 2015. Anti-CD81 but not anti-SR-BI blocks *Plasmodium falciparum* liver infection in a humanized mouse model. *J Antimicrob Chemother* **70:** 1784–1787.

Fowler RE, Margos G, Mitchell GH. 2004. The cytoskeleton and motility in apicomplexan invasion. *Adv Parasitol* **56:** 213–263.

Frevert U, Sinnis P, Cerami C, Shreffler W, Takacs B, Nussenzweig V. 1993. Malaria circumsporozoite protein binds to heparan sulfate proteoglycans associated with the surface membrane of hepatocytes. *J Exp Med* **177:** 1287–1298.

Gonzalez V, Combe A, David V, Malmquist NA, Delorme V, Leroy C, Blazquez S, Menard R, Tardieux I. 2009. Host cell entry by apicomplexa parasites requires actin polymerization in the host cell. *Cell Host Microbe* **5:** 259–272.

Graewe S, Rankin KE, Lehmann C, Deschermeier C, Hecht L, Froehlke U, Stanway RR, Heussler V. 2011. Hostile takeover by *Plasmodium*: Reorganization of parasite and host cell membranes during liver stage egress. *PLoS Pathog* **7:** e1002224.

Grutzke J, Rindte K, Goosmann C, Silvie O, Rauch C, Heuer D, Lehmann MJ, Mueller AK, Brinkmann V, Matuschewski K, et al. 2014. The spatiotemporal dynamics and

Cite this article as *Cold Spring Harb Perspect Med* doi: 10.1101/cshperspect.a025486

membranous features of the *Plasmodium* liver stage tubovesicular network. *Traffic* **15**: 362–382.

Hanson KK, Mair GR. 2014. Stress granules and *Plasmodium* liver stage infection. *Biol Open* **3**: 103–107.

Haussig JM, Matuschewski K, Kooij TW. 2011. Inactivation of a *Plasmodium* apicoplast protein attenuates formation of liver merozoites. *Mol Microbiol* **81**: 1511–1525.

Inacio P, Zuzarte-Luis V, Ruivo MTG, Falkard B, Nagaraj N, Rooijers K, Mann M, Mair G, Fidock D, Mota MM. 2015. A role for ER stress during *Plasmodium* liver stage infection. *EMBO Rep* **16**: 955–964.

Ishino T, Chinzei Y, Yuda M. 2005. Two proteins with 6-cys motifs are required for malarial parasites to commit to infection of the hepatocyte. *Mol Microbiol* **58**: 1264–1275.

Ishino T, Boisson B, Orito Y, Lacroix C, Bischoff E, Loussert C, Janse C, Menard R, Yuda M, Baldacci P. 2009. LISP1 is important for the egress of *Plasmodium berghei* parasites from liver cells. *Cell Microbiol* **11**: 1329–1339.

Itoe MA, Sampaio JL, Cabal GG, Real E, Zuzarte-Luis V, March S, Bhatia SN, Frischknecht F, Thiele C, Shevchenko A, et al. 2014. Host cell phosphatidylcholine is a key mediator of malaria parasite survival during liver stage infection. *Cell Host Microbe* **16**: 778–786.

Jayabalasingham B, Bano N, Coppens I. 2010. Metamorphosis of the malaria parasite in the liver is associated with organelle clearance. *Cell Res* **20**: 1043–1059.

Jayabalasingham B, Voss C, Ehrenman K, Romano JD, Smith ME, Fidock DA, Bosch J, Coppens I. 2014. Characterization of the ATG8-conjugation system in 2 *Plasmodium* species with special focus on the liver stage: Possible linkage between the apicoplastic and autophagic systems? *Autophagy* **10**: 269–284.

Jobe O, Lumsden J, Mueller AK, Williams J, Silva-Rivera H, Kappe SH, Schwenk RJ, Matuschewski K, Krzych U. 2007. Genetically attenuated *Plasmodium berghei* liver stages induce sterile protracted protection that is mediated by major histocompatibility complex class I–dependent interferon-γ-producing CD8⁺ T cells. *J Infect Dis* **196**: 599–607.

Kaiser K, Camargo N, Kappe SH. 2003. Transformation of sporozoites into early exo-erythrocytic malaria parasites does not require host cells. *J Exp Med* **197**: 1045–1050.

Kappe S, Bruderer T, Gantt S, Fujioka H, Nussenzweig V, Menard R. 1999. Conservation of a gliding motility and cell invasion machinery in Apicomplexan parasites. *J Cell Biol* **147**: 937–944.

Kaushansky A, Metzger PG, Douglass AN, Mikolajczak SA, Lakshmanan V, Kain HS, Kappe SH. 2013a. Malaria parasite liver stages render host hepatocytes susceptible to mitochondria-initiated apoptosis. *Cell Death Dis* **4**: e762.

Kaushansky A, Ye AS, Austin LS, Mikolajczak SA, Vaughan AM, Camargo N, Metzger PG, Douglass AN, Macbeath G, Kappe SH. 2013b. Suppression of host p53 is critical for *Plasmodium* liver-stage infection. *Cell Rep* **3**: 630–637.

Kaushansky A, Douglass AN, Arang N, Vigdorovich V, Dambrauskas N, Kain HS, Austin LS, Sather DN, Kappe SH. 2015. Malaria parasites target the hepatocyte receptor EphA2 for successful host infection. *Science* **350**: 1089–1092.

Krotoski WA, Collins WE, Bray RS, Garnham PC, Cogswell FB, Gwadz RW, Killick-Kendrick R, Wolf R, Sinden R, Koontz LC, et al. 1982. Demonstration of hypnozoites in sporozoite-transmitted *Plasmodium vivax* infection. *Am J Trop Med Hyg* **31**: 1291–1293.

Labaied M, Harupa A, Dumpit RF, Coppens I, Mikolajczak SA, Kappe SH. 2007. *Plasmodium yoelii* sporozoites with simultaneous deletion of P52 and P36 are completely attenuated and confer sterile immunity against infection. *Infect Immun* **75**: 3758–3768.

Labaied M, Jayabalasingham B, Bano N, Cha SJ, Sandoval J, Guan G, Coppens I. 2011. *Plasmodium* salvages cholesterol internalized by LDL and synthesized de novo in the liver. *Cell Microbiol* **13**: 569–586.

Liehl P, Mota MM. 2012. Innate recognition of malarial parasites by mammalian hosts. *Int J Parasitol* **42**: 557–566.

Liehl P, Zuzarte-Luis V, Chan J, Zillinger T, Baptista F, Carapau D, Konert M, Hanson KK, Carret C, Lassnig C, et al. 2014. Host-cell sensors for *Plasmodium* activate innate immunity against liver-stage infection. *Nat Med* **20**: 47–53.

Lindner SE, Sartain MJ, Hayes K, Harupa A, Moritz RL, Kappe SH, Vaughan AM. 2014. Enzymes involved in plastid-targeted phosphatidic acid synthesis are essential for *Plasmodium yoelii* liver-stage development. *Mol Microbiol* **91**: 679–693.

Lopes da Silva M, Thieleke-Matos C, Cabrita-Santos L, Ramalho JS, Wavre-Shapton ST, Futter CE, Barral DC, Seabra MC. 2012. The host endocytic pathway is essential for *Plasmodium berghei* late liver stage development. *Traffic* **13**: 1351–1363.

March S, Ng S, Velmurugan S, Galstian A, Shan J, Logan DJ, Carpenter AE, Thomas D, Sim BK, Mota MM, et al. 2013. A microscale human liver platform that supports the hepatic stages of *Plasmodium falciparum* and vivax. *Cell Host Microbe* **14**: 104–115.

Mazier D, Landau I, Druilhe P, Miltgen F, Guguen-Guillouzo C, Baccam D, Baxter J, Chigot JP, Gentilini M. 1984. Cultivation of the liver forms of *Plasmodium vivax* in human hepatocytes. *Nature* **307**: 367–369.

Mazier D, Beaudoin RL, Mellouk S, Druilhe P, Texier B, Trosper J, Miltgen F, Landau I, Paul C, Brandicourt O, et al. 1985. Complete development of hepatic stages of *Plasmodium falciparum* in vitro. *Science* **227**: 440–442.

Meis JF, Verhave JP, Jap PH, Sinden RE, Meuwissen JH. 1983. Malaria parasites—Discovery of the early liver form. *Nature* **302**: 424–426.

Mikolajczak SA, Jacobs-Lorena V, MacKellar DC, Camargo N, Kappe SH. 2007. L-FABP is a critical host factor for successful malaria liver stage development. *Int J Parasitol* **37**: 483–489.

Mikolajczak SA, Sacci JB Jr, De La Vega P, Camargo N, VanBuskirk K, Krzych U, Cao J, Jacobs-Lorena M, Cowman AF, Kappe SH. 2011. Disruption of the *Plasmodium falciparum* liver-stage antigen-1 locus causes a differentiation defect in late liver-stage parasites. *Cell Microbiol* **13**: 1250–1260.

Mikolajczak SA, Lakshmanan V, Fishbaugher M, Camargo N, Harupa A, Kaushansky A, Douglass AN, Baldwin M, Healer J, O'Neill M, et al. 2014. A next-generation genetically attenuated *Plasmodium falciparum* parasite created by triple gene deletion. *Mol Ther* **22:** 1707–1715.

Mikolajczak SA, Vaughan AM, Kangwanrangsan N, Roobsoong W, Fishbaugher M, Yimamnuaychok N, Rezakhani N, Lakshmanan V, Singh N, Kaushansky A, et al. 2015. *Plasmodium vivax* liver stage development and hypnozoite persistence in human liver-chimeric mice. *Cell Host Microbe* **17:** 526–535.

Miller JL, Harupa A, Kappe SH, Mikolajczak SA. 2012. *Plasmodium yoelii* macrophage migration inhibitory factor is necessary for efficient liver-stage development. *Infect Immun* **80:** 1399–1407.

Miller JL, Sack BK, Baldwin M, Vaughan AM, Kappe SH. 2014. Interferon-mediated innate immune responses against malaria parasite liver stages. *Cell Rep* **7:** 436–447.

Molina-Cruz A, Garver LS, Alabaster A, Bangiolo L, Haile A, Winikor J, Ortega C, van Schaijk BC, Sauerwein RW, Taylor-Salmon E, et al. 2013. The human malaria parasite Pfs47 gene mediates evasion of the mosquito immune system. *Science* **340:** 984–987.

Mueller AK, Camargo N, Kaiser K, Andorfer C, Frevert U, Matuschewski K, Kappe SH. 2005a. *Plasmodium* liver stage developmental arrest by depletion of a protein at the parasite-host interface. *Proc Natl Acad Sci* **102:** 3022–3027.

Mueller AK, Labaied M, Kappe SH, Matuschewski K. 2005b. Genetically modified *Plasmodium* parasites as a protective experimental malaria vaccine. *Nature* **433:** 164–167.

Nagel A, Prado M, Heitmann A, Tartz S, Jacobs T, Deschermeier C, Helm S, Stanway R, Heussler V. 2013. A new approach to generate a safe double-attenuated *Plasmodium* liver stage vaccine. *Int J Parasitol* **43:** 503–514.

Ng S, Schwartz RE, March S, Galstian A, Gural N, Shan J, Prabhu M, Mota MM, Bhatia SN. 2015. Human iPSC-derived hepatocyte-like cells support *Plasmodium* liver-stage infection in vitro. *Stem Cell Rep* **4:** 348–359.

Nussenzweig RS, Vanderberg J, Most H, Orton C. 1967. Protective immunity produced by the injection of x-irradiated sporozoites of *Plasmodium berghei*. *Nature* **216:** 160–162.

Orito Y, Ishino T, Iwanaga S, Kaneko I, Kato T, Menard R, Chinzei Y, Yuda M. 2013. Liver-specific protein 2: A *Plasmodium* protein exported to the hepatocyte cytoplasm and required for merozoite formation. *Mol Microbiol* **87:** 66–79.

Pei Y, Tarun AS, Vaughan AM, Herman RW, Soliman JM, Erickson-Wayman A, Kappe SH. 2010. *Plasmodium* pyruvate dehydrogenase activity is only essential for the parasite's progression from liver infection to blood infection. *Mol Microbiol* **75:** 957–971.

Ploemen IH, Croes HJ, van Gemert GJ, Wijers-Rouw M, Hermsen CC, Sauerwein RW. 2012. *Plasmodium berghei* Deltap52&p36 parasites develop independent of a parasitophorous vacuole membrane in Huh-7 liver cells. *PLoS ONE* **7:** e50772.

Pradel G. 2007. Proteins of the malaria parasite sexual stages: Expression, function and potential for transmission blocking strategies. *Parasitology* **134:** 1911–1929.

Prado M, Eickel N, De Niz M, Heitmann A, Agop-Nersesian C, Wacker R, Schmuckli-Maurer J, Caldelari R, Janse CJ, Khan SM, et al. 2015. Long-term live imaging reveals cytosolic immune responses of host hepatocytes against

Plasmodium infection and parasite escape mechanisms. *Autophagy* **11:** 1561–1579.

Rieckmann KH, Carson PE, Beaudoin RL, Cassells JS, Sell KW. 1974. Letter: Sporozoite induced immunity in man against an Ethiopian strain of *Plasmodium falciparum*. *Trans R Soc Trop Med Hyg* **68:** 258–259.

Rijpma SR, van der Velden M, Gonzalez-Pons M, Annoura T, van Schaijk BC, van Gemert GJ, van den Heuvel JJ, Ramesar J, Chevalley-Maurel S, Ploemen IH, et al. 2016. Multidrug ATP-binding cassette transporters are essential for hepatic development of *Plasmodium* sporozoites. *Cell Microbiol* **18:** 369–383.

Risco-Castillo V, Topcu S, Son O, Briquet S, Manzoni G, Silvie O. 2014. CD81 is required for rhoptry discharge during host cell invasion by *Plasmodium yoelii* sporozoites. *Cell Microbiol* **16:** 1533–1548.

Sacci JB Jr, Alam U, Douglas D, Lewis J, Tyrrell DL, Azad AF, Kneteman NM. 2006. *Plasmodium falciparum* infection and exo-erythrocytic development in mice with chimeric human livers. *Int J Parasitol* **36:** 353–360.

Sack BK, Miller JL, Vaughan AM, Douglass A, Kaushansky A, Mikolajczak S, Coppi A, Gonzalez-Aseguinolaza G, Tsuji M, Zavala F, et al. 2014. Model for in vivo assessment of humoral protection against malaria sporozoite challenge by passive transfer of monoclonal antibodies and immune serum. *Infect Immun* **82:** 808–817.

Sack BK, Keitany GJ, Vaughan AM, Miller JL, Wang R, Kappe SH. 2015. Mechanisms of stage-transcending protection following immunization of mice with late liver stage-arresting genetically attenuated malaria parasites. *PLoS Pathog* **11:** e1004855.

Sahu T, Boisson B, Lacroix C, Bischoff E, Richier Q, Formaglio P, Thiberge S, Dobrescu I, Menard R, Baldacci P. 2014. ZIPCO, a putative metal ion transporter, is crucial for *Plasmodium* liver-stage development. *EMBO Mol Med* **6:** 1387–1397.

Sala KA, Nishiura H, Upton LM, Zakutansky SE, Delves MJ, Iyori M, Mizutani M, Sinden RE, Yoshida S, Blagborough AM. 2015. The *Plasmodium berghei* sexual stage antigen PSOP12 induces anti-malarial transmission blocking immunity both in vivo and in vitro. *Vaccine* **33:** 437–445.

Sattabongkot J, Yimamnuaychoke N, Leelaudomlipi S, Rasameesoraj M, Jenwithisuk R, Coleman RE, Udomsangpetch R, Cui L, Brewer TG. 2006. Establishment of a human hepatocyte line that supports in vitro development of the exo-erythrocytic stages of the malaria parasites *Plasmodium falciparum* and *P. vivax*. *Am J Trop Med Hyg* **74:** 708–715.

Seder RA, Chang LJ, Enama ME, Zephir KL, Sarwar UN, Gordon IJ, Holman LA, James ER, Billingsley PF, Gunasekera A, et al. 2013. Protection against malaria by intravenous immunization with a nonreplicating sporozoite vaccine. *Science* **341:** 1359–1365.

Silvie O, Goetz K, Matuschewski K. 2008. A sporozoite asparagine-rich protein controls initiation of *Plasmodium* liver stage development. *PLoS Pathog* **4:** e1000086.

Silvie O, Rubinstein E, Franetich JF, Prenant M, Belnoue E, Renia L, Hannoun L, Eling W, Levy S, Boucheix C, et al. 2003. Hepatocyte CD81 is required for *Plasmodium falciparum* and *Plasmodium yoelii* sporozoite infectivity. *Nat Med* **9:** 93–96.

Silvie O, Charrin S, Billard M, Franetich JF, Clark KL, van Gemert GJ, Sauerwein RW, Dautry F, Boucheix C, Mazier D, et al. 2006. Cholesterol contributes to the organization of tetraspanin-enriched microdomains and to CD81-dependent infection by malaria sporozoites. *J Cell Sci* **119:** 1992–2002.

Spring M, Murphy J, Nielsen R, Dowler M, Bennett JW, Zarling S, Williams J, de la Vega P, Ware L, Komisar J, et al. 2013. First-in-human evaluation of genetically attenuated *Plasmodium falciparum* sporozoites administered by bite of *Anopheles* mosquitoes to adult volunteers. *Vaccine* **31:** 4975–4983.

Stanway RR, Witt T, Zobiak B, Aepfelbacher M, Heussler VT. 2009. GFP-targeting allows visualization of the apicoplast throughout the life cycle of live malaria parasites. *Biol Cell* **101:** 415–430.

Stanway RR, Mueller N, Zobiak B, Graewe S, Froehlke U, Zessin PJ, Aepfelbacher M, Heussler VT. 2011. Organelle segregation into *Plasmodium* liver stage merozoites. *Cell Microbiol* **13:** 1768–1782.

Sturm A, Amino R, van de Sand C, Regen T, Retzlaff S, Rennenberg A, Krueger A, Pollok JM, Menard R, Heussler VT. 2006. Manipulation of host hepatocytes by the malaria parasite for delivery into liver sinusoids. *Science* **313:** 1287–1290.

Sturm A, Graewe S, Franke-Fayard B, Retzlaff S, Bolte S, Roppenser B, Aepfelbacher M, Janse C, Heussler V. 2009. Alteration of the parasite plasma membrane and the parasitophorous vacuole membrane during exoerythrocytic development of malaria parasites. *Protist* **160:** 51–63.

Tardif KD, Siddiqui A. 2003. Cell surface expression of major histocompatibility complex class I molecules is reduced in hepatitis C virus subgenomic replicon-expressing cells. *J Virol* **77:** 11644–11650.

Tarun AS, Baer K, Dumpit RF, Gray S, Lejarcegui N, Frevert U, Kappe SH. 2006. Quantitative isolation and in vivo imaging of malaria parasite liver stages. *Int J Parasitol* **36:** 1283–1293.

Tarun AS, Dumpit RF, Camargo N, Labaied M, Liu P, Takagi A, Wang R, Kappe SH. 2007. Protracted sterile protection with *Plasmodium yoelii* pre-erythrocytic genetically attenuated parasite malaria vaccines is independent of significant liver-stage persistence and is mediated by CD8[+] T cells. *J Infect Dis* **196:** 608–616.

Tarun AS, Peng X, Dumpit RF, Ogata Y, Silva-Rivera H, Camargo N, Daly TM, Bergman LW, Kappe SH. 2008. A combined transcriptome and proteome survey of malaria parasite liver stages. *Proc Natl Acad Sci* **105:** 305–310.

Templeton TJ, Kaslow DC. 1999. Identification of additional members define a *Plasmodium falciparum* gene superfamily which includes Pfs48/45 and Pfs230. *Mol Biochem Parasitol* **101:** 223–227.

Thieleke-Matos C, da Silva ML, Cabrita-Santos L, Pires CF, Ramalho JS, Ikonomov O, Seixas E, Shisheva A, Seabra MC, Barral DC. 2014. Host PI(3,5)P2 activity is required for *Plasmodium berghei* growth during liver stage infection. *Traffic* **15:** 1066–1082.

VanBuskirk KM, O'Neill MT, De La Vega P, Maier AG, Krzych U, Williams J, Dowler MG, Sacci JB Jr, Kangwanrangsan N, Tsuboi T, et al. 2009. Pre-erythrocytic, live-attenuated *Plasmodium falciparum* vaccine candidates by design. *Proc Natl Acad Sci* **106:** 13004–13009.

van de Sand C, Horstmann S, Schmidt A, Sturm A, Bolte S, Krueger A, Lutgehetmann M, Pollok JM, Libert C, Heussler VT. 2005. The liver stage of *Plasmodium berghei* inhibits host cell apoptosis. *Mol Microbiol* **58:** 731–742.

van Dijk MR, Douradinha B, Franke-Fayard B, Heussler V, van Dooren MW, van Schaijk B, van Gemert GJ, Sauerwein RW, Mota MM, Waters AP, et al. 2005. Genetically attenuated, P36p-deficient malarial sporozoites induce protective immunity and apoptosis of infected liver cells. *Proc Natl Acad Sci* **102:** 12194–12199.

van Dijk MR, van Schaijk BC, Khan SM, van Dooren MW, Ramesar J, Kaczanowski S, van Gemert GJ, Kroeze H, Stunnenberg HG, Eling WM, et al. 2010. Three members of the 6-cys protein family of *Plasmodium* play a role in gamete fertility. *PLoS Pathog* **6:** e1000853.

van Schaijk BC, Janse CJ, van Gemert GJ, van Dijk MR, Gego A, Franetich JF, van de Vegte-Bolmer M, Yalaoui S, Silvie O, Hoffman SL, et al. 2008. Gene disruption of *Plasmodium falciparum* p52 results in attenuation of malaria liver stage development in cultured primary human hepatocytes. *PLoS ONE* **3:** e3549.

van Schaijk BC, Kumar TR, Vos MW, Richman A, van Gemert GJ, Li T, Eappen AG, Williamson KC, Morahan BJ, Fishbaugher M, et al. 2014a. Type II fatty acid biosynthesis is essential for *Plasmodium falciparum* sporozoite development in the midgut of *Anopheles* mosquitoes. *Eukaryot Cell* **13:** 550–559.

van Schaijk BC, Ploemen IH, Annoura T, Vos MW, Foquet L, van Gemert GJ, Chevalley-Maurel S, van de Vegte-Bolmer M, Sajid M, Franetich JF, et al. 2014b. A genetically attenuated malaria vaccine candidate based on *P. falciparum* b9/slarp gene-deficient sporozoites. *eLife* **3:** e03582.

Vaughan AM, O'Neill MT, Tarun AS, Camargo N, Phuong TM, Aly AS, Cowman AF, Kappe SH. 2009. Type II fatty acid synthesis is essential only for malaria parasite late liver stage development. *Cell Microbiol* **11:** 506–520.

Vaughan AM, Mikolajczak SA, Wilson EM, Grompe M, Kaushansky A, Camargo N, Bial J, Ploss A, Kappe SH. 2012. Complete *Plasmodium falciparum* liver-stage development in liver-chimeric mice. *J Clin Invest* **122:** 3618–3628.

Vaughan AM, Pinapati RS, Cheeseman IH, Camargo N, Fishbaugher M, Checkley LA, Nair S, Hutyra CA, Nosten FH, Anderson TJ, et al. 2015. *Plasmodium falciparum* genetic crosses in a humanized mouse model. *Nat Methods* **12:** 631–633.

Vinetz JM. 2005. *Plasmodium* ookinete invasion of the mosquito midgut. *Curr Top Microbiol Immunol* **295:** 357–382.

Yalaoui S, Huby T, Franetich JF, Gego A, Rametti A, Moreau M, Collet X, Siau A, van Gemert GJ, Sauerwein RW, et al. 2008. Scavenger receptor BI boosts hepatocyte permissiveness to *Plasmodium* infection. *Cell Host Microbe* **4:** 283–292.

Yu M, Kumar TR, Nkrumah LJ, Coppi A, Retzlaff S, Li CD, Kelly BJ, Moura PA, Lakshmanan V, Freundlich JS, et al. 2008. The fatty acid biosynthesis enzyme FabI plays a key role in the development of liver-stage malarial parasites. *Cell Host Microbe* **4:** 567–578.

Molecular Signaling Involved in Entry and Exit of Malaria Parasites from Host Erythrocytes

Shailja Singh[1,2] and Chetan E. Chitnis[1,3]

[1]Department of Parasites and Insect Vectors, Institut Pasteur, 75015 Paris, France

[2]Shiv Nadar University, Gautam Buddha Nagar, Uttar Pradesh 201314, India

[3]Malaria Group, International Centre for Genetic Engineering and Biotechnology (ICGEB), New Delhi 110067, India

Correspondence: cchitnis@gmail.com

During the blood stage, *Plasmodium* spp. merozoites invade host red blood cells (RBCs), multiply, exit, and reinvade uninfected RBCs in a continuing cycle that is responsible for all the clinical symptoms associated with malaria. Entry into (invasion) and exit from (egress) RBCs are highly regulated processes that are mediated by an array of parasite proteins with specific functional roles. Many of these parasite proteins are stored in specialized apical secretory vesicles, and their timely release is critical for successful invasion and egress. For example, the discharge of parasite protein ligands to the apical surface of merozoites is required for interaction with host receptors to mediate invasion, and the timely discharge of proteases and pore-forming proteins helps in permeabilization and dismantling of limiting membranes during egress. This review focuses on our understanding of the signaling mechanisms that regulate apical organelle secretion during host cell invasion and egress by malaria parasites. The review also explores how understanding key signaling mechanisms in the parasite can open opportunities to develop novel strategies to target *Plasmodium* parasites and eliminate malaria.

*P*lasmodium falciparum has a complex life cycle involving multiple stages in two hosts, namely, the vertebrate human host and the invertebrate *Anopheles* mosquito, which also serves as the vector for transmission. *P. falciparum* sporozoites are introduced into the human host following a bite by an infected female *Anopheles* mosquito in search of a blood meal. The injected sporozoites traverse through the bloodstream to the liver where they infect hepatocytes, multiply, and differentiate into merozoites. The merozoites are released into the bloodstream in membrane-bound packets called merosomes, which protect the parasite from host immune mechanisms. Merozoites emerge from merosomes in the bloodstream and go on to invade host red blood cells (RBCs) within which they develop and multiply by schizogeny over a period of 36–48 hours. Once the next generation of merozoites has developed, the mature schizont ruptures and merozoites egress in a highly synchronized manner. Merozoite egress requires disruption of the RBC cytoskeleton and rupture of multiple limiting membranes (Salmon et al. 2001; Wickham et al. 2003). Key parasite effectors that mediate egress include proteases as well as perforin-like proteins (Blackman 2008; Roiko and Carruthers 2009, 2013; Agarwal et al. 2012; Garg et al. 2013). Many of these effectors are localized in apical organelles and are secreted in a timely, regulated manner to initiate egress of merozoites from mature schizonts. The released merozoites go on to invade uninfected erythrocytes to continue blood-stage multiplication.

Invasion of host erythrocytes by *P. falciparum* merozoites is also a complex multistep process that involves initial attachment, apical reorientation, junction formation, development of a nascent vacuole, and movement of the parasite into the vacuole, followed by resealing of the vacuole so that the parasite is surrounded by a vacuolar membrane at the end of invasion (Dvorak et al. 1975; Aikawa et al. 1978; Cowman and Crabb 2006; Gilson and Crabb 2009; Riglar et al. 2011; Baum 2013). Many of the parasite ligands that bind host receptors to mediate these steps during invasion are initially localized in the micronemes and rhoptries at the apical end of merozoites. They are secreted to the surface of the merozoite in a highly regulated manner to enable receptor binding and invasion (Singh et al. 2010; Gaur and Chitnis 2011; Riglar et al. 2011; Singh and Chitnis 2012; Sharma and Chitnis 2013).

Here, we will review our current understanding of the signals and signaling mechanisms that regulate the highly coordinated processes of parasite egress and host cell invasion. This review will focus on our understanding of the key signaling mechanisms that trigger the release of parasite proteins from apical organelles to mediate parasite egress and invasion. We will include information from both malaria parasites as well as the related apicomplexan parasite, *Toxoplasma gondii*, which shares many common features in the process of host cell invasion. Finally, we will discuss how a better understanding of signaling processes during invasion and egress may provide novel targets for intervention to interrupt the malaria parasite life cycle and eliminate malaria.

MOLECULAR PLAYERS AND SIGNALS FOR EGRESS OF *Plasmodium falciparum* MEROZOITES FROM MATURE SCHIZONTS

Egress of *P. falciparum* merozoites from RBCs requires breaching of multiple barriers including the parasitophorous vacuole membrane (PVM), the host cytoskeleton, and the host plasma membrane (HPM). Parasite egress is synchronized with completion of its replicative cycle when next generation of invasive parasites have developed fully. Several parasite proteases have been identified as key effectors of the egress process in apicomplexan blood-stage parasites (Blackman 2008; Roiko and Carruthers 2009). In addition, perforin-like proteins with homology with mammalian perforins are involved in egress by *T. gondii* tachyzoites (TgPLP) as well as *P. falciparum* merozoites (PfPLP) (Kafsack et al. 2009, 2010; Garg et al. 2013). The PLPs and the subtilisin-like protease, PfSub1, which mediate egress, are located in micronemes and exonemes, respectively (Yeoh et al. 2007; Agarwal et al. 2012; Garg et al. 2013). What are the signals and signaling mechanisms that trigger release of these effectors to initiate egress?

The phytohormone abscisic acid (ABA) was identified as the internal signal that triggers egress of *T. gondii* tachyzoites (Nagamune et al. 2008). In plants, ABA acts as a hormone that mediates growth and responses to environmental cues through cyclic ADP-ribose (cADPR) and calcium (Ca^{2+}) fluxes (Wu et al. 1997). In *T. gondii*, ABA induces the production of cADPR, which activates Ca^{2+} release from an internal membrane-bound pool (probably the endoplasmic reticulum [ER]) leading to secretion of microneme proteins such as TgPLP (Chini et al. 2005; Nagamune et al. 2008). Although the parasite genome has candidate genes for ABA synthesis, the presence of the entire biosynthetic pathway remains to be confirmed. Reflecting its plant heritage, ABA is most likely synthesized in the apicoplast, an organelle found in apicomplexans that is derived from an algal endosymbiont. Interestingly, ABA levels spike late in schizogeny just before parasite egress. Thus, the steep increase in production of ABA at the end of the replicative cycle might

Cite this article as *Cold Spring Harb Perspect Med* doi: 10.1101/cshperspect.a026815

serve as an intrinsic cue for egress. The herbicide fluridone, which inhibits ABA synthesis, blocks egress of *T. gondii* tachyzoites (Nagamune et al. 2008). Furthermore, mice treated with fluridone survive inoculation with a lethal dose of *Toxoplasma*. Fluridone also blocks Ca^{2+}-mediated egress of *P. falciparum* merozoites from mature schizonts (S Singh and CE Chitnis, unpubl.), suggesting a conserved role for ABA in regulating egress in apicomplexan parasites (Fig. 1).

Rupture of limiting membranes during egress exposes *T. gondii* tachyzoites to a drop in the concentration of K^+ ($[K^+]$), which activates tachyzoite motility leading to rapid exit of mature tachyzoites (Moudy et al. 2001). Precisely how the tachyzoite senses $[K^+]$ is not known, although phospholipase C (PLC), cytosolic $[Ca^{2+}]$ levels, and several Ca^{+2}-responsive proteins are thought to play a role (Moudy et al. 2001). The levels of $[K^+]$ in the environment may be a natural external cue for tachyzoite egress at the end of the replicative cycle. However, parasites have also been observed to exit host cells in the absence of parasite motility or low $[K^+]$ (Lavine and Arrizabalaga 2008; Abkarian et al. 2011). In case of malaria parasites, osmotic stress and host cell membrane tension may induce egress (Abkarian et al. 2011). Under normal circumstances, however, it is likely that the parasite uses intrinsic as well as extrinsic cues such as ABA and $[K^+]$, respectively, as signals to trigger escape.

Several recent studies have provided compelling evidence for a role for proteases in egress of *Plasmodium* spp. merozoites (Blackman 2004, 2008). Protease inhibitors have proved invaluable tools in analyzing the role of proteases in *Plasmodium* biology and have shown that egress is a protease-dependent function. Although multiple models for merozoite egress have been proposed, evidence is accumulating in support of a model in which the PVM is disrupted before the RBC membrane (RBCM) (Winograd et al. 1999; Wickham et al. 2003). Further evidence for a model in which the parasite egresses in a stepwise manner came from observations that disruption of each limiting membrane is sensitive to different protease in-

hibitors (Salmon et al. 2001; Wickham et al. 2003; Soni et al. 2005; Millholland et al. 2011). Whereas the cysteine and serine protease inhibitors, leupeptin and antipain, block RBCM disruption, the cysteine protease inhibitor E-64 blocks PVM disruption (Glushakova et al. 2008). The targets of these inhibitors, however, remain to be determined.

Other proteases involved in egress include DPAP3, a cathepsin-C like cysteine protease, which is required for maturation of PfSUB1, a subtilisin-like protease implicated in egress (Arastu-Kapur et al. 2008). PfSUB1 is an essential protein that is expressed in late-blood-stage parasites and is secreted into the PV from apical merozoite organelles called exonemes before egress (Yeoh et al. 2007). Once in the PV, PfSUB1 processes serine-rich antigen 5 (SERA5) and potentially other serine-repeat antigen (SERA) proteins (Yeoh et al. 2007; Arastu-Kapur et al. 2008). The SERAs are PV proteins with papain-like putative protease domains. Although evidence of proteolytic activity has yet to be shown by SERAs, it is possible that PfSub1 processing of SERA5 and other SERAs results in their activation and proteolysis of host cytoskeletal proteins to aid in parasite egress (Yeoh et al. 2007). Alternatively, SERAs might activate other parasite or host proteins that promote parasite egress. PfSERA5 processing from a precursor to mature form is linked to egress because this putative activation step occurs coincident with parasite exit from the erythrocyte (Blackman 2008). Inhibition of PfSERA5 by a cyclical peptide halts late-stage development of intraerythrocytic parasites possibly by blocking egress (Fairlie et al. 2008).

A host calcium-dependent protease, calpain-1, is also required for efficient parasite egress of *Plasmodium* spp. merozoites and *Toxoplasma* tachyzoites (Olaya and Wasserman 1991; Chandramohanadas et al. 2009). Treatment of *P. falciparum* infected erythrocytes with an irreversible cysteine protease inhibitor, DCG04, did not affect parasite maturation but prevented parasite release from the host cell (Chandramohanadas et al. 2009). Selective extraction of treated cells identified host calpain-1 as the target of the inhibitor. Calpain-1 was observed in

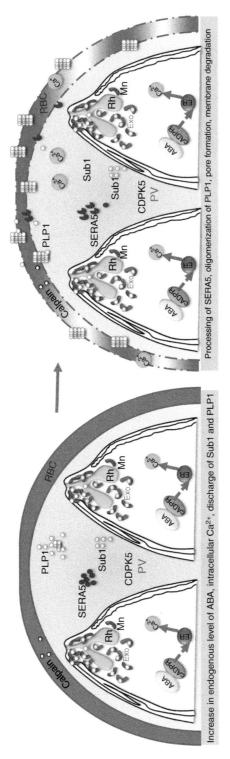

Figure 1. Regulation of merozoites' egress from host erythrocyte. An increase in abscisic acid (ABA) in schizonts leads to release of Ca²⁺ from the endoplasmic reticulum (ER) through the cADPR pathway. Increase in cytosolic Ca²⁺ triggers release of microneme (Mn) proteins such as PfPLP1 and exoneme (Exo) proteins such as PfSub1. Following secretion, PfPLP1 relocalizes to the limiting membranes and permeabilizes them to facilitate egress. Following its discharge to the parasitophorous vacuole (PV), PfSub1 mediates the processing of PfSERA5, leading to membrane degradation and egress.

the cytoplasm of the infected host cell until the schizont stage of parasite growth, when it relocated to the membrane following binding to Ca^{2+} and activation. Calpain-1 depletion from erythrocytes prevented parasite egress and led to growth arrest in the schizont stage, whereas reconstitution with recombinant calpain-1 restored normal growth development (Chandramohanadas et al. 2009). Human host cells treated with siRNA for host calpains (calpains 1 and 2) showed that it was required for *T. gondii* egress (Chandramohanadas et al. 2009).

ROLE OF APICAL ORGANELLE DISCHARGE IN REGULATION OF PARASITE EGRESS

Until recently, micronemes, the tubular shaped secretory organelles at the apical end of apicomplexan parasites, were thought to primarily contain adhesins that bind to cognate receptors on host cells during invasion. However, recently it has been shown that they also contain proteins that may be involved in parasite egress such as the pore-forming *T. gondii* perforin-like protein (TgPLP1) (Kafsack et al. 2009, 2010). It has been known for some time that microneme secretion is triggered by elevation of cytosolic Ca^{2+}. More recently, Ca^{2+} has also been implicated in regulating microneme secretion, which is required for parasite egress (Kafsack et al. 2009; Garg et al. 2013). Some of the molecular players in the calcium signaling pathway that play key roles in microneme secretion include TgCDPK1 and TgCDPK3, members of the calcium-dependent protein kinase family (Lourido et al. 2010). In a parallel study, using whole genome sequencing of *Toxoplasma* egress mutants, TgCDPK3 was found to be an essential factor for Ca^{2+}-induced egress from host cells. Because TgCDPK3 localizes to the periphery of the parasite, TgCDPK3 is proposed to be part of a signaling pathway that senses changes in the environment leading to egress (Lourido et al. 2012; McCoy et al. 2012). In case of *P. falciparum,* PfCDPK1 has been shown to play a role in microneme secretion (Bansal et al. 2013). In addition, although conditional deletion of PfCDPK5 results in a block in *P. falciparum* merozoite egress from mature schizonts, loss of PfCDPK5 does not

impair RBC invasion (Dvorin et al. 2010). Whether PfCDPK5 is responsible for regulating release of an apical organelle that is required for egress remains to be determined.

The activation of cGMP-dependent protein kinase G (TgPKG) has also been shown to induce microneme secretion and egress. Compound 1, a selective apicomplexan PKG inhibitor, was used to establish the role of TgPKG in microneme secretion and egress (Wiersma et al. 2004). Treatment of *P. falciparum* schizonts with compound 1 results in a block in schizont rupture, which does not occur when transgenic parasites with a gatekeeper mutation are treated with compound 1 (Taylor et al. 2010; Collins et al. 2013). Phosphoproteomic analysis of merozoites with and without treatment with Compound 1 suggests that a cGMP-dependent kinase serves as a signaling hub that regulates key processes in invasion and egress of *P. falciparum* merozoites (Alam et al. 2015). Interestingly, in contrast to PfCDPK5 knockdown parasites, Compound 1-treated merozoites were not invasive (Dvorin et al. 2010). Collectively, these findings describe the complex signaling pathways that regulate egress and suggest that the different pathways cross talk with each other enabling the parasite to respond to multiple signals to orchestrate a timely escape from host cells.

MOLECULAR PLAYERS FOR ERYTHROCYTE INVASION BY *Plasmodium* spp. MEROZOITES

Following egress and release from mature schizonts, *Plasmodium* merozoites go on to invade uninfected erythrocytes to initiate another round of intracellular replication. Erythrocyte invasion by *Plasmodium spp.* merozoites has been studied extensively by live cell imaging and electron microscopy (Dvorak et al. 1975; Aikawa et al. 1978; Riglar et al. 2011; Hanssen et al. 2013). After attachment to erythrocytes, merozoites reorient and develop a tight junction between their apical ends and target erythrocytes (Aikawa et al. 1978; Besteiro et al. 2011; Riglar et al 2011). These steps are mediated by multiple interactions between parasite protein ligands and host receptors (Gaur and Chitnis 2011; Cowman et al. 2012). The identity of host receptors involved in erythrocyte invasion came initially from studies that used genetically deficient erythrocytes or enzyme-treated erythrocytes for invasion studies. The first report on essentiality of a molecular interaction between *Plasmodium* spp. merozoites and erythrocytes during invasion was based on the observation that Duffy negativity in West Africa was associated with the absence of *P. vivax* infection (Miller et al. 1976). It was shown that *P. vivax* is dependent on interaction with the Duffy blood group antigen (also known as Duffy antigen receptor for chemokines [DARC]) to establish a blood-stage infection in humans (Miller et al. 1976; Horuk et al. 1993). However, recent studies have identified *P. vivax* strains in Kenya, Brazil, and Madagascar that can infect Duffy-negative individuals suggesting that *P. vivax* may invade using alternative invasion pathways (Ryan et al. 2006; Cavasini et al. 2007; Ménard et al. 2010). In case of *P. falciparum*, glycophorins A, B, C (GPA, GPB, GPC) were identified as receptors for invasion (Gaur and Chitnis 2011). However, no human erythrocyte lacking an individual receptor has been found to be completely refractory to invasion by *P. falciparum* indicating redundancy in invasion pathways. Following identification of host receptors, a family of erythrocyte-binding proteins (EBPs) that includes *P. vivax* and *P. knowlesi* Duffy-binding proteins (PvDBP and PkDBP) and *P. falciparum* erythrocyte-binding antigens, EBA-175, EBA-140, EBA-181, and EBL-1, were identified (Gaur and Chitnis 2011). GPA, GPB, and GPC have been shown to bind EBA-175, EBA-140, and EBL-1, respectively (Gaur and Chitnis 2011).

Another *P. falciparum* multigene family, which shares homology with *P. vivax* reticulocyte-binding proteins and binds erythrocytes, is the PfRH family of *P. falciparum* proteins (Gaur and Chitnis 2011). The PfRH protein family includes PfRH1a, PfRH1b PfRH2a, PfRH2b, PfRH4, and PfRH5. Genetic knockout studies have confirmed that PfRH2a/b and PfRH4 mediate sialic acid independent invasion pathways (Cowman et al. 2012). Complement receptor 1

(CR1) has recently been shown to serve as the erythrocyte receptor for PfRH4 (Tham et al. 2010). PfRH5 has also been shown to mediate invasion of Aotus erythrocytes by *P. falciparum* (Hayton et al. 2008). Basigin has been recently shown to be a receptor for PfRH5 binding (Crosnier et al. 2011). Other merozoite proteins implicated in invasion include thrombospondin-related anonymous protein (TRAP) homologs such as MTRAP and PTRAMP that contain the characteristic thrombospondin repeat (TSR) adhesive domains (Bartholdson et al. 2012; Siddiqui et al. 2013). Recent work has shown that the conserved apical membrane antigen-1 (PfAMA1) in complex with the rhoptry neck proteins (PfRON2 and PfRON4) localizes to the junction (Richard et al. 2010; Besteiro et al. 2011; Srinivasan et al. 2011). The exported PfRON2 protein is inserted into the erythrocyte membrane and interacts with secreted PfAMA1 during invasion. Other invasion-related proteins include two protein complexes, the high-molecular-weight (HMW) complex composed of RhopH1, RhopH2, and RhopH3 and the low-molecular-weight (LMW) complex composed of RAP1, RAP2, and RAP3. Apart from these adhesins and their interacting parasite ligands, *Plasmodium* spp. merozoites have a conserved molecular machinery for motility, which comprises of a central actin–myosin motor located in the pellicle of the parasite that is linked with both a surface adhesin and the inner membrane complex (IMC) and is likely to drive the invasion process (Sharma and Chitnis 2013). Recent work has shown that PfRON2-PfAMA1 interaction may not be essential for junction formation and there may be alternative pathways for invasion that are not dependent on the actin–myosin motor (Bargieri et al. 2014).

MOLECULAR SIGNALS THAT REGULATE APICAL ORGANELLE DISCHARGE DURING INVASION

As discussed above, many of the parasite proteins that bind erythrocyte receptors to mediate different steps in the invasion process are localized to the micronemes and rhoptries and must be translocated to the merozoite surface in a regulated manner to enable receptor engagement and invasion. For example, PfAMA1 and PfEBA175 are localized in the micronemes, whereas PfRON2, and PfRON4 are localized in the rhoptry neck and PfRH2, PfRH5, PfRAP1-3, and PfRhop1-3 are localized in the rhoptry bulb. The timely discharge of microneme and rhoptry proteins is essential for successful invasion by *P. falciparum* merozoites (Singh et al. 2010; Riglar et al. 2011; Hanssen et al. 2013).

What are the external signals and internal signaling pathways that mediate discharge of microneme and rhoptry proteins in *Plasmodium* merozoites and *Toxoplasma* tachyzoites during invasion? Studies with *T. gondii* tachyzoites first revealed that the levels of free cytosolic Ca^{2+} are high in tachyzoites during the process of gliding and are restored to basal levels following attachment to target cells during invasion (Carruthers and Sibley 1999; Carruthers et al. 1999; Lovett et al. 2002; Moreno and Docampo 2003). Similarly, cytosolic Ca^{2+} levels are high in *P. falciparum* merozoites and are restored to basal levels following attachment to target erythrocytes during invasion indicating that Ca^{2+} may regulate processes such as vesicular secretion during invasion (Singh et al. 2010). Indeed, treatment of *P. falciparum* merozoites with A23187 triggers an increase in cytosolic Ca^{2+} and secretion of microneme proteins such as PfAMA1 and PfEBA-175 but has no effect on secretion of rhoptry proteins (Singh et al. 2010). Importantly, the Ca^{2+} ionophore, A23187, induces microneme secretion in absence of extracellular Ca^{2+}, which indicates that Ca^{2+} from intracellular stores is sufficient for secretion of microneme proteins (Singh et al. 2010). Ethanol and other short-chain alcohols elevate cytosolic Ca^{2+} in *T. gondii* tachyzoites to stimulate microneme secretion (Carruthers and Sibley 1999; Carruthers et al. 1999). Treatment of tachyzoites with thapsigargin, which inhibits sarcoplasmic/endoplasmic reticulum calcium ATPase (SERCA) and blocks pumping of Ca^{2+} from the cytosol back to the endoplasmic reticulum (ER), increases cytosolic $[Ca^{2+}]$ levels and triggers secretion of microneme proteins. In contrast, chelation of cytosolic Ca^{2+} by treatment of

T. gondii tachyzoites or *P. falciparum* merozoites with BAPTA-AM inhibits microneme release and invasion of host cells (Singh et al. 1990; Carruthers and Sibley 1999; Carruthers et al. 1999). Ca^{2+} is stored in organelles such as the ER, mitochondria, and acidocalcisomes in apicomplexan parasites (Garcia 1999; Alleva and Kirk 2001). Treatment of *T. gondii* tachyzoites with ethanol raises levels of intracellular inositol triphosphate (IP_3), which trigger Ca^{2+} release by binding to IP_3-receptor gated Ca^{2+} channels (IP_3R) on the ER. Furthermore, xestospongin C, an IP_3R antagonist, inhibits ethanol-triggered release of Ca^{2+} and microneme secretion in *T. gondii* suggesting the presence of IP_3R (Lovett et al. 2002). The presence of PLC has been shown in *T. gondii* and PLC transcripts have been detected in *P. falciparum* blood-stage parasites. Moreover, an inhibitor of PLC has been shown to block Ca^{2+} release in *T. gondii* and *P. falciparum* providing further evidence for the presence of an IP_3-mediated pathway for Ca^{2+} release in these parasites (Carruthers and Sibley 1999; Carruthers et al. 1999; Lovett et al. 2002; Moreno et al. 2003; Vaid et al. 2008; Singh et al. 2010). Treatment of *T. gondii* with ryanodine or caffeine, which are agonists of the ryanodine receptor (RyR)-gated Ca^{2+} channel on ER, also leads to an increase in cytosolic Ca^{2+} and microneme secretion (Lovett et al. 2002). The ER thus appears to be the primary intracellular store from which Ca^{2+} is mobilized. Endogenous cyclic ADP ribose (cADPR), which can bind RyR to induce calcium release, was detected in *T. gondii* extracts suggesting that it may also play a role as a second messenger to regulate calcium levels and microneme secretion (Chini et al. 2005). Moreover, treatment of *T. gondii* tachyzoites with RyR antagonists, 8-bromo-cADPR and ruthenium red, blocks microneme secretion (Chini et al. 2005). Although use of modulators has provided pharmacological evidence for the presence of both IP_3R and RyR in both *P. falciparum* and *T. gondii*, the genes encoding IP_3R and RyR have not yet been identified.

The increase in cytosolic $[Ca^{2+}]$ levels activates *P. falciparum* calcium-dependent protein kinase 1 (PfCDPK1) and *T. gondii* CDPK1

(TgCDPK1), which play central roles in orchestrating many of the processes required for invasion of host cells, including microneme release and the activation of the actin–myosin motor (Green et al. 2008; Kato et al. 2008b; Lourido et al. 2010; Bansal et al. 2013). Recently, a screen for molecules required for invasion of host cells by *T. gondii* identified a DOC2 protein that is required for microneme secretion, presumably by mediating Ca^{2+}-dependent vesicular docking activity (Farrell et al. 2012). The *P. falciparum* ortholog of this protein is also required for the invasion of red blood cells and release of micronemes (Farrell et al. 2012). Independent of Ca^{2+} release, chemical genetic and phosphoproteomics evidence suggests that cyclic guanosine monophosphate (cGMP) and the cGMP-dependent kinase, PKG, also play an essential role in microneme release and invasion (Moon et al. 2009; Alam et al. 2015).

What might be the external signals that trigger secretion of microneme and rhoptry proteins during invasion? We have shown that exposure of *P. falciparum* merozoites to a low-$[K^+]$ environment as found in blood plasma can serve as a natural signal that triggers an increase in cytosolic $[Ca^{2+}]$ through the PLC pathway leading to secretion of microneme proteins such as PfEBA175 and PfAMA1 to the merozoite surface (Singh et al. 2010). Following translocation to the merozoite surface, binding of EBA175 to GPA restores basal $[Ca^{2+}]$ levels and triggers release of rhoptry proteins such as PfRH2b, Clag3.1, and PfTRAMP (Singh et al. 2010; Siddiqui et al. 2013). Secretion of microneme and rhoptry proteins to the merozoite surface is thus a two-step process as shown in Figure 2. Microneme proteins have also been shown to play a role in rhoptry secretion in *T. gondii*. Deletion of microneme protein MIC8 resulted in a block in rhoptry secretion and parasite growth (Kessler et al. 2008). The cytoplasmic domain of microneme proteins was implicated in playing a role to trigger rhoptry secretion (Kessler et al. 2008).

The pathway by which a low-$[K^+]$ environment triggers an increase in cytosolic $[Ca^{2+}]$ in *P. falciparum* merozoites is regulated by another ubiquitous second messenger, namely, 3′-5′ cyclic adenosine monophosphate (cAMP) (Dawn et al. 2014). The transfer of *P. falciparum* merozoites to a low-$[K^+]$ medium activates the parasite carbonic anhydrase (PfCA), which produces H^+ ions and bicarbonate (HCO_3^-) to balance cytosolic pH (Dawn et al. 2014). Increase in cytosolic bicarbonate levels activates bicarbonate-sensitive soluble adenylate cyclase, PfACβ leading to an increase in cAMP levels, which activates protein kinase A (PfPKA) as well as the cAMP responsive GTP exchange protein called exchange protein activated by cAMP (PfEPAC) (Fig. 2) (Dawn et al. 2014). In other eukaryotic cells, activated EPAC transfers GTP to Rap1 GTPase, which then activates PLC (Gloerich and Bos 2010). Use of specific agonists as well as inhibitors has shown that the EPAC pathway for activation of PLC following an increase in cAMP is present and is responsible for the increase in $[Ca^{2+}]$ when merozoites are exposed to a low-$[K^+]$ environment following egress from schizonts. In addition to regulating levels of free $[Ca^{2+}]$ in merozoites, cAMP also directly regulates microneme secretion by activating PKA (Dawn et al. 2014).

A recent study describes a different mechanism for elevation of cytosolic $[Ca^{2+}]$ in merozoites leading to microneme release. This study suggests the interaction of rhoptry protein PfRh1 to host RBCs triggers a surge in cytosolic $[Ca^{2+}]$ levels in merozoites leading to release of microneme proteins. However, this model does not explain what triggers the release of PfRh1 from the rhoptries to the merozoite surface in the first place and implies that rhoptry secretion may precede microneme secretion (Gao et al. 2013).

The identification of some of the key players involved in signaling pathways leading to microneme and rhoptry discharge during invasion provides novel targets for intervention. For example, targeting PfCDPK1 with small molecule inhibitors will block release of key invasion-related microneme proteins to inhibit blood-stage parasite growth (Bansal et al. 2013). Given that enzymes such as PfCDPK1, which contain both the calmodulin-like Ca^{2+}-binding domain and kinase domain, are of plant origin and are not found in mammalian cells suggests that it should be possible to design specific inhibitors

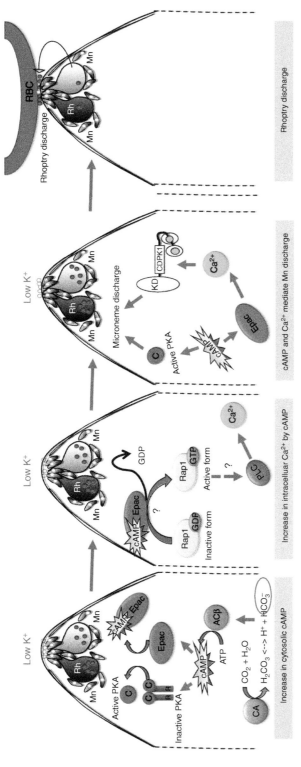

Figure 2. Model for cyclic adenosine monophosphate (cAMP) and Ca^{2+}-mediated signaling pathways that regulate apical organelle discharge in *Plasmodium falciparum* merozoites. Exposure of *P. falciparum* merozoites to a low-K^+ environment as present in blood plasma leads to production of H^+ and HCO_3^- ions by carbonic anhydrase (CA) to maintain pH. HCO_3^- ions activate soluble adeylate cyclase (PfACβ) leading to increase in levels of cAMP. Elevation of cAMP activates its downstream effectors, protein kinase A (PKA) and exchange protein activated by cAMP (EPAC). PKA plays a direct role in regulating microneme secretion. EPAC activates Rap1 GTPase by transferring GTP to Rap1. Rap1-GTP activates phospholipase C (PLC) leading to an increase in cytosolic Ca^{2+} levels, which leads to activation of calcium–dependent protein kinase 1 (PfCDPK1) and secretion of microneme proteins such as EBA175. Engagement of EBA175 with its receptor glycophorin A (GlyA) restores basal $[Ca^{2+}]$ levels and triggers discharge of rhoptry proteins such as PfClag3.1. Mn, Micronemes; Rh, rhoptries.

S. Singh and C.E. Chitnis

that block activation of PfCDPK1 following binding to Ca^{2+}. Similarly other *P. falciparum* enzymes such as carbonic anhydrase (PfCA) or adenylate cyclase (PfACβ) could also be targeted to block production of second messengers required for transduction of signals that trigger microneme release to block blood-stage growth. The signaling pathways that lead to release of rhoptry proteins remain to be defined. Targeting both signaling pathways that are involved in microneme and rhoptry release may provide synergy to efficiently block erythrocyte invasion by apicomplexan pathogens.

FUTURE PERSPECTIVES

Significant progress has been made toward understanding the molecular basis of key steps in the biology of blood-stage malaria parasites such as RBC invasion and merozoite egress following replication in schizonts. As we identify the key parasite ligands involved in invasion, it is clear that it is unlikely that a single merozoite antigen will hold the key to the invasion process. Instead, we have learned that the invasion process is complex and has multiple steps with redundancies built into each step. So, there will be no key parasite ligand that can be targeted to block invasion. It is more likely that we will find combinations of antigens that are critical for invasion and yield synergy to block invasion with high efficiency when targeted together with a combination of specific antibodies. Such combinations may yield high rates of growth inhibition across diverse parasite strains and may provide the basis of highly effective blood-stage vaccines. Such vaccines may have an impact not only on blood-stage parasitemia but also on gametocyte densities leading to a reduction in transmission potential. Such vaccines that interrupt malaria transmission (VIMT) may be useful in elimination strategies in endemic regions in addition to providing protection against malaria.

The regulated secretion of key effector molecules from merozoite apical organelles plays an important role in the complex processes of host cell invasion and egress. A clear understanding of the complete signaling cascades that regulate

apical organelle secretion is likely to reveal targets for small molecule inhibitors that can block invasion or egress. Such targets may provide attractive points for intervention to block blood-stage parasite growth. Some of the signaling pathways may be common to different stages. For example, development of gametes from gametocytes is also regulated by calcium and requires secretion of effectors such as perforin-like protein PfPLP2 for gamete egress. The signaling pathways that regulate processes such as gametocyte activation and gamete egress are not understood. If the signaling pathways that regulate steps such as vesicular secretion leading to egress of sexual-stage parasites are similar to those in blood stages, it may be possible to target both blood-stage growth and malaria transmission. Such interventions can not only protect against malaria but also assist in elimination of malaria by reducing malaria transmission.

CONCLUDING REMARKS

During blood-stage infection *Plasmodium* spp. merozoites repeatedly invade, multiply, exit, and reinvade host RBCs. The key steps of exit from mature schizonts and reinvasion of RBCs by merozoites requires timely regulation of key cellular processes such as apical organelle discharge, which is regulated by cAMP and Ca^{2+}-dependent signal transduction pathways. The internal and external signals that regulate levels of second messengers such as cAMP and Ca^{2+} have been identified and some of the key players of the signaling pathways are known. A complete understanding of the signaling pathways that regulate the process of apical organelle secretion will enable the design of novel intervention strategies that block parasite egress or invasion to block blood-stage parasite growth. Some of the signaling pathways that regulate processes such as vesicular discharge in the blood stage may be common to other stages as well. It may thus be possible to target pathways that are common to both the blood and sexual stages to provide protection against malaria as well as block malaria transmission to eventually eliminate malaria.

 Cite this article as *Cold Spring Harb Perspect Med* doi: 10.1101/cshperspect.a026815

ACKNOWLEDGMENTS

We apologize to researchers whose work could not be cited because of space constraints. Work on erythrocyte invasion in our laboratories has been supported by the Department of Biotechnology (DBT), Government of India and European Commission (MalSig and EVIMalaR grants). S.S. is a recipient of the Innovative Young Biotechnology Award Grant from DBT.

REFERENCES

Abkarian M, Massiera G, Berry L, Roques M, Braun-Breton C. 2011. A novel mechanism for egress of malarial parasites from red blood cells. *Blood* **117**: 4118–4124.

Agarwal S, Singh MK, Garg S, Chitnis CE, Singh S. 2012. Ca²⁺-mediated exocytosis of subtilisin-like protease 1: A key step in egress of *Plasmodium falciparum* merozoites. *Cell Microbiol* **15**: 910–921.

Aikawa M, Miller LH, Johnson J, Rabbege J. 1978. Erythrocyte entry by malarial parasites. A moving junction between erythrocyte and parasite. *J Cell Biol* **77**: 72–82.

Alam MM, Solyakov L, Bottrill AR, Flueck C, Siddiqui FA, Singh S, Mistry S, Viskaduraki M, Lee K, Hopp CS, et al. 2015. Phosphoproteomics reveals malaria parasite Protein Kinase G as a signalling hub regulating egress and invasion. **6**: 7285.

Alleva LM, Kirk K. 2001. Calcium regulation in the intraerythrocytic malaria parasite *Plasmodium falciparum*. *Mol Biochem Parasitol* **117**: 121–128.

Arastu-Kapur S, Ponder EL, Fonović UP, Yeoh S, Yuan F, Fonović M, Grainger M, Phillips CI, Powers JC, Bogyo M. 2008. Identification of proteases that regulate erythrocyte rupture by the malaria parasite *Plasmodium falciparum*. *Nature Chem Biol* **4**: 203–213.

Bansal A, Singh S, More KR, Hans D, Nangalia K, Yogavel M, Sharma A, Chitnis CE. 2013. Characterization of *Plasmodium falciparum* calcium-dependent protein kinase 1 (PfCDPK1) and its role in microneme secretion during erythrocyte invasion. *J Biol Chem* **18**: 1590–1602.

Bargieri D, Lagal V, Andenmatten N, Tardieux I, Meissner M, Ménard R. 2014. Host cell invasion by apicomplexan parasites: The junction conundrum. *PLoS Pathog* **10**: e1004273.

Bartholdson SJ, Bustamante LY, Crosnier C, Johnson S, Lea S, Rayner JC, Wright GJ. 2012. Semaphorin-7A is an erythrocyte receptor for *P. falciparum* merozoite-specific TRAP homolog MTRAP. *PLoS Pathog* **8**: e1003031.

Baum J. 2013. A complete molecular understanding of malaria parasite invasion of the human erythrocyte: Are we there yet? *Pathog Glob Health* **107**: 107–110.

Besteiro S, Dubremetz JF, Lebrun M. 2011. The moving junction of apicomplexan parasites: A key structure for invasion. *Cell Microbiol* **13**: 797–805.

Blackman MJ. 2004. Proteases in host cell invasion by the malaria parasite. *Cell Microbiol* **6**: 893–903.

Blackman MJ. 2008. Malarial proteases and host cell egress: An "emerging" cascade. *Cell Microbiol* **10**: 1925–1934.

Carruthers VB, Sibley LD. 1999. Mobilization of intracellularcalcium stimulates microneme discharge in *Toxoplasma gondii*. *Mol Microbiol* **31**: 421–428.

Carruthers VB, Moreno SNJ, Sibley LD. 1999. Ethanol and acetaldehyde elevate intracellular [Ca²⁺] and stimulate microneme discharge in *Toxoplasma gondii*. *Biochem J* **342**: 379–386.

Cavasini CE, Mattos LC, Couto AA, Bonini-Domingos CR, Valencia SH, Neiras WC, Alves RT, Rossit AR, Castilho L, Machado RL. 2007. *Plasmodium vivax* infection among Duffy antigen-negative individuals from the Brazilian Amazon region: An exception? *Trans R Soc Trop Med Hyg* **101**: 1042–1044.

Chandramohanadas R, Davis PH, Beiting DP, Harbut MB, Darling C, Velmourougane G, Lee MY, Greer PA, Roos DS, Greenbaum DC. 2009. Apicomplexan parasites co-opt host calpains to facilitate their escape from infected cells. *Science* **314**: 794–797.

Chini EN, Nagamune K, Wetzel DM, Sibley LD. 2005. Evidence that the cADPR signalling pathway controls calcium-mediated microneme secretion in *Toxoplasma gondii*. *Biochem J* **389**: 269–277.

Collins CR, Hackett F, Strath M, Penzo M, Withers-Martinez C, Baker DA, Blackman MJ. 2013. Malaria parasite cGMP-dependent protein kinase regulates blood stage merozoite secretory organelle discharge and egress. *PLoS Pathog* **9**: e1003344.

Cowman AF, Crabb BS. 2006. Invasion of red blood cells by malaria parasites. *Cell* **124**: 755–766.

Cowman AF, Berry D, Baum J. 2012. The cellular and molecular basis for malaria parasite invasion of the human red blood cell. *J Cell Biol* **198**: 961–971.

Crosnier C, Bustamante LY, Bartholdson SJ, Bei AK, Theron M, Uchikawa M, Mboup S, Ndir O, Kwiatkowski DP, Duraisingh MT, et al. 2011. Basigin is a receptor essential for erythrocyte invasion by *Plasmodium falciparum*. *Nature* **480**: 534–537.

Dawn A, Singh S, More KR, Siddiqui FA, Pachikara N, Ramdani G, Langsley G, Chitnis CE. 2014. The central role of cAMP in regulating *Plasmodium falciparum* merozoite invasion of human erythrocytes. *PLoS Pathog* **10**: e1004520.

Dvorak JA, Miller LH, Whitehouse WC, Shiroishi T. 1975. Invasion of erythrocytes by malaria merozoites. *Science* **187**: 748–750.

Dvorin JD, Martyn DC, Patel SD, Grimley JS, Collins CR, Hopp CS, Bright AT, Westenberger S, Winzeler E, Blackman MJ, et al. 2010. A plant-like kinase in *Plasmodium falciparum* regulates parasite egress from erythrocytes. *Science* **328**: 910–912.

Fairlie WD, Spurck TP, McCoubrie JE, Gilson PR, Miller SK, McFadden GI, Malby R, Crabb BS, Hodder AN. 2008. Inhibition of malaria parasite development by a cyclic peptide that targets the vital parasite protein SERA5. *Infect Immun* **76**: 4332–4344.

Farrell A, Thirugnanam S, Lorestani A, Dvorin JD, Eidell KP. 2012. A DOC2 protein identified by mutational profiling is essential for apicomplexan parasite exocytosis. *Science* **335**: 218–221.

Gao X, Gunalan K, Yap SS, Preiser PR. 2013. Triggers of key calcium signals during erythrocyte invasion by *Plasmodium falciparum. Nat Commun* **4:** 2862.

Garcia CR. 1999. Ca^{2+} homeostasis and signaling in the blood-stage malaria parasite. *Parasitol Today* **15:** 488–491.

Garg S, Agarwal S, Kumar S, Shams Yazdani S, Chitnis CE, Singh S. 2013. Calcium-dependent permeabilization of erythrocytes by a perforin-like protein during egress of malaria parasites. *Nat Commun* **4:** 1736.

Gaur D, Chitnis CE. 2011. Molecular interactions and signaling mechanisms during erythrocyte invasion by malaria parasites. *Curr Opin Microbiol* **14:** 422–428.

Gilson PR, Crabb BS. 2009. Morphology and kinetics of the three distinct phases of red blood cell invasion by *Plasmodium falciparum* merozoites. *Int J Parasitol* **39:** 91–96.

Gloerich M, Bos JL. 2010. Epac: Defining a new mechanism for cAMP action. *Annu Rev Pharmacol Toxicol* **50:** 355–375.

Glushakova S, Mazar J, Hohmann-Marriott MF, Hama E, Zimmerberg J. 2008. Irreversible effect of cysteine protease inhibitors on the release of malaria parasites from infected erythrocytes. *Cell Microbiol* **11:** 95–105.

Green JL, Rees-Channer RR, Howell SA, Martin SR, Knuepfer E, Taylor HM, Grainger M, Holder AA. 2008. The motor complex of *Plasmodium falciparum*: Phosphorylation by a Ca^{2+} dependent protein kinase. *J Biol Chem* **283:** 30980–30989.

Hanssen E, Dekiwadia C, Riglar DT, Rug M, Lemgruber L, Cowman AF, Cyrklaff M, Kudryashev M, Frischknecht F, Baum J, et al. 2013. Electron tomography of *Plasmodium falciparum* merozoites reveals core cellular events that underpin erythrocyte invasion. *Cell Microbiol* **15:** 1457–1472.

Hayton K, Gaur D, Liu A, Takahashi J, Henschen B, Singh S, Lambert L, Furuya T, Bouttenot R, Doll M. 2008. Erythrocyte binding protein PfRH5 polymorphisms determine species-specific pathways of *Plasmodium falciparum* invasion. *Cell Host Microbe* **4:** 40–51.

Horuk R, Chitnis CE, Darbonne WC, Colby TJ, Rybicki A, Hadley TJ, Miller LH. 1993. A receptor for the malarial parasite *Plasmodium vivax*: The erythrocyte chemokine receptor. *Science* **261:** 1182–1184.

Kafsack BF, Carruthers VB. 2010. Apicomplexan perforin-like proteins. *Commun Integr Biol* **3:** 18–23.

Kafsack BF, Pena JD, Coppens I, Ravindran S, Boothroyd JC, Carruthers VB. 2009. Rapid membrane disruption by a perforin-like protein facilitates parasite exit from host cells. *Science* **323:** 530–533.

Kato N, Sakata T, Breton G, Roch KGL, Nagle A, Andersen C, Bursulaya B, Henson K, Johnson J, Kumar KA, et al. 2008b. Gene expression signatures and small-molecule compounds link a protein kinase to *Plasmodium falciparum* motility. *Nat Chem Biol* **4:** 347–356.

Kessler H, Herm-Götz A, Hegge S, Rauch M, Soldati-Favre D, Frischknecht F, Meissner M. 2008. Microneme protein 8—A new essential invasion factor in *Toxoplasma gondii*. *J Cell Sci* **121:** 947e956.

Lavine MD, Arrizabalaga G. 2008. Exit from host cells by the pathogenic parasite *Toxoplasma gondii* does not require motility. *Eukaryot Cell* **7:** 131–140.

Lourido S, Shuman J, Zhang C, Shokat KM, Hui R, Sibley LD. 2010. Calcium-dependent protein kinase 1 is an essential regulator of exocytosis in *Toxoplasma. Nature* **465:** 359–362.

Lourido S, Tang K, Sibley LD. 2012. Distinct signalling pathways control *Toxoplasma* egress and host-cell invasion. *EMBO J* **31:** 4524–4534.

Lovett JL, Marchesini N, Moreno SNJ, Sibley LD. 2002. *Toxoplasma gondii* microneme secretion involves intracellular Ca^{2+} release from IP3/ryanodine sensitive stores. *J Biol Chem* **277:** 25870–25876.

McCoy JM, Whitehead L, van Dooren GG, Tonkin CJ. 2012. TgCDPK3 regulates calcium-dependent egress of *Toxoplasma gondii* from host cells. *PLoS Pathog* **8:** e1003066.

Ménard D, Barnadas C, Bouchier C, Henry-Halldin C, Gray LR, Ratsimbasoa A, Thonier V, Carod JF, Domarle O, Colin Y. 2010. *Plasmodium vivax* clinical malaria is commonly observed in Duffy-negative Malagasy people. *Proc Natl Acad Sci* **107:** 5967–5971.

Miller LH, Mason SJ, Clyde DF, McGinniss MH. 1976. The resistance factor to *Plasmodium vivax* in blacks. The Duffy-blood-group genotype, FyFy. *N Engl J Med* **295:** 302–304.

Millholland MG, Chandramohanadas R, Pizzarro A, Wehr A, Shi H, Darling C, Lim CT, Greenbaum DC. 2011. The malaria parasite progressively dismantles the host erythrocyte cytoskeleton for efficient egress. *Mol Cell Proteomics* **10:** M111.010678.

Moon RW, Taylor CJ, Bex C, Schepers R, Goulding D, Janse CJ, Waters AP, Baker DA, Billker O. 2009. A cyclic GMP signalling module that regulates gliding motility in a malaria parasite. *PLoS Pathog* **5:** e1000599.

Moreno SN, Docampo R. 2003. Calcium regulation in protozoan parasites. *Curr Opin Microbiol* **6:** 359–364.

Moudy R, Manning TJ, Beckers CJ. 2001. The loss of cytoplasmic potassium upon host cell breakdown triggers egress of *Toxoplasma gondii. J Biol Chem* **276:** 41492–41501.

Nagamune K, Hicks LM, Fux B, Brossier F, Chini EN, Sibley LD. 2008. Abscisic acid controls calcium-dependent egress and development in *Toxoplasma gondii. Nature* **451:** 207–210.

Olaya P, Wasserman M. 1991. Effect of calpain inhibitors on the invasion of human erythrocytes by the parasite *Plasmodium falciparum. Biochim Biophys Acta* **1096:** 217–221.

Richard D, MacRaild CA, Riglar DT, Chan JA, Foley M, Baum J, Ralph SA, Norton RS, Cowman AF. 2010. Interaction between *Plasmodium falciparum* apical membrane antigen 1 and the rhoptry neck protein complex defines a key step in the erythrocyte invasion process of malaria parasites. *J Biol Chem* **285:** 14815–14822.

Riglar DT, Richard D, Wilson DW, Boyle MJ, Dekiwadia C, Turnbull L, Angrisano F, Marapana DS, Rogers KL, Whitchurch CB, et al. 2011. Super-resolution dissection of coordinated events during malaria parasite invasion of the human erythrocyte. *Cell Host Microbe* **9:** 9–20.

Roiko MS, Carruthers VB. 2009. New roles for perforins and proteases in apicomplexan egress. *Cell Microbiol* **11:** 1444–14452.

Cite this article as *Cold Spring Harb Perspect Med* doi: 10.1101/cshperspect.a026815

Roiko MS, Carruthers VB. 2013. Functional dissection of *Toxoplasma gondii* perforin-like protein 1 reveals a dual domain mode of membrane binding for cytolysis and parasite egress. *J Biol Chem* **288:** 8712–8725.

Ryan JR, Stoute JA, Amon J, Dunton RF, Mtalib R, Koros J, Owuor B, Luckhart S, Wirtz RA, Barnwell JW. 2006. Evidence for transmission of *Plasmodium vivax* among a Duffy antigen negative population in Western Kenya. *Am J Trop Med Hyg* **75:** 575–581.

Salmon BL, Oksman A, Goldberg DE. 2001. Malaria parasite exit from the host erythrocyte: A two-step process requiring extraerythrocytic proteolysis. *Proc Natl Acad Sci* **98:** 271–276.

Sharma P, Chitnis CE. 2013. Key molecular events during host cell invasion by Apicomplexan pathogens. *Curr Opin Microbiol* **16:** 432–437.

Siddiqui FA, Dhawan S, Singh S, Singh B, Gupta P, Pandey A, Mohmmed A, Gaur D, Chitnis CE. 2013. A thrombospondin structural repeat containing rhoptry protein from *Plasmodium falciparum* mediates erythrocyte invasion. *Cell Microbiol* **15:** 1341–1356.

Singh S, Chitnis CE. 2012. Signaling mechanism involved in apical organelle discharge during invasion of apicomplexan parasites. *Microbes Infect* **10:** 820–824.

Singh S, Alam MM, Pal-Bhowmick I, Brzostowski JA, Chitnis CE. 2010. Distinct external signals trigger sequential release of apical organelles during erythrocyte invasion by malaria parasites. *PLoS Pathog* **6:** e1000746.

Soni S, Dhawan S, Rosen KM, Chafel M, Chishti AH, Hanspal M. 2005. Characterization of events preceding the release of malaria parasite from the host red blood cell. *Blood Cells Mol Dis* **35:** 201–211.

Srinivasan P, Beatty WL, Diouf A, Herrera R, Ambroggio X, Moch JK, Tyler JS, Narum DL, Pierce SK, Boothroyd JC,

et al. 2011. Binding of Plasmodium merozoite proteins RON2 and AMA1 triggers commitment to invasion. *Proc Natl Acad Sci* **108:** 13275–13280.

Taylor HM, McRobert L, Grainger M, Sicard A, Dluzewski AR, Hopp CS, Holder AA, Baker DA. 2010. The malaria parasite cyclic GMP-dependent protein kinase plays a central role in blood-stage schizogony. *Eukaryot Cell* **9:** 37–45.

Tham WH, Wilson DW, Lopaticki S, Schmidt CQ, Tetteh-Quarcoo PB, Barlow PN, Richard D, Corbin JE, Beeson JG, Cowman AF. 2010. Complement receptor 1 is the host erythrocyte receptor for *Plasmodium falciparum* PfRh4 invasion ligand. *Proc Natl Acad Sci* **107:** 17327–17332.

Vaid A, Thomas DC, Sharma P. 2008. Role of Ca^{2+}/CaM-PfPKB signaling pathway in erythrocyte invasion by *Plasmodium falciparum*. *J Biol Chem* **283:** 5589–5597.

Wickham ME, Culvenor JG, Cowman AF. 2003. Selective inhibition of a two step egress of malaria parasites from the host erythrocyte. *J Biol Chem* **278:** 37658–37663.

Wiersma HI, Galuska SE, Tomley FM, Sibley LD, Liberator PA, Donald RG. 2004. A role for coccidian cGMP-dependent protein kinase in motility and invasion. *Int J Parasitol* **34:** 369–380.

Winograd E, Clavijo CA, Bustamante LY, Jaramillo M. 1999. Release of merozoites from *Plasmodium falciparum*−infected erythrocytes could be mediated by a non-explosive event. *Parasitol Res* **85:** 621–624.

Wu Y, Kuzma J, Maréchal E, Graeff R, Lee HC, Foster R, Chua NH. 1997. Abscisic acid signaling through cyclic ADP-ribose in plants. *Science* **278:** 2126–2130.

Yeoh S, O'Donnell RA, Koussis K, Dluzewski AR, Ansell KH, et al. 2007. Subcellular discharge of a serine protease mediates release of invasive malaria parasites from host erythrocytes. *Cell* **131:** 1072–1083.

Host Cell Tropism and Adaptation of Blood-Stage Malaria Parasites: Challenges for Malaria Elimination

Caeul Lim,[1,2] Selasi Dankwa,[1,2] Aditya S. Paul,[1] and Manoj T. Duraisingh[1]

[1]Harvard T.H. Chan School of Public Health, Boston, Massachusetts 02115

Correspondence: mduraisi@hsph.harvard.edu

Plasmodium falciparum and *Plasmodium vivax* account for most of the mortality and morbidity associated with malaria in humans. Research and control efforts have focused on infections caused by *P. falciparum* and *P. vivax*, but have neglected other malaria parasite species that infect humans. Additionally, many related malaria parasite species infect nonhuman primates (NHPs), and have the potential for transmission to humans. For malaria elimination, the varied and specific challenges of all of these *Plasmodium* species will need to be considered. Recent advances in molecular genetics and genomics have increased our knowledge of the prevalence and existing diversity of the human and NHP *Plasmodium* species. We are beginning to identify the extent of the reservoirs of each parasite species in humans and NHPs, revealing their origins as well as potential for adaptation in humans. Here, we focus on the red blood cell stage of human infection and the host cell tropism of each human *Plasmodium* species. Determinants of tropism are unique among malaria parasite species, presenting a complex challenge for malaria elimination.

More than 60% of known infectious organisms are zoonotic, and they account for 75% of emerging human diseases (Taylor et al. 2001; Jones et al. 2008). The predominant species of malaria parasites infecting humans, *Plasmodium falciparum* and *Plasmodium vivax*, are anthroponotic in human populations; however, these species also originated from a transmission event from African great apes to humans (Liu et al. 2010, 2014). In addition, four other malaria parasite species from the genus *Plasmodium* infect humans: *Plasmodium malariae*, *Plasmodium ovale curtisi*, *Plasmodium ovale wallikeri*, thought to be transmitted within humans, and *Plasmodium knowlesi*, a zoonosis of humans from macaque monkeys. All *Plasmodium* species are characterized by a complex life cycle with several stages of differentiation through its anopheline mosquito vector and the vertebrate host. In humans, following a primary stage of infection and multiplication in the liver, parasites are released into the bloodstream. The clinical symptoms of malaria are associated with the blood stage, when parasites proliferate asexually by invasion of red blood cells (RBCs), replication, egress from the infected cell, and reinvasion of an uninfected cell in a cyclical fashion. A subset of parasites can leave this asexual cycle to develop into sexual forms known as gametocytes, which are taken up by mosquitoes,

---

[2]These authors contributed equally to this work.

Cite this article as *Cold Spring Harb Perspect Med* doi: 10.1101/cshperspect.a025494

in which sexual recombination and development occur to form parasites that can be reintroduced into the host, completing the life cycle.

In contrast to *Plasmodium* species that infect lizards and birds, the host range for primate *Plasmodium* species was thought to be highly restricted with only rare instances of zoonotic transmission. Recently, however, this dogma of strict host tropism in nature has been challenged, particularly with the emergence of *P. knowlesi* in the human population. Restrictions to infection of the host can occur at many points throughout the life cycle of *Plasmodium* parasites. Because host and vector habitat and behavior are difficult to study in natural settings, host–cell tropism at the RBC invasion step has been the most studied at the molecular and cellular level. Furthermore, with advances in molecular genomic and genetic tools, we now have a greater understanding of parasite species diversity present also in animal host populations. This increased knowledge raises several questions and concerns as the research agenda shifts toward the eradication of malaria. How large and deep is the repertoire of existing *Plasmodium* species? Is the range of *Plasmodium* species to which humans are susceptible fully known? Is the zoonotic reservoir significant today as a means of transmission?

Here, we review the molecular determinants at the RBC invasion step that regulate host-cell tropism, discussing how these factors may influence the ability of *Plasmodium* parasites to breach species barriers and expand host range, impeding efforts to eliminate malaria.

MOLECULAR MEDIATORS OF RBC INVASION AND TROPISM

For successful RBC invasion, an extracellular *Plasmodium* parasite must initiate and execute a complex, well-ordered series of molecular interactions with the plasma membrane surface of the host cell. At each step of invasion, parasite proteins or invasion ligands bind to native receptors on the RBC surface or secreted parasite receptors (Cowman et al. 2012). The two superfamilies of *Plasmodium* invasion ligands that mediate the most specific interactions with

receptors on the RBC surface, and therefore thought to be primary determinants of tropism, are the Duffy-binding protein ligand (DBL) family and the reticulocyte-binding protein homolog (RBL) family (Fig. 1) (Cowman and Crabb 2006; Tham et al. 2012; Wright and Rayner 2014; Paul et al. 2015).

The DBL invasion ligands all contain a well-characterized Duffy-binding-like receptor-binding domain, named for the founding members of this family—the *P. vivax* Duffy-binding protein (PvDBP) (Wertheimer and Barnwell 1989) and the orthologous *P. knowlesi* Duffy-binding protein α (PkDBPα) (Haynes et al. 1988). The interaction of PvDBP or PkDBPα with the RBC Duffy antigen receptor for chemokines (DARC) is the major determinant of human infection by these *Plasmodium* species (Miller et al. 1975; Singh et al. 2005). *P. falciparum* has an even larger repertoire of DBL invasion ligands, all of which use sialic acid–containing receptors on the human RBC surface to mediate invasion. At least one of these invasion ligands, PfEBA-175 has previously been implicated in host tropism (Martin et al. 2005).

The *P. vivax* proteins PvRBP1 and PvRBP2, for which the RBL family is named, are thought to restrict *P. vivax* to reticulocytes by virtue of their specific binding to reticulocytes (Galinski et al. 1992). Despite the kinship between the two species, the RBL ligands in *P. knowlesi*, PkNBPXa and PkNBPXb, are strongly divergent from their *P. vivax* counterparts (Mayer et al. 2009); their role in human infection is not known. In *P. falciparum*, PfRh proteins have been shown to underlie preferences for specific receptor repertoires (PfRh4; Stubbs et al. 2005; Gaur et al. 2006), as well as preference of RBCs from different host species (Rh5; Hayton et al. 2008, 2013).

A more detailed review of factors involved in invasion of host RBCs by the parasites can be found in Singh and Chitnis (2016).

Plasmodium knowlesi: AN ESTABLISHED ZOONOSIS

A Zoonosis Happening Today

P. knowlesi is currently the only clearly zoonotic malaria parasite. Although the first natural case

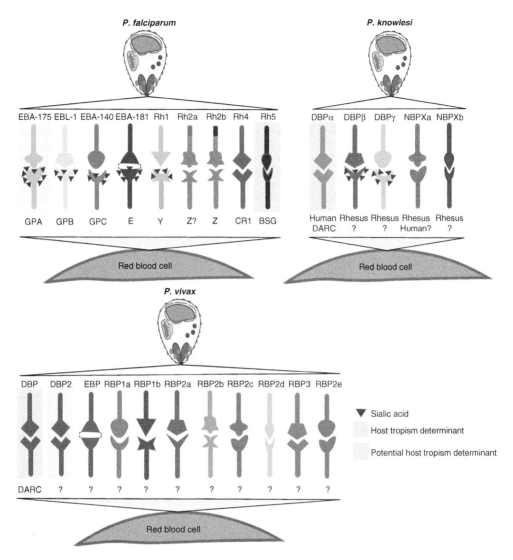

Figure 1. Specific ligand–receptor interactions mediate *Plasmodium* invasion of red blood cells (RBCs) that can determine host tropism. Parasite invasion ligands and their cognate RBC receptors are shown for *Plasmodium falciparum*, *Plasmodium vivax*, and *Plasmodium knowlesi*. A question mark or letter indicates receptors that are yet to be identified. Orange shading highlights known host tropism determinants, whereas grey shading indicates potential host tropism determinants. The triangles on some RBC receptors denote sialic acid residues. For *P. vivax*, DBP2 represents the duplicated DBP that has been implicated in *P. vivax* invasion of Duffy antigen receptor for chemokines (DARC)-negative individuals (Ménard et al. 2013). The expanded RBP family identified through whole-genome sequencing (WGS) of the *P. vivax* SalI reference strain (Carlton et al. 2008) comprises RBP1a, RBP1b, RBP2a, RBP2b, RBP2c, RBP2d, and RBP3, whereas EBP and RBP2e represent the predicted Duffy-binding protein ligand (DBL) and reticulocyte-binding protein homolog (RBL) orthologs identified through WGS of a *P. vivax* field isolate (Hester et al. 2013). *P. knowlesi* DBPα-DARC invasion pathway functions in invasion of macaque RBCs; however, it does not appear to be a tropism determinant for the macaque host population. NBPXa has been shown to bind human RBCs in vitro, but its role in invasion of human RBCs remains to be defined.

of *P. knowlesi* malaria was reported as early as 1965 (Chin et al. 1965), it was only in 2004 that Singh et al. conclusively showed that the majority, if not all, of cases diagnosed as *P. malariae* on the basis of morphology in the Kapit division of Malaysia from 2000 to 2002 were in fact *P. knowlesi* (Singh et al. 2004). A follow-up study examined archival blood films from 1996 and confirmed that misdiagnosis of *P. knowlesi* for *P. malariae* had been common earlier than realized. The investigators also speculated that an earlier survey conducted in 1952 may also have misidentified *P. knowlesi* cases as *P. malariae*, challenging the idea that it is a newly emerging zoonosis (Lee et al. 2009). Since then, cases have been reported in various regions of Southeast Asia and *P. knowlesi* is now the leading cause of malaria in some parts of Malaysia (Singh and Daneshvar 2013). Although there is significant evidence suggesting that most transmission is zoonotic (Singh et al. 2004; Daneshvar et al. 2009), a recent study reports cases, albeit limited, of infection within families, without notable interaction with potential zoonotic hosts (Barber et al. 2012). Intriguingly, another recent study suggests that the prevalence may be higher than previously thought, with a potentially large asymptomatic population harboring the parasite (Fornace et al. 2015). In any case, human encroachment on macaque habitats (Cox Singh and Culleton 2015) will only increase the opportunity for the parasite to evolve and adapt to humans. To date, there is little evidence of direct transmission among humans (Singh et al. 2004; Daneshvar et al. 2009).

P. knowlesi Diversity

Considerable diversity has been found within *P. knowlesi* strains isolated in human populations. Parasitemia and disease severity in human patients were found to be associated with a specific allele of the PkNBPXb invasion ligand (Ahmed et al. 2014). A subsequent whole-genome study found dimorphism in the natural *P. knowlesi* population (Pinheiro et al. 2015). A larger study soon supported the possibility of two distinct *P. knowlesi* populations in circulation (Assefa et al. 2015; Divis et al. 2015). These studies, comprising isolates from two natural macaque hosts (long-tailed and pig-tailed macaques), as well as humans, showed that there are two distinct sympatric clusters of *P. knowlesi* matching to the two natural macaque hosts. The genetic diversity between these clusters was great enough to suspect subspeciation. Strikingly, although interaction between the clusters is likely limited because of different geographical and ecological niches of the macaque hosts, both of the clusters are found in humans. Introgression between subspecies provides opportunities for a parasite to adapt to a new environment and potentially new host organisms. The possibility of hybridization in the human host was speculated, based on genetic mosaicism observed across the genome. Further, through genomic analyses of human isolates several genes were found to be under strong positive selection in the human population. These data indicate the potential for *P. knowlesi* to adapt and evolve within the human population.

Adaptation of *P. knowlesi* to Human RBCs

Consistent with *P. knowlesi* being a zoonosis of humans derived by transmission from macaque monkeys, in vitro culture of *P. knowlesi* has always been performed in macaque blood, because the low replication rate in human blood has impeded continuous propagation (Kocken et al. 2002). Interestingly, it was found that *P. knowlesi* parasites used in malaria therapy of neurosyphilis human patients resulted in high parasitemia infections and pathogenesis with increased passage through humans, suggesting an adaptation toward virulence (van Rooyen and Pile 1935; Ciuca et al. 1955). Recently, both our group and another group successfully obtained *P. knowlesi* lines adapted to grow efficiently in human RBCs (Lim et al. 2013; Moon et al. 2013). In both cases, the parental *P. knowlesi* H strain was in culture for an extended period of time in a mixture of human and macaque RBCs, until it was able to be maintained in purely human RBCs. The increased invasion efficiency observed in the human-adapted lines remains reliant on the PkDBPα–DARC interaction (Moon et al. 2013). Interestingly, we found that although the parental strain showed a strong preference for the very young fraction of circulating human RBCs, the human-adapted line had circumvented this specific tropism, permitting invasion of an expanded pool of RBCs of varying age (Lim et al. 2013). Whether this mechanism mirrors the natural mode of adaptation in the field is yet to be determined. Increased numbers of human infections, particularly those of high density, may serve as a sentinel of increased adaptation of *P. knowlesi* to the human population.

P. vivax: STRENGTH IN DIVERSITY

Diversity and Origin of *P. vivax*

Despite being the most widely distributed of the human malaria parasites, *P. vivax* has long been considered benign and has not received as much attention as the demonstrably lethal *P. falciparum*. It is becoming apparent that *P. vivax* parasites are considerably more diverse than *P. falciparum* (Rosenberg et al. 1989; Qari et al. 1991, 1992; Cui et al. 2003; Neafsey et al. 2012; Carlton et al. 2013). In a recent study, next-generation sequencing of four geographically distinct *P. vivax* isolates (Neafsey et al. 2012) revealed a high rate of single-nucleotide polymorphisms (SNPs). *P. vivax* therefore has a larger effective population size compared with *P. falciparum* that has not gone through a recent bottleneck or drug-driven sweep in selection.

Analysis of a growing number of samples from different geographical locations has also led to the discovery of "*P. vivax*–like" parasites such as *Plasmodium simium* (Coatney et al. 1971; Costa et al. 2014). *P. simium*, found in New World monkeys, is considered to be morphologically and genetically indistinguishable from *P. vivax* (Collins et al. 1969; Coatney et al. 1971; Deane 1988). A recent study showed that wild monkeys infected with *P. simium* showed high levels of seropositivity against *P. vivax* antigens (Camargos Costa et al. 2015). Sequencing of the PsDBP gene revealed only four polymorphic sites compared with PvDBP, highlighting the remarkable similarity between *P. vivax* and *P. simium* and suggesting a poten-

tially large sylvatic reservoir for *P. vivax* or *P. vivax*–like parasites.

Two other *Plasmodium* species closely related to *P. vivax* have also been identified—*Plasmodium cynomolgi* and *Plasmodium simiovale*. Antibodies against the circumsporozoite protein of *P. simiovale* were detected in human population studies (Qari et al. 1993; Udhayakumar et al. 1994; Marrelli et al. 1998); however, an independent study could not confirm the presence of *P. simiovale* in the human population (Gopinath et al. 1994) and experimental infection of humans with *P. simiovale* in an early study was not successful (Dissanaike 1965). A recent analysis of the sequence of merozoite surface protein 9 (MSP-9) from diverse *Plasmodium* species suggests that *P. simiovale* and the macaque parasite, *Plasmodium fieldi*, form a clade, whereas *P. vivax* and *P. cynomolgi* form another (Chenet et al. 2013), arguing for a more in-depth phylogenetic analysis of this species. Interestingly, a case of *P. cynomolgi* human infection has been reported recently in Malaysia, showing the biological ability of this parasite to naturally infect humans (Ta et al. 2014).

Where does *P. vivax* originally come from? The position of *P. vivax* within a clade of related parasites that includes *P. cynomolgi*, which infects Asian primates, led to the widely held view that *P. vivax* originated in Asia. This theory, however, was at odds with the near-fixation of the DARC-negative allele in sub-Saharan Africa, which largely confers protection against *P. vivax* (Young et al. 1955; Miller et al. 1975). Several recent studies have identified *P. vivax*–like parasites in African great apes (Kaiser et al. 2010; Krief et al. 2010; Prugnolle et al. 2010). A large-scale study by Liu et al. (2014) found a much greater diversity of *P. vivax* in African great apes than found within the human population. The extant African ape reservoir of *P. vivax* likely descended from an ancient parasite pool, which served as a source for a single zoonotic transfer that has given rise to modern human *P. vivax*. Interestingly, the ape *P. vivax*–like parasites can infect both gorillas and chimpanzees alike, suggesting frequent transmission between these species. The reduced diversity of extant human *P. vivax* likely results from a bottlenecked lineage that spread from Africa, where, thereafter, it became severely restricted within Africa as DARC negativity spread among the human population.

The PvDBP–DARC Interaction: Indispensable for *P. vivax*?

Three invasion ligands had been identified for *P. vivax* (PvDBP, PvRBP1, and PvRBP2) (Wertheimer and Barnwell 1989; Galinski et al. 1992) before the assembly of the full genome, which thereafter revealed the presence of several more members of the RBL family (Fig. 1) (Carlton et al. 2008). The interaction of PvDBP with the DARC receptor, however, had been shown to be essential for human infection (Miller et al. 1975; Wertheimer and Barnwell 1989).

De novo assembly of additional *P. vivax* isolates revealed that the SalI reference strain, which had been extensively passaged in vivo in monkey models, was missing several large genomic regions including loci for putative invasion ligands of both the RBL and DBL family (Hester et al. 2013). In addition, a duplication of PvDBP (Ménard et al. 2013) was observed in several field isolates, an apparently recent event, based on the similarity of the two DBP loci. In any case, *P. vivax* possesses a large set of invasion ligands that could be used to confer phenotypic diversity.

A number of reports have recently documented *P. vivax* infection in several DARC-negative individuals (Ménard et al. 2010a,b; Woldearegai et al. 2013). Additionally, cases of high parasitemia and severe disease caused by *P. vivax* have been increasing over the past decade (White et al. 2014). These discoveries suggest a diversity in the ability of *P. vivax* isolates to infect human RBCs.

A Hidden Pool of *P. vivax* in Plain Sight?

P. vivax can consistently be detected in the few DARC-positive individuals that are surveyed in largely DARC-negative populations (Culleton and Carter 2012). DARC-negative individuals also show significant exposure in populations of almost exclusive DARC negativity. Strikingly, samples collected by passive case detection from 13% of individuals attending a clinic in the Republic of Congo had antibodies to the preerythrocytic stage of *P. vivax* (Culleton et al. 2009). These studies support the hypothesis that there is ongoing transmission of *P. vivax* in sub-Saharan Africa, although the extent of this "transmission" has not been fully assessed. It has been suggested that the small population of DARC-positive individuals ($<5\%$) may be sufficient to sustain this highly transmissible species. Further, it is possible that there exists a large reservoir of *P. vivax* in humans with a very low circulating parasitemia, which, nevertheless, can be transmitted to humans. The growing number of *P. vivax* cases in DARC-negative individuals adds yet another challenge. The discovery of *P. vivax* in gorillas and chimpanzees now provides the additional complexity of an animal reservoir. In fact, an expanded NHP reservoir could exist in many geographical areas as *P. vivax* and related species have also been found in various South American monkeys, including howler monkeys (Costa et al. 2014). A human traveler from the Central African Republic infected with ape *P. vivax* (Prugnolle et al. 2013), the lone case of a modern zoonotic transfer of this parasite species, suggests that if interaction between the human and NHP populations increases, risk of animal-borne *P. vivax* may increase in the human population.

Challenges for Establishing a *P. vivax* Blood-Stage Vaccine

Efforts to develop preventative measures against malaria have been heavily skewed toward *P. falciparum* (discussed later in this review) (Reyes-Sandoval 2013). It is becoming apparent that this lag in research in *P. vivax* control and prevention will be a major and persistent challenge in our goal toward malaria elimination (WHO 2015). The search for an ideal blood-stage vaccine target has centered on PvDBP because of its necessity in invading human RBCs. Antibodies raised against the binding region of PvDBP, called region II (RII), have been shown to be efficient at inhibiting the binding of PvDBP to DARC (Chitnis and Sharma 2008).

     Cite this article as *Cold Spring Harb Perspect Med* doi: 10.1101/cshperspect.a025494

PvRII has also shown promise in preclinical trials in animal models (Mueller et al. 2009). However, the high diversity among *P. vivax* strains and in the PvDBP alleles has led to conflicting reports on whether a PvRII-based vaccine would confer protection against all strains (de Sousa et al. 2014). Although there are a few more antigens under consideration as blood-stage vaccine targets (such as merozoite surface protein 1 [MSP-1] and apical membrane antigen 1 [AMA-1]), there is clearly a need to screen a larger set of antigens to find a more suitable one (Valencia et al. 2011). In addition, as the community decides how and where to concentrate vaccine development resources, several unique features of *P. vivax* should be considered, such as its higher transmissibility compared with *P. falciparum* (Brown et al. 2009) and its tendency to cause relapse in patients as a result of the elusive hypnozoite stage. Other life-cycle stages such as the preerythrocytic or transmission stages may thus be better to target in developing an efficient vaccine for *P. vivax*; indeed, efforts to interrupt these stages have been more successful (Reyes-Sandoval 2013).

P. falciparum: THE MALIGNANT MALARIA

Origin of *P. falciparum*

The origin of the deadly *P. falciparum* has been the subject of intense study. Until recently, the only identified parasite species closely related to *P. falciparum* in the *Laverania* sublineage was the chimpanzee parasite *Plasmodium reichenowi*. There were various hypotheses offered about the origin of *P. falciparum* with genetic evidence suggesting that it arose from *P. reichenowi*, likely by a single host transfer from chimpanzees to humans (Rich et al. 2009). Subsequent studies identified two other *P. falciparum*–related chimpanzee parasites *Plasmodium gaboni* (Ollomo et al. 2009) and *Plasmodium billcollinsi* (Krief et al. 2010). Nevertheless, seminal work by Liu et al. (2010), revealed that *P. falciparum* originated from a single host transfer from gorillas and not chimpanzees. *P. falciparum* was found to be most closely related to a

Plasmodium species isolated from Western gorillas, later termed *Plasmodium praefalciparum* (Rayner et al. 2011). This study, which relied on amplification of mitochondrial sequences from single copies of *Plasmodium* genomes from ape fecal samples, also revealed a diversity of closely related *Laverania* species displaying specificity for either gorilla or chimpanzee hosts (Fig. 2).

The potential for closely related great ape parasites such as *P. praefalciparum* to infect humans does not presently appear to be significant (Sundararaman et al. 2013; Délicat-Loembet et al. 2015), with *P. falciparum* clearly emerging from a single ancient transmission event. Conversely, *P. falciparum* has been found to infect bonobos and gorillas as an anthroponosis, which raises concerns about potential animal reservoirs of *P. falciparum*. However, most of the *P. falciparum*–infected great apes were captive and living in close proximity to humans (Krief et al. 2010; Prugnolle et al. 2010), suggesting that such a threat is low and will not undermine elimination efforts, as long as humans continue to live apart from great apes or treat captive apes with antimalarials.

Diversity in Invasion Ligands

A comparison of the *P. reichenowi* and *P. falciparum* genome sequences implicates RBL and DBL invasion ligands as factors associated with adaptation to a host species. Although the two genomes are highly similar, the loci for several orthologous invasion ligands in the two species are extensively differentiated between species, as evidenced by pseudogenization, disruptions in gene synteny, and sequence divergence (Otto et al. 2014). Variant expression of invasion ligands in laboratory-adapted and field strains has shown the differential usage of ligand–receptor interactions between *P. falciparum* isolates for the invasion of RBCs (Reed et al. 2000; Duraisingh et al. 2003a,b; Nery et al. 2006; Bei et al. 2007; Jennings et al. 2007; Gomez-Escobar et al. 2010). The use of diverse ligand–receptor pairs is thought to be both a mechanism of immune evasion and a means to invade diverse RBC subtypes within an individ-

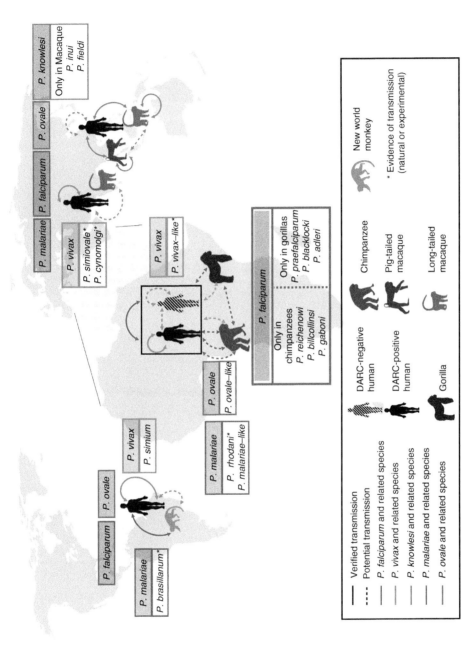

Figure 2. Global distribution and transmission of *Plasmodium* species in human and animal populations. *Plasmodium falciparum* (red), *Plasmodium vivax* (green), *Plasmodium malariae* (purple) and the two species of *Plasmodium ovale* (blue) is found in Southeast Asia. Arrows between the different hosts indicate established transmission of the different parasite species within the human population, and/or between or from nonhuman primates. The dotted arrows show potential transmission of parasites to look out for, based on population surveys. All arrows are similarly color-coded. *Plasmodium* species related to the main human species are in boxes in corresponding colors and species for which cases of human infection have been observed (experimentally or naturally) are marked with an asterisk. DARC, Duffy antigen receptor for chemokines.

ual, between individuals, and even potentially between host species.

Sialic Acid and Host Specificity

The sialic acid on RBCs appears to be key to the binding of many invasion ligands of *P. falciparum*, including the DBL invasion ligands, PfEBA-175, PfEBL-1, PfEBA-140, and PfEBA-181, and the RBL invasion ligand Rh1 (Orlandi et al. 1992; Gilberger 2003; Lobo 2003; Maier et al. 2003; Triglia et al. 2005; Mayer et al. 2009). Some strains are highly dependent on the presence of sialic acid for successful invasion, whereas other strains can invade in a sialic acid–independent fashion (Stubbs et al. 2005; Gaur et al. 2006). Humans express only the *N*-acetylneuraminic acid (Neu5Ac) form of sialic acid, because of an inactivating mutation in the enzyme cytidine monophosphate *N*-acetyl-neuraminic acid hydroxylase (CMAH), which otherwise converts Neu5Ac to *N*-glycolylneuraminic acid (Neu5Gc) (Chou et al. 1998; Irie et al. 1998; Hayakawa et al. 2001). In contrast to humans, all great apes have an intact *CMAH* gene and express a high degree of Neu5Gc on their RBC surface (Muchmore et al. 1998).

It has been postulated that this chemical difference in sialic acid between humans and other great apes might influence the specificity of *Laverania* parasites for their hosts. Chimpanzees can be experimentally infected with *P. falciparum* (Blacklock and Adler 1922; Daubersies et al. 2000); however, natural infections of wild-living chimpanzees have not been observed (Liu et al. 2010). Evidence to date suggests that *P. reichenowi* does not infect humans (Blacklock and Adler 1922; Bruce-Chwatt et al. 1970). One study showed that PfEBA-175 and *P. reichenowi* EBA-175 preferentially bind to RBCs of their own host species and erythroid-like cells expressing the host-specific sialic acid (Martin et al. 2005). The investigators further showed that *Aotus* monkeys, which serve as model organisms for *P. falciparum* (Herrera et al. 2002) express Neu5Ac, potentially explaining their susceptibility to *P. falciparum* infection. However, it was subsequently observed that PfEBA-175 binds to both Neu5Ac and

Neu5Gc (Wanaguru et al. 2013), contradicting previous findings (Martin et al. 2005), but potentially providing an explanation for the ability of Neu5Gc to potently inhibit binding of PfEBA-175 to human RBCs (Orlandi et al. 1992). Indeed, homologs of EBA-175 from *P. reichenowi* and *P. billcollinsi*, another chimpanzee parasite, bind human RBCs as well as human glycophorin A with similar affinities, suggesting that perhaps EBA-175 is not a major tropism determinant for these species (Wanaguru et al. 2013).

PfRh5 as a Host Restriction Factor

Of the RBL and DBL invasion ligands, PfRh5 is the only established invasion ligand that has been found to be essential for RBC invasion by all *P. falciparum* strains tested to date (Crosnier et al. 2011). Interestingly, polymorphisms in this molecule are associated with invasion into *Aotus* RBCs, through mapping using the progeny of a genetic cross (Hayton et al. 2008, 2013). Subsequently, it was found that PfRh5 binds chimpanzee and gorilla basigin (BSG) at much reduced levels compared with human BSG, suggesting that the molecule might be critical in defining the specificity of *P. falciparum* for human RBCs. Specific amino acid residues in BSG were identified that contribute to recognition of human BSG by PfRh5. Notably, two of these residues, F27 and K191, were identified as targets of positive selection in a study using population genetics and phylogenetics (Forni et al. 2015), providing further evidence that this key receptor is under selection pressure both within the human lineage and during NHP evolution.

Targeting the Tropism Ligands of *P. falciparum* for Vaccine Development

Sterile immunity to *P. falciparum* infection—the ultimate goal of a malaria vaccine—does not occur in naturally exposed human populations. Instead, individuals acquire partial immunity with age (Persson et al. 2008; Badiane et al. 2013), likely a result of continual exposure to *Plasmodium* infections and gradual acquisition of antibodies against parasite antigens, including many invasion ligands. The merozoite invasion ligands have been proposed as vaccine candidates. However, inclusion of multiple antigens in an invasion-blocking vaccine would be necessary to effectively counter the ability of *P. falciparum* to use different invasion pathways and overcome sequence polymorphism of invasion ligands (Nery et al. 2006; Bowyer et al. 2015; Mensah-Brown et al. 2015). Many studies have reported the presence of invasion-inhibitory antibodies acquired toward *P. falciparum* DBL ligands, (PfEBA-175, PfEBA-140, PfEBA-181) and RBL ligands (PfRh2 and PfRh4) (Ford et al. 2007; Persson et al. 2008; Reiling et al. 2010; Reiling et al. 2012; Badiane et al. 2013). Recent studies have shown that simultaneous blockade of multiple invasion ligand–receptor interactions can synergistically inhibit invasion (Lopaticki et al. 2011; Williams et al. 2012; Pandey et al. 2013), showing the potential of such a vaccine strategy. Recently, several in vitro–based culture studies have shown the strong potential of the essential invasion ligand PfRh5 as an antigenic target for inhibition (Douglas et al. 2011, 2014; Patel et al. 2013; Reddy et al. 2014). Additionally, administration of a PfRh5-based experimental vaccine blocks *P. falciparum* infection in *Aotus* monkeys following parasite inoculation (Douglas et al. 2015). It is possible that a major challenge to elimination of *P. falciparum* by vaccine strategies targeting invasion ligands is the polymorphism and redundancy that might allow the parasites to persist in reservoirs such as young RBCs that can be invaded using hitherto unidentified ligand–receptor interactions.

THE OTHER *PLASMODIA*: AN UNEXPECTED DIVERSITY

Although *P. ovale* and *P. malariae* are understudied relative to other human malaria parasites, they contribute significantly to the global malaria burden. The distribution of *P. ovale* is thought to be limited to some tropical areas in Africa, New Guinea, and parts of the Philippines and Indonesia (Mueller et al. 2007). Its global burden may, however, be an underesti-

mation, as *P. ovale* presents with low parasitemia and is easy to miss or misdiagnose as the morphologically similar and more prevalent *P. vivax*. Diagnosis became more sensitive and accurate with the development of a species-specific polymerase chain reaction (PCR) method (Snounou et al. 1993). However, some cases identified as *P. ovale* by light microscopy could not be detected by this method because of strong genetic variation (Tachibana et al. 2002; Win et al. 2004; Calderaro et al. 2007) among analyzed samples. It took several years after these observations for Sutherland et al. (2010) to show that the "classic" and "variant" types of *P. ovale* are in fact two distinct subspecies that are nonrecombining but sympatric in endemic regions.

Similarly, variant forms of *P. malariae*, not detectable through the standard species-specific PCR, have been observed in distinct endemic regions, such as China and Southeast Asia (Kawamoto et al. 1999). The same variant sequence was found in distinct geographical regions, indicating the presence of a stable and common form of *P. malariae*. Further investigation will determine whether this is another existing or ongoing speciation event.

Both *P. ovale*–like and *P. malariae*–like species have been detected in African great apes, albeit at a much lower frequency than the *Laverania* clade, in the study conducted by Liu and colleagues (2010). This discovery warrants further investigation to determine whether these neglected species are also more widely prevalent than assumed. In addition, historical observations suggest that *P. malariae* may be able to infect a larger range of host species; *P. brasilianum*, a parasite in South American monkeys and *P. rhodaini*, found in African chimpanzees are morphologically similar to *P. malariae* and show similar disease progression. They can both be transmitted to humans experimentally, and it has been suggested that this species might indeed be *P. malariae* (Coatney 1968; Rayner 2015). Genetic analysis now suggests that *P. malariae* can infect Old and New World monkeys as well as humans, presenting a formidable zoonotic reservoir for *P. malariae* (Lalremruata et al. 2015).

PERSPECTIVES: WHAT WILL WE NEED TO REACH ELIMINATION?

Defining the Extent of Zoonotic Reservoirs: Continuous Surveying and Sampling

Emergence of new zoonoses would rely on a number of criteria being favorable, including the probability of contact between human and animal host, shared mosquito vectors, and RBC-stage infectivity. This is well-discussed in a review, in which J.K. Baird, writing before the discovery of multiple *Laverania* species, assesses the risk of 18 non-*Laverania* NHP species and one *Laverania* species found in different geographic regions to cause human infection (Baird 2009). He concludes that only three species have great potential to be zoonotic—*P. knowlesi*, which is already well established as a human parasite, *P. cynomolgi*, for which there has been one report of a natural human infection (Ta et al. 2014), and *Plasmodium inui*, which is often found in the same natural hosts and vectors as *P. knowlesi*.

Today, our knowledge of the extent to which we are exposed to *Plasmodium* species has come primarily from direct surveys of individuals, animal hosts, and mosquito vectors in malaria-endemic regions. Modern-day efforts to determine the bounds of the *P. knowlesi* zoonotic reservoir have relied on sampling of wild macaques (Lee et al. 2011; Moyes et al. 2014), which helps prioritize areas of high-transmission risk, but as the investigators note, the animal reservoir may extend beyond the known natural hosts. It is also important to obtain whole-genome sequences of *P. knowlesi* from macaque reservoirs to fully detect evidence of selection and potential host switching. Although *Laverania* parasites, appear to have limited potential to cause zoonotic infections in the populations studied (Sundararaman et al. 2013; Délicat-Loembet et al. 2015), longitudinal surveys covering wider regions may provide more definitive evidence. Further sensitive and specific detection methods will be crucial in defining the extent of the reservoir.

Although not discussed in this review, vector surveys and studies will also be required to provide evidence for transmission to hu-

mans under favorable conditions (Vythilingam 2010; Paupy et al. 2013; Maeno et al. 2015).

Critical Review of Hospital Records and Case Studies for Early Detection of Unusual Cases

Although host and vector sampling are very useful in assessing the risk of zoonotic infections, they require extensive resources and can be impractical. Hospital records have proven invaluable in documenting cases of interest. Indeed, case reports and hospital records have led to many of the important reevaluations of dogma discussed in this review, including cases of *P. vivax* in DARC-negative individuals (Rubio et al. 1999), possible zoonotic *P. vivax* (Prugnolle et al. 2013), and the first case of *P. cynomolgi* human infection (Ta et al. 2014). Many of these findings, however, rely on correct diagnosis on site. Diagnosis based on morphology is prone to mistakes (*P. knowlesi* misdiagnosed as *P. malariae,* or *P. ovale* and possibly *P. cynomolgi* as *P. vivax*) and it is critical that molecular tools be used to definitively identify *Plasmodium* species. Increased awareness of the presence of these parasites in endemic regions will be important in early detection of unusual cases. This should also be accompanied with development of new rapid diagnostic tests that can detect and discriminate a larger range of species, as well as training of local public health staff.

The Promise of In Vitro Experimental Advances

The robust in vitro culture system accounts for our disproportionately greater knowledge of *P. falciparum* above other human *Plasmodium* species. Although advances in genomic tools are lending greater insight into the more neglected species, in vitro experiments will remain the gold standard to understand the mechanisms of invasion and host tropism. There have been substantial advances in studying *P. vivax* ex vivo (Russell et al. 2012) and even potential for genetic manipulation in vivo (Moraes Barros et al. 2014). There are reports of short-term culture of *P. vivax* in vitro (Golenda et al. 1997) and of *P. malariae* (Lingnau et al. 1994), but efforts to

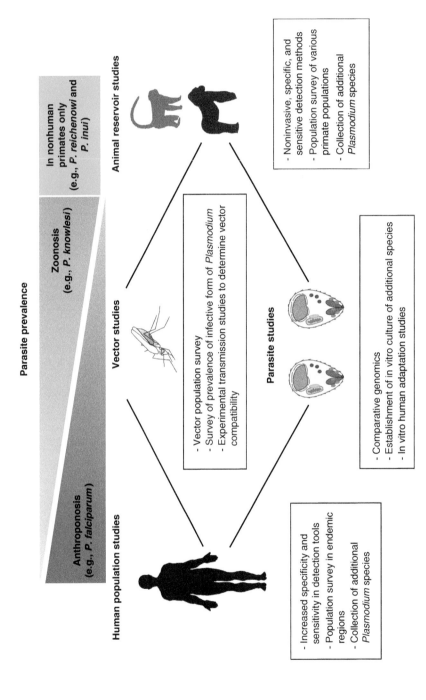

Figure 3. Toward reaching the goal of malaria elimination. Studies addressing several aspects of the ecology and biology of *Plasmodium* parasites can shed light on their evolving tropism and host adaptation. Vector, human host, and animal host population studies can help determine the diversity of *Plasmodium* species to which humans are exposed. Experimental studies can determine compatibility between parasites and hosts and elucidate the molecular mechanisms behind differences in cell tropism.

establish a reliable in vitro culture system should be renewed for these species, as well as *P. ovale*. In vitro culture will also facilitate initial screening of blood-stage vaccine targets for *P. vivax* and help identify promising candidates to pursue further. The success of adapting *P. knowlesi* to human blood has opened new doors in investigating mechanisms of host switch and adaptation relevant in the field, and has also provided the community with a more accessible tool for genetic manipulation because it obviates the need for macaque blood (Lim et al. 2013; Moon et al. 2013). Isolation of the newly identified parasites will be a daunting task but will provide a much-needed resource as we hopefully approach control if not eradication of the human *Plasmodium* species. Figure 3 summarizes studies that in conjunction will provide the necessary information for more efficient and relevant eradication strategies.

CONCLUDING REMARKS

Control of malaria has been a goal for the scientific community for several decades, while there is now a renewed emphasis on elimination. Most effort to date has focused mainly on *P. falciparum* and *P. vivax*, leaving the burden and prevalence of the lesser-studied species unclear. Having been comparatively understudied, the true extent of these parasites in humans and potential zoonotic reservoirs is not known. Expansion of current surveillance efforts to include all potential reservoirs might be needed. Methodologies with increased sensitivity will be essential for the detection of low parasitemia infections that are associated with the less-studied *Plasmodium* species. Continuous and more sensitive sampling and sequencing of human and animal *Plasmodium* species will keep us informed on the existing diversity and influence the elimination strategies to implement. *Plasmodium* parasites are continuously evolving, and molecular determinants leading to changes and expansion in host tropism will be key factors to investigate, which in some cases might identify critical molecules for development as vaccine candidates. Finally, it is also important to consider that human development is dramatically changing the ecology of infection, as human encroachment may create new and greater opportunities for potential animal reservoirs to transmit *Plasmodium* parasites.

ACKNOWLEDGMENTS

We thank James H. Mullen for his assistance with the figures.

REFERENCES

*Reference is also in this collection.

Ahmed AM, Pinheiro MM, Divis PC, Siner A, Zainudin R, Wong IT, Lu CW, Singh-Khaira SK, Millar SB, Lynch S, et al. 2014. Disease progression in *Plasmodium knowlesi* malaria is linked to variation in invasion gene family members. *PLoS Negl Trop Dis* **8**: e3086.

Assefa S, Lim C, Preston MD, Duffy CW, Nair MB, Adroub SA, Kadir KA, Goldberg JM, Neafsey DE, Divis P, et al. 2015. Population genomic structure and adaptation in the zoonotic malaria parasite *Plasmodium knowlesi*. *Proc Natl Acad Sci* **112**: 13027–13032.

Badiane AS, Bei AK, Ahouidi AD, Patel SD, Salinas N, Ndiaye D, Sarr O, Ndir O, Tolia NH, Mboup S, et al. 2013. Inhibitory humoral responses to the *Plasmodium falciparum* vaccine candidate EBA-175 are independent of the erythrocyte invasion pathway. *Clin Vaccine Immunol* **20**: 1238–1245.

Baird JK. 2009. Malaria zoonoses. *Travel Med Infect Dis* **7**: 269–277.

Barber BE, William T, Dhararaj P, Anderios F, Griff MJ, Yeo TW, Anstey NM. 2012. Epidemiology of *Plasmodium knowlesi* malaria in north-east Sabah, Malaysia: Family clusters and wide age distribution. *Malaria J* **11**: 401.

Bei AK, Membi CD, Rayner JC, Mubi M, Ngasala B, Sultan AA, Premji Z, Duraisingh MT. 2007. Variant merozoite protein expression is associated with erythrocyte invasion phenotypes in *Plasmodium falciparum* isolates from Tanzania. *Mol Biochem Parasitol* **153**: 66–71.

Blacklock B, Adler S. 1922. A parasite resembling *Plasmodium falciparum* in a chimpanzee. *Ann Trop Med Parasitol* **16**: 99–106.

Bowyer PW, Stewart LB, Aspeling-Jones H, Mensah-Brown HE, Ahouidi AD, Amambua-Ngwa A, Awandare GA, Conway DJ. 2015. Variation in *Plasmodium falciparum* erythrocyte invasion phenotypes and merozoite ligand gene expression across different populations in areas of malaria endemicity. *Infect Immun* **83**: 2575–2582.

Brown GV, Moorthy VS, Reed Z, Mendis K, Arévalo-Herrera M, Alonso P; WHO MALVAC Committee. 2009. Priorities in research and development of vaccines against *Plasmodium vivax* malaria. *Vaccine* **27**: 7228–7235.

Bruce-Chwatt LJ, Garnham PC, Shute PG, Draper CC. 1970. Induced double infection with *Plasmodium vivax* and *P. falciparum* in a splenectomized chimpanzee. *Trans R Soc Trop Med Hyg* **64**: 2.

Calderaro A, Piccolo G, Perandin F, Gorrini C, Peruzzi S, Zuelli C, Ricci L, Manca N, Dettori G, Chezzi C, et al. 2007. Genetic polymorphisms influence *Plasmodium ovale* PCR detection accuracy. *J Clin Microbiol* **45**: 1624–1627.

Camargos Costa D, Pereira de Assis GM, de Souza Silva FA, Araújo FC, de Souza Junior JC, Braga Hirano ZM, Satiko Kano F, Nóbrega de Sousa T, Carvalho LH, Ferreira Alves de Brito C. 2015. *Plasmodium simium*, a *Plasmodium vivax*-related malaria parasite: Genetic variability of Duffy binding protein II and the Duffy antigen/receptor for chemokines. *PLoS ONE* **10**: e0131339.

Carlton JM, Silva JC, Bidwell SL, Adams JH, Silva JC, Bidwell SL, Lorenzi H, Caler E, Crabtree J, Angiuoli SV, Merino EF, Amedeo P, et al. 2008. Comparative genomics of the neglected human malaria parasite *Plasmodium vivax*. *Nature* **455**: 757–763.

Carlton JM, Das A, Escalante AA. 2013. Genomics, population genetics and evolutionary history of *Plasmodium vivax*. *Adv Parasitol* **81**: 203–222.

Chenet SM, Pacheco MA, Bacon DJ, Collins WE, Barnwell JW, Escalante AA. 2013. The evolution and diversity of a low complexity vaccine candidate, merozoite surface protein 9 (MSP-9), in *Plasmodium vivax* and closely related species. *Infect Genet Evol* **20**: 239–248.

Chin W, Contacos PG, Coatney GR, Kimball HR. 1965. A naturally acquired quotidian-type malaria in man transferable to monkeys. *Science* **149**: 865–865.

Chitnis CE, Sharma A. 2008. Targeting the *Plasmodium vivax* Duffy-binding protein. *Trends Parasitol* **24**: 29–34.

Chou HH, Takematsu H, Diaz S, Iber J, Nickerson E, Wright KL, Muchmore EA, Nelson DL, Warren ST, Varki A. 1998. A mutation in human CMP-sialic acid hydroxylase occurred after the *Homo-Pan* divergence. *Proc Natl Acad Sci* **95**: 11751–11756.

Ciuca M, Chelarescu M, Sofletea A, Constantenescu P, Teriteanu E, Cortez P, Balanovschi G, Ilies M. 1955. *Contribution expérimentale a l'étude de l'immunité dans le paludisme*. L'Academia, Bucharest, Romania.

Coatney GR. 1968. Simian malarias in man: Facts, implications, and predictions. *Am J Trop Med Hyg* **17**: 147–155.

Coatney GR, Collins WE, Contacos PG. 1971. The primate malarias. U.S. National Institute of Allergy and Infectious Diseases, Washington, DC.

Collins WE, Contacos PG, Guinn EG. 1969. Observations on the sporogonic cycle and transmission of *Plasmodium simium* Da Fonseca. *J Parasitol* **55**: 814–816.

Costa DC, da Cunha VP, de Assis GM, de Souza Junior JC, Hirano ZM, de Arruda ME, Kano FS, Carvalho LH, de Brito CF. 2014. *Plasmodium simium/Plasmodium vivax* infections in southern brown howler monkeys from the Atlantic Forest. *Mem Inst Oswaldo Cruz* **109**: 641–653.

Cowman AF, Crabb BS. 2006. Invasion of red blood cells by malaria parasites. *Cell* **124**: 755–766.

Cowman AF, Berry D, Baum J. 2012. The cell biology of disease: The cellular and molecular basis for malaria parasite invasion of the human red blood cell. *J Cell Biol* **198**: 961–971.

Cox Singh J, Culleton R. 2015. *Plasmodium knowlesi*: From severe zoonosis to animal model. *Trends Parasitol* **31**: 232–238.

Crosnier C, Bustamante LY, Bartholdson SJ, Bei AK, Theron M, Uchikawa M, Mboup S, Ndir O, Kwiatkowski DP, Duraisingh MT, et al. 2011. Basigin is a receptor essential for erythrocyte invasion by *Plasmodium falciparum*. *Nature* **480**: 534–537.

Cui L, Escalante AA, Imwong M, Snounou G. 2003. The genetic diversity of *Plasmodium vivax* populations. *Trends Parasitol* **19**: 220–226.

Culleton R, Carter R. 2012. African *Plasmodium vivax*: Distribution and origins. *Int J Parasitol* **42**: 1091–1097.

Culleton R, Ndounga M, Zeyrek FY, Coban C, Casimiro PN, Takeo S, Tsuboi T, Yadava A, Carter R, Tanabe K. 2009. Evidence for the transmission of *Plasmodium vivax* in the Republic of the Congo, West Central Africa. *J Infect Dis* **200**: 1465–1469.

Daneshvar C, Davis TM, Cox-Singh J, Rafa'ee MZ, Zakaria SK, Divis PC, Singh B. 2009. Clinical and laboratory features of human *Plasmodium knowlesi* infection. *Clin Infect Dis* **49**: 852–860.

Daubersies P, Thomas AW, Millet P, Brahimi K, Langermans JA, Ollomo B, BenMohamed L, Slierendregt B, Eling W, Van Belkum A, et al. 2000. Protection against *Plasmodium falciparum* malaria in chimpanzees by immunization with the conserved pre-erythrocytic liver-stage antigen 3. *Nat Med* **6**: 1258–1263.

Deane LM. 1988. Malaria studies and control in Brazil. *Am J Trop Med Hyg* **38**: 223–230.

Délicat-Loembet L, Rougeron V, Ollomo B, Arnathau C, Roche B, Elguero E, Moukodoum ND, Okougha AP, Mve Ondo B, Boundenga L, et al. 2015. No evidence for ape *Plasmodium* infections in humans in Gabon. *PLoS ONE* **10**: e0126933.

de Sousa TN, Kano FS, de Brito CFA, Carvalho LH. 2014. The Duffy binding protein as a key target for a *Plasmodium vivax* vaccine: Lessons from the Brazilian Amazon. *Mem Inst Oswaldo Cruz* **109**: 608–617.

Dissanaike AS. 1965. Simian malaria parasites of Ceylon. *Bull World Health Organ* **32**: 593–597.

Divis PCS, Singh B, Anderios F, Hisam S, Matusop A, Kocken CH, Assefa SA, Duffy CW, Conway DJ. 2015. Admixture in humans of two divergent *Plasmodium knowlesi* populations associated with different macaque host species. *PLoS Pathog* **11**: e1004888–17.

Douglas AD, Williams AR, Illingworth JJ, Kamuyu G, Biswas S, Goodman AL, Wyllie DH, Crosnier C, Miura K, Wright GJ, et al. 2011. The blood-stage malaria antigen PfRH5 is susceptible to vaccine-inducible cross-strain neutralizing antibody. *Nat Commun* **2**: 601–619.

Douglas AD, Williams AR, Knuepfer E, Illingworth JJ, Furze JM, Crosnier C, Choudhary P, Bustamante LY, Zakutansky SE, Awuah DK, et al. 2014. Neutralization of *Plasmodium falciparum* merozoites by antibodies against PfRH5. *J Immunol* **192**: 245–258.

Douglas AD, Baldeviano GC, Lucas CM, Lugo-Roman LA, Crosnier C, Bartholdson SJ, Diouf A, Miura K, Lambert LE, Ventocilla JA, et al. 2015. A PfRH5-based vaccine is efficacious against heterologous strain blood-stage *Plasmodium falciparum* infection in *Aotus* monkeys. *Cell Host Microbe* **17**: 130–139.

Duraisingh MT, Triglia T, Ralph SA, Rayner JC, Barnwell JW, McFadden GI, Cowman AF. 2003a. Phenotypic variation of *Plasmodium falciparum* merozoite proteins directs receptor targeting for invasion of human erythrocytes. *EMBO J* **22:** 1047–1057.

Duraisingh MT, Maier AG, Triglia T, Cowman AF. 2003b. Erythrocyte-binding antigen 175 mediates invasion in *Plasmodium falciparum* utilizing sialic acid-dependent and -independent pathways. *Proc Natl Acad Sci* **100:** 4796–4801.

Ford L, Lobo CA, Rodriguez M, Zalis MG, Machado RL, Rossit AR, Cavasini CE, Couto AA, Enyong PA, Lustigman S. 2007. Differential antibody responses to *Plasmodium falciparum* invasion ligand proteins in individuals living in malaria-endemic areas in Brazil and Cameroon. *Am J Trop Med Hyg* **77:** 977–983.

Fornace KM, Nuin NA, Betson M, Grigg MJ, William T, Anstey NM, Yeo TW, Cox J, Ying LT, Drakeley CJ. 2015. Asymptomatic and submicroscopic carriage of *Plasmodium knowlesi* malaria in household and community members of clinical cases in Sabah, Malaysia. *J Infect Dis* **213:** 784–787.

Forni D, Pontremoli C, Cagliani R, Pozzoli U, Clerici M, Sironi M. 2015. Positive selection underlies the species-specific binding of *Plasmodium falciparum* RH5 to human basigin. *Mol Ecol* **24:** 4711–4722.

Galinski MRM, Medina CCC, Ingravallo PP, Barnwell JWJ. 1992. A reticulocyte-binding protein complex of *Plasmodium vivax* merozoites. *Cell* **69:** 1213–1226.

Gaur D, Furuya T, Mu J, Jiang LB, Su XZ, Miller LH. 2006. Upregulation of expression of the reticulocyte homology gene 4 in the *Plasmodium falciparum* clone Dd2 is associated with a switch in the erythrocyte invasion pathway. *Mol Biochem Parasitol* **145:** 205–215.

Gilberger TW, Thompson JK, Triglia T, Good RT, Duraisingh MT, Cowman AF. 2003. A novel erythrocyte binding antigen-175 paralogue from *Plasmodium falciparum* defines a new trypsin-resistant receptor on human erythrocytes. *J Biol Chem* **278:** 14480–14486.

Golenda CF, Li J, Rosenberg R. 1997. Continuous in vitro propagation of the malaria parasite *Plasmodium vivax*. *Proc Natl Acad Sci* **94:** 6786–6791.

Gomez-Escobar N, Amambua Ngwa A, Walther M, Okebe J, Ebonyi A, Conway DJ. 2010. Erythrocyte invasion and merozoite ligand gene expression in severe and mild *Plasmodium falciparum* malaria. *J Infect Dis* **201:** 444–452.

Gopinath R, Wongsrichanalai C, Cordón-Rosales C, Mirabelli L, Kyle D, Kain KC. 1994. Failure to detect a *Plasmodium vivax*–like malaria parasite in globally collected blood samples. *J Infect Dis* **170:** 1630–1633.

Hayakawa T, Satta Y, Gagneux P, Varki A, Takahata N. 2001. *Alu*-mediated inactivation of the human CMP-*N*-acetylneuraminic acid hydroxylase gene. *Proc Natl Acad Sci* **98:** 11399–11404.

Haynes JD, Dalton JP, Klotz FW, McGinniss MH, Hadley TJ, Hudson DE, Miller LH. 1988. Receptor-like specificity of a *Plasmodium knowlesi* malarial protein that binds to Duffy antigen ligands on erythrocytes. *J Exp Med* **167:** 1873–1881.

Hayton K, Gaur D, Liu A, Takahashi J, Henschen B, Singh S, Lambert L, Furuya T, Bouttenot R, Doll M, et al. 2008. Erythrocyte binding protein PfRH5 polymorphisms determine species-specific pathways of *Plasmodium falciparum* invasion. *Cell Host Microbe* **4:** 40–51.

Hayton K, Dumoulin P, Henschen B, Liu A, Papakrivos J, Wellems TE. 2013. Various PfRH5 polymorphisms can support *Plasmodium falciparum* invasion into the erythrocytes of owl monkeys and rats. *Mol Biochem Parasitol* **187:** 103–110.

Herrera S, Perlaza BL, Bonelo A, Arévalo-Herrera M. 2002. *Aotus* monkeys: Their great value for anti-malaria vaccines and drug testing. *Int J Parasitol* **32:** 1625–1635.

Hester J, Chan ER, Menard D, Mercereau-Puijalon O, Barnwell J, Zimmerman PA, Serre D. 2013. De novo assembly of a field isolate genome reveals novel *Plasmodium vivax* erythrocyte invasion genes. *PLoS Negl Trop Dis* **7:** e2569.

Irie A, Koyama S, Kozutsumi Y, Kawasaki T, Suzuki A. 1998. The molecular basis for the absence of *N*-glycolylneuraminic acid in humans. *J Biol Chem* **273:** 15866–15871.

Jennings CV, Ahouidi AD, Zilversmit M, Bei AK, Rayner J, Sarr O, Ndir O, Wirth DF, Mboup S, Duraisingh MT. 2007. Molecular analysis of erythrocyte invasion in *Plasmodium falciparum* isolates from Senegal. *Infect Immun* **75:** 3531–3538.

Jones KE, Patel NG, Levy MA, Storeygard A, Balk D, Gittleman JL, Daszak P. 2008. Global trends in emerging infectious diseases. *Nature* **451:** 990–993.

Kaiser M, Löwa A, Ulrich M, Ellerbrok H, Goffe AS, Blasse A, Zommers Z, Couacy-Hymann E, Babweteera F, Zuberbühler K, et al. 2010. Wild chimpanzees infected with 5 *Plasmodium* species. *Emerg Infect Dis* **16:** 1956–1959.

Kawamoto F, Liu Q, Ferreira MU, Tantular IS. 1999. How prevalent are *Plasmodium ovale* and *P. malariae* in East Asia? *Parasitol Today* **15:** 422–426.

Kocken CH, Ozwara H, van der Wel A, Beetsma AL, Mwenda JM, Thomas AW. 2002. *Plasmodium knowlesi* provides a rapid in vitro and in vivo transfection system that enables double-crossover gene knockout studies. *Infect Immun* **70:** 655–660.

Krief S, Escalante AA, Pacheco MA, Mugisha L, André C, Halbwax M, Fischer A, Krief JM, Kasenene JM, Crandfield M, et al. 2010. On the diversity of malaria parasites in African apes and the origin of *Plasmodium falciparum* from Bonobos. *PLoS Pathog* **6:** e1000765.

Lalremruata A, Magris M, Vivas-Martínez S, Koehler M, Esen M, Kempaiah P, Jeyaraj S, Perkins DJ, Mordmüller B, Metzger WG. 2015. Natural infection of *Plasmodium brasilianum* in humans: Man and monkey share quartan malaria parasites in the Venezuelan Amazon. *EBioMedicine* **2:** 1186–1192.

Lee KS, Cox-Singh J, Brooke G, Matusop A, Singh B. 2009. *Plasmodium knowlesi* from archival blood films: Further evidence that human infections are widely distributed and not newly emergent in Malaysian Borneo. *Int J Parasitol* **39:** 1125–1128.

Lee KS, Divis PCS, Zakaria SK, Matusop A, Julin RA, Conway DJ, Cox-Singh J, Singh B. 2011. *Plasmodium knowlesi*: Reservoir hosts and tracking the emergence in humans and macaques. *PLoS Pathog* **7:** e1002015.

Lim C, Hansen E, DeSimone TM, Moreno Y, Junker K, Bei A, Brugnara C, Buckee CO, Duraisingh MT. 2013. Expansion of host cellular niche can drive adaptation of a zoonotic malaria parasite to humans. *Nat Commun* **4:** 1638–1639.

Lingnau A, Doehring-Schwerdtfeger E, Maier WA. 1994. Evidence for 6-day cultivation of human *Plasmodium malariae*. *Parasitol Res* **80:** 265–266.

Liu W, Li Y, Learn GH, Rudicell RS, Robertson JD, Keele BF, Ndjango JB, Sanz CM, Morgan DB, et al. 2010. *Proc Natl Acad Sci* **102:** 12819–12824.

Liu W, Li Y, Shaw KS, Learn GH, Plenderleith LJ, Malenke JA, Sundararaman SA, Ramirez MA, Crystal PA, Smith AG, et al. 2014. African origin of the malaria parasite *Plasmodium vivax*. *Nat Commun* **5:** 1–10.

Lobo CA, Rodriguez M, Reid M, Lustigman S. 2003. Glycophorin C is the receptor for the *Plasmodium falciparum* erythrocyte binding ligand PfEBP-2(baebl). *Blood* **101:** 4628–4631.

Lopaticki S, Maier AG, Thompson J, Wilson DW, Tham WH, Triglia T, Gout A, Speed TP, Beeson JG, Healer J, et al. 2011. Reticulocyte and erythrocyte binding-like proteins function cooperatively in invasion of human erythrocytes by malaria parasites. *Infect Immun* **79:** 1107–1117.

Maeno Y, Quang NT, Culleton R, Kawai S, Masuda G, Nakazawa S, Marchand RP. 2015. Humans frequently exposed to a range of non-human primate malaria parasite species through the bites of *Anopheles dirus* mosquitoes in South-central Vietnam. *Parasit Vectors* **8:** 376.

Maier AG, Duraisingh MT, Reeder JC, Patel SS, Kazura JW, Zimmerman PA, Cowman AF. 2003. *Plasmodium falciparum* erythrocyte invasion through glycophorin C and selection for Gerbich negativity in human populations. *Nat Med* **9:** 87–92.

Marrelli MT, Branquinho MS, Hoffmann EH, Taipe-Lagos CB, Natal D, Kloetzel JK. 1998. Correlation between positive serology for *Plasmodium vivax*–like/*Plasmodium simiovale* malaria parasites in the human and anopheline populations in the State of Acre, Brazil. *Trans R Soc Trop Med Hyg* **92:** 149–151.

Martin MJ, Rayner JC, Gagneux P, Barnwell JW, Varki A. 2005. Evolution of human-chimpanzee differences in malaria susceptibility: Relationship to human genetic loss of *N*-glycolylneuraminic acid. *Proc Natl Acad Sci* **102:** 12819–12824.

Mayer DC, Cofie J, Jiang L, Hartl DL, Tracy E, Kabat J, Mendoza LH, Miller LH. 2009. Glycophorin B is the erythrocyte receptor of *Plasmodium falciparum* erythrocyte-binding ligand, EBL-1. *Proc Natl Acad Sci* **106:** 5348–5352.

Ménard D, Barnadas C, Bouchier C, Henry-Halldin C, Gray LR, Ratsimbasoa A, Thonier V, Carod JF, Domarle O, Colin Y, Locatelli S, et al. 2010a. Origin of the human malaria parasite *Plasmodium falciparum* in gorillas. *Nature* **467:** 420–425.

Ménard D, Barnadas C, Bouchier C, Henry-Halldin C, Gray LR, Ratsimbasoa A, Thonier V, Carod JF, Domarle O, Colin Y, et al. 2010b. *Plasmodium vivax* clinical malaria is commonly observed in Duffy-negative Malagasy people. *Proc Natl Acad Sci* **107:** 5967–5971.

Ménard D, Chan ER, Benedet C, Ratsimbasoa A, Kim S, Chim P, Do C, Witkowski B, Durand R, Thellier M, et al. 2013. Whole genome sequencing of field isolates reveals a common duplication of the Duffy binding protein gene in Malagasy *Plasmodium vivax* strains. *PLoS Negl Trop Dis* **7:** e2489.

Mensah-Brown HE, Amoako N, Abugri J, Stewart LB, Agongo G, Dickson EK, Ofori MF, Stoute JA, Conway DJ, Awandare GA. 2015. Analysis of erythrocyte invasion mechanisms of *Plasmodium falciparum* clinical isolates across 3 malaria-endemic areas in Ghana. *J Infect Dis* **212:** 1288–1297.

Miller LH, Mason SJ, Dvorak JA, McGinniss MH, Rothman IK. 1975. Erythrocyte receptors for (*Plasmodium knowlesi*) malaria: Duffy blood group determinants. *Science* **189:** 561–563.

Moon RW, Hall J, Rangkuti F, Ho YS, Almond N, Mitchell GH, Pain A, Holder AA, Blackman MJ. 2013. Adaptation of the genetically tractable malaria pathogen *Plasmodium knowlesi* to continuous culture in human erythrocytes. *Proc Natl Acad Sci* **110:** 531–536.

Moraes Barros RR, Straimer J, Sa JM, Salzman RE, Melendez-Muniz VA, Mu J, Fidock DA, Wellems TE. 2014. Editing the *Plasmodium vivax* genome, using zinc-finger nucleases. *J Infect Dis* **211:** 125–129.

Moyes CL, Henry AJ, Golding N, Huang Z, Singh B, Baird JK, Newton PN, Huffman M, Duda KA, Drakeley CJ, et al. 2014. Defining the geographical range of the *Plasmodium knowlesi* reservoir. *PLoS Negl Trop Dis* **8:** e2780.

Muchmore EA, Diaz S, Varki A. 1998. A structural difference between the cell surfaces of humans and the great apes. *Am J Phys Anthropol* **107:** 187–198.

Mueller I, Zimmerman PA, Reeder JC. 2007. *Plasmodium malariae* and *Plasmodium ovale*—The "bashful" malaria parasites. *Trends Parasitol* **23:** 278–283.

Mueller I, Galinski MR, Baird JK, Carlton JM, Kochar DK, Alonso PL, del Portillo HA. 2009. Key gaps in the knowledge of *Plasmodium vivax*, a neglected human malaria parasite. *Lancet Infect Dis* **9:** 555–566.

Neafsey DE, Galinsky K, Jiang RH, Young L, Sykes SM, Saif S, Gujja S, Goldberg JM, Young S, Zeng Q, et al. 2012. The malaria parasite *Plasmodium vivax* exhibits greater genetic diversity than *Plasmodium falciparum*. *Nature* **44:** 1046–1050.

Nery S, Deans AM, Mosobo M, Marsh K, Rowe JA, Conway DJ. 2006. Expression of *Plasmodium falciparum* genes involved in erythrocyte invasion varies among isolates cultured directly from patients. *Mol Biochem Parasitol* **149:** 208–215.

Ollomo B, Durand P, Prugnolle F, Douzery E, Arnathau C, Nkoghe D, Leroy E, Renaud. 2009. A new malaria agent in African hominids. *PLoS Pathog* **5:** e1000446.

Orlandi PA, Klotz FW, Haynes JD. 1992. A malaria invasion receptor, the 175-kilodalton erythrocyte binding antigen of *Plasmodium falciparum* recognizes the terminal Neu5Ac(α2-3)Gal- sequences of glycophorin A. *J Cell Biol* **116:** 901–909.

Otto TD, Rayner JC, Böhme U, Pain A, Spottiswoode N, Sanders M, Quail M, Ollomo B, Renaud F, Thomas AW, et al. 2014. Genome sequencing of chimpanzee malaria parasites reveals possible pathways of adaptation to human hosts. *Nat Commun* **5:** 4754.

Pandey AK, Reddy KS, Sahar T, Gupta S, Singh H, Reddy EJ, Asad M, Siddiqui FA, Gupta P, Singh B, et al. 2013. Identification of a potent combination of key *Plasmodium falciparum* merozoite antigens that elicit strain-transcending parasite-neutralizing antibodies. *Infect Immun* **81:** 441–451.

Patel SD, Ahouidi AD, Bei AK, Dieye TN, Mboup S, Harrison SC, Duraisingh MT. 2013. *Plasmodium falciparum* merozoite surface antigen, PfRH5, elicits detectable levels of invasion-inhibiting antibodies in humans. *J Infect Dis* **208:** 1679–1687.

Paul AS, Egan ES, Duraisingh MT. 2015. Host–parasite interactions that guide red blood cell invasion by malaria parasites. *Curr Opin Hematol* **22:** 220–226.

Paupy C, Makanga B, Ollomo B, Rahola N, Durand P, Magnus J, Willaume E, Renaud F, Rontenille D, Prugnolle F. 2013. *Anopheles moucheti* and *Anopheles vinckei* are candidate vectors of ape *Plasmodium* parasites, including *Plasmodium praefalciparum* in Gabon. *PLoS ONE* **8:** e57294.

Persson KE, McCallum FJ, Reiling L, Lister NA, Stubbs J, Cowman AF, Marsh K, Beeson JG. 2008. Variation in use of erythrocyte invasion pathways by *Plasmodium falciparum* mediates evasion of human inhibitory antibodies. *J Clin Invest* **118:** 342–351.

Pinheiro MM, Ahmed MA, Millar SB, Sanderson T, Otto TD, Lu WC, Krishna S, Rayner JC, Cox-Singh J. 2015. *Plasmodium knowlesi* genome sequences from clinical isolates reveal extensive genomic dimorphism. *PLoS ONE* **10:** e0121303.

Prugnolle F, Durand P, Neel C, Ollomo B, Ayala FJ, Arnathau C, Etienne L, Mpoudi-Ngole E, Nkoghe D, Leroy E, et al. 2010. African great apes are natural hosts of multiple related malaria species, including *Plasmodium falciparum*. *Proc Natl Acad Sci* **107:** 1458–1463.

Prugnolle F, Rougeron V, Becquart P, Berry A, Makanga B, Rahola N, Arnathau C, Ngoubangoye B, Ménard S, Willaume E, et al. 2013. Diversity, host switching and evolution of *Plasmodium vivax* infecting African great apes. *Proc Natl Acad Sci* **110:** 8123–8128.

Qari SH, Goldman IF, Povoa MM, Oliveira S, Alpers MP, Lal AA. 1991. Wide distribution of the variant form of the human malaria parasite *Plasmodium vivax*. *J Biol Chem* **266:** 16297–16300.

Qari SH, Goldman IF, Povoa MM, di Santi S, Alpers MP, Lal AA. 1992. Polymorphism in the circumsporozoite protein of the human malaria parasite *Plasmodium vivax*. *Mol Biochem Parasitol* **55:** 105–113.

Qari SH, Shi YP, Goldman IF, Udhayakumar V, Alpers MP, Collins WE, Lal AA. 1993. Identification of *Plasmodium vivax*–like human malaria parasite. *Lancet* **341:** 780–783.

Rayner JC. 2015. *Plasmodium malariae* malaria: From monkey to man? *EBioMedicine* **2:** 1023–1024.

Rayner JC, Liu W, Peeters M, Sharp PM, Hahn BH. 2011. A plethora of *Plasmodium* species in wild apes: A source of human infection? *Trends Parasitol* **27:** 222–229.

Reddy KS, Pandey AK, Singh H, Sahar T, Emmanuel A, Chitnis CE, Chauhan VS, Gaur D. 2014. Bacterially expressed full-length recombinant *Plasmodium falciparum* RH5 protein binds erythrocytes and elicits potent strain-transcending parasite-neutralizing antibodies. *Infect Immun* **82:** 152–164.

Reed MB, Caruana SR, Batchelor AH, Thompson JK, Crabb BS, Cowman AF. 2000. Targeted disruption of an erythrocyte binding antigen in *Plasmodium falciparum* is associated with a switch toward a sialic acid-independent pathway of invasion. *Proc Natl Acad Sci* **97:** 7509–7514.

Reiling L, Richards JS, Fowkes FJ, Barry AE, Triglia T, Chokejindachai W, Michon P, Tavul L, Siba PM, Cowman AF, et al. 2010. Target of protective immunity against *Plasmodium falciparum* malaria. *J Immunol* **185:** 6157–6167.

Reiling L, Richards JS, Fowkes FJ, Wilson DW, Chokejindachai W, Barry AE, Tham WH, Stubbs J, Langer C, Donelson J, et al. 2012. The *Plasmodium falciparum* erythrocyte invasion ligand Pfrh4 as a target of functional and protective human antibodies against malaria. *PLoS ONE* **7:** e45253.

Reyes-Sandoval A. 2013. *Plasmodium vivax* malaria vaccines: Why are we where we are? *Hum Vaccin Immunother* **9:** 2558–2565.

Rich SM, Leendertz FH, Xu G, LeBreton M, Djoko CF, Aminake MN, Takang EE, Diffo JL, Pike BL, Rosenthal BM, et al. 2009. The origin of malignant malaria. *Proc Natl Acad Sci* **106:** 14902–14907.

Rosenberg R, Wirtz RA, Lanar DE, Sattabongkot J, Hall T, Waters AP, Prasittisuk C. 1989. Circumsporozoite protein heterogeneity in the human malaria parasite *Plasmodium vivax*. *Science* **245:** 973–976.

Rubio JM, Benito A, Roche J, Berzosa PJ, García ML, Micó M, Edú M, Alvar J. 1999. Semi-nested, multiplex polymerase chain reaction for detection of human malaria parasites and evidence of *Plasmodium vivax* infection in Equatorial Guinea. *Am J Trop Med Hyg* **60:** 183–187.

Russell B, Suwanarusk R, Malleret B, Costa FT, Snounou G, Kevin Baird J, Nosten F, Rénia L. 2012. Human ex vivo studies on asexual *Plasmodium vivax*: The best way forward. *Int J Parasitol* **42:** 1063–1070.

* Singh S, Chitnis CE. 2016. Molecular signaling involved in entry and exit of malaria parasites from host erythrocytes. *Cold Spring Harb Perspect Med* doi: 10.1101/cshperspect.a026815.

Singh B, Daneshvar C. 2013. Human infections and detection of *Plasmodium knowlesi*. *Clin Microbiol Rev* **26:** 165–184.

Singh B, Sung LK, Matusop A, Radhakrishnan A, Shamsul SS, Cox-Singh J, Thomas A, Conway DJ. 2004. A large focus of naturally acquired *Plasmodium knowlesi* infections in human beings. *Lancet* **363:** 1017–1024.

Singh AP, Ozwara H, Kocken CH, Puri SK, Thomas AW, Chitnis CE. 2005. Targeted deletion of *Plasmodium knowlesi* Duffy binding protein confirms its role in junction formation during invasion. *Mol Microbiol* **55:** 1925–1934.

Snounou G, Viriyakosol S, Zhu XP, Jarra W, Pinheiro L, do Rosario VE, Thaithong S, Brown KN. 1993. High sensitivity of detection of human malaria parasites by the use of nested polymerase chain reaction. *Mol Biochem Parasitol* **61:** 315–320.

Stubbs J, Simpson KM, Triglia T, Plouffe D, Tonkin CJ, Duraisingh MT, Maier AG, Winzeler EA, Cowman AF. 2005. Molecular mechanism for switching of P. falciparum invasion pathways into human erythrocytes. *Science* **309:** 1384–1387.

Sundararaman SA, Liu W, Keele BF, Learn GH, Bittinger K, Mouacha F, Ahuka-Mundeke S, Manske M, Sherrill-Mix S, Li Y, et al. 2013. *Plasmodium falciparum*–like parasites infecting wild apes in southern Cameroon do not represent a recurrent source of human malaria. *Proc Natl Acad Sci* **110:** 7020–7025.

Sutherland CJ, Tanomsing N, Nolder D, Oguike M, Jennison C, Pukrittayakamee S, Dolecek C, Hien TT, do Rosário VE, Arez AP, et al. 2010. Two nonrecombining sympatric forms of the human malaria parasite *Plasmodium ovale* occur globally. *J Infect Dis* **201**: 1544–1550.

Ta TH, Hisam S, Lanza M, Jiram Al, Ismail N, Rubio JM. 2014. First case of a naturally acquired human infection with *Plasmodium cynomolgi*. *Malaria J* **13**: 1–7.

Tachibana M, Tsuboi T, Kaneko O, Khuntirat B, Torii M. 2002. Two types of *Plasmodium ovale* defined by SSU rRNA have distinct sequences for ookinete surface proteins. *Mol Biochem Parasitol* **122**: 223–226.

Taylor LH, Latham SM, Woolhouse ME. 2001. Risk factors for human disease emergence. *Philos Trans R Soc B Biol Sci* **356**: 983–989.

Tham WH, Healer J, Cowman AF. 2012. Erythrocyte and reticulocyte binding-like proteins of *Plasmodium falciparum*. *Trends Parasitol* **28**: 23–30.

Triglia T, Duraisingh MT, Good RT, Cowman AF. 2005. Reticulocyte-binding protein homologue 1 is required for sialic acid-dependent invasion into human erythrocytes by *Plasmodium falciparum*. *Mol Microbiol* **55**: 162–174.

Udhayakumar V, Qari SH, Patterson P, Collins WE, Lal AA. 1994. Monoclonal antibodies to the circumsporozoite protein repeats of a *Plasmodium vivax*–like human malaria parasite and *Plasmodium simiovale*. *Infect Immun* **62**: 2098–2100.

Valencia SH, Rodríguez DC, Acero DL, Ocampo V, Arévalo-Herrera M. 2011. Platform for *Plasmodium vivax* vaccine discovery and development. *Mem Inst Oswaldo Cruz* **106**: 179–192.

van Rooyen CE, Pile GR. 1935. Observations on infection by *Plasmodium knowlesi* (ape malaria) in the treatment of general paralysis of the insane. *Br Med J* **2**: 662–666.

Vythilingam I. 2010. *Plasmodium knowlesi* in humans: A review on the role of its vectors in Malaysia. *Trop Biomed* **27**: 1–12.

Wanaguru M, Crosnier C, Johnson S, Rayner JC, Wright GJ. 2013. Biochemical analysis of the *Plasmodium falciparum* erythrocyte-binding antigen-175 (EBA175)-glycophorin-A interaction: Implications for vaccine design. *J Biol Chem* **288**: 32106–32117.

Wertheimer SP, Barnwell JW. 1989. *Plasmodium vivax* interaction with the human Duffy blood group glycoprotein: Identification of a parasite receptor-like protein. *Exp Parasitol* **69**: 340–350.

White NJ, Pukrittayakamee S, Hien TT, Faiz MA, Mokuolu OA, Dondorp AM. 2014. Malaria. *Lancet* **383**: 723–735.

Williams AR, Douglas AD, Miura K, Illingworth JJ, Choudhary P, Murungi LM, Furze JM, Diouf A, Miotto O, Crosnier C, et al. 2012. Enhancing blockade of *Plasmodium falciparum* erythrocyte invasion: Assessing combinations of antibodies against PfRH5 and other merozoite antigens. *PLoS Pathog* **8**: e1002991.

Win TT, Jalloh A, Tantular IS, Tsuboi T, Ferreira MU, Kimura M, Kawamoto F. 2004. Molecular analysis of *Plasmodium ovale* variants. *Emerg Infect Dis* **10**: 1235–1240.

Woldearegai TG, Kremsner PG, Kun JFJ, Mordmuller B. 2013. *Plasmodium vivax* malaria in Duffy-negative individuals from Ethiopia. *Trans R Soc Trop Med Hyg* **107**: 328–331.

WHO. 2015. World malaria report 2015. World Health Organization, Geneva, pp. 1–280.

Wright GJ, Rayner JC. 2014. *Plasmodium falciparum* erythrocyte invasion: Combining function with immune evasion. *PLoS Pathog* **10**: ve1003943.

Young MD, Eyles DE, Burgess RW, Jeffery GM. 1955. Experimental testing of the immunity of Negroes to *Plasmodium vivax*. *J Parasitol* **41**: 315–318.

Cite this article as *Cold Spring Harb Perspect Med* doi: 10.1101/cshperspect.a025494

Immune Responses in Malaria

Carole A. Long[1] and Fidel Zavala[2]

[1]Laboratory of Malaria and Vector Research, National Institute of Allergy and Infectious Diseases, National Institute of Health, Rockville, Maryland 20852

[2]Departmentof Molecular Microbiology and Immunology, Bloomberg School of Public Health, Johns Hopkins University, Baltimore, Maryland 21205

Correspondence: clong@niaid.nih.gov; fzavala1@jhu.edu

Evidence accumulated through the years clearly indicates that antiparasite immune responses can efficiently control malaria parasite infection at all development stages, and under certain circumstances they can prevent parasite infection. Translating these findings into vaccines or immunotherapeutic interventions has been difficult in part because of the extraordinary biological complexity of this parasite, which has several developmental stages expressing unique sets of stage-specific genes and multiple antigens, most of which are antigenically diverse. Nevertheless, in the last 30 years major advances have resulted in characterization of a number of vaccine candidates, exploration of the repertoire of host immune responses to the various parasite stages, and also identification of significant hurdles that need to be overcome. Most important, these advances strengthened the concept that the induction of host immune responses that target all developmental stages of *Plasmodium* can efficiently control or abrogate *Plasmodium* infections and strongly support the notion that an effective vaccine can be developed. This vaccine would be a critical component for programs aimed at controlling or eradicating malaria.

In this review, we address immune responses to the various stages of parasite development—preerythrocytic, asexual stages in red cells, and sexual and mosquito stages. Our expanding understanding of these responses and their targets provides a foundation for the development of vaccines directed at the three major developmental stages of malaria parasites.

IMMUNE RESPONSES TO PREERYTHROCYTIC (PE) ANTIGENS

Antibody Responses to PE Antigens

Early studies in rodent malaria showed that immunization with attenuated *Plasmodium ber-* *ghei* sporozoites induced antibodies that recognized the sporozoite surface and neutralized their infectivity (Nussenzweig et al. 1967). Subsequent studies in which humans were immunized with attenuated *Plasmodium falciparum* sporozoites confirmed the protective efficacy of the sporozoite-induced immune responses (Rieckmann et al. 1979). Humans naturally exposed to parasite infection in endemic areas also develop antisporozoite responses, as indicated by studies in malaria-endemic areas of Africa and Asia, which reported that antisporozoite antibodies are most frequently detected in individuals older than 50 years and in only a minority of children (Nardin et al. 1979; Tapchaisri et al. 1983; Druilhe et al. 1986). In vitro assays with sera from endemic areas showed that sporozoite-reactive sera inhibit sporozoite invasion of hepatocytes in vitro (Hollingdale et al. 1984; Hoffman et al. 1986; Mellouk et al. 1986; Hollingdale et al. 1989).

The antibodies that bind to sporozoites recognize different antigens. Among these, the circumsporozoite protein (CSP) was the first antigen identified in rodent and human malaria sporozoites (Nussenzweig and Nussenzweig 1989). A CSP-based vaccine (RTS,S) has undergone a phase III vaccine trial, and is discussed in detail in Healer et al. (2016). Anti-CSP antibodies bind the entire surface of sporozoites and induce the shedding of the CSP (Stewart et al. 1986). Most of them recognize the repeat domain of this protein, which is conserved in all strains of *P. falciparum* (Zavala et al. 1985a). Most importantly, they inhibit sporozoite infectivity in vivo and in vitro (Zavala et al. 1985b; Persson et al. 2002). Longitudinal studies, focused on antibodies specific for the CSP repeats showed an age-dependent distribution of antibodies as had been observed using an immunofluorescence antibody (IFA) assay (Zavala et al. 1985b; Del Giudice et al. 1987, 1990).

Studies in endemic areas revealed that the presence of anti-CSP antibodies correlated with transmission exposure and increased with age (Campbell et al. 1987; Esposito et al. 1988; Marsh et al. 1988). Studies on the carboxy- and amino-terminal regions flanking the repeat domain indicate that they contain important functional domains that enable sporozoite infectivity (Coppi et al. 2011). Sera from endemic areas contain antibodies against nonrepeat regions of the CSP, and the presence of *P. falciparum* amino-terminal-specific antibodies has been associated with the development of clinical immunity (Bongfen et al. 2009). Recently, it was shown that antibodies against this amino-terminal region strongly inhibit sporozoite infectivity in vivo (Espinosa et al. 2015).

Thrombospondin-related adhesive protein (TRAP) (Robson et al. 1988) is a parasite antigen also considered as a vaccine candidate. This is a transmembrane protein containing adhesive domains that enable the motility of sporozoites

in mosquitoes and vertebrate hosts, mediating their migration from skin to the liver. Early studies showed that sera from individuals immunized with *P. falciparum* sporozoites had antibodies against TRAP and these antibodies inhibited sporozoite infection of hepatocytes in vitro (Rogers et al. 1992). In Mali, the presence of antibodies against TRAP was associated with lower parasitemia, protection against infection (Scarselli et al. 1993; John et al. 2003), and protection against cerebral malaria (Dolo et al. 1999). Antibodies against TRAP are short lived in children, waning significantly during the dry season (John et al. 2003), as also observed with anti-CSP antibodies (Marsh et al. 1988).

LSA1 is a 197-Kd molecule consisting of a large number of repeated sequences, expressed exclusively in *P. falciparum* during early liver stages and no ortholog exists in rodent parasites (Guerin-Marchand et al. 1987; Zhu and Hollingdale 1991). This antigen is widely recognized by sera from individuals living in endemic areas (Fidock et al. 1994; Kurtis et al. 2001). Studies using sera from children in Gabon reported an association between anti-LSA1 titers and partial resistance to infection (Domarle et al. 1999). Another antigen, CelTOS (cell-traversal protein for ookinetes and sporozoites) (Kariu et al. 2006) is a conserved protein present in two different motile stages and appears to elicit cross-species protection (Bergmann-Leitner et al. 2010). Limited epidemiologic information on CelTOS indicates that individuals living in endemic areas develop cellular and humoral responses against this antigen (Anum et al. 2015).

Studies in Kenya that evaluated antibody responses to CSP, LSA-1, and TRAP, indicated that antibody levels against these three antigens, instead of a single antigen, displayed a stronger correlation with lower incidence and reduced risk of clinical malaria, as well as with diminished severity of disease (John et al. 2005, 2008). Recent studies using high-throughput assays to screen hundreds of *Plasmodium* antigens revealed that, compared to blood-stage reactivity, there was an infrequent reactivity to preerythrocytic antigens (Doolan et al. 2008; Crompton et al. 2010). These studies associated pro-

Cite this article as *Cold Spring Harb Perspect Med* doi: 10.1101/cshperspect.a025577

tection with the breadth of antigens recognized instead of responses to single antigens.

Overall, studies with sera from individuals living in endemic areas and volunteers immunized with irradiated sporozoites indicate that the development of antibodies against sporozoite antigens is clearly age and dose dependent, and their magnitude is limited. There is a consensus that antibodies induced by natural exposure may in some areas correlate with partial protection but they do not confer sterile immunity.

T-Cell Responses to Preerythrocytic (PE) Antigens

The notion that T cells can be an effective antiparasite immune mechanism derives from studies in rodent models showing that $CD8^+$ and $CD4^+$ T cells inhibit the development of malaria liver stages (Tsuji and Zavala 2003). Studies in endemic areas indicate that naturally exposed individuals are able to mount specific $CD8^+$ T-cell responses to CSP and TRAP, but these responses are low in magnitude and detectable only in a minority of individuals (Doolan et al. 1993; Flanagan et al. 2003). Studies in some endemic areas failed to detect $CD8^+$ T-cell responses against any of the overlapping peptides representing the entire CSP sequence, including most of the variant isolates (Doolan et al. 1991). A study in Kenya suggested a degree of protection against anemia among individuals that produced interferon γ (IFN-γ) in response to TRAP peptides (Ong'echa et al. 2003). Human vaccine trials using recombinant viruses as immunogens have shown the induction of $CD8^+$ T-cell responses against these antigens and an association with partial protection (Ewer et al. 2013).

$CD4^+$ T cells against CSP are also found in individuals living in endemic areas. Early studies showed that several epitopes are recognized in both the CSP of *Plasmodium vivax* and *P. falciparum,* and these responses appear to be more frequent against polymorphic epitopes (Good et al. 1988; Zevering et al. 1994) The presence of CSP-specific $CD4^+$ T cells in individuals living in endemic areas did not show correlation with clinical immunity (de Groot et al. 1989; Riley et al. 1990; Esposito et al. 1992). T-cell responses against other antigens such as HEP17 (Doolan et al. 1996) and STARP (Fidock et al. 1994) have also been identified; however, these antigens are expressed in liver and asexual stages and therefore the target of their potential protective effect remains to be defined.

The difficulties in detecting robust T-cell responses against PE antigens in individuals living in endemic areas contrasts with the relative ease at which these responses are detected in volunteers immunized with attenuated sporozoites (Seder et al. 2013) or subunit vaccines (Ewer et al. 2013). This indicates that natural exposure to parasite antigens may not be sufficient to induce robust T-cell responses. Taken together, naturally acquired antibody and T-cell responses against PE antigens are of low magnitude and infrequent, particularly in children. Although some studies indicate an association of naturally induced immune responses with clinical immunity, these responses may never confer sterile protection. This is likely because of low antigen inoculum received by individuals as mosquitoes inject only a few sporozoites (10–100) and this may not be sufficient to induce strong immune responses. Indeed, anti-PE responses induced in humans after immunization with attenuated sporozoites can confer a high degree of sterile protection, but this requires exposure to 1000 infective bites (Herrington et al. 1991) or the intravenous injection of several hundred thousand sporozoites (Seder et al. 2013). Decades of studies on the CSP protein laid the groundwork for the development and testing of the RTS,S vaccine, which is based on this protein using a platform of a hepatitis B particle (discussed in Healer et al. 2016). However, this vaccine is only partially effective and its longevity is limited. The development of a more efficient PE vaccine that could effectively contribute to eradication efforts will require a better understanding of the immune mechanisms operating in sporozoite-induced immunity, the identification of additional target antigens, and the design of a new generation of vaccines capable of inducing not only high antibody titers but also strong cell-mediated immune protection.

IMMUNE RESPONSES TO ASEXUAL ERYTHROCYTIC STAGES

The asexual stages of malaria parasites have been intensively investigated because they are most accessible to investigators in the blood of an infected person and because they are responsible for the pathology associated with this disease. It is known that those living in malaria-endemic areas progressively develop partial resistance to infection with *P. falciparum*, although this takes many years to attain (reviewed in Beeson et al. 2008; Langhorne et al. 2008; Crompton et al. 2014). The classic depiction of the natural history of immunity to malaria as a function of age was provided by long-term studies in Kenya (Marsh and Kinyanjui 2006). As illustrated in Marsh and Kinyanjui (2006), these studies revealed that young children are likely to have the highest parasitemias and also are more likely to develop severe malaria pathology (Milner 2016). As children age, they are still susceptible to infection accompanied by clinical symptoms but are less likely to develop severe disease. This pattern continues into adolescence and adulthood with even fewer clinical symptoms but still the periodic presence of parasites. Studies on the acquisition of immunity to *P. vivax* indicate that resistance may be acquired more rapidly than with *P. falciparum* (reviewed in Mueller 2013).

Perhaps the most important finding in our understanding of this naturally acquired immunity to *P. falciparum* malaria was published in 1961 (Cohen et al. 1961). That study established that pooled IgG antibodies from African adults living in a malaria-endemic area could dramatically drive down parasitemias when passively transferred to children with malaria. It was later confirmed and extended using IgGs from Africans transferred to Asians failing chemotherapy for malaria (Sabchareon et al. 1991). Its functionality, despite the geographic distance, provided evidence that the protective antibodies either recognized conserved determinants or a very broad range of allelic types. These experi-

ments have provided the experimental foundation for efforts to develop a malaria vaccine, historically with the main goal of protecting children against severe disease and death. Despite all this time we are not certain of the antigenic targets of those protective antibodies nor are we certain of the effector mechanisms involved in the reduction of parasite burden. Further, we do not know the contribution of T cells (beyond helper function) or other cells of the immune system to these responses. The large number of parasite-encoded proteins (approximately 5400 genes) and the allelic diversity of many of those proteins have complicated the identification of targets of protective immune responses as well as efforts to develop vaccines that elicit broadly reactive protective responses. Nevertheless, the fact that people living in endemic areas become at least partially immune to malaria provides evidence that a vaccine against this disease should be possible. Overall, progress has been slow and results of phase II clinical trials testing several blood-stage vaccine candidates have been disappointing (Healer et al. 2016). Thus, there is significant impetus for identification of new potential vaccine candidates and combinations of candidates from blood stages, expanded efforts to understand the important cells and effector mechanisms to be targeted, and exploration of immunization strategies that would elicit these responses.

Effector Mechanisms and Assays

Selection of malaria vaccine candidates and their rapid evaluation has been hampered by numerous problems, including difficulties encountered in expressing novel malaria proteins in recombinant protein expression systems in a correct configuration and the lack of assays and markers, which predict protection in vivo. Many investigators have shown that those infected with malaria parasites produce an array of antibodies against many different asexual-stage proteins and these have usually been examined one at a time. More recent studies have extended these results using microarrays with *Escherichia coli* produced proteins (Gray et al. 2007; Doolan et al. 2008; Crompton et al. 2010).

It has been difficult to correlate responses to individual parasite proteins with protection, although it has been proposed that cytophilic IgG1 and IgG3 isotypes are more correlated with protective responses (Bouharoun-Tayoun and Druilhe 1992).

Assessing these antibodies has ranged from direct enzyme-linked immunosorbent assay (ELISA) measurements to evaluation of functional activity using assays such as in vitro parasite growth inhibition, opsonization with antibodies and leukocytes, complement fixation, measuring antibodies to proteins on the erythrocyte surface by flow cytometry or agglutination tests, and antibody-dependent cellular cytotoxicity assays. However, it has been difficult to correlate any single assay with clinical protection, so the relative contribution of these antibody effector functions in vivo is not established.

Merozoite Proteins

Merozoite proteins have been the focus of most studies of immune responses to the asexual stages of infection and work in Cowman et al. (2012) discusses the architecture of a merozoite as well as its organelles and some of the proteins involved in invasion. One of the first merozoite proteins to be investigated was the merozoite surface protein 1 (MSP1), one of a number of MSP molecules, which provide a surface coating for merozoites and likely contribute to the invasion process. Monoclonal antibodies to the carboxyl terminus of this large protein were able to protect mice passively against lethal challenge with the rodent parasite *Plasmodium yoelii* (Majarian et al. 1984; Burns et al. 1989), and subsequent studies established that both mice and Aotus monkeys could be immunized against a lethal parasite challenge using either the *P. yoelii* or *P. falciparum* MSP1 carboxyl terminus (Daly and Long 1993; Stowers et al. 2001). Later efforts to move this candidate into human clinical trials in Africa proved disappointing (Ogutu et al. 2009). Humans living in malaria-endemic areas do develop antibodies to MSP1, and in some cases these responses have been associated with protection. Apical

membrane antigen 1 (AMA1) (Deans et al. 1982; reviewed in Remarque et al. 2008) is a micronemal protein, which is translocated to the merozoite surface during invasion and, in conjunction with RON2, contributes to the moving junction on the red cell during invasion (Lamarque et al. 2011); it is also present in sporozoites. Its critical central role during erythrocyte invasion has made it a target for both vaccines and drugs, and immunization-challenge studies with PfAMA1 in Aotus monkeys showed protective responses (Stowers et al. 2002). Further, antibodies to AMA1 from a variety of animal species strongly inhibit red cell invasion in vitro, and antibodies to it are commonly found in those living in endemic areas, including young children. Nevertheless, this has presented significant problems for investigators because of the allelic diversity found in different strains of *P. falciparum* (Thomas et al. 1990), and success in human clinical trials has been limited (Sagara et al. 2009; Thera et al. 2011). However, several groups have shown in preclinical studies that immunization with a mixture of four to five alleles elicits antibodies with greater cross-strain specificity (Dutta et al. 2013; Miura et al. 2013b; Terheggen et al. 2014), and immunization with AMA1 combined with RON2 may elicit more effective responses (Srinivasan et al. 2014).

Other merozoite proteins involved in erythrocyte binding have been examined as possible targets of protective host immune responses. Most can be categorized as erythrocyte binding-like (EBL) or reticulocyte binding-like (RBL or Rh) (reviewed in Tham et al. 2012). These are located in the apical organelles and some have been shown to be targets of invasion-inhibiting antibodies. However, the existence of multiple parasite-encoded ligands has allowed these organisms to use redundant invasion pathways and potentially escape host immune responses (reviewed by Wright and Rayner 2014).

One of these proteins, PfRh5 (reticulocyte-binding protein homolog), has been identified as a critical merozoite component because of its binding to basigin on the red cell membrane (Crosnier et al. 2011). PfRh5 also interacts with two other parasite molecules, PfRipr (Chen et al. 2011) and CyRPA (Reddy et al. 2015).

Although people living in a malaria-endemic area generally develop low levels of antibody to PfRh5 (Douglas et al. 2011; Tran et al. 2014), animals immunized with this antigen can produce antibodies with significant growth inhibition activity (Douglas et al. 2014) and, in the case of nonhuman primates, show protective immune responses even against heterologous parasites (Douglas et al. 2015).

Parasite Proteins on the Infected Red Cell Surface

There are several multigene families encoding important proteins exported to the infected red cell membrane. Perhaps the most important are the complex VAR proteins encoded by the large, polymorphic PfEMP1 (erythrocyte membrane protein) gene family with approximately 60 members with different *var* repertoires in different parasite strains (reviewed in Chan et al. 2014; Hviid and Jensen 2015). These large proteins have multiple variant domains, which bind ligands such as CD36 and ICAM-1 on host tissues and contribute to sequestration of *P. falciparum* parasites on the vascular endothelium (see Smith 2014 for review of adhesion domains). This has resulted in some variants being associated with specific disease pathogenesis such as cerebral malaria (Milner 2016). PfEMP1 proteins are displayed on the surface of the infected red cell for many hours and would be excellent targets for host immune responses, but their complexity, antigenic heterogeneity, and ability to switch from one PfEMP1 protein to another are daunting for vaccinology. However, it is clear that those living in malaria-endemic areas develop antibodies to the surfaces of infected red cells and these responses have been implicated in naturally acquired immunity, perhaps by sequential acquisition of antibodies caused by infection with various parasite strains (Bull et al. 1998; Mackintosh et al. 2008; Chan et al. 2012).

The most defined member of this family is VAR2CSA, a member of the PfEMP1 family, which has been implicated in pregnancy-associated malaria because of its binding to chondroitin-sulfate A (CSA) found in the placenta (Fried and Duffy 2016). Multiparous women develop antibodies to VAR2CSA and these antibodies appear to contribute to their resistance to placental malaria after the first pregnancy (reviewed in Ataide et al. 2014). Localization of important target epitopes within this large molecule, producing correct conformation of specific domains, and some allelic variation have all complicated studies with this molecule.

Two other polymorphic gene families are the *rifins* (repetitive interspersed family) and the *stevors* (subtelomeric variant open reading frame), which encode the RIFINS and STEVOR protein families. Much less is known about these proteins and immune responses to them, although recent evidence has indicated that both the RIFINS (Goel et al. 2015) and the STEVORS (Niang et al. 2014) can promote rosetting of red blood cells; this is an aggregation of infected and uninfected red cells, which in some studies has been suggested to contribute to malaria pathogenesis (Carlson et al. 1990).

Protective Immune Responses

Given the wide array of humoral immune responses to various antigens associated with asexual stages, a meta-analysis of the literature was conducted to try to associate antibodies to specific merozoite proteins with incidence of *P. falciparum* malaria (Fowkes et al. 2010). Some limited associations were noted with proteins such as MSP3 and MSP1–19, but it is unclear whether these are cause-and-effect relationships. Overall, evidence has accumulated based on results in model systems that high levels of antibodies to merozoite antigens are likely to be required to achieve protection in humans. This is thought to be because of the short window available to attack extracellular merozoites before they enter a new red cell. Further, the major clinical trials of blood-stage vaccines have been performed with single antigens and it is likely that combinations of antigens will be required. In this context, protection from clinical malaria has been reported to be associated with both the breadth and magnitude of the antibody responses to merozoite antigens (Osier et al. 2008).

Other potential targets of naturally acquired immunity are the variant surface antigens present on the membranes of infected red cells. It has been suggested that this immunity depends on acquisition of antibodies to these antigens and that the complexity and variability of protein families such as PfEMP1 requires the progressive accumulation of antibodies to different variants over time (reviewed in Chan et al. 2014; Smith 2014; Hviid and Jensen 2015). It may be that robust antibody responses to both merozoite and cell surface antigens are required to attain naturally acquired clinical immunity although there is limited data on this possibility and replicating it in vaccines remains a challenge.

In the context of elimination/eradication, the question has been raised as to the rationale for asexual-stage vaccines, especially given that they may be only partially effective. However, there are still large numbers of children susceptible to serious disease caused by malaria. Moreover, as malaria continues to decline, much larger numbers of adolescents and adults will not have the benefit of naturally acquired immunity and will be susceptible to serious illness if malaria resurges. Having a vaccine that can provide protection to these people will continue to be of relevance in malaria immunity.

Impact of Malaria Infection on the Immune System

Infection by asexual stages of plasmodia triggers an array of signals and responses in both the innate and adaptive host immune systems. Whether these responses contribute to protection or pathology or both has been difficult to evaluate, particularly in human studies. Although the evidence for a protective role of B cells and antibodies has been noted, the direct contribution of CD4[+] T cells in protection against blood stages beyond a helper function for CD4[+] T cells has mainly derived from rodent models of malaria. For example, it has been shown that CD4[+] T cells can dramatically reduce infection with *Plasmodium chabaudi* in the absence of B cells (Grun and Weidanz 1981). Many other cell types have been implicated in these complex responses as well.

Innate immune cells can be activated by various pathogen-associated molecular patterns (PAMPs); some of the PAMPs implicated include hemozoin, parasite DNA, and the glycosylphosphatidylinositol anchors of malaria proteins (reviewed in Gazzinelli et al. 2014). Receptor activation results in the release of various proinflammatory cytokines and chemokines, including TNF-α and interleukin 1β (IL-1β), leading to systemic pathology and many of the symptoms of malaria such as paroxysms of fever (see Milner 2016).

The long period required for acquisition of natural immunity to malaria and the lack of "sterile" immunity to this infection have led to the suggestion that dysregulation of the host immune system contributes to this incomplete immunity. In addition, reports that antibodies to some parasite antigens are short-lived has led to the suggestion that there are deficiencies in the generation and maintenance of memory B cells in malaria-infected individuals (Portugal et al. 2013; Scholzen and Sauerwein 2013). However, whether this is responsible for the slow development of naturally acquired immunity has been questioned (Hviid et al. 2015). It has also been observed that malaria-exposed individuals have a larger proportion of atypical memory B cells (Weiss et al. 2009), although their specificity is not known and this has not been directly linked with malaria infection. Additional investigations of different B-cell populations, immunologic memory, and protective immune mechanisms will be required to illuminate these issues.

IMMUNE RESPONSES TO SEXUAL AND MOSQUITO-STAGE PARASITES

Characterization of Parasite Sexual Stages

Although asexual stages are responsible for the clinical symptoms of malaria, its transmission requires differentiation to sexual stages, which can be picked up and transmitted by anopheline mosquitoes (Nilsson et al. 2015; Mitchell and Catteruccia 2016). Sexual stages II−IV are sequestered from the peripheral circulation, but eventually stage-V male and female gametocytes reemerge into the bloodstream where they can be engulfed by mosquitoes taking a blood meal. Markers of the various gametocyte stages, as well as proteins specific to male or female gametocytes, have been sought for some time. However, mature gametocytes no longer present *var* gene products on the red cell surface and other surface markers have not been definitively identified (Sutherland 2009). Once in the mosquito, the male and female gametocytes emerge from the red cells in the mosquito midgut as gametes where fertilization occurs. At this point, the gametes, zygotes, and ookinetes are accessible to antibodies, leukocytes, or other factors, such as complement, which may be present in the blood meal.

Initial evidence that vertebrate immune responses can interfere with sexual-stage development and mosquito infection led to the concept of transmission-blocking vaccines (reviewed in Stowers and Carter 2001; Sinden 2010). The first studies were conducted in avian models of malaria when birds were immunized with killed blood containing gametocytes, making them less infectious to mosquitoes than controls (Huff et al. 1958). Almost two decades later, it was shown that chickens immunized with inactivated *Plasmodium gallinaceum* gametocytes produced a transmission-blocking activity found in the serum (Carter and Chen 1976; Gwadz 1976). Interestingly, these serum effectors did not affect the gametocytes directly but rather acted on the parasites in the mosquito. Transmission-blocking immunity was also reported with rodent and nonhuman primate malaria parasites (Gwadz and Green 1978; Mendis and Targett 1979). Identification of monoclonal antibodies with transmission-blocking activity in mosquito-feeding experiments facilitated identification of parasite antigens that were the targets of transmission-blocking activity and also established the critical role of antibodies in blocking transmission (Kaushal et al. 1983; Rener et al. 1983). These studies also resulted in a method to evaluate antibodies to sexual stages, viz., the standard mosquito membrane feeding assay (SMFA). In this assay, cultured gametocytes are incubated with antibodies and the mixture fed to anopheline mosquitoes; 1 week later, the oocysts on the mosquito midgut are enumerated. Recent efforts to qualify the SMFA and to analyze data derived from this assay have increased its applicability to transmission-blocking studies (Churcher et al. 2012; Miura et al. 2013a).

Such antibodies with transmission-blocking activity were then used to identify the parasite antigens they targeted, primarily revealing molecules of 25, 48/45, and 230 kDa (Rener et al. 1983). More recently, efforts have been made to exploit the sequencing of plasmodial genomes as well as transcriptional and proteomic analysis to identify sexual-stage proteins or mRNAs for such proteins found in these stages and the mosquito (Hall et al. 2005; Khan et al. 2005; Silvestrini et al. 2005; Young et al. 2005). These would be possible targets for antibodies or drugs targeting gametocytes.

Identification and Investigations of Pre- and Postfertilization Proteins

For convenience, immune responses to parasite antigens have been divided into prefertilization and postfertilization proteins (reviewed in Pradel 2007; Nikolaeva et al. 2015; Wu et al. 2015).

Prefertilization Antigens

Most studies have focused on a limited set of parasite proteins and considerable difficulties have been encountered in expressing many of them in recombinant platforms, particularly antigens such as Pfs230 and Pfs48/45, which are members of the 6-cysteine protein family. These proteins are characterized by repeating motifs of six conserved cysteine residues, which are coexpressed in gametocytes and have been implicated in the process of fertilization of male and female gametes. Interestingly, activity of antibodies to Pfs230 in the SMFA is enhanced by serum complement, which apparently retains some activity in the blood meal (Read et al. 1994). Although presenting difficulties in expression, inclusion of such proteins in a transmission-blocking vaccine has the potential for boosting by natural infection, which is not the case for proteins expressed only in the mosquito vector. In addition, although some polymorphism has been reported for these molecules, it is less than that of many asexual-stage antigens (Niederwieser et al. 2001). Similarly, evidence

Cite this article as *Cold Spring Harb Perspect Med* doi: 10.1101/cshperspect.a025577

has been presented that the *P. vivax* protein (Pvs230) can also elicit transmission-blocking activity (Tachibana et al. 2012).

Postfertilization Antigens

Because proteins such as Pfs25 and Pvs25 have limited or no expression in the vertebrate host, they are not subject to selection by the vertebrate immune system and consequently are generally quite conserved (Tsuboi et al. 1998). However, as noted, this limits the possibility of boosting of vaccine-induced immune responses by natural infection. The best studied of the postfertilization proteins is Pfs25 and to a lesser extent its homolog in *P. vivax* (Pvs25). Each is found on the surface of the ookinete and includes four epidermal growth factor (EGF)-like domains. Structural studies have revealed Pvs25 to be a flat triangular molecule that could tile the surface of ookinetes; residues forming the triangle are conserved in P25 molecules from all plasmodial species (Saxena et al. 2006). The report of anti-Pfs25 monoclonal antibodies and polyclonal antibodies, which have transmission-blocking activity in SMFA experiments have supported its candidacy as a potential transmission-blocking vaccine (Kaslow et al. 1988). Whether effector antibodies prevent ookinete crossing of the midgut or have other roles in reducing oocyst numbers is not yet clear. Further, estimates of specific antibody concentration required to attain 50% inhibition of oocyst density in the SMFA indicate that relatively high antibody concentrations, approximately 100 μg/ml, will be required (Cheru et al. 2010), and eliciting high, long-lasting antibody titers in humans remains a challenge.

Two recent studies have sought to compare immune responses to different transmission-blocking antigens using the SMFA (Miura et al. 2013c; Kapulu et al. 2015). In one study, proteins were produced in the wheat germ cell-free expression system and antibodies generated in mice. Detailed analysis of SMFA results showed that Pfs25 elicited IgGs with higher inhibition than anti-Pfs230 or anti-HAP2. This was the first demonstration that *P. falciparum* HAP2, a protein also involved in fertilization, could elicit antibodies with transmission-blocking activity. In the second study (Kapulu et al. 2015), viral vectors encoding parasite proteins were used to immunize mice and the resultant antibodies compared; both anti-Pfs230-C and anti-Pfs25 gave very high levels of blockade in the SMFA.

Other postfertilization proteins, some of which have been investigated as potential transmission-blocking vaccine candidates, include micronemal proteins of the ookinete, proteins found in the cytoplasmic crystalloid organelle, as well as the enzymes such as enolase and chitinase produced by the parasite (reviewed by Pradel 2007; Nikolaeva et al. 2015; Wu et al. 2015). Many of these proteins are likely to have important roles in exodus from the blood meal, attachment to the midgut wall, invasion of the midgut, protection of the parasite, and oocyst development but have not been well studied in terms of immune responses.

Host Immune Responses to Sexual-Stage Parasites

Host immune responses to gametocyte surface membranes have been examined in some individuals from malaria-endemic areas to explore the hypothesis that such natural immune responses could either reduce gametocyte sequestration, gametocyte density in vivo, or infectivity to mosquitoes (Bousema and Drakeley 2011). However, it has proven difficult to show recognition of stage-V-specific proteins on the surface of infected red cells. Some data have been presented that sera from African children recognize these cells by flow cytometry (Saeed et al. 2008); another study reported seroreactivity to gametocytes by IFA, which correlated with reduction of gametocyte density (Baird et al. 1991). Detailed investigation of the gametocyte surface at various stages of differentiation will be important future activities.

With regard to specific antigens present in gametes or zygotes, several studies have reported antibodies in those living in malaria-endemic areas to Pfs230 (Graves et al. 1988; Healer et al. 1999; Bousema et al. 2010; Miura et al. 2013c; Jones et al. 2015) and to Pfs48/45 (Roeffen et al. 1996; Bousema et al. 2010; Jones et al. 2015). Some of these responses have been correlated with transmission-reducing activity as measured by SMFA in the same sera. Evidence for the presence of antibodies to Pfs25 in human populations is inconsistent, perhaps depending on the methodology used (Riley et al. 1994; Miura et al. 2013c).

In addition to the immune responses of the vertebrate host, it is clear that the mosquito vector has an innate immune system, which can also affect the outcome of infection by plasmodia. Those responses are beyond the scope of this review but are discussed in Crompton et al. (2014).

FUTURE PERSPECTIVES

Overall, studies on antiparasite immune responses of the vertebrate host have identified a repertoire of potential immune effector mechanisms and a number of antigens as candidates for vaccine development. In the process these studies have also identified some of the many challenges that lie ahead.

The positive results obtained in the phase III trial of the RTS,S vaccine have established that a malaria vaccine is potentially feasible. Given these results, the next 5 years should see major efforts to develop a more advanced formulation, an effort that will require a more nuanced understanding of the interactions between the host and the infecting sporozoite. Characterizing the specificities and affinities of anti-CSP protective antibodies, identifying optimal immunization strategies, and addressing issues of allelic polymorphism in the CSP protein should contribute to improvements in the vaccine In addition, expanded efforts should be made to identify other important PE antigens and to develop methodologies that can elicit antigen-specific CD8$^+$ T cells in humans.

As discussed previously, the adoptive transfer of antibodies from individuals living in endemic areas drastically reduced parasitemia in *P. falciparum*–infected children. The antiparasite phenotype of naturally acquired immunity is clearly attributable to the inhibitory effect of antibodies on the progressive development of asexual stages. To date, vaccine studies with asexual stages have focused mostly on single antigens with a likely functional role in parasite replication. Although this may be a sensible approach, there is no evidence that protective immunity is restricted to the recognition of only a few antigens. In fact, it is possible that vaccines inducing broad, multiantigen immune responses may be more effective and long lasting. Also, although the prospect is daunting, we need to pursue efforts to identify conserved targets on the surface of the infected red cell. It is therefore urgent to develop extensive programs to design vaccines consisting of multiple antigens from different parasite stages. This is a major challenge as multispecific immune responses may not be easy to induce, as it is not uncommon to find antigen competition/interference when using combination vaccines. Moreover, it is not clear that there exist sensitive methodologies that can show the occurrence of additive or synergistic effects of the induced immune responses.

The extensive antigenic diversity in antigens from PE and asexual stages, which are currently studied for vaccine development is a significant hurdle. However, this should not be considered an insurmountable obstacle, as new biotechnological advances should make possible the development of multiallelic vaccine constructs. Finally, recent evidence indicating that individuals exposed to parasite infection undergo immune exhaustion and a possible inability to develop an efficient immunological memory is a matter of concern. It is unclear the extent to which these immune dysfunctions may impair the development of immune responses induced by vaccines or if it may decrease vaccine efficacy.

Resurgent interest in the sexual stages of parasites and in malaria transmission in the field has generated interest in the possibility of a transmission-blocking component of a multistage vaccine. Whether the current antigens identified or other parasite or mosquito antigens can elicit sufficiently high titers of antibodies in humans to affect transmission to the mosquito will be an important question to answer in the next 5 years. Also, we must seek vaccine formulations and expression platforms that generate longer lasting humoral immune responses, because responses to some transmission reducing parasite proteins may not be boosted by natural infection. Finally, issues of what level of responses in a population are required to reduce transmission in a given area and how to determine that level must be approached. Nevertheless, a component of a vaccine that could aid in reducing transmission below a critical threshold would be an important contribution to malaria vaccine development.

CONCLUDING REMARKS

Characterization of immune responses induced by natural exposure to parasites has facilitated the identification of mechanisms of immunity that provide partial protection, particularly for immune responses to asexual stages. These studies show that naturally acquired immune responses against asexual stages are effective against parasites and that these responses reduce morbidity, even though they do not cause full parasite clearance. In contrast, naturally acquired immune responses against PE and sexual stages are of low magnitude and there is no clear evidence that they have a protective effect or mediate clinical immunity. The interest in immune responses to PE and sexual stages and the antigens they recognize derives from experimental vaccine studies in animal models or in human trials in the case of attenuated sporozoites, which showed the development of sterilizing immunity. The challenge now is to transform these findings into a highly effective vaccine for malaria.

Considerable advances have been made in reducing malaria in many parts of the world over the past decade using existing tools. However, the logistics and financing required to retain and to expand these advances in the face of antimalarial drug resistance and declining efficacy of insecticides will be challenging. As we consider moving beyond the current situation into an era of malaria eradication, the development and deployment of a highly effective malaria vaccine is still a critically important but unrealized component in the portfolio of responses to this global challenge. Pursuing a more complete and detailed view of the immunologic interface between host and the various parasite stages should enhance the opportunities for developing such a vaccine.

ACKNOWLEDGMENTS

We gratefully acknowledge all the scientists and study volunteers over many decades who have contributed to our knowledge of immune responses in malaria. Many of these publications could not be included because of space limitations, and in some cases we have used reviews of various topics. C.A.L. acknowledges support from the Intramural Research Program of the National Institute of Allergy and Infectious Diseases, National Institutes of Health (NIH). F.Z. is supported by NIH/National Institute of Allergy and Infectious Diseases (NIAID) Grant R01 AI44375. We also thank Ms. Daria Nikolaeva for assistance with the sexual-stage references.

REFERENCES

*Reference is also in this collection.

Anum D, Kusi KA, Ganeshan H, Hollingdale MR, Ofori MF, Koram KA, Gyan BA, Adu-Amankwah S, Badji E, Huang J, et al. 2015. Measuring naturally acquired ex vivo IFN-γ responses to *Plasmodium falciparum* cell-traversal protein for ookinetes and sporozoites (CelTOS) in Ghanaian adults. *Malaria J* **14:** 20.

Ataide R, Mayor A, Rogerson SJ. 2014. Malaria, primigravidae, and antibodies: Knowledge gained and future perspectives. *Trends Parasitol* **30:** 85–94.

Baird JK, Jones TR, Purnomo, Masbar S, Ratiwayanto S, Leksana B. 1991. Evidence for specific suppression of gametocytemia by *Plasmodium falciparum* in residents of hyperendemic Irian Jaya. *Am J Trop Med Hyg* **44:** 183–190.

Beeson JG, Osier FH, Engwerda CR. 2008. Recent insights into humoral and cellular immune responses against malaria. *Trends Parasitol* **24:** 578–584.

Bergmann-Leitner ES, Mease RM, De La Vega P, Savranskaya T, Polhemus M, Ockenhouse C, Angov E. 2010. Immunization with pre-erythrocytic antigen CelTOS from *Plasmodium falciparum* elicits cross-species protection against heterologous challenge with *Plasmodium berghei*. *PLoS ONE* **5:** e12294.

Bongfen SE, Ntsama PM, Offner S, Smith T, Felger I, Tanner M, Alonso P, Nebie I, Romero JF, Silvie O, et al. 2009. The N-terminal domain of *Plasmodium falciparum* circumsporozoite protein represents a target of protective immunity. *Vaccine* **27:** 328–335.

Bouharoun-Tayoun H, Druilhe P. 1992. *Plasmodium falciparum* malaria: Evidence for an isotype imbalance which may be responsible for delayed acquisition of protective immunity. *Infect Immun* **60:** 1473–1481.

Bousema T, Drakeley C. 2011. Epidemiology and infectivity of *Plasmodium falciparum* and *Plasmodium vivax* gametocytes in relation to malaria control and elimination. *Clin Microbiol Rev* **24:** 377–410.

Bousema T, Roeffen W, Meijerink H, Mwerinde H, Mwakalinga S, van Gemert GJ, van de Vegte-Bolmer M, Mosha F, Targett G, Riley EM, et al. 2010. The dynamics of naturally acquired immune responses to *Plasmodium falciparum* sexual stage antigens Pfs230 and Pfs48/45 in a low endemic area in Tanzania. *PLoS ONE* **5:** e14114.

Bull PC, Lowe BS, Kortok M, Molyneux CS, Newbold CI, Marsh K. 1998. Parasite antigens on the infected red cell surface are targets for naturally acquired immunity to malaria. *Nat Med* **4:** 358–360.

Burns JM Jr, Majarian WR, Young JF, Daly TM, Long CA. 1989. A protective monoclonal antibody recognizes an epitope in the carboxyl-terminal cysteine-rich domain in the precursor of the major merozoite surface antigen of the rodent malarial parasite, *Plasmodium yoelii. J Immunol* **143:** 2670–2676.

Campbell GH, Collins FH, Brandling-Bennett AD, Schwartz IK, Roberts JM. 1987. Age-specific prevalence of antibody to a synthetic peptide of the circumsporozoite protein of *Plasmodium falciparum* in children from three villages in Kenya. *Am J Trop Med Hyg* **37:** 220–224.

Carlson J, Helmby H, Hill AV, Brewster D, Greenwood BM, Wahlgren M. 1990. Human cerebral malaria: Association with erythrocyte rosetting and lack of anti-rosetting antibodies. *Lancet* **336:** 1457–1460.

Carter R, Chen DH. 1976. Malaria transmission blocked by immunisation with gametes of the malaria parasite. *Nature* **263:** 57–60.

Chan JA, Howell KB, Reiling L, Ataide R, Mackintosh CL, Fowkes FJ, Petter M, Chesson JM, Langer C, Warimwe GM, et al. 2012. Targets of antibodies against *Plasmodium falciparum*–infected erythrocytes in malaria immunity. *J Clin Invest* **122:** 3227–3238.

Chan JA, Fowkes FJ, Beeson JG. 2014. Surface antigens of *Plasmodium falciparum*–infected erythrocytes as immune targets and malaria vaccine candidates. *Cell Mol Life Sci* **71:** 3633–3657.

Chen L, Lopaticki S, Riglar DT, Dekiwadia C, Uboldi AD, Tham WH, O'Neill MT, Richard D, Baum J, Ralph SA, et al. 2011. An EGF-like protein forms a complex with PfRh5 and is required for invasion of human erythrocytes by *Plasmodium falciparum. PLoS Pathog* **7:** e1002199.

Cheru L, Wu Y, Diouf A, Moretz SE, Muratova OV, Song G, Fay MP, Miller LH, Long CA, Miura K. 2010. The IC$_{50}$ of anti-Pfs25 antibody in membrane-feeding assay varies among species. *Vaccine* **28:** 4423–4429.

Churcher TS, Blagborough AM, Delves M, Ramakrishnan C, Kapulu MC, Williams AR, Biswas S, Da DF, Cohuet A, Sinden RE. 2012. Measuring the blockade of malaria transmission—An analysis of the standard membrane feeding assay. *Int J Parasitol* **42:** 1037–1044.

Cohen S, McGregor IA, Carrington S. 1961. γ-Globulin and acquired immunity to human malaria. *Nature* **192:** 733–737.

Coppi A, Natarajan R, Pradel G, Bennett BL, James ER, Roggero MA, Corradin G, Persson C, Tewari R, Sinnis P. 2011. The malaria circumsporozoite protein has two functional domains, each with distinct roles as sporozoites journey from mosquito to mammalian host. *J Exp Med* **208:** 341–356.

Crompton PD, Kayala MA, Traore B, Kayentao K, Ongoiba A, Weiss GE, Molina DM, Burk CR, Waisberg M, Jasinskas A, et al. 2010. A prospective analysis of the Ab response to *Plasmodium falciparum* before and after a malaria season by protein microarray. *Proc Natl Acad Sci* **107:** 6958–6963.

Crompton PD, Moebius J, Portugal S, Waisberg M, Hart G, Garver LS, Miller LH, Barillas-Mury C, Pierce SK. 2014. Malaria immunity in man and mosquito: Insights into unsolved mysteries of a deadly infectious disease. *Annu Rev Immunol* **32:** 157–187.

Crosnier C, Bustamante LY, Bartholdson SJ, Bei AK, Theron M, Uchikawa M, Mboup S, Ndir O, Kwiatkowski DP, Duraisingh MT, et al. 2011. Basigin is a receptor essential for erythrocyte invasion by *Plasmodium falciparum. Nature* **480:** 534–537.

Daly TM, Long CA. 1993. A recombinant 15-kilodalton carboxyl-terminal fragment of *Plasmodium yoelii yoelii* 17XL merozoite surface protein 1 induces a protective immune response in mice. *Infect Immun* **61:** 2462–2467.

Deans JA, Alderson T, Thomas AW, Mitchell GH, Lennox ES, Cohen S. 1982. Rat monoclonal antibodies which inhibit the in vitro multiplication of *Plasmodium knowlesi. Clin Exp Immunol* **49:** 297–309.

de Groot AS, Johnson AH, Maloy WL, Quakyi IA, Riley EM, Menon A, Banks SM, Berzofsky JA, Good MF. 1989. Human T cell recognition of polymorphic epitopes from malaria circumsporozoite protein. *J Immunol* **142:** 4000–4005.

Dolo A, Modiano D, Doumbo O, Bosman A, Sidibe T, Keita MM, Naitza S, Robson KJ, Crisanti A. 1999. Thrombospondin related adhesive protein (TRAP), a potential malaria vaccine candidate. *Parassitologia* **41:** 425–428.

Domarle O, Migot-Nabias F, Mvoukani JL, Lu CY, Nabias R, Mayombo J, Tiga H, Deloron P. 1999. Factors influencing resistance to reinfection with *Plasmodium falciparum. Am J Trop Med Hyg* **61:** 926–931.

Doolan DL, Houghten RA, Good MF. 1991. Location of human cytotoxic T cell epitopes within a polymorphic domain of the *Plasmodium falciparum* circumsporozoite protein. *Int Immunol* **3:** 511–516.

Doolan DL, Khamboonruang C, Beck HP, Houghten RA, Good MF. 1993. Cytotoxic T lymphocyte (CTL) low-responsiveness to the *Plasmodium falciparum* circumsporozoite protein in naturally-exposed endemic populations: Analysis of human CTL response to most known variants. *Int Immunol* **5:** 37–46.

Doolan DL, Hedstrom RC, Rogers WO, Charoenvit Y, Rogers M, de la Vega P, Hoffman SL. 1996. Identification and characterization of the protective hepatocyte erythrocyte protein 17 kDa gene of *Plasmodium yoelii*, homolog of *Plasmodium falciparum* exported protein 1. *J Biol Chem* **271:** 17861–17868.

Doolan DL, Mu Y, Unal B, Sundaresh S, Hirst S, Valdez C, Randall A, Molina D, Liang X, Freilich DA, et al. 2008. Profiling humoral immune responses to *P. falciparum* infection with protein microarrays. *Proteomics* **8**: 4680–4694.

Douglas AD, Williams AR, Illingworth JJ, Kamuyu G, Biswas S, Goodman AL, Wyllie DH, Crosnier C, Miura K, Wright GJ, et al. 2011. The blood-stage malaria antigen PfRH5 is susceptible to vaccine-inducible cross-strain neutralizing antibody. *Nat Commun* **2**: 601.

Douglas AD, Williams AR, Knuepfer E, Illingworth JJ, Furze JM, Crosnier C, Choudhary P, Bustamante LY, Zakutansky SE, Awuah DK, et al. 2014. Neutralization of *Plasmodium falciparum* merozoites by antibodies against PfRH5. *J Immunol* **192**: 245–258.

Douglas AD, Baldeviano GC, Lucas CM, Lugo-Roman LA, Crosnier C, Bartholdson SJ, Diouf A, Miura K, Lambert LE, Ventocilla JA, et al. 2015. A PfRH5-based vaccine is efficacious against heterologous strain blood-stage *Plasmodium falciparum* infection in aotus monkeys. *Cell Host Microbe* **17**: 130–139.

Druilhe P, Pradier O, Marc JP, Miltgen F, Mazier D, Parent G. 1986. Levels of antibodies to *Plasmodium falciparum* sporozoite surface antigens reflect malaria transmission rates and are persistent in the absence of reinfection. *Infect Immun* **53**: 393–397.

Dutta S, Dlugosz LS, Drew DR, Ge X, Ababacar D, Rovira YI, Moch JK, Shi M, Long CA, Foley M, et al. 2013. Overcoming antigenic diversity by enhancing the immunogenicity of conserved epitopes on the malaria vaccine candidate apical membrane antigen-1. *PLoS Pathog* **9**: e1003840.

Espinosa DA, Gutierrez GM, Rojas-Lopez M, Noe AR, Shi L, Tse SW, Sinnis P, Zavala F. 2015. Proteolytic cleavage of the *Plasmodium falciparum* circumsporozoite protein is a target of protective antibodies. *J Infect Dis* **212**: 1111–1119.

Esposito F, Lombardi S, Modiano D, Zavala F, Reeme J, Lamizana L, Coluzzi M, Nussenzweig RS. 1988. Prevalence and levels of antibodies to the circumsporozoite protein of *Plasmodium falciparum* in an endemic area and their relationship to resistance against malaria infection. *Trans R Soc Trop Med Hyg* **82**: 827–832.

Esposito F, Lombardi S, Modiano D, Habluetzel A, Del Nero L, Lamizana L, Pietra V, Rotigliano G, Corradin G, Ravot E, et al. 1992. In vitro immune recognition of synthetic peptides from the *Plasmodium falciparum* CS protein by individuals naturally exposed to different sporozoite challenge. *Immunol Lett* **33**: 187–199.

Ewer KJ, O'Hara GA, Duncan CJ, Collins KA, Sheehy SH, Reyes-Sandoval A, Goodman AL, Edwards NJ, Elias SC, Halstead FD, et al. 2013. Protective CD8$^+$ T-cell immunity to human malaria induced by chimpanzee adenovirus-MVA immunisation. *Nat Commun* **4**: 2836.

Fidock DA, Gras-Masse H, Lepers JP, Brahimi K, Benmohamed L, Mellouk S, Guerin-Marchand C, Londono A, Raharimalala L, Meis JF, et al. 1994. *Plasmodium falciparum* liver stage antigen-1 is well conserved and contains potent B and T cell determinants. *J Immunol* **153**: 190–204.

Flanagan KL, Mwangi T, Plebanski M, Odhiambo K, Ross A, Sheu E, Kortok M, Lowe B, Marsh K, Hill AV. 2003. Ex vivo interferon-γ immune response to thrombospondin-related adhesive protein in coastal Kenyans: Longevity

and risk of *Plasmodium falciparum* infection. *Am J Trop Med Hyg* **68**: 421–430.

Fowkes FJ, Richards JS, Simpson JA, Beeson JG. 2010. The relationship between anti-merozoite antibodies and incidence of *Plasmodium falciparum* malaria: A systematic review and meta-analysis. *PLoS Med* **7**: e1000218.

* Fried M, Duffy PE. 2016. Malaria during pregnancy. *Cold Spring Harb Perspect Med* doi: 10.1101/cshperspect. a025551.

Gazzinelli RT, Kalantari P, Fitzgerald KA, Golenbock DT. 2014. Innate sensing of malaria parasites. *Nat Rev Immunol* **14**: 744–757.

Goel S, Palmkvist M, Moll K, Joannin N, Lara P, Akhouri RR, Moradi N, Ojemalm K, Westman M, Angeletti D, et al. 2015. RIFINs are adhesins implicated in severe *Plasmodium falciparum* malaria. *Nat Med* **21**: 314–317.

Good MF, Pombo D, Quakyi IA, Riley EM, Houghten RA, Menon A, Alling DW, Berzofsky JA, Miller LH. 1988. Human T-cell recognition of the circumsporozoite protein of *Plasmodium falciparum*: Immunodominant T-cell domains map to the polymorphic regions of the molecule. *Proc Natl Acad Sci* **85**: 1199–1203.

Graves PM, Carter R, Burkot TR, Quakyi IA, Kumar N. 1988. Antibodies to *Plasmodium falciparum* gamete surface antigens in Papua New Guinea sera. *Parasite Immunol* **10**: 209–218.

Gray JC, Corran PH, Mangia E, Gaunt MW, Li Q, Tetteh KK, Polley SD, Conway DJ, Holder AA, Bacarese-Hamilton T, et al. 2007. Profiling the antibody immune response against blood stage malaria vaccine candidates. *Clin Chem* **53**: 1244–1253.

Guerin-Marchand C, Druilhe P, Galey B, Londono A, Patarapotikul J, Beaudoin RL, Dubeaux C, Tartar A, Mercereau-Puijalon O, Langsley G. 1987. A liver-stage-specific antigen of *Plasmodium falciparum* characterized by gene cloning. *Nature* **329**: 164–167.

Gwadz RW. 1976. Successful immunization against the sexual stages of *Plasmodium gallinaceum*. *Science* **193**: 1150–1151.

Gwadz RW, Green I. 1978. Malaria immunization in Rhesus monkeys. A vaccine effective against both the sexual and asexual stages of *Plasmodium knowlesi*. *J Exp Med* **148**: 1311–1323.

Hall N, Karras M, Raine JD, Carlton JM, Kooij TW, Berriman M, Florens L, Janssen CS, Pain A, Christophides GK, et al. 2005. A comprehensive survey of the *Plasmodium* life cycle by genomic, transcriptomic, and proteomic analyses. *Science* **307**: 82–86.

Healer J, McGuinness D, Carter R, Riley E. 1999. Transmission-blocking immunity to *Plasmodium falciparum* in malaria-immune individuals is associated with antibodies to the gamete surface protein Pfs230. *Parasitology* **119**: 425–433.

* Healer J, Cowman AF, Kaslow DC, Birkett AJ. 2016. Vaccines to accelerate malaria elimination and eventual eradication. *Cold Spring Harb Perspect Med* doi: 10.1101/ cshperspect.a025627.

Herrington D, Davis J, Nardin E, Beier M, Cortese J, Eddy H, Losonsky G, Hollingdale M, Sztein M, Levine M, et al. 1991. Successful immunization of humans with irradiated malaria sporozoites: Humoral and cellular responses of the protected individuals. *Am J Trop Med Hyg* **45:** 539–547.

Hoffman SL, Wistar R Jr, Ballou WR, Hollingdale MR, Wirtz RA, Schneider I, Marwoto HA, Hockmeyer WT. 1986. Immunity to malaria and naturally acquired antibodies to the circumsporozoite protein of *Plasmodium falciparum*. *N Engl J Med* **315:** 601–606.

Hollingdale MR, Nardin EH, Tharavanij S, Schwartz AL, Nussenzweig RS. 1984. Inhibition of entry of *Plasmodium falciparum* and *P. vivax* sporozoites into cultured cells; An in vitro assay of protective antibodies. *J Immunol* **132:** 909–913.

Hollingdale MR, Hogh B, Petersen E, Wirtz RA, Bjorkmann A. 1989. Age-dependent occurrence of protective anti-*Plasmodium falciparum* sporozoite antibodies in a holoendemic area of Liberia. *Trans R Soc Trop Med Hyg* **83:** 322–324.

Huff CG, Marchbank DF, Shiroishi T. 1958. Changes in infectiousness of malarial gametocytes. II: Analysis of the possible causative factors. *Exp Parasitol* **7:** 399–417.

Hviid L, Jensen AT. 2015. PfEMP1—A parasite protein family of key importance in *Plasmodium falciparum* malaria immunity and pathogenesis. *Adv Parasitol* **88:** 51–84.

Hviid L, Barfod L, Fowkes FJ. 2015. Trying to remember: Immunological B cell memory to malaria. *Trends Parasitol* **31:** 89–94.

John CC, Zickafoose JS, Sumba PO, King CL, Kazura JW. 2003. Antibodies to the *Plasmodium falciparum* antigens circumsporozoite protein, thrombospondin-related adhesive protein, and liver-stage antigen 1 vary by ages of subjects and by season in a highland area of Kenya. *Infect Immun* **71:** 4320–4325.

John CC, Moormann AM, Pregibon DC, Sumba PO, McHugh MM, Narum DL, Lanar DE, Schluchter MD, Kazura JW. 2005. Correlation of high levels of antibodies to multiple pre-erythrocytic *Plasmodium falciparum* antigens and protection from infection. *Am J Trop Med Hyg* **73:** 222–228.

John CC, Tande AJ, Moormann AM, Sumba PO, Lanar DE, Min XM, Kazura JW. 2008. Antibodies to pre-erythrocytic *Plasmodium falciparum* antigens and risk of clinical malaria in Kenyan children. *J Infect Dis* **197:** 519–526.

Jones S, Grignard L, Nebie I, Chilongola J, Dodoo D, Sauerwein R, Theisen M, Roeffen W, Singh SK, Singh RK, et al. 2015. Naturally acquired antibody responses to recombinant Pfs230 and Pfs48/45 transmission blocking vaccine candidates. *J Infect* **71:** 117–127.

Kapulu MC, Da DF, Miura K, Li Y, Blagborough AM, Churcher TS, Nikolaeva D, Williams AR, Goodman AL, Sangare I, et al. 2015. Comparative assessment of transmission-blocking vaccine candidates against *Plasmodium falciparum*. *Sci Rep* **5:** 11193.

Kariu T, Ishino T, Yano K, Chinzei Y, Yuda M. 2006. CelTOS, a novel malarial protein that mediates transmission to mosquito and vertebrate hosts. *Mol Microbiol* **59:** 1369–1379.

Kaslow DC, Quakyi IA, Syin C, Raum MG, Keister DB, Coligan JE, McCutchan TF, Miller LH. 1988. A vaccine candidate from the sexual stage of human malaria that contains EGF-like domains. *Nature* **333:** 74–76.

Kaushal DC, Carter R, Rener J, Grotendorst CA, Miller LH, Howard RJ. 1983. Monoclonal antibodies against surface

determinants on gametes of *Plasmodium gallinaceum* block transmission of malaria parasites to mosquitoes. *J Immunol* **131:** 2557–2562.

Khan SM, Franke-Fayard B, Mair GR, Lasonder E, Janse CJ, Mann M, Waters AP. 2005. Proteome analysis of separated male and female gametocytes reveals novel sex-specific *Plasmodium* biology. *Cell* **121:** 675–687.

Kurtis JD, Hollingdale MR, Luty AJ, Lanar DE, Krzych U, Duffy PE. 2001. Pre-erythrocytic immunity to *Plasmodium falciparum*: The case for an LSA-1 vaccine. *Trends Parasitol* **17:** 219–223.

Lamarque M, Besteiro S, Papoin J, Roques M, Vulliez-Le Normand B, Morlon-Guyot J, Dubremetz JF, Fauquenoy S, Tomavo S, Faber BW, et al. 2011. The RON2-AMA1 interaction is a critical step in moving junction-dependent invasion by apicomplexan parasites. *PLoS Pathog* **7:** e1001276.

Langhorne J, Ndungu FM, Sponaas AM, Marsh K. 2008. Immunity to malaria: More questions than answers. *Nat Immunol* **9:** 725–732.

Mackintosh CL, Mwangi T, Kinyanjui SM, Mosobo M, Pinches R, Williams TN, Newbold CI, Marsh K. 2008. Failure to respond to the surface of *Plasmodium falciparum* infected erythrocytes predicts susceptibility to clinical malaria amongst African children. *Int J Parasitol* **38:** 1445–1454.

Majarian WR, Daly TM, Weidanz WP, Long CA. 1984. Passive immunization against murine malaria with an IgG3 monoclonal antibody. *J Immunol* **132:** 3131–3137.

Marsh K, Kinyanjui S. 2006. Immune effector mechanisms in malaria. *Parasite Immunol* **28:** 51–60.

Marsh K, Hayes RH, Carson DC, Otoo L, Shenton F, Byass P, Zavala F, Greenwood BM. 1988. Anti-sporozoite antibodies and immunity to malaria in a rural Gambian population. *Trans R Soc Trop Med Hyg* **82:** 532–537.

Mellouk S, Mazier D, Druilhe P, Berbiguier N, Danis M. 1986. In vitro and in vivo results suggesting that anti-sporozoite antibodies do not totally block *Plasmodium falciparum* sporozoite infectivity. *N Engl J Med* **315:** 648.

Mendis KN, Targett GA. 1979. Immunisation against gametes and asexual erythrocytic stages of a rodent malaria parasite. *Nature* **277:** 389–391.

* Milner DA. 2016. Malaria pathogenesis. *Cold Spring Harb Perspect Med* doi: 10.1101/cshperspect.a025569.

* Mitchell SN, Catteruccia F. 2016. Anopheline reproductive biology: Impacts on vectorial capacity and potential avenues for malaria control. *Cold Spring Harb Perspect Med* doi: 10.1101/cshperspect.a025593.

Miura K, Deng B, Tullo G, Diouf A, Moretz SE, Locke E, Morin M, Fay MP, Long CA. 2013a. Qualification of standard membrane-feeding assay with *Plasmodium falciparum* malaria and potential improvements for future assays. *PLoS ONE* **8:** e57909.

Miura K, Herrera R, Diouf A, Zhou H, Mu J, Hu Z, MacDonald NJ, Reiter K, Nguyen V, Shimp RL Jr, et al. 2013b. Overcoming allelic specificity by immunization with five allelic forms of *Plasmodium falciparum* apical membrane antigen 1. *Infect Immun* **81:** 1491–1501.

Miura K, Takashima E, Deng B, Tullo G, Diouf A, Moretz SE, Nikolaeva D, Diakite M, Fairhurst RM, Fay MP, et al. 2013c. Functional comparison of *Plasmodium falciparum* transmission-blocking vaccine candidates by the standard membrane-feeding assay. *Infect Immun* **81:** 4377–4382.

Nardin EH, Nussenzweig RS, McGregor IA, Bryan JH. 1979. Antibodies to sporozoites: Their frequent occurrence in individuals living in an area of hyperendemic malaria. *Science* **206:** 597–599.

Niang M, Bei AK, Madnani KG, Pelly S, Dankwa S, Kanjee U, Gunalan K, Amaladoss A, Yeo KP, Bob NS, et al. 2014. STEVOR is a *Plasmodium falciparum* erythrocyte binding protein that mediates merozoite invasion and rosetting. *Cell Host Microbe* **16:** 81–93.

Niederwieser I, Felger I, Beck HP. 2001. Limited polymorphism in *Plasmodium falciparum* sexual-stage antigens. *Am J Trop Med Hyg* **64:** 9–11.

Nikolaeva D, Draper SJ, Biswas S. 2015. Toward the development of effective transmission-blocking vaccines for malaria. *Expert Rev Vaccines* **14:** 653–680.

Nilsson SK, Childs LM, Buckee C, Marti M. 2015. Targeting human transmission biology for malaria elimination. *PLoS Pathog* **11:** e1004871.

Nussenzweig V, Nussenzweig RS. 1989. Rationale for the development of an engineered sporozoite malaria vaccine. *Adv Immunol* **45:** 283–334.

Nussenzweig RS, Vanderberg J, Most H, Orton C. 1967. Protective immunity produced by the injection of x-irradiated sporozoites of *Plasmodium berghei*. *Nature* **216:** 160–162.

Ogutu BR, Apollo OJ, McKinney D, Okoth W, Siangla J, Dubovsky F, Tucker K, Waitumbi JN, Diggs C, Wittes J, et al. 2009. Blood stage malaria vaccine eliciting high antigen-specific antibody concentrations confers no protection to young children in Western Kenya. *PLoS ONE* **4:** e4708.

Ong'echa JM, Lal AA, Terlouw DJ, Ter Kuile FO, Kariuki SK, Udhayakumar V, Orago AS, Hightower AW, Nahlen BL, Shi YP. 2003. Association of interferon-γ responses to pre-erythrocytic stage vaccine candidate antigens of *Plasmodium falciparum* in young Kenyan children with improved hemoglobin levels. XV: Asembo Bay Cohort Project. *Am J Trop Med Hyg* **68:** 590–597.

Osier FH, Fegan G, Polley SD, Murungi L, Verra F, Tetteh KK, Lowe B, Mwangi T, Bull PC, Thomas AW, et al. 2008. Breadth and magnitude of antibody responses to multiple *Plasmodium falciparum* merozoite antigens are associated with protection from clinical malaria. *Infect Immun* **76:** 2240–2248.

Persson C, Oliveira GA, Sultan AA, Bhanot P, Nussenzweig V, Nardin E. 2002. Cutting edge: A new tool to evaluate human pre-erythrocytic malaria vaccines: Rodent parasites bearing a hybrid *Plasmodium falciparum* circumsporozoite protein. *J Immunol* **169:** 6681–6685.

Portugal S, Pierce SK, Crompton PD. 2013. Young lives lost as B cells falter: What we are learning about antibody responses in malaria. *J Immunol* **190:** 3039–3046.

Pradel G. 2007. Proteins of the malaria parasite sexual stages: Expression, function and potential for transmission blocking strategies. *Parasitology* **134:** 1911–1929.

Read D, Lensen AH, Begarnie S, Haley S, Raza A, Carter R. 1994. Transmission-blocking antibodies against multiple, non-variant target epitopes of the *Plasmodium fal-*

ciparum gamete surface antigen Pfs230 are all complement-fixing. *Parasite Immunol* **16:** 511–519.

Reddy KS, Amlabu E, Pandey AK, Mitra P, Chauhan VS, Gaur D. 2015. Multiprotein complex between the GPI-anchored CyRPA with PfRH5 and PfRipr is crucial for *Plasmodium falciparum* erythrocyte invasion. *Proc Natl Acad Sci* **112:** 1179–1184.

Remarque EJ, Faber BW, Kocken CH, Thomas AW. 2008. Apical membrane antigen 1: A malaria vaccine candidate in review. *Trends Parasitol* **24:** 74–84.

Rener J, Graves PM, Carter R, Williams JL, Burkot TR. 1983. Target antigens of transmission-blocking immunity on gametes of *Plasmodium falciparum*. *J Exp Med* **158:** 976–981.

Rieckmann KH, Beaudoin RL, Cassells JS, Sell KW. 1979. Use of attenuated sporozoites in the immunization of human volunteers against falciparum malaria. *Bull World Health Organ* **57:** 261–265.

Riley EM, Allen SJ, Bennett S, Thomas PJ, O'Donnell A, Lindsay SW, Good MF, Greenwood BM. 1990. Recognition of dominant T cell-stimulating epitopes from the circumsporozoite protein of *Plasmodium falciparum* and relationship to malaria morbidity in Gambian children. *Trans R Soc Trop Med Hyg* **84:** 648–657.

Riley EM, Bennett S, Jepson A, Hassan-King M, Whittle H, Olerup O, Carter R. 1994. Human antibody responses to Pfs 230, a sexual stage-specific surface antigen of *Plasmodium falciparum*: Non-responsiveness is a stable phenotype but does not appear to be genetically regulated. *Parasite Immunol* **16:** 55–62.

Robson KJ, Hall JR, Jennings MW, Harris TJ, Marsh K, Newbold CI, Tate VE, Weatherall DJ. 1988. A highly conserved amino-acid sequence in thrombospondin, properdin and in proteins from sporozoites and blood stages of a human malaria parasite. *Nature* **335:** 79–82.

Roeffen W, Mulder B, Teelen K, Bolmer M, Eling W, Targett GA, Beckers PJ, Sauerwein R. 1996. Association between anti-Pfs48/45 reactivity and *P. falciparum* transmission-blocking activity in sera from Cameroon. *Parasite Immunol* **18:** 103–109.

Rogers WO, Malik A, Mellouk S, Nakamura K, Rogers MD, Szarfman A, Gordon DM, Nussler AK, Aikawa M, Hoffman SL. 1992. Characterization of *Plasmodium falciparum* sporozoite surface protein 2. *Proc Natl Acad Sci* **89:** 9176–9180.

Sabchareon A, Burnouf T, Ouattara D, Attanath P, Bouharoun-Tayoun H, Chantavanich P, Foucault C, Chongsuphajaisiddhi T, Druilhe P. 1991. Parasitologic and clinical human response to immunoglobulin administration in falciparum malaria. *Am J Trop Med Hyg* **45:** 297–308.

Saeed M, Roeffen W, Alexander N, Drakeley CJ, Targett GA, Sutherland CJ. 2008. *Plasmodium falciparum* antigens on the surface of the gametocyte-infected erythrocyte. *PLoS ONE* **3:** e2280.

Sagara I, Dicko A, Ellis RD, Fay MP, Diawara SI, Assadou MH, Sissoko MS, Kone M, Diallo AI, Saye R, et al. 2009. A randomized controlled phase 2 trial of the blood stage AMA1-C1/Alhydrogel malaria vaccine in children in Mali. *Vaccine* **27:** 3090–3098.

Saxena AK, Singh K, Su HP, Klein MM, Stowers AW, Saul AJ, Long CA, Garboczi DN. 2006. The essential mosquito-stage P25 and P28 proteins from *Plasmodium* form tile-like triangular prisms. *Nat Struct Mol Biol* **13**: 90–91.

Scarselli E, Tolle R, Koita O, Diallo M, Muller HM, Fruh K, Doumbo O, Crisanti A, Bujard H. 1993. Analysis of the human antibody response to thrombospondin-related anonymous protein of *Plasmodium falciparum*. *Infect Immun* **61**: 3490–3495.

Scholzen A, Sauerwein RW. 2013. How malaria modulates memory: Activation and dysregulation of B cells in *Plasmodium* infection. *Trends Parasitol* **29**: 252–262.

Seder RA, Chang LJ, Enama ME, Zephir KL, Sarwar UN, Gordon IJ, Holman LA, James ER, Billingsley PF, Gunasekera A, et al. 2013. Protection against malaria by intravenous immunization with a nonreplicating sporozoite vaccine. *Science* **341**: 1359–1365.

Silvestrini F, Bozdech Z, Lanfrancotti A, Di Giulio E, Bultrini E, Picci L, Derisi JL, Pizzi E, Alano P. 2005. Genome-wide identification of genes upregulated at the onset of gametocytogenesis in *Plasmodium falciparum*. *Mol Biochem Parasitol* **143**: 100–110.

Sinden RE. 2010. A biologist's perspective on malaria vaccine development. *Hum Vaccin* **6**: 3–11.

Smith JD. 2014. The role of PfEMP1 adhesion domain classification in *Plasmodium falciparum* pathogenesis research. *Mol Biochem Parasitol* **195**: 82–87.

Srinivasan P, Ekanem E, Diouf A, Tonkin ML, Miura K, Boulanger MJ, Long CA, Narum DL, Miller LH. 2014. Immunization with a functional protein complex required for erythrocyte invasion protects against lethal malaria. *Proc Natl Acad Sci* **111**: 10311–10316.

Stewart MJ, Nawrot RJ, Schulman S, Vanderberg JP. 1986. *Plasmodium berghei* sporozoite invasion is blocked in vitro by sporozoite-immobilizing antibodies. *Infect Immun* **51**: 859–864.

Stowers A, Carter R. 2001. Current developments in malaria transmission-blocking vaccines. *Expert Opin Biol Ther* **1**: 619–628.

Stowers AW, Cioce V, Shimp RL, Lawson M, Hui G, Muratova O, Kaslow DC, Robinson R, Long CA, Miller LH. 2001. Efficacy of two alternate vaccines based on *Plasmodium falciparum* merozoite surface protein 1 in an Aotus challenge trial. *Infect Immun* **69**: 1536–1546.

Stowers AW, Kennedy MC, Keegan BP, Saul A, Long CA, Miller LH. 2002. Vaccination of monkeys with recombinant *Plasmodium falciparum* apical membrane antigen 1 confers protection against blood-stage malaria. *Infect Immun* **70**: 6961–6967.

Sutherland CJ. 2009. Surface antigens of *Plasmodium falciparum* gametocytes—A new class of transmission-blocking vaccine targets? *Mol Biochem Parasitol* **166**: 93–98.

Tachibana M, Sato C, Otsuki H, Sattabongkot J, Kaneko O, Torii M, Tsuboi T. 2012. *Plasmodium vivax* gametocyte protein Pvs230 is a transmission-blocking vaccine candidate. *Vaccine* **30**: 1807–1812.

Tapchaisri P, Chomcharn Y, Poonthong C, Asavanich A, Limsuwan S, Maleevan O, Tharavanij S, Harinasuta T. 1983. Anti-sporozoite antibodies induced by natural infection. *Am J Trop Med Hyg* **32**: 1203–1208.

Terheggen U, Drew DR, Hodder AN, Cross NJ, Mugyenyi CK, Barry AE, Anders RF, Dutta S, Osier FH, Elliott SR, et al. 2014. Limited antigenic diversity of *Plasmodium fal-*

ciparum apical membrane antigen 1 supports the development of effective multi-allele vaccines. *BMC Med* **12**: 183.

Tham WH, Healer J, Cowman AF. 2012. Erythrocyte and reticulocyte binding-like proteins of *Plasmodium falciparum*. *Trends Parasitol* **28**: 23–30.

Thera MA, Doumbo OK, Coulibaly D, Laurens MB, Ouattara A, Kone AK, Guindo AB, Traore K, Traore I, Kouriba B, et al. 2011. A field trial to assess a blood-stage malaria vaccine. *N Engl J Med* **365**: 1004–1013.

Thomas AW, Waters AP, Carr D. 1990. Analysis of variation in PF83, an erythrocytic merozoite vaccine candidate antigen of *Plasmodium falciparum*. *Mol Biochem Parasitol* **42**: 285–287.

Tran TM, Ongoiba A, Coursen J, Crosnier C, Diouf A, Huang CY, Li S, Doumbo S, Doumtabe D, Kone Y, et al. 2014. Naturally acquired antibodies specific for *Plasmodium falciparum* reticulocyte-binding protein homologue 5 inhibit parasite growth and predict protection from malaria. *J Infect Dis* **209**: 789–798.

Tsuboi T, Kaslow DC, Gozar MM, Tachibana M, Cao YM, Torii M. 1998. Sequence polymorphism in two novel *Plasmodium vivax* ookinete surface proteins, Pvs25 and Pvs28, that are malaria transmission-blocking vaccine candidates. *Mol Med* **4**: 772–782.

Tsuji M, Zavala F. 2003. T cells as mediators of protective immunity against liver stages of *Plasmodium*. *Trends Parasitol* **19**: 88–93.

Weiss GE, Crompton PD, Li S, Walsh LA, Moir S, Traore B, Kayentao K, Ongoiba A, Doumbo OK, Pierce SK. 2009. Atypical memory B cells are greatly expanded in individuals living in a malaria-endemic area. *J Immunol* **183**: 2176–2182.

Wright GJ, Rayner JC. 2014. *Plasmodium falciparum* erythrocyte invasion: Combining function with immune evasion. *PLoS Pathog* **10**: e1003943.

Wu Y, Sinden RE, Churcher TS, Tsuboi T, Yusibov V. 2015. Development of malaria transmission-blocking vaccines: From concept to product. *Adv Parasitol* **89**: 109–152.

Young JA, Fivelman QL, Blair PL, de la Vega P, Le Roch KG, Zhou Y, Carucci DJ, Baker DA, Winzeler EA. 2005. The *Plasmodium falciparum* sexual development transcriptome: A microarray analysis using ontology-based pattern identification. *Mol Biochem Parasitol* **143**: 67–79.

Zavala F, Masuda A, Graves PM, Nussenzweig V, Nussenzweig RS. 1985a. Ubiquity of the repetitive epitope of the CS protein in different isolates of human malaria parasites. *J Immunol* **135**: 2790–2793.

Zavala F, Tam JP, Hollingdale MR, Cochrane AH, Quakyi I, Nussenzweig RS, Nussenzweig V. 1985b. Rationale for development of a synthetic vaccine against *Plasmodium falciparum* malaria. *Science* **228**: 1436–1440.

Zevering Y, Khamboonruang C, Rungruengthanakit K, Tungviboonchai L, Ruengpipattanapan J, Bathurst I, Barr P, Good MF. 1994. Life-spans of human T-cell responses to determinants from the circumsporozoite proteins of *Plasmodium falciparum* and *Plasmodium vivax*. *Proc Natl Acad Sci* **91**: 6118–6122.

Zhu J, Hollingdale MR. 1991. Structure of *Plasmodium falciparum* liver stage antigen-1. *Mol Biochem Parasitol* **48**: 223–226.

Cite this article as *Cold Spring Harb Perspect Med* doi: 10.1101/cshperspect.a025577

Malaria Pathogenesis

Danny A. Milner, Jr.

Harvard T.H. Chan School of Public Health, American Society for Clinical Pathology, Center for Global Health, Chicago, Illinois 60603

Correspondence: dmilner@ascp.org

In the mosquito–human life cycle, the six species of malaria parasites infecting humans (*Plasmodium falciparum, Plasmodium vivax, Plasmodium ovale wallickeri, Plasmodium ovale curtisi, Plasmodium malariae*, and *Plasmodium knowlesi*) undergo 10 or more morphological states, replicate from single to 10,000+ cells, and vary in total population from one to many more than 10^6 organisms. In the human host, only a small number of these morphological stages lead to clinical disease and the vast majority of all malaria-infected patients in the world produce few (if any) symptoms in the human. Human clinical disease (e.g., fever, anemia, coma) is the result of the parasite preprogrammed biology in concert with the human pathophysiological response. Caveats and corollaries that add variation to this host–parasite interaction include parasite genetic diversity of key proteins, coinfections, comorbidities, delays in treatment, human polymorphisms, and environmental determinants.

Pathogenesis, the manner of development of a disease, for a human malaria clinical illness is a complex story that has many players, settings, and potential outcomes. As with any truly successful parasite, the observed outcome of evolution in malaria is the undisturbed transition from mosquito to human to mosquito with little impact on the vector and host. Although impact of malaria can be seen at the individual, community, country, and global level, from the parasite's perspective, a healthy host serving as two blood meals with a bit of fever in between is the norm. In fact, human clinical disease is quite rare relative to the global interaction network of mosquitoes and humans.

The biology of *Plasmodium falciparum* malaria parasites, as measured in vitro, is finite, predictable, and easily experimentally perturbed during the 48-hour life cycle (Bozdech et al. 2003a,b; Llinas and DeRisi 2004). In the mosquito–human life cycle, however, this parasite, along with the other five species infecting humans (*Plasmodium vivax, Plasmodium ovale wallickeri, Plasmodium ovale curtisi, Plasmodium malariae*, and *Plasmodium knowlesi*), undergoes 10 or more morphological states, replicate from a single to 10,000+ cells, and vary in total population from one to many more than 10^6 organisms (Liu et al. 2011; Cator et al. 2012; Dixon et al. 2012; Mohandas and An 2012; Antinori et al. 2013; Wright and Rayner 2014; Cui et al. 2015; Josling and Llinas 2015; Stone et al. 2015). In addition, all of these parasites (with the exception of *P. knowlesi* in humans) have been exposed for thousands of millennia to the physical, immunological, and more recently chemotherapeutic barriers in mosquitoes and humans, which places tremendous selection pressure across the species (Sabeti et al. 2002; Volkman et al. 2007; Bañuls et al. 2013; Perry 2014). It is clearly a finely tuned, well-rehearsed, and deftly executed program.

A similar selection pressure has been placed on humans and resulted in such fascinating evolutionary outcomes as sickle cell disease, hemoglobinopathies, cytokine mutations, and enzyme deficiency, which confer, as a conceptual group, the ability to survive to maturity and reproduction (Bañuls et al. 2013; Perry 2014). Death from malaria at an age less than 6 years (the current most common demographic) cannot be a goal of the parasite (speaking teleologically) and, thus, its occurrence should be cause for concern and investigation. However, the rarity of this event (438,000 out of 214,000,000 clinical cases or ~0.2%) leaves the unfortunate mortality as an aberrant footnote in the overall biology of the species as a whole (WHO 2015). We should not, however, accept even one death from a preventable and treatable disease.

When we turn to the parasite inside the human host, only a small number of these morphological stages lead to clinical disease and the vast majority of all malaria-infected patients in the world produce few (if any) symptoms in the human (WHO 2015). This is a crucial point of the biology that is often missed or ignored by experimentalists and "single-mechanism" focused scientists. Every person who is infected with malaria (regardless of whether or not they show symptoms) has the parasite go through the exact same life-cycle morphological changes and human–parasite interactions. Disease, thus, must be the result of exaggeration of this baseline interaction, which, as mentioned, is beneficial to neither the parasite nor the human. Further evidence for this lies, obviously, within the overall rarity of such events. Moreover, there are relatively few physiological states the parasite can achieve inside the human host—all of this biology is accomplished with a meager 6000 genes, most of which have no known function (Bozdech et al. 2003a,b; Daily et al. 2007; Milner et al. 2012).

Human clinical disease is, thus, the result of the interaction of the parasite preprogrammed biology in concert with the human pathophys-

iological response. Caveats and corollaries that add variation to this host–parasite interaction include parasite genetic diversity of key proteins, coinfections, comorbidities, delays in treatment, human polymorphisms, and environmental determinants (Goncalves et al. 2014). The final clinical disease result includes a spectrum of fever, anemia, and coma, among many others (Hafalla et al. 2011; Oakley et al. 2011; Grau and Craig 2012).

When one questions, "how do we get rid of cerebral malaria?" (one of the more common causes of death), it is surprising to no one to hear the answer, "reduce the overall burden of malaria disease." This may seem simple but, in fact, is a complex answer. Interventions with rapid drug treatment for anyone with a fever will drastically reduce the burden of mortality (sometimes to zero) in a given location (Clark et al. 2010). The treatment probably not only staves off a prolonged acute disease state (which may be a component of cerebral malaria [CM]) but also provides an antigen source to the immune system to create antibody and other responses that may quiet future infections. This effect, however, only lasts as long as the diversity of the parasite is stable (a result of endemicity) and the drug access continues (a result of infrastructure stability). In a world where eradication is a goal for malaria, the incidence of CM with multiple interventions may decrease or even vanish in the current at-risk population (children less than 6 years of age in sub-Saharan Africa). However, the risk of CM may simply shift to these same children at a later stage (or their children) as a region moves from high endemicity to low endemicity. During this entire process, however, the biology of the parasite will remain relatively stable and, thus, the risk for any of the currently observed diseases states will still exist. How, where, and why these disease states emerge (or vanish) is a product of many factors beyond the parasite, the vast majority of which are within our control.

UNCOMPLICATED MALARIA

Within the geographic regions where the human population is at risk for malaria infection

(2.5 billion), annually 215,000,000 clinical infections occur for which patients have symptoms and seek medical attention. Patient illness represents, however, a subset of all individuals who have been bitten by infected mosquitoes and a much larger portion of the "at-risk" population would show a positive malaria smear or other diagnostic test if they were screened (asymptomatic infection, true number variable and difficult to estimate) (malERA Consultative Group on Diagnoses and Diagnostics 2011; McMorrow et al. 2011; Laishram et al. 2012; Babiker et al. 2013; Lin et al. 2014; Stone et al. 2015). The exact malaria parasite biology within these two groups is probably very similar with the essential differences being due to the human immune response, number of prior infections, and exposure profile (Doolan and Martinez-Alier 2006; Dzikowski et al. 2006; Marsh and Kinyanjui 2006; De Leenheer and Pilyugin 2008; Punsawad 2013; de Souza 2014; Krzych et al. 2014). The symptoms of malaria infection can only begin in any ill patient with the first liver schizont rupture and release of merozoites into the peripheral circulation—this event is silent for the vast majority of patients who will become clinically ill. As the parasites continue through their asexual life cycle of merozoite reinvasion, trophozoite development, and schizont rupture over 24 to 48 hours, the level of parasitemia parallels the level of human response (i.e., fever, C-reactive protein [CRP], and tumor necrosis factor α [TNF-α]) until the patient crosses a threshold of awareness and "feels ill" (Oakley et al. 2011). Uncomplicated malaria is defined as symptoms present (fever) but no clinical or laboratory signs to indicate severity or vital organ dysfunction (WHO 2015).

Within the human host during an initial infection, macrophage ingestion of merozoites, ruptured schizonts, or antigen-presenting trophozoites in the circulation or spleen leads to release of TNF-α (Chakravorty et al. 2008; Randall and Engwerda 2010). The molecule, along with others in a cascade, is responsible for fever during infection. Other important molecules found during active infection include interleukin 10 (IL-10) and interferon γ (IFN-γ) among others (Clark et al. 2008; McCall and Sauerwein 2010; Freitas do Rosario and Langhorne 2012; Gun et al. 2014; Hunt et al. 2014). In subsequent infections, some degree of antibody production produced by the prior macrophage–T-cell–B-cell axis of the immune system confers additional macrophage activity leading to a more efficient clearance of parasites and production of new antibodies (Wykes and Good 2006; Freitas do Rosario and Langhorne 2012; Krzych et al. 2014; Hviid et al. 2015). As the human host immune system works its way through the continuously presented parasite protein repertoire, additional antibodies develop conferring additional protection.

Uncomplicated malaria is easily treated during each symptomatic episode with antimalarias specific to the parasite and the vast majority of patients easily clear the infection when treated with proper compliance.

P. falciparum

P. falciparum (Pf) modifies the surface of the infected red blood cell and creates an adhesive phenotype, which removes the parasite from circulation for nearly half of the asexual life cycle, a unique time frame among the malaria parasites (Grau and Craig 2012). The binding of the infected erythrocytes can occur with endothelium, platelets, or uninfected red blood cells (Fairhurst and Wellems 2006; Kraemer and Smith 2006; Smith et al. 2013). The parasite accomplishes this cytoadherant ("sticky cell") state through the *P. falciparum* erythrocyte membrane protein 1 (PfEMP1), which is the product of *var* gene transcription (Smith et al. 2013). Within a given Pf parasite, there are ∼60 copies of the *var* gene, each highly variable and different from the others. These genes represent some of the most diverse within the parasite's genome and within the total parasite population. Their expression is driven by several mechanisms including immune selection pressure and epigenetics. This aspect of the parasites's biology (*var* gene expression) occurs in all infections including asymptomatic and uncomplicated malaria. The potential of this human–parasite interaction to cause disease in humans has a definite spectrum discussed below (Smith et al. 2013). Regardless of the disease variability, the sequestration (temporary removal of the parasite from circulation through red cell surface binding) of Pf occurs during every human infection for half of the asexual life cycle. Thus, in a low-level infection in which a single mosquito bite has introduced a single brood of synchronous parasites, patients may show negative peripheral blood smears. This may be especially true in the traveler or residents of low-endemicity regions. In highly endemic settings, however, patients are bitten repeatedly and can present with a continuous fever and an accompanying consistently positive blood smear during the first decades of life. As a local immunity to the Pf population evolves in a given host, smears may again drop to very low levels and even become undetectable despite ongoing transmission.

P. vivax

P. vivax (Pv) is the most common malaria parasite causing clinical disease outside of Africa (WHO 2015). Unlike Pf, but like all other human malaria parasites, Pv does not show a prolonged period of sequestration during infection (Costa et al. 2011). The parasite is, thus, probably more frequently exposed to clearance by the spleen and more commonly seen on a peripheral blood smear during an infection. One of the unique features of Pv is the red cell preference for reticulocytes and the use of predominantly the Duffy antigen for invasion although not absolutely (Moreno-Pérez et al. 2013; Zimmerman et al. 2013). This leads to a clinical infection with a lower level of parasitemia than is seen in Pf. Because reticulocytes are larger than mature red cells, the infected cells appear larger than the cells around them on peripheral blood smear. Characteristic Schuffner's dots, which are caveola–vesicle structures, are seen in both Pv and *P. ovale* (Udagama et al. 1988). The diagnostic form of Pv is the amoeboid form where the cytoplasm, unique to Pv, has finger-like projections without a typical round-to-oval structure.

Clinically, patients present almost identically to other malaria infections with fever plus a constellation of other possible symptoms. Unlike Pf and *P. malariae* (which have a single liver schizont rupture even shortly after sporozoite invasion), Pv, and Po may "reemerge" when hypnozoites (quiescent forms that last months to years in the liver from a single sporozoite exposure) release merozoites. Thus, the clinical timing of a disease (many months or years after exposure) could be a clue to one of these organisms.

P. ovale

P. ovale (Po) was shown to be two distinct species (*P. ovale curtisi* and *P. ovale wallikeri*), which only differ by a shorter latency period in *P. ovale wallikeri* and genetic sequence differences (Oguike et al. 2011). Thus, these two sympatric organisms are impossible to distinguish, present with the same clinical syndrome, and respond to the same therapy. Although their behavior is similar to Pv, Po does not require the Duffy blood group antigen for invasion of red blood cells. On peripheral blood smear, the diagnostic forms of Po are the comet form of the trophozoite as well as the oval appearance of infected red blood cells and the presence of fimbria or finger-like projects of the red cell membrane. The ring, schizont, and gametocyte stages of Po are very similar to Pv.

P. malariae

P. malariae (Pm) is the most benign form of malaria infection with several distinct clinical features (Collins and Jeffery 2007; Mueller et al. 2007; Das 2008). Patients have fever every 72 hours during an infection due to the longer parasite life cycle (Collins and Jeffery 2007). The number of merozoites produced with each schizont rupture is lower and, thus, the parasitemias are lower overall in these patient compared with others types of malaria (Collins and Jeffery 2007). This long life cycle and low level of infection leads to a more robust immune response. Thus, Pm is often considered to cause a chronic malaria they may last decades. One unique outcome of Pm is the deposition of immune complexes in the kidneys that can result in nephritis (Das 2008). On peripheral blood smear, the parasite shows the classic and diagnostic "band" form as well as a schizont with few merozoites and a central pigment globule (golden in color) refer to as a "daisy" form.

Clinically, patients who are ill with malaria symptoms and show forms suggestive of Pm should be evaluated for *P. knowlesi* as well as Pf because the detection of symptoms and/or the likelihood of co-infection is higher than a truly symptomatic Pm patient (Singh and Daneshvar 2013).

P. knowlesi

P. knowlesi (Pk) is found in a limited distribution in Malaysian/Indonesian Borneo with cases reported in other southeast Asian countries, including Vietnam, Singapore, Myanmar, Cambodia, Thailand, and the Philippines (Muller and Schlagenhauf 2014). Exposure to mosquitoes that feed on long-tailed and/or pigtailed macaques (Singh and Daneshvar 2013) is required for transmission as no human-to-human (via mosquito) transmission has been reported. In vitro work has shown that the parasites prefer young red blood cells but can, over time, adapt to infect older human red blood cells, a phenomenon that currently limits rapid spread of the infection beyond the human:monkey milieu (Lim et al. 2013). The disease presents like other malarias with fever/chills and headache with uncommon features like nausea/vomiting, myalgia/arthralgia, upper respiratory symptoms, and jaundice (Muller and Schlagenhauf 2014). Although rare, fatal complications of Pk have occurred and do so with higher frequency than seen in Pv and Pf proportionally (Singh and Daneshvar 2013) owing to the new emergence in humans (zoonosis) and absence of sufficient time for human adaptability. Although Pk is not unique among the nonhuman vertebrate malarias that have been transmitted to humans, the current emergence of a large population distribution of a disease with high mortality has not been previously reported and warrants careful attention (Ta et al. 2014).

SEVERE MALARIA

P. vivax

During an infection with only Pv and no other comorbidities, death from the disease is exceedingly rare (if not unheard of). However, in the presence of comorbidities, severe disease and fatal outcomes are reported. Because of the relapsing phenotype of the liver, chronic disease can lead to severe anemia and malnutrition, which predispose to coinfections and a poor immune response (Dumas et al. 2009; Anstey et al. 2012; Costa et al. 2012). Like severe Pf and Pk (and any severe infection), the final common pathway can include respiratory distress, hepatorenal failure, and shock (Anstey et al. 2012). Coma has been reported rarely in Pv infection but the cause of this coma is not the same as is seen in Pf (in which parasite sequestration to a high level in the brain is seen in fatal cases).

P. knowlesi

The rate of severe disease in Pk is higher (~8%), proportionally, than is seen in Pf or Pv and has higher mortality (3%) (Antinori et al. 2013). Similar to severe Pf malaria in adults, Pk-severe disease typically presents with the same initial constellation of fever, etc., and progresses in severe disease to include hypotension, respiratory distress, acute renal failure, hyperbilirubinemia, and shock (Rajahram et al. 2012; Antinori et al. 2013). Coma, as is required for a Pf cerebral malaria diagnosis, is not always seen in Pk fatal cases. The "common pathway" of any severe infection (i.e., may be seen in Pf, bacterial sepsis, etc.) is the result of an exaggerated human immune response in the presence of an untreated or delayed in treatment infection and probably not a result of specific mechanisms of the organisms. In fact, Pk as a cause of other morbid conditions (Gram-negative sepsis) has been reported. Pathologically, where Pf shows intense sequestration in the brain along with congestion and possibly brain swelling, Pk has a similar appearance in tissue with a curious lack of ICAM-1 in the brain (Cox-Singh et al. 2010; Menezes et al. 2012). The Pk family of genes homologous to Pf *var* genes is the SICAvars, which are larger in structure (12 vs. two exons) and quantity ($>$200 vs. 60) than the *var* genes of Pf (Lapp et al. 2009). The exact mechanism and interactions of Pk with human endothelium to produce sequestration are yet to be elucidated.

PLACENTAL MALARIA

The Pf parasite can uniquely cause a range of pathological changes in the setting of pregnancy due to the ability of the parasite to sequester paired with the large sink of novel placental molecules such as chondroitin sulfate (CSA). The parasite's PfEMP1 proteins that are products of the *var2CSA* genes bind to CSA as the parasites pass through the placenta, removing them from circulation, whereas non-CSA-binding parasites continue circulating. Maternal antibody that has developed to malaria in previous infections appears to destroy the non-CSA-binding parasites, whereas the placenta acts as a protected space for propagation. In addition to the direct effects of placental binding, mononuclear cell infiltrates may also be present and in very high numbers. Depending on when the malaria infection occurs during pregnancy, the placenta at examination may show pigment trapped in fibrin (older infection) or parasites and/or mononuclear cells (active infection). In addition to Pf, Pv has been reported to be associated with complications in pregnancy, including anemia, miscarriage, low birth weight, and congenital malaria (Anstey et al. 2012; Costa et al. 2012). The placental pathology in Pv, however, does not show the same degree of parasite or monocyte involvement and remains to be elucidated.

SEVERE MALARIA ANEMIA

The pediatric population in areas of high transmission is uniquely susceptible to severe malarial anemia (SMA) during the first 2 years of life. When the children present, blood transfusion can be life-saving along with antimalarial drugs. The exact mechanisms of the pathways that lead to SMA are not well understood. The disruption of the immune response of monocytes and lymphocytes in the presence of hemozoin may lead to an inappropriate regulation of erythropoietin (through IL-6, regulated on activation, normal T-cell expressed, and secreted [RANTES], and macrophage inflammatory protein 1s [MIP-1s]) (Perkins et al. 2011). The removal of red cell membrane and red cells completely by the spleen in an accelerated fashion due to the presence of malaria has also been suggested.

ACIDOSIS

Acidosis is a complex metabolic state with a range of etiologies (Planche and Krishna 2006; Taylor et al. 2012). Within malaria, acidosis is caused by a combination of several factors. The malaria parasite produces *Plasmodium* lactate dehydrogenase (pLDH), which creates lactic acid leading to decreased pH. Respiratory distress is a common feature of severe malaria and, through sequestration, somnolence, and/or brain swelling, direct central suppression of the respiratory centers leads to irregular breathing patterns in the setting of acidosis, which may contribute to the pH imbalance. Supportive therapy to protect the airway and more aggressively rebalance the pH may decrease mortality (Cheng and Yansouni 2013).

CEREBRAL MALARIA

The unique ability of *P. falciparum* to bind to endothelium produces the clinicopathological syndrome of CM in both children and adults. In highly endemic settings, children under 5 years are at highest risk for the disease with a mortality of 10% to 20%. In low-endemic settings, all ages are at risk and mortality can be higher in adults. In the nonimmune population (e.g., travelers, military, etc.), a low level of infection ($<$1% parasitemia) can result in clinical signs of CM and be life-threatening. The clinical manifestations of CM may start with a typical malaria presentation and quickly (over minutes to hours) degenerate to a comatose state. After exclusion of other possibly causes of coma (e.g., postictal state, hypoglycemia, meningitis, bacterial sepsis, head trauma/cerebral bleed, etc.), a clinical diagnosis of CM can be made, which is

Cite this article as *Cold Spring Harb Perspect Med* doi: 10.1101/cshperspect.a025569

best confirmed by examination of the retinal for signs of malaria retinopathy (Seydel et al. 2015). In any case, the diagnostic pathological feature of the disease—at autopsy—is the presence of *P. falciparum* parasites in greater than 20% of capillaries in the brain by either tissue smear or histological sections (Taylor et al. 2004). Other pathological features that are variably present include fibrin thrombi, ring hemorrhages, discoloration of the brain, axonal injury, and capillary leakage (Dorovini-Zis et al. 2011). Brain vessels will appear congested in all cases with brain swelling more prominent in acute deaths such as African pediatric patients ($<$48 hours). Multiorgan failure and acute respiratory distress syndrome with diffuse alveolar damage is more common in adult patients, particularly those that have a prolonged course of disease (Hanson et al. 2010, 2014; Medana et al. 2011; Ponsford et al. 2012; Prapansilp et al. 2013; Maude et al. 2014).

The pathobiology of CM is not completely understood but a large body of evidence from both clinical and pathological studies has implicated a series of events and pathways at work within the disease landscape. Endothelial activation to a more "sticky" state is the first step. During the early phases of any malaria infection, macrophage stimulation leads to TNF-α production, the increase of which stimulates display of adherence molecules in the brain endothelium like intracellular adhesion molecule 1 (ICAM-1). Other such stimulations lead to a variety of other up-regulation events as summarized in Figure 1. A large number of malaria parasites can bind, through PfEMP1, to ubiquitous molecules such as CD36 (platelets and endothelium outside of the brain), which logically explains both the thrombocytopenia of malaria infection as well as the very low incidence of CM compared with all malaria infections. In the African child under 5 years of age, the combination of factors leading to the increase in the "sticky" phenotype is most likely a delay in treatment of a malarial infection paired with a lack of well-developed protective specific antibodies in the setting of poor general health (e.g., malnutrition). For infected individuals outside of this setting, the total lack of immunity drives the disease. The ca-

pacity of the human immune system to clear a disease, which relies almost exclusively on macrophage phagocytosis is the macrophage compartment. Antibodies speed this process by increased uptake efficiency. In autopsy studies of children, the spleen, the primary site of clearance of the parasites in most CM patients shows a large burden of malaria pigment and macrophages but no parasites. This suggests that the clearance ability of the spleen is high and efficient. Where the process of clearance breaks down may be in the capacity of circulating monocytes/macrophages to keep up with the sequestration and parasite life cycle (every 48 hours).

OVERLAP IN SEVERE DISEASE

Severe malaria in African children is often a monosyndromic presentation with little, if any, overt complications beyond coma, anemia, and/or acidosis. Studies suggest that in adult patients, the disease has multiple modalities at play in fatal cases including respiratory, hepatic, renal, and vascular complications. Equivalent studies in pediatric cases suggest that evidence of early changes in these same pathways may be at work; however, the rapid pace from presentation to either death or recovery does not allow these additional processes to manifest. In pediatric patients in Africa, an overlap of SMA, acidosis, and/or CM can occur, which may lead to higher mortality in overlap groups. CM, as there is not current ancillary treatment beyond antimalarias and supportive therapy, remains a key factor in mortality outcomes.

CONCLUDING REMARKS

Malaria pathogenesis has a broad and narrow context depending on the frame of reference. For fatal disease, the sequestration of Pf in tissues along with up-regulation of cytokines, toxic substances, and a lack of adequate, timely therapy, are key features of the process. For the remainder of malaria infections, the negative aspects of the disease are results of imbalance in the parasite–human interaction for a given species with the exception of Pk, a true zoonosis. As eradication moves from a goal to a ra-

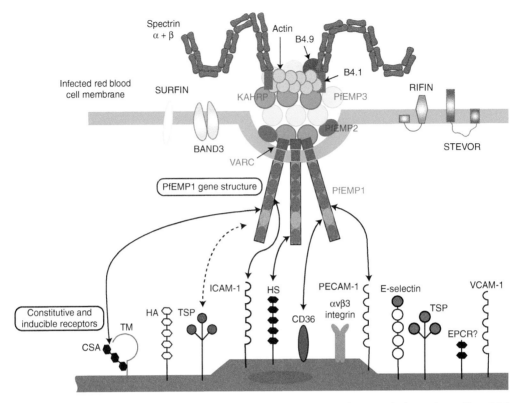

Figure 1. A model of the interactions between *Plasmodium* parasites (predominantly from *Plasmodium falciparum, top*) and the human endothelium (*bottom*) is shown. The prominent feature is the *P. falciparum* erythrocyte membrane protein 1 (PfEMP1) molecules that protrude from the raised knob structures, which in themselves are made of a combination of human and parasite proteins in a tight complex. Surfins, rifins, and stevors from the parasite are also located in the red cell membrane. On the human side, a range of molecules, depending on tissue, are involved infected parasite interactions, including those that are always present on endothelium (e.g., CD36, outside of the brain and on platelets), are present during activation (e.g., intracellular adhesion molecule 1 [ICAM-1]), and are activated during interaction with other molecules (e.g., endothelial protein C receptor [EPCR] and thrombospondin [TSP]). Special tissue situations include chondroitin sulfate (CSA) in the placenta and CR-1 on uninfected red blood cells (which mediates rosette formation).

tional plan of action, a firm understanding of the pathogenesis of malaria in all patient groups is required to not only predict where disease (especially severe disease) will occur but be able to prevent it.

ACKNOWLEDGMENTS

We thank the citizens of Malawi for their enormous contribution to understanding the pathogenesis of malaria in both pediatric and placental disease as well as the ongoing contributions from the citizens and our colleagues in Southeast Asia for their paramount work. Every

illness with malaria affects the person, their family, and their society and our hope through this review is to bring us many steps closer to an end to malaria for everyone.

REFERENCES

Anstey NM, Douglas NM, Poespoprodjo JR, Price RN. 2012. *Plasmodium vivax*: Clinical spectrum, risk factors and pathogenesis. *Adv Parasitol* **80:** 151–201.

Antinori S, Galimberti L, Milazzo L, Corbellino M. 2013. *Plasmodium knowlesi*: The emerging zoonotic malaria parasite. *Acta Tropica* **125:** 191–201.

Babiker HA, Gadalla AA, Ranford-Cartwright LC. 2013. The role of asymptomatic *P. falciparum* parasitaemia in the evolution of antimalarial drug resistance in areas of seasonal transmission. *Drug Resist Updat* **16:** 1–9.

Bañuls AL, Thomas F, Renaud F. 2013. Of parasites and men. *Infect Genet Evol* **20:** 61–70.

Bozdech Z, Llinas M, Pulliam BL, Wong ED, Zhu J, DeRisi JL. 2003a. The transcriptome of the intraerythrocytic developmental cycle of *Plasmodium falciparum*. *PLoS Biol* **1:** E5.

Bozdech Z, Zhu J, Joachimiak MP, Cohen FE, Pulliam B, DeRisi JL. 2003b. Expression profiling of the schizont and trophozoite stages of *Plasmodium falciparum* with a long-oligonucleotide microarray. *Genome Biol* **4:** R9.

Cator LJ, Lynch PA, Read AF, Thomas MB. 2012. Do malaria parasites manipulate mosquitoes? *Trends Parasitol* **28:** 466–470.

Chakravorty SJ, Hughes KR, Craig AG. 2008. Host response to cytoadherence in *Plasmodium falciparum*. *Biochem Soc Trans* **36:** 221–228.

Cheng MP, Yansouni CP. 2013. Management of severe malaria in the intensive care unit. *Crit Care Clin* **29:** 865–885.

Clark IA, Alleva LM, Budd AC, Cowden WB. 2008. Understanding the role of inflammatory cytokines in malaria and related diseases. *Travel Med Infect Dis* **6:** 67–81.

Clark TD, Njama-Meya D, Nzarubara B, Maiteki-Sebuguzi C, Greenhouse B, Staedke SG, Kamya MR, Dorsey G, Rosenthal PJ. 2010. Incidence of malaria and efficacy of combination antimalarial therapies over 4 years in an urban cohort of Ugandan children. *PLoS ONE* **5:** e11759.

Collins WE, Jeffery GM. 2007. *Plasmodium malariae*: Parasite and disease. *Clin Microbiol Rev* **20:** 579–592.

Costa FT, Lopes SC, Ferrer M, Leite JA, Martin-Jaular L, Bernabeu M, Nogueira PA, Mourao MP, Fernandez-Becerra C, Lacerda MV, et al. 2011. On cytoadhesion of *Plasmodium vivax*: Raison d'etre? *Mem Inst Oswaldo Cruz* **106:** 79–84.

Costa FT, Lopes SC, Albrecht L, Ataide R, Siqueira AM, Souza RM, Russell B, Renia L, Marinho CR, Lacerda MV. 2012. On the pathogenesis of *Plasmodium vivax* malaria: Perspectives from the Brazilian field. *Int J Parasitol* **42:** 1099–1105.

Cox-Singh J, Hiu J, Lucas SB, Divis PC, Zulkarnaen M, Chandran P, Wong KT, Adem P, Zaki SR, Singh B, et al. 2010. Severe malaria—A case of fatal *Plasmodium knowlesi* infection with post-mortem findings: A case report. *Malaria J* **9:** 10.

Cui L, Lindner S, Miao J. 2015. Translational regulation during stage transitions in malaria parasites. *Ann NY Acad Sci* **1342:** 1–9.

Daily JP, Scanfeld D, Pochet N, Le Roch K, Plouffe D, Kamal M, Sarr O, Mboup S, Ndir O, Wypij D, et al. 2007. Distinct physiological states of *Plasmodium falciparum* in malaria-infected patients. *Nature* **450:** 1091–1095.

Das BS. 2008. Renal failure in malaria. *J Vector Borne Dis* **45:** 83–97.

De Leenheer P, Pilyugin SS. 2008. Immune response to a malaria infection: Properties of a mathematical model. *J Biol Dyn* **2:** 102–120.

de Souza JB. 2014. Protective immunity against malaria after vaccination. *Parasite Immunol* **36:** 131–139.

Dixon MW, Dearnley MK, Hanssen E, Gilberger T, Tilley L. 2012. Shape-shifting gametocytes: How and why does *P. falciparum* go banana-shaped? *Trends Parasitol* **28:** 471–478.

Doolan DL, Martinez-Alier N. 2006. Immune response to pre-erythrocytic stages of malaria parasites. *Curr Mol Med* **6:** 169–185.

Dorovini-Zis K, Schmidt K, Huynh H, Fu W, Whitten RO, Milner D, Kamiza S, Molyneux M, Taylor TE. 2011. The neuropathology of fatal cerebral malaria in Malawian children. *Am J Pathol* **178:** 2146–2158.

Dumas JF, Simard G, Flamment M, Ducluzeau PH, Ritz P. 2009. Is skeletal muscle mitochondrial dysfunction a cause or an indirect consequence of insulin resistance in humans? *Diabetes Metab* **35:** 159–167.

Dzikowski R, Templeton TJ, Deitsch K. 2006. Variant antigen gene expression in malaria. *Cell Microbiol* **8:** 1371–1381.

Fairhurst RM, Wellems TE. 2006. Modulation of malaria virulence by determinants of *Plasmodium falciparum* erythrocyte membrane protein-1 display. *Curr Opin Hematol* **13:** 124–130.

Freitas do Rosario AP, Langhorne J. 2012. T cell-derived IL-10 and its impact on the regulation of host responses during malaria. *Int J Parasitol* **42:** 549–555.

Goncalves RM, Lima NF, Ferreira MU. 2014. Parasite virulence, co-infections and cytokine balance in malaria. *Pathog Glob Health* **108:** 173–178.

Grau GE, Craig AG. 2012. Cerebral malaria pathogenesis: Revisiting parasite and host contributions. *Future Microbiol* **7:** 291–302.

Gun SY, Claser C, Tan KS, Renia L. 2014. Interferons and interferon regulatory factors in malaria. *Mediators Inflamm* **2014:** 243713.

Hafalla JC, Silvie O, Matuschewski K. 2011. Cell biology and immunology of malaria. *Immunol Rev* **240:** 297–316.

Hanson J, Lee SJ, Mohanty S, Faiz MA, Anstey NM, Charunwatthana P, Yunus EB, Mishra SK, Tjitra E, Price RN, et al. 2010. A simple score to predict the outcome of severe malaria in adults. *Clin Infect Dis* **50:** 679–685.

Hanson J, Anstey NM, Bihari D, White NJ, Day NP, Dondorp AM. 2014. The fluid management of adults with severe malaria. *Crit Care* **18:** 642.

Hunt NH, Ball HJ, Hansen AM, Khaw LT, Guo J, Bakmiwewa S, Mitchell AJ, Combes V, Grau GE. 2014. Cerebral malaria: γ-Interferon redux. *Front Cell Infect Microbiol* **4:** 113.

Hviid L, Barfod L, Fowkes FJ. 2015. Trying to remember: Immunological B cell memory to malaria. *Trends Parasitol* **31:** 89–94.

Josling GA, Llinas M. 2015. Sexual development in *Plasmodium* parasites: Knowing when it's time to commit. *Nat Rev Microbiol* **13:** 573–587.

Kraemer SM, Smith JD. 2006. A family affair: *var* genes, PfEMP1 binding, and malaria disease. *Curr Opin Microbiol* **9:** 374–380.

Krzych U, Zarling S, Pichugin A. 2014. Memory T cells maintain protracted protection against malaria. *Immunol Lett* **161:** 189–195.

Laishram DD, Sutton PL, Nanda N, Sharma VL, Sobti RC, Carlton JM, Joshi H. 2012. The complexities of malaria disease manifestations with a focus on asymptomatic malaria. *Malaria J* **11**: 29.

Lapp SA, Korir CC, Galinski MR. 2009. Redefining the expressed prototype *SICAvar* gene involved in *Plasmodium knowlesi* antigenic variation. *Malaria J* **8**: 181.

Lim C, Hansen E, DeSimone TM, Moreno Y, Junker K, Bei A, Brugnara C, Buckee CO, Duraisingh MT. 2013. Expansion of host cellular niche can drive adaptation of a zoonotic malaria parasite to humans. *Nat Commun* **4**: 1638.

Lin JT, Saunders DL, Meshnick SR. 2014. The role of submicroscopic parasitemia in malaria transmission: What is the evidence? *Trends Parasitol* **30**: 183–190.

Liu Z, Miao J, Cui L. 2011. Gametocytogenesis in malaria parasite: Commitment, development and regulation. *Future Microbiol* **6**: 1351–1369.

Llinas M, DeRisi JL. 2004. Pernicious plans revealed: *Plasmodium falciparum* genome wide expression analysis. *Curr Opin Microbiol* **7**: 382–387.

malERA Consultative Group on Diagnoses and Diagnostics. 2011. A research agenda for malaria eradication: Diagnoses and diagnostics. *PLoS Med* **8**: e1000396.

Marsh K, Kinyanjui S. 2006. Immune effector mechanisms in malaria. *Parasite Immunol* **28**: 51–60.

Maude RJ, Barkhof F, Hassan MU, Ghose A, Hossain A, Abul Faiz M, Choudhury E, Rashid R, Abu Sayeed A, Charunwatthana P, et al. 2014. Magnetic resonance imaging of the brain in adults with severe falciparum malaria. *Malaria J* **13**: 177.

McCall MB, Sauerwein RW. 2010. Interferon-γ—Central mediator of protective immune responses against the pre-erythrocytic and blood stage of malaria. *J Leukocyte Biol* **88**: 1131–1143.

McMorrow ML, Aidoo M, Kachur SP. 2011. Malaria rapid diagnostic tests in elimination settings—Can they find the last parasite? *Clin Microbiol Infect* **17**: 1624–1631.

Medana IM, Day NP, Sachanonta N, Mai NT, Dondorp AM, Pongponratn E, Hien TT, White NJ, Turner GD. 2011. Coma in fatal adult human malaria is not caused by cerebral oedema. *Malaria J* **10**: 267.

Menezes RG, Pant S, Kharoshah MA, Senthilkumaran S, Arun M, Nagesh KR, Bhat NB, Mahadeshwara Prasad DR, Karki RK, Subba SH, et al. 2012. Autopsy discoveries of death from malaria. *Legal Med* **14**: 111–115.

Milner DA Jr, Pochet N, Krupka M, Williams C, Seydel K, Taylor TE, Van de Peer Y, Regev A, Wirth D, Daily JP, et al. 2012. Transcriptional profiling of *Plasmodium falciparum* parasites from patients with severe malaria identifies distinct low vs. high parasitemic clusters. *PLoS ONE* **7**: e40739.

Mohandas N, An X. 2012. Malaria and human red blood cells. *Med Microbiol Immunol* **201**: 593–598.

Moreno-Pérez DA, Ruíz JA, Patarroyo MA. 2013. Reticulocytes: *Plasmodium vivax* target cells. *Biol Cell* **105**: 251–260.

Mueller I, Zimmerman PA, Reeder JC. 2007. *Plasmodium malariae* and *Plasmodium ovale*—The "bashful" malaria parasites. *Trends Parasitol* **23**: 278–283.

Muller M, Schlagenhauf P. 2014. *Plasmodium knowlesi* in travellers, update 2014. *Int J Infect Dis* **22**: 55–64.

Oakley MS, Gerald N, McCutchan TF, Aravind L, Kumar S. 2011. Clinical and molecular aspects of malaria fever. *Trends Parasitol* **27**: 442–449.

Oguike MC, Betson M, Burke M, Nolder D, Stothard JR, Kleinschmidt I, Proietti C, Bousema T, Ndounga M, Tanabe K, et al. 2011. *Plasmodium ovale curtisi* and *Plasmodium ovale wallikeri* circulate simultaneously in African communities. *Int J Parasitol* **41**: 677–683.

Perkins DJ, Were T, Davenport GC, Kempaiah P, Hittner JB, Ong'echa JM. 2011. Severe malarial anemia: Innate immunity and pathogenesis. *Int J Biol Sci* **7**: 1427–1442.

Perry GH. 2014. Parasites and human evolution. *Evol Anthropol* **23**: 218–228.

Planche T, Krishna S. 2006. Severe malaria: Metabolic complications. *Curr Mol Med* **6**: 141–153.

Ponsford MJ, Medana IM, Prapansilp P, Hien TT, Lee SJ, Dondorp AM, Esiri MM, Day NP, White NJ, Turner GD. 2012. Sequestration and microvascular congestion are associated with coma in human cerebral malaria. *J Infect Dis* **205**: 663–671.

Prapansilp P, Medana I, Mai NT, Day NP, Phu NH, Yeo TW, Hien TT, White NJ, Anstey NM, Turner GD. 2013. A clinicopathological correlation of the expression of the angiopoietin-Tie-2 receptor pathway in the brain of adults with *Plasmodium falciparum* malaria. *Malaria J* **12**: 50.

Punsawad C. 2013. Effect of malaria components on blood mononuclear cells involved in immune response. *Asian Pac J Trop Biomed* **3**: 751–756.

Rajahram GS, Barber BE, William T, Menon J, Anstey NM, Yeo TW. 2012. Deaths due to *Plasmodium knowlesi* malaria in Sabah, Malaysia: Association with reporting as *Plasmodium malariae* and delayed parenteral artesunate. *Malaria J* **11**: 284.

Randall LM, Engwerda CR. 2010. TNF family members and malaria: Old observations, new insights and future directions. *Exp Parasitol* **126**: 326–331.

Sabeti PC, Reich DE, Higgins JM, Levine HZ, Richter DJ, Schaffner SF, Gabriel SB, Platko JV, Patterson NJ, McDonald GJ, et al. 2002. Detecting recent positive selection in the human genome from haplotype structure. *Nature* **419**: 832–837.

Seydel KB, Kampondeni SD, Valim C, Potchen MJ, Milner DA, Muwalo FW, Birbeck GL, Bradley WG, Fox LL, Glover SJ, et al. 2015. Brain swelling and death in children with cerebral malaria. *N Engl J Med* **372**: 1126–1137.

Singh B, Daneshvar C. 2013. Human infections and detection of *Plasmodium knowlesi*. *Clin Microbiol Rev* **26**: 165–184.

Smith JD, Rowe JA, Higgins MK, Lavstsen T. 2013. Malaria's deadly grip: Cytoadhesion of *Plasmodium falciparum*-infected erythrocytes. *Cell Microbiol* **15**: 1976–1983.

Stone W, Goncalves BP, Bousema T, Drakeley C. 2015. Assessing the infectious reservoir of falciparum malaria: Past and future. *Trends Parasitol* **31**: 287–296.

Ta TH, Hisam S, Lanza M, Jiram AI, Ismail N, Rubio JM. 2014. First case of a naturally acquired human infection with *Plasmodium cynomolgi*. *Malaria J* **13**: 68.

Taylor TE, Fu WJ, Carr RA, Whitten RO, Mueller JS, Fosiko NG, Lewallen S, Liomba NG, Molyneux ME. 2004. Differentiating the pathologies of cerebral malaria by postmortem parasite counts. *Nat Med* **10**: 143–145.

Cite this article as *Cold Spring Harb Perspect Med* doi: 10.1101/cshperspect.a025569

Taylor WR, Hanson J, Turner GD, White NJ, Dondorp AM. 2012. Respiratory manifestations of malaria. *Chest* **142:** 492–505.

Udagama PV, Atkinson CT, Peiris JS, David PH, Mendis KN, Aikawa M. 1988. Immunoelectron microscopy of Schuffner's dots in *Plasmodium vivax*–infected human erythrocytes. *Am J Pathol* **131:** 48–52.

Volkman SK, Sabeti PC, DeCaprio D, Neafsey DE, Schaffner SF, Milner DA Jr, Daily JP, Sarr O, Ndiaye D, Ndir O, et al. 2007. A genome-wide map of diversity in *Plasmodium falciparum*. *Nat Genet* **39:** 113–119.

WHO. 2015. World malaria report 2015. World Health Organization, Geneva.

Wright GJ, Rayner JC. 2014. *Plasmodium falciparum* erythrocyte invasion: Combining function with immune evasion. *PLoS Pathog* **10:** e1003943.

Wykes M, Good MF. 2006. Memory B cell responses and malaria. *Parasite Immunol* **28:** 31–34.

Zimmerman PA, Ferreira MU, Howes RE, Mercereau-Puijalon O. 2013. Red blood cell polymorphism and susceptibility to *Plasmodium vivax*. *Adv Parasitol* **81:** 27–76.

Malaria during Pregnancy

Michal Fried and Patrick E. Duffy

Laboratory of Malaria Immunology and Vaccinology, NIAID, NIH, Bethesda, MD 20892

Correspondence: michal.fried@nih.gov; duffype@niaid.nih.gov

One hundred and twenty-five million women in malaria-endemic areas become pregnant each year (see Dellicour et al. *PLoS Med* **7:** e1000221 [2010]) and require protection from infection to avoid disease and death for themselves and their offspring. Chloroquine prophylaxis was once a safe approach to prevention but has been abandoned because of drug-resistant parasites, and intermittent presumptive treatment with sulfadoxine–pyrimethamine, which is currently used to protect pregnant women throughout Africa, is rapidly losing its benefits for the same reason. No other drugs have yet been shown to be safe, tolerable, and effective as prevention for pregnant women, although monthly dihydroartemisinin–piperaquine has shown promise for reducing poor pregnancy outcomes. Insecticide-treated nets provide some benefits, such as reducing placental malaria and low birth weight. However, this leaves a heavy burden of maternal, fetal, and infant morbidity and mortality that could be avoided. Women naturally acquire resistance to *Plasmodium falciparum* over successive pregnancies as they acquire antibodies against parasitized red cells that bind chondroitin sulfate A in the placenta, suggesting that a vaccine is feasible. Pregnant women are an important reservoir of parasites in the community, and women of reproductive age must be included in any elimination effort, but several features of malaria during pregnancy will require special consideration during the implementation of elimination programs.

Pregnant women and women of childbearing age will require special consideration during mass campaigns for malaria elimination. Malaria susceptibility increases during pregnancy, making these women an important parasite reservoir in the community. Meanwhile, the biology and clinical presentations of *Plasmodium falciparum* in semi-immune women interfere with diagnosis during pregnancy, rendering targeted interventions ineffective for control (Fig. 1). Furthermore, concerns for teratogenicity and embryotoxicity complicate the proposed application of any drugs, vaccines, or antivector measures among women of reproductive age, greatly hindering mass campaign planning. For example, primaquine is the leading drug being assessed as a gametocytocidal agent to block parasite transmission to mosquitoes, but is contraindicated in pregnancy because the glucose-6-phosphate dehydrogenase status and hence hemolysis risk of the fetus would be unknown. This chapter reviews malaria during pregnancy, including its epidemiology and disease burden, molecular pathogenesis, naturally acquired immunity and potential for vaccines, diagnostic dilemmas, and drugs being used or

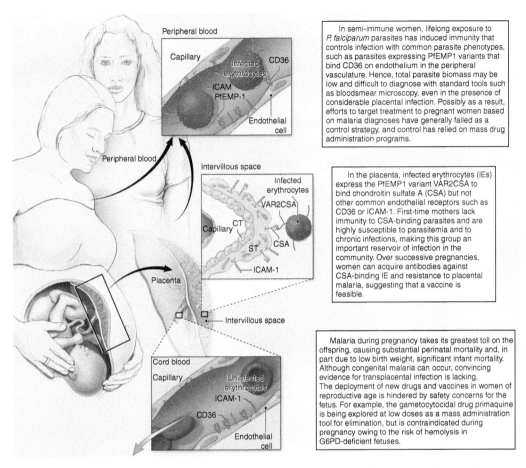

In semi-immune women, lifelong exposure to *P. falciparum* parasites has induced immunity that controls infection with common parasite phenotypes, such as parasites expressing PfEMP1 variants that bind CD36 on endothelium in the peripheral vasculature. Hence, total parasite biomass may be low and difficult to diagnose with standard tools such as bloodsmear microscopy, even in the presence of considerable placental infection. Possibly as a result, efforts to target treatment to pregnant women based on malaria diagnoses have generally failed as a control strategy, and control has relied on mass drug administration programs.

In the placenta, infected erythrocytes (IEs) express the PfEMP1 variant VAR2CSA to bind chondroitin sulfate A (CSA) but not other common endothelial receptors such as CD36 or ICAM-1. First-time mothers lack immunity to CSA-binding parasites and are highly susceptible to parasitemia and to chronic infections, making this group an important reservoir of infection in the community. Over successive pregnancies, women can acquire antibodies against CSA-binding IE and resistance to placental malaria, suggesting that a vaccine is feasible.

Malaria during pregnancy takes its greatest toll on the offspring, causing substantial perinatal mortality and, in part due to low birth weight, significant infant mortality. Although congenital malaria can occur, convincing evidence for transplacental infection is lacking. The deployment of new drugs and vaccines in women of reproductive age is hindered by safety concerns for the fetus. For example, the gametocytocidal drug primaquine is being explored at low doses as a mass administration tool for elimination, but is contraindicated during pregnancy owing to the risk of hemolysis in G6PD-deficient fetuses.

Figure 1. Malaria during pregnancy features several unique host–parasite interactions that require special attention for elimination strategies. Although malaria is more common in pregnant women than other adults, it is difficult to diagnose and therefore to control. The few drugs known to be safe during pregnancy are losing efficacy to drug-resistant *Plasmodium falciparum* parasites, and the use of new drugs or other interventions is hindered by concerns for fetal safety. Based on the knowledge of malaria immunity during pregnancy, vaccine approaches appear promising for the control of PM, but first-generation candidates are only now entering clinical trials and it is unclear whether these products will interrupt malaria transmission in pregnant women.

considered for prevention and treatment, to envision future approaches for malaria elimination that might be applied to women who may be pregnant.

EPIDEMIOLOGY AND BURDEN OF DISEASE

Pregnancy malaria looks very different in areas of low and unstable transmission versus high and stable transmission, although overall disease burden in different transmission zones may be similarly heavy in the absence of preventive measures. Where malaria transmission is low and unstable, women are infected infrequently but therefore have low immunity and often rapidly progress to severe disease syndromes when infected. These women have higher risks of severe malaria and death than their nonpregnant counterparts during *P. falciparum* infection (Duffy and Desowitz 2001) and are more likely to develop syndromes like respiratory distress and cerebral malaria (Nosten et al. 1991). In low transmission areas, women of all parities have increased susceptibility to malaria (Nosten et al.

1991). Women in these areas should be routinely screened and promptly treated for infection to prevent the risk of severe disease and death.

In areas of stable *P. falciparum* malaria transmission, where approximately 50 million pregnancies occur each year, women are semi-immune and often carry their infections with few or no symptoms. Disease for mother and offspring often develops as an insidious process, and this can make it difficult to relate outcomes such as severe maternal anemia or low birth weight (LBW) back to the infection that caused these sequelae. In areas of stable transmission, primigravid women are at greatest risk, and over successive pregnancies women naturally acquire resistance to *P. falciparum* that reduces parasite density and prevents disease. Resistance has been associated with antibodies against the parasitized red cells that bind chondroitin sulfate A (CSA) in the placenta (Fried et al. 1998a). In communities in which malaria control has improved and the incidence of malaria decreases, the incidence of *P. falciparum* pregnancy malaria also decreases, but malaria-specific antibodies wane and the parasite burden and sequelae during any individual infection increase (Mayor et al. 2015).

In areas of stable transmission, interventional studies have provided evidence to estimate the burden of disease. Chemoprophylaxis with pyrimethamine/dapsone (Maloprim) in The Gambia provided significant benefits to primigravid (Greenwood et al. 1992) and grandmulti-gravid (parity >7) women (Greenwood et al. 1989; Menendez et al. 1994): primigravidae on prophylaxis had lower rates of parasitemia and higher hematocrits. The latter is an important effect, because maternal anemia increases risks of LBW, preterm delivery (PTD), perinatal mortality, and neonatal mortality in low- and middle-income countries (Rahman et al. 2016). In a recent meta-analysis, chemoprevention reduced the risk of moderate-to-severe maternal anemia in first- and second-time mothers by ~40% in malaria-endemic areas (Radeva-Petrova et al. 2014); severe maternal anemia is a major risk factor for maternal mortality when women suffer postpartum hemorrhage, a common event in low-income countries (Tort et al. 2015).

Malaria prevention similarly improves child outcomes, both before and after delivery. In a meta-analysis of interventional trials, relative risk of perinatal mortality when mothers received prevention was 0.73 (95% CI, 0.53–0.99) (Garner and Gulmezoglu 2006). Effective prophylaxis reduces the risk of LBW newborns, and LBW is a strong predictor for infant mortality: extrapolating from this reduction in LBW, malaria prevention was estimated to reduce the mortality of neonates born to Gambian primigravidae by 42%, and the postneonatal mortality by 18% (Greenwood et al. 1992). In an observational birth cohort study, placental malaria (PM) in Tanzanian primigravidae was directly related to increased postneonatal mortality: 9.3% mortality for offspring of infected first-time mothers, compared with 2.6% for offspring of uninfected first-time mothers (Duffy and Fried 2011). PM in multigravid women did not significantly increase mortality risk of their offspring. In this community, the population attributable risk percent (PAR%) of postneonatal infant mortality owing to PM was 29.2% for first pregnancies.

The direct measurement of postneonatal mortality exceeds the estimates of mortality that would result from LBW, suggesting that other PM-related mechanisms might contribute to infant deaths. Several studies have related PM to increased risks of malaria infection (Schwarz et al. 2008; Goncalves et al. 2014) and to severe malaria (Goncalves et al. 2014) in offspring during infancy, but this relationship has not been observed in other studies (Awine et al. 2016). Interestingly, PM appears to influence immune responses and milieu in the offspring, which could influence their malaria susceptibility. Fetal sensitization to malaria antigens is common (Fievet et al. 1996; King et al. 2002; Malhotra et al. 2005). Some newborns of infected mothers display a "tolerant" phenotype, and have an increased risk of infection and lower hemoglobin levels during early life (Malhotra et al. 2009). Plasma cytokine levels at birth predict levels measured later during infancy, particularly for interleukin 1β (IL-1β) and tumor necrosis factor α (TNF-α), and also predict the risks of malaria infection and severe disease (Kabyemela et al. 2013); however, a relationship between PM and cord cytokine profiles has not been defined. More work is needed to understand whether and how PM in the mother may continue to influence malaria outcomes in her child.

Mixed malaria infections such as *P. falciparum* and *Plasmodium vivax* might also alter pregnancy malaria outcomes, but many mixed infections appear to be mono-infections when diagnosed by peripheral blood smear (BS). *P. vivax*, like *P. falciparum*, is associated with poor pregnancy outcomes, but, unlike *P. falciparum*, sequelae may be more common in multigravid pregnancies (reviewed in Duffy 2001). Non-falciparum infections were infrequent and did not appear to impact pregnancy outcomes in West Africa, where *P. vivax* was absent outside Mali (Williams et al. 2016). In *P. vivax*–endemic areas, women should be actively screened and treated, but management is complicated because primaquine is contraindicated due to fetal hemolysis risk and, therefore, liver hypnozoite parasite forms remain and cause relapses in the mother.

MOLECULAR PATHOGENESIS

In stable transmission zones, malaria during pregnancy has a unique epidemiology characterized by parity-dependent susceptibility: primigravid women are infected more frequently and with higher placental parasite densities than multigravid women. A prominent feature of *P. falciparum* malaria during pregnancy is the accumulation of parasites in the placenta, whereas parasite density in the peripheral circulation is low or undetectable (Brabin 1983; McGregor 1984). For decades, the increased susceptibility to malaria during pregnancy was attributed to immunological changes associated with pregnancy, but this could not explain the reduction in infection rate and placental parasite burden over successive pregnancies.

An alternative molecular model to explain parity-dependent susceptibility is based on the ability of *P. falciparum* infected erythrocytes (IEs) to adhere to receptors on the vascular endothelium and thereby sequester in deep vascular beds. During pregnancy, IEs accumulate in the intervillous spaces or bind to the surface of the syncytiotrophoblast in the placenta. In this model, the placenta presents a new receptor for IE adhesion, thereby selecting a parasite subpopulation to which women are naïve before their first pregnancy, making first-time mothers most susceptible. Analyses of the binding profile of placental IE have shown that this parasite subpopulation adheres to placental CSA, and not to CD36, which commonly supports the binding of IE from nonpregnant individuals (Fried and Duffy 1996). With successive pregnancies, women develop specific antibodies to CSA binding and placental IEs that enable them to better control the infection (Fried et al. 1998a); immunoepidemiology studies that support this model are discussed below. Following the identification of CSA as the unique receptor that supports parasite adhesion in the placenta, additional studies conducted at different sites have confirmed this binding phenotype (Fried et al. 1998a, 2006; Beeson et al. 1999; Maubert et al. 2000; Muthusamy et al. 2007).

CSA is a glycosaminoglycan comprising repeats of the disaccharide D-glucoronic acid and *N*-acetyl-D-galactosamine (GalNAc). CSA is sulfated at the C4 position of GalNAc. The closely related glycosaminoglycans chondroitin sulfate B and chondroitin sulfate C do not support placental IE adhesion. CSA chains vary in their length and degree of sulfation, and further characterization has shown that a low-sulfated CSA (Achur et al. 2000; Alkhalil et al. 2000; Fried et al. 2000; Andrews et al. 2005) of at least six disaccharide repeats (Alkhalil et al. 2000) is optimal to support placental IE adhesion.

IE sequestration in the placenta is followed by the accumulation of macrophages and B cells in the intervillous spaces. The intensity of the inflammatory immune infiltrate varies between women and is inversely related to acquired immunity: macrophages are more commonly observed in placentas from primigravidae who lack specific immunity to placental IE than in those from multigravidae (Garnham 1938; Muehlenbachs et al. 2007).

The cytokine milieu in a healthy uninfected placenta displays a bias toward type 2 cytokines.

PM leads to marked changes in the cytokine milieu, including increased levels of TNF-α, interferon γ (IFN-γ), IL-10, monocyte chemoattractant protein 1, macrophage inflammatory protein 1 (MIP-1α and MIP-1β), CXC ligand 8, CXC ligand 9, and CXC ligand 13 (Fried et al. 1998b; Moormann et al. 1999; Abrams et al. 2003; Chaisavaneeyakorn et al. 2003; Rogerson et al. 2003; Suguitan et al. 2003a,b; Kabyemela et al. 2008; Dong et al. 2012). Increased levels of the cytokines TNF-α and IFN-γ, and the chemokine CXCL9 that is regulated by IFN-γ, have been associated with LBW deliveries, especially among primigravid women (Fried et al. 1998b; Rogerson et al. 2003; Kabyemela et al. 2008; Dong et al. 2012). Similarly, transcript levels for the chemokines CXCL13, CXCL9, and CCL18 negatively correlate with birth weight, and up-regulation of IL-8 and TNF-α transcription in the placenta has been associated with intrauterine growth retardation (Moormann et al. 1999; Muehlenbachs et al. 2007). These studies support but do not prove that these inflammatory mediators contribute to PM sequelae. Animal models that reproduce placental sequestration and inflammation are needed for mechanistic studies to better understand disease pathogenesis.

IMMUNITY AND VACCINES

Parity-Dependent Acquisition of Antibodies

The unique epidemiology of pregnancy malaria is characterized by parity-dependent susceptibility. Different approaches to evaluate parity-dependent humoral immunity have included serum or plasma reactivity to the IE surface by flow cytometry, adhesion-blocking activity, agglutination of IE, and opsonizing activity (Table 1). Regardless of assay, parity-dependent acquisition of antibody against placental parasites or CSA-binding laboratory isolates has been consistently observed across many studies. Levels of antibodies that surface-react are higher in multigravidae compared with primigravidae in many different countries (Fried et al. 1998a; Ricke et al. 2000; Staalsoe et al. 2001, 2004; Tuikue Ndam et al. 2004; Megnekou et al. 2005; Fievet et al.

2006; Feng et al. 2009; Aitken et al. 2010; Mayor et al. 2011). Adhesion-blocking antibody levels are significantly higher among multigravid than primigravid women (Fried et al. 1998a; O'Neil-Dunne et al. 2001; Jaworowski et al. 2009; Ndam et al. 2015). Although agglutination of placental parasites is uncommon (Beeson et al. 1999), the proportion of serum samples with agglutinating antibodies was significantly higher among multigravidae than primigravidae (Beeson et al. 1999; Maubert et al. 1999). Similarly, opsonic phagocytosis increased with parity (Keen et al. 2007; Jaworowski et al. 2009). Thus, antibodies to CSA-binding IE or placental parasites provide a robust correlate of parity-dependent resistance, regardless of assay.

Antibodies to Placental Parasites and Infection Status or Infection Risk

Garnham (1938) described three phases of PM based on histology. In the acute or active infection phase, IE accumulate in the intervillous spaces. In the next phase, now called chronic infection, maternal inflammatory cells accumulate, notably monocytes−macrophages containing malaria pigment (hemozoin). After IE are cleared, parasite pigment remains in the intervillous fibrin, sometimes persisting for months, depending on the parasite burden and corresponding amount of pigment (McGready et al. 2002; Muehlenbachs et al. 2010). This last phase of the infection is referred to as past infection. This chronology of PM is typical for primigravidae, but not for multigravidae who usually clear placental parasites quickly and do not progress beyond the active infection phase. Poor outcomes related to PM, such as LBW and maternal anemia, are most strongly associated with the chronic phase of infection (Ordi et al. 1998; Ismail et al. 2000; Shulman et al. 2001; Muehlenbachs et al. 2010).

The relationship of antibodies to infection status or infection risk has varied between studies (Table 2). This may be due, in part, to the heterogeneous chronology of placental infections, and in part to the effect of infection to boost antibodies. In three of four studies, antiadhesion antibodies have been associated with a

Table 1. Studies of naturally acquired antiparasite antibodies and parity

Reference/study (year)	Test	Parasite tested	Plasma/sera collected at	n	Results
Ricke et al. 2000	Surface proteins by flow	CSA-selected	Third trimester	P: 30 S: 30 M: 103	Increase with parity
Staalsoe et al. 2001, 2004	Surface proteins by flow	CSA-selected	Third trimester; delivery	P: 78 S: 105	Increase with parity
Megnekou et al. 2005	Surface proteins by flow	CSA-selected	Combined second–third trimesters	P: 101 S/M: 114	Increase with parity
Fievet et al. 2006	Surface proteins by flow	Placental parasites	Second trimester	P: 62 S: 50 M: 153	Increase with parity
Feng et al. 2009	Surface proteins by flow	CSA-selected	Second trimester	P: 80 S: 16 M: 45	Increase with parity
Aitken et al. 2010	Surface proteins by flow	CSA-selected	Second and third trimesters	P: 131 S: 108 M: 310	Increase with parity
Brolin et al. 2010	Surface proteins by flow	CSA-selected	Third trimester	P: 189 S: 21 M: 72	Increase with parity
Mayor et al. 2011	Surface proteins by flow	CSA-selected, placental parasites	Delivery	P: 30 M: 60	PM^-: M > P PM^+: M > P for placental isolates
Fried et al. 1998a	Anti-adhesion	Placental parasites	Delivery	P: 51 S: 62 M: 84	Increase with parity
O'Neil-Dunne et al. 2001	Anti-adhesion	CSA-selected	During pregnancy	P: 45 S/M: 84	Increase with parity at gestational age of 12–20 wk
Jaworowski et al. 2009	Anti-adhesion	CSA-selected	Third trimester	P: 44 M: 29	Increase with parity
Beeson et al. 1999, 2004	Agglutination	Placental parasites	Second trimester	P: 12 M:12	Increase with parity
Maubert et al. 1999	Agglutination	CSA-selected, placental parasites	Delivery	P: 13–76[a] M: 17–143[a]	PM^+: Increase with parity for 2/4 isolates
Keen et al. 2007	Opsonizing activity	CSA-selected	Postpartum	P: 21 M: 16	Increase with parity
Jaworowski et al. 2009	Opsonizing activity	CSA-selected	Third trimester	P: 44 M: 29	Increase with parity
Feng et al. 2009	Opsonizing activity	CSA-selected	Second trimester	P: 80 S: 16 M: 45	Increase with parity

Only studies that analyzed more than five subjects per group are included.

P, Primigravidae; S, secundigravidae; M, multigravidae; PM^+, malaria-infected; $PM-$, uninfected; CSA, chondroitin sulfate A.

[a]Number of plasma samples analyzed vary among tested isolates.

Cite this article as *Cold Spring Harb Perspect Med* doi: 10.1101/cshperspect.a025551

Table 2. Studies of naturally acquired antiparasite antibodies and malaria infection status

Reference/study (year)	Test	Parasite tested	Plasma/sera collected at	n	Results
Staalsoe et al. 2001	Surface proteins by flow	CSA-selected	Third trimester	P: 55 M: 58	Multigravid: inverse correlation between Abs and parasite density
Staalsoe et al. 2004	Surface proteins by flow	CSA-selected	Delivery	All 477	Chronic and past infection > PM^- and acute infection, regardless of parity
Beeson et al. 2004	Surface proteins by flow	CSA-selected	Delivery	P: 54 M: 54	Primigravid: $PM^+ > PM^-$ Multigravid: no differences
Elliott et al. 2005	Surface proteins by flow	CSA-selected	Delivery	P: 46 M: 20	Primigravid: $PM^+ > PM^-$ for IgG1, IgG3 Multigravid: no differences
Ataide et al. 2010	Surface proteins by flow	CSA-selected	Third trimester	P: 268	Primigravid: $PM^+ > PM^-$
Ataide et al. 2011	Surface proteins by flow	CSA-selected	Third trimester	S: 187	Secundigravid: $PM^+ > PM^-$
Tutterrow et al. 2012a	Surface proteins by flow	CSA-selected	Second–third trimester	Total 27	$PM^- > PM^+$
Mayor et al. 2011, 2013	Surface proteins by flow	Placental parasites	Delivery	Total 293	Acute, chronic, and past infections > PM^-, regardless of parity
Fried et al. 1998	Anti-adhesion	Placental parasites	Delivery	P: 29 S: 68 M: 46	Secundigravid: $PM^- > PM^+$ Primigravid: low activity, no differences Multigravid: high activity, no differences
O'Neil-Dunne et al. 2001	Anti-adhesion	CSA-selected	Delivery	Total 97	Inverse correlation between Abs and placental parasite density
Beeson et al. 2004	Anti-adhesion	CSA-selected	Delivery	P: 54 M: 54	Primigravid: $PM^+ > PM^-$ Multigravid: no differences
Ndam et al. 2015	Anti-adhesion	CSA-selected	Delivery	Total 266	$PM^- > PM^+$
Beeson et al. 2004	Agglutination	CSA-selected placental parasites	Delivery	P:54 M:54	Primigravid and multigravid: $PM^+ > PM^-$
Ataide et al. 2010	Opsonizing activity	CSA-selected	Third trimester	P:268	Primigravid: $PM^+ > PM^-$
Ataide et al. 2011	Opsonizing activity	CSA-selected	Third trimester	S: 187	Secundigravid: $PM^+ > PM^-$

PM^+, Placental malaria positive, defined by the presence of parasites in the placenta; PM^-, no parasites or the evidence of past infection by histology; CSA, chondroitin sulfate A.

reduced risk of infection, or to reduced parasite densities in infected women, supporting a role in protection. Opsonizing activity, agglutinating activity, and IE surface reactivity are elevated during and after an infection, which confounds efforts to assess their relationship with protection against infection. Because naturally acquired immunity to malaria controls infection but does not confer sterile resistance that completely prevents infection, infections also occur in semi-immune multigravidae, and infection boosts their antibody levels (Table 2). As a consequence, increased levels of antibodies, including those that agglutinate, opsonize, or react to the surface of IE, can reflect current or recent exposure to the parasite and thereby confound efforts to find correlates of protection (Ataide et al. 2010).

Immune Responses and Pregnancy Outcomes

PM commonly leads to severe maternal anemia and LBW deliveries, especially among primigravidae. The association between naturally acquired antibodies and pregnancy outcomes has been seen in some but not all studies, and notably the target population and antibody assay have differed between studies (Table 3). Among Kenyan women with chronic malaria, low serum reactivity to the surface of CSA-binding laboratory IE was associated with lower hemoglobin level and reduced birth weight (Staalsoe et al. 2004). Among 141 malaria-infected women in Malawi (Feng et al. 2009), serum reactivity to the IE surface during the second trimester was lower among the women who presented with anemia (hemoglobin <11 g/dL) at the time of delivery (Feng et al. 2009). Opsonic activity among malaria-infected secundigravid women in Malawi was associated with increased birth weight, and opsonic activity was higher among nonanemic than anemic malaria-infected multigravidae (Jaworowski et al. 2009; Ataide et al. 2011). Among Mozambican women who had been infected during pregnancy, high serum reactivity to both placental and children's IE at the time of delivery was associated with increased birth weight and ges-

tational age (Mayor et al. 2013). In Kenya, levels of anti-adhesion antibodies to placental IE were associated with increased birth weight and gestational age among offspring of secundigravidae (Duffy and Fried 2003). In Benin, anti-adhesion antibodies reduced the likelihood of LBW deliveries (Ndam et al. 2015). Among multigravid women, anti-adhesion antibodies have not been associated with risks of maternal anemia and LBW (Duffy and Fried 2003; Jaworowski et al. 2009), presumably because as a group these women enjoy protective immunity. Together, these studies provide strong support for the idea that antibodies to placental IE confer protection, but do not indicate which antibody effector mechanism(s) is primarily responsible.

PREGNANCY MALARIA VACCINE DEVELOPMENT

Currently, the leading candidate for a vaccine to prevent pregnancy malaria is VAR2CSA, a member of the *var* gene or PfEMP1 protein family that is up-regulated in placental parasites as well as CSA-selected laboratory parasites (Salanti et al. 2003; Tuikue Ndam et al. 2005). VAR2CSA is a large protein of $\sim$350 kDa comprising six extracellular Duffy-binding-like (DBL) domains and is too large to manufacture as an intact molecule. Therefore, immunogens being considered for product development incorporate one or a few domains, with or without adjacent interdomain regions.

Several studies compared primigravid to multigravid women for their seroreactivity with different VAR2CSA domains (Table 4). Parity-dependent acquisition of VAR2CSA domain-specific antibody has varied between studies. This could reflect differences in the recombinant proteins based on expression system, allelic variant, or domain boundaries, or differences in study populations such as transmission intensity, gestational age, or prevalence of infection at the time of serum sampling.

Antibody boosting during infection can confound attempts to distinguish between protective antibodies and markers of exposure. Perhaps, for this reason, VAR2CSA antibodies have

Table 3. Studies of naturally acquired antiparasite antibodies and pregnancy outcomes

Reference/study (year)	Test	Parasite tested	Results
Staalsoe et al. 2004	Surface proteins by flow	CSA-selected	Among women with chronic malaria, high IgG associated to increased maternal HGB and BW
Beeson et al. 2004	Surface proteins by flow	CSA-selected	No association to BW or maternal HGB
Feng et al. 2009	Surface proteins by flow	CSA-selected	PM^+: Abs at weeks 14–26 associated to decreased maternal anemia (HGB < 10 g/dL)
Aitken et al. 2010	Surface proteins by flow	CSA-selected	No association to maternal anemia, BW, and GA
Serra-Casas et al. 2010	Surface proteins by flow	CSA-selected	No association to LBW, GA, and maternal anemia
Ataide et al. 2010	Surface proteins by flow	CSA-selected	Primigravid: no association to LBW or anemia
Ataide et al. 2011	Surface proteins by flow	CSA-selected	Secundigravid PM^+: no correlation with BW or maternal HGB
Mayor et al. 2013	Surface proteins by flow	Placental parasites	High Abs to placental and child isolates associated to increased BW
Duffy and Fried 2003	Anti-adhesion	Placental parasites	Anti-adhesion Abs associated to increased BW, GA
Beeson et al. 2004	Anti-adhesion	CSA-selected	No association to BW or maternal HGB
Jaworowski et al. 2009	Anti-adhesion	CSA-selected	Multigravid: no association to maternal HGB or BW
Ndam et al. 2015	Anti-adhesion	CSA-selected	Anti-adhesion Abs associated to decreased LBW and SGA
Beeson et al. 2004	Agglutination	CSA-selected	No association to BW or maternal HGB
Feng et al. 2009	Opsonizing activity	CSA-selected	PM^+: Abs at weeks 14–26 associated to decreased maternal anemia (HGB < 11 g/dL)
Jaworowski et al. 2009	Opsonizing activity	CSA-selected	Multigravid PM^+: lower opsonic activity in anemic (HGB < 11 g/dL); no association to BW
Ataide et al. 2010	Opsonizing activity	CSA-selected	Primigravid: no association to LBW or maternal anemia
Ataide et al. 2011	Opsonizing activity	CSA-selected	Secundigravid PM^+: correlated with BW

P, Primigravidae; S, secundigravidae; M, multigravidae; CSA, chondroitin sulfate A; PM^+, malaria-infected; PM^-, uninfected; HGB, hemoglobin; BW, birth weight; LBW, low birth weight; GA, gestational age.

not been related to protection from infection in many studies. After measuring antibody levels to individual DBL domains and domain combinations, Tutterrow et al. (2012a) concluded that antibodies to multiple domains and alleles are needed to reduce PM risk. In Benin, high levels of VAR2CSA-DBL3x antibody during the first two trimesters reduced the risk of PM, although a similar trend was observed with antibody to an unrelated VAR domain (Ndam et al. 2015).

Relationships between VAR2CSA antibodies and pregnancy outcomes have also varied between studies. Among Kenyan women with

Table 4. Studies of naturally acquired VAR2CSA antibodies and parity

Domain	Parity effect	Abs measured at	Study site year, transmission pattern	References
DBL1	Yes	Delivery	2001–2005, Muheza-Tanzania, perennial	Oleinikov et al. 2007
	No	Enrollment[a] and delivery	2001, Thiadiaye-Senegal, seasonal	Tuikue Ndam et al. 2006
DBL1–DBL2	Yes	Enrollment[a] and delivery	2008–2010, Comé-Benin, perennial	Ndam et al. 2015
DBL2	No	Enrollment[a] and delivery	2001, Thiadiaye-Senegal, seasonal	Dechavanne et al. 2015
	Yes	Delivery	2003–2006, Manhica-Mozambique, perennial	Mayor et al. 2013
ID1-ID2a	No	All trimesters	1994–1996 and 2001–2005, Ngali II and Yaoundé Cameroon, high transmission and low transmission	Babakhanyan et al. 2014
DBL3	Yes	Delivery	2001–2005, Muheza-Tanzania, holoendemic	Oleinikov et al. 2007
		Enrollment[a] and delivery	2008–2010, Comé-Benin, perennial	Ndam et al. 2015
	No	Third trimester	2000–2002, Blantyre-Malawi, perennial	Brolin et al. 2010
		Delivery	2003–2006, Manhica-Mozambique, perennial	Mayor et al. 2013
DBL4	Yes	Delivery	2008–2010, Comé-Benin, perennial	Ndam et al. 2015
	No	Delivery	2001–2005, Muheza-Tanzania, perennial	Oleinikov et al. 2007
		Enrollment[a]	2008–2010, Comé-Benin, perennial	Ndam et al. 2015
DBL5	Yes	Delivery	Ghana[b], seasonal	Salanti et al. 2004
		Enrollment[a] and delivery	2001, Thiadiaye-Senegal, seasonal	Tuikue Ndam et al. 2006
		Third trimester	2000–2002, Blantyre-Malawi, perennial	Brolin et al. 2010
		During pregnancy[c]	2005–2008, Ouidah-Benin, perennial	Gnidehou et al. 2010
		Delivery	2003–2006, Manhica-Mozambique, perennial	Mayor et al. 2013
		Enrollment[a]	2008–2010, Comé-Benin, perennial	Ndam et al. 2015
	No	Delivery	2001–2005, Muheza-Tanzania, perennial	Oleinikov et al. 2007
		Enrollment[a] and delivery	2001, Thiadiaye-Senegal, seasonal	Dechavanne et al. 2015
		Delivery	2008–2010, Comé-Benin, perennial	Ndam et al. 2015
DBL6	Yes	Enrollment[a] and delivery	2001, Thiadiaye-Senegal, seasonal	Tuikue Ndam et al. 2006
		Delivery	2001–2005, Muheza-Tanzania, perennial	Oleinikov et al. 2007
		Delivery	2003–2006, Manhica-Mozambique, perennial	Mayor et al. 2013
	No	Third trimester	2000–2002, Blantyre-Malawi, perennial	Brolin et al. 2010
		Enrollment[a] and delivery	2001, Thiadiaye-Senegal, seasonal	Dechavanne et al. 2015

[a]Samples collected at enrollment at any time during the first 6 months of gestation.
[b]Study year and site information not available.
[c]Samples collected during pregnancy, but timing not specified.

Cite this article as *Cold Spring Harb Perspect Med* doi: 10.1101/cshperspect.a025551

acute or chronic malaria infection, higher DBL5 antibody levels reduced the risk of LBW delivery (Salanti et al. 2004). Among Mozambican women infected at least once during their pregnancy, above-the-median antibody levels to DBL3X and DBL6ε, as well as the unrelated merozoite antigen AMA1, were associated with increased birth weight and gestational age (Mayor et al. 2013). In Benin, high DBL1-ID1-DBL2 antibody levels during the first two trimesters reduced the risk of LBW (Ndam et al. 2015). Additional studies that define relationships between specific antibody and protection are needed to advance the development of a vaccine to prevent malaria during pregnancy.

DIAGNOSIS

Despite its large burden of disease, *P. falciparum* infection can be difficult to diagnose during pregnancy, particularly in semi-immune women who often are asymptomatic during infection. Although IEs accumulate in the placenta, parasite density in peripheral blood can be too low for detection by routine BS microscopy. BS is the gold standard for malaria diagnosis and is ideal for discriminating the different human malaria parasite species; however, quality varies substantially, and the requirement for microscope and trained microscopist limits BS availability or quality in many places. Paradoxically, although pregnancy malaria is difficult to recognize and diagnose, many women in endemic areas unnecessarily receive antimalarial treatments in the absence of infection. In Mozambique, BS was negative in more than 70% of pregnant women with clinical symptoms of malaria (Bardaji et al. 2008). Because antimalarials are often prescribed on the basis of clinical and not laboratory criteria, many pregnant women receive unnecessary treatment with drugs that have an unclear safety profile especially in the first trimester.

Rapid diagnostic tests (RDTs) are a more recent tool that is gaining wider acceptance for diagnosis in the general population. RDTs use immunochromatographic approaches to detect soluble *Plasmodium* antigens, including histidine-rich protein-2 (HRP-2), aldolase, and parasite lactate dehydrogenase (pLDH). The OptiMAL test, based on pLDH detection, gave varying results when compared with peripheral BS in different studies of pregnant women, with sensitivity ranging from 15% to 97% and specificity from 91% to 98% (Mankhambo et al. 2002; VanderJagt et al. 2005; Tagbor et al. 2008). The sensitivity of the OptiMAL test increases with parasite density, and all samples with parasite density < 100 per μl were misdiagnosed in one study (VanderJagt et al. 2005). In a larger study (Tagbor et al. 2008), OptiMal had 100% sensitivity and 93% specificity for parasite densities > 50 per μl blood, but sensitivity of only 57% at lower densities. RDTs that detect pLDH have the advantage that they are designed to detect only live parasites; however, gametocytemia in the absence of asexual blood stage parasites can still produce positive results.

In general, RDTs that detect HRP-2 have a higher sensitivity than those that detect pLDH. In one study, RDT-HRP-2 sensitivity was greater than 90% when compared with peripheral BS, and 80%–95% when compared with placental BS with specificity between 61% and 94% (Leke et al. 1999; Mockenhaupt et al. 2002; Singer et al. 2004; Mayor et al. 2012). In a multicenter study in West Africa, RDTs that combine the detection of pLDH and HRP-2 showed similar good sensitivity at some but not all sites (range 63.6%–95.1% in primigravidae) when compared with diagnoses using BS and PCR at first antenatal visits, but not at subsequent visits or at delivery in Ghanaian women (<60% sensitivity in all parity groups at delivery) (Williams et al. 2015). In Papua New Guinea, HRP-2/pLDH RDTs were deemed insufficiently sensitive for intermittent screening of asymptomatic anemic women (Umbers et al. 2015). A weakness of RDT-HRP-2 tests is the prolonged half-life of the antigen. HRP-2 can be identified in plasma samples several weeks after parasite clearance, and therefore cannot distinguish current from recent infection (Wongsrichanalai et al. 1999; Mayxay et al. 2001; Tjitra et al. 2001). In Burkina Faso, 2/32 parasitemic pregnant women continued to have detectable HRP-2 antigen 28 d after receiving artemisinin combination therapy (Kattenberg et al. 2012). These shortcomings hinder the use of existing RDTs for managing malaria or monitoring treatment efficacy during pregnancy.

DRUGS FOR PREVENTION AND TREATMENT

Intermittent Presumptive Treatment (IPTp)

PM is associated with maternal anemia, LBW deliveries, PTD, and fetal loss. Severe maternal anemia increases the risk of maternal death, and both LBW and PTD increase the risk of infant death. To avoid these poor outcomes, measures to prevent PM have been recommended by the World Health Organization (WHO). The first agent used to prevent PM was weekly choloroquine (CQ) at a prophylaxis dose. However, the emergence of CQ-resistant parasites in sub-Saharan Africa during the 1980s prompted the search for new strategies. A 1992 study in Malawi showed that two treatment doses of SP given during the second and early third trimester significantly reduced the prevalence of PM compared with CQ (Schultz et al. 1994). A subsequent trial in Kenya confirmed that two SP treatment doses reduced PM prevalence in HIV-infected women (Table 5) (Parise et al. 1998).

In the early 2000s, WHO recommended intermittent presumptive treatment (IPTp) for pregnant women in malaria-endemic regions, with at least two curative doses of the antimalarial drug SP, one dose in the second and the other dose in the third trimester of pregnancy. In 2012, WHO updated the recommendation, increasing the number to three or more SP doses. In practice, women in areas of moderate–high malaria transmission should receive SP at each antenatal care visit during the second and third trimesters (because four visits are recommended), with 1 mo intervals between doses (www.who.int/malaria/areas/preventive_thera pies/pregnancy/en).

Owing to the spread of SP resistance in sub-Saharan Africa, artemisinin-based combinations (ACTs) were adopted as the first-line treatment for uncomplicated malaria in the 2000s (Eastman and Fidock 2009). Even as the general population was switching to ACT as treatment policy, the IPTp-SP strategy was being widely adopted for pregnant women. At present, WHO continues to recommend IPTp-SP, even in areas with high levels of SP resistance and treatment failure. Here, we summarize studies that have examined the associations between IPTp-SP and malaria parasitemia detected in maternal peripheral blood or placental blood (Table 5). We do not include studies that only reported an association between IPTp-SP and other pregnancy outcomes because the main goal of IPTp-SP is to improve pregnancy outcomes by preventing PM. Improved outcomes without an effect on parasitological measures are difficult to interpret.

During the years 1992–2002, IPTp-SP significantly reduced PM in studies conducted across Africa. However, most data collected after 2001–2002 in East and Southeast Africa indicate that IPTp-SP lost its efficacy to reduce PM prevalence and/or parasite density. This trend has progressed to West Africa, where one site in Ghana reported that IPTp-SP did not reduce PM prevalence (van Spronsen et al. 2012).

SP resistance results from accumulating mutations in *dhfr* and *dhps* genes. The quintuple *P. falciparum* mutations (three in *Pfdhfr* and two mutations in *Pfdhps*) have been associated with treatment failure (Kublin et al. 2002; Naidoo and Roper 2013), and increased placental parasite density with an increasing number of *Pfdhfr* mutations (Mockenhaupt et al. 2007). A WHO document published in November 2015 (www.who.int/malaria/publications/atoz/istp - and - act - in - pregnancy.pdf) stated that "An association between sextuple mutant haplotypes of *P. falciparum* and decreased birth weight has been reported in observational studies in a few sites in East Africa. Further studies are required to assess this and to devise the best and most cost-effective prevention strategies in areas of very high SP resistance." The policy of continuing IPTp-SP in areas of high resistance is puzzling and inconsistent with WHO directives for malaria treatment (Nosten and McGready 2015), as well as studies that strongly relate *dhfr*/*dhps* mutations to treatment failure.

Currently, IPTp-SP remains efficacious for reducing the rate of PM and/or parasite burden at some sites in West Africa. However, even in

Table 5. Studies of IPTp-SP efficacy[a]

References	Study site	Study years	n	Study design	Outcome
Schultz et al. 1994	Mangochi district, Malawi, high transmission	1992	357 (placental BS $n = 159$)	Assigned to one of three arms: (1) weekly CQ, (2) one dose SP followed by weekly CQ, (3) two doses SP	Two doses significantly reduced the rate of peripheral and placental parasitemia
Verhoeff et al. 1998	Chikwawa district, Malawi, high transmission	1993–1994	1837 delivery data: 575	Observational, enrollment at first ANC visit, outcomes measured at delivery	At delivery, no differences in prevalence of placental or peripheral parasitemia between one and two doses
Parise et al. 1998	Kisumu, Kenya, high transmission	1994–1996	2077	Assigned to one of three arms: (1) two doses SP, (2) monthly doses of SP between enrollment and gestational week 34, (3) case management with SP	Two doses or monthly SP significantly reduced the prevalence of infection detected in peripheral and placental samples
Shulman et al. 1999	Kilifi, Kenya, hypertholoendemic and mesoendemic sites	1996–1997	1264	Double-blind, randomized, controlled; number of SP doses (1–3) based on gestational age at enrollment	At gestational week 34, $\geq$ one dose of IPTp-SP significantly reduced the prevalence of peripheral parasitemia; PM: significantly higher proportion of negative by histology in the treatment group; no differences by BS
Feng et al. 2010	Blantyre, Malawi, low transmission	1997–2006	8131	Observational, enrollment at delivery	1997–2001: number of IPTp-SP doses associated with protection from PM 2002–2006: IPTp-SP not associated with a reduction in PM
Harrington et al. 2009	Muheza, Tanzania, high transmission	2002–2005	880	Observational, enrollment at delivery	No IPTp versus $\geq$ one dose: SP usage associated with increased placental parasite density
Gies et al. 2009	Boromo, Burkina Faso, seasonal, high transmission	2004–2006	915 (peripheral blood) 878 (placental blood)	Substudy of larger study to evaluate IPTp	None to one versus > two doses: reduction in the prevalence of infection detected in peripheral and placental blood

Continued

Table 5. *Continued*

References	Study site	Study years	n	Study design	Outcome
Tiono et al. 2009	Bousse district, Burkina Faso, seasonal, high transmission	2004–2005	648	Randomized, three treatment arms: (1) IPTp-SP, (2) weekly CQ, (3) IPTp-CQ	At delivery, the prevalence of maternal peripheral parasitemia significantly lower in IPTp-SP than CQ group; significant reduction in PM in IPTp-SP versus weekly CQ but not versus IPTp-CQ
Menendez et al. 2008	Manhica district, Mozambique, moderate transmission	2003–2005	1030	Double-blind, randomized, placebo-controlled	Placebo + ITN versus SP + ITN: no difference in placental infection Reduction in the prevalence of peripheral blood parasitemia and active placental infection
Ndyomugyenyi et al. 2011	Kabale district, Uganda, low and unstable transmission	2004–2007	5328	Randomized, placebo-controlled, blinded for SP versus placebo but not for ITN use	IPTp versus ITN versus IPTp + ITN: no differences in infection rate at gestational weeks 36–40 and at delivery
Hommerich et al. 2007	Agogo, Ghana, hyper- to holoendemic	2006	226	Observational, enrollment at delivery	No IPTp versus $\geq$ one SP dose: SP associated with decreased placental infection detected by RDT and PCR but not by microscopy
Diakite et al. 2011	Bla district, Mali, seasonal, high transmission	2006–2008	814	Randomized to two treatment arms: (1) two SP does, (2) three SP doses	PM reduced by half after three doses versus two doses
Vanga-Bosson et al. 2011	Côte d'Ivoire, six sites (four urban, two semiurban) in three regions	2008	2044	Observational, enrollment at delivery	None versus one to two doses: reduction in PM
Wilson et al. 2011	Accra, Ghana, moderate transmission	2009	363	Observational, enrollment at ANC (third trimester)	Prior use of IPTp significantly reduced maternal infection
Gutman et al. 2013	Machinga, Malawi, high transmission	2010	703	Observational, enrollment at delivery	None to one dose versus $\geq$ two doses: number of doses had no effect on placental and peripheral parasitemia
Gutman et al. 2015	Machinga and Blantyre, Malawi, high and low transmission	Machinga: 2010 Blantyre: 2009–2011	Machinga: 710 Blantyre: 1141	Observational, enrollment at delivery	Sextuple mutated haplotype in Pfdhfr/Pfdhps associated with significant increase in placental and peripheral parasitemia and parasite density

Cite this article as *Cold Spring Harb Perspect Med* doi: 10.1101/cshperspect.a025551

	Location, transmission	Year	N	Study design	Findings
Mace et al. 2015	Mansa, Zambia, high transmission	2009–2011	435	Observational, enrollment at delivery	<two versus ≥ two doses: no difference in PM, a decrease in any infection (placental including past infection and peripheral blood) among primigravidae
Toure et al. 2014	Côte d'Ivoire, six sites (three rural, three urban), perennial transmission with seasonal peaks	2009–2010	1317	Observational, enrollment at delivery	None versus one versus ≥ two doses: no differences in PM
Cisse et al. 2014	Bobo-Dioulasso, Burkina Faso, seasonal, high transmission	2010	579	Observational, enrollment during routine ANC visit	No association between SP usage and malaria infection prevalence during pregnancy; lower parasite density in women that used SP
Coulibaly et al. 2014	Kita and Kayes regions, Mali; Ziniaré, Burkina Faso, seasonal high transmission	2009–2010 2010–2011	268 (Mali) 312 (BF)	IPTp-SP for clearing asymptomatic infection during pregnancy	Low treatment failure: 1.1% at day 42, PCR adjusted
van Spronsen et al. 2012	Gushegu, Ghana, high transmission	2010	145	Observational, enrollment at delivery	No association between IPTp usage, number of SP doses, and PM
Tonga et al. 2013	Sanaga-Maritime Littoral region, Cameroon, hyperendemic	2011–2012	201	Observational, enrollment at delivery	None to one versus > two doses IPTp: no difference in PM rate
Arinaitwe et al. 2013	Tororo, Uganda, high transmission	2011	566	Observational, enrollment at delivery	<two versus ≥ two doses: no differences in PM rate or parasite density
Braun et al. 2015	Fort Portal, western Uganda, mesoendemic	2013	728	Observational, enrollment at delivery	None versus one to two doses: no differences in placental or peripheral infection rate
Mpogoro et al. 2014	Geita region, Tanzania, high transmission	2014	431	Observational, enrollment at delivery	<three versus ≥ three SP doses: ≥three doses associated with a reduction in PM (26/431 received ≥three doses)

SP, Sulfadoxine–pyrimethamine; CQ, chloroquine; BW, birth weight; LBW, low birth weight; PTD, preterm delivery; SGA, small for gestational age; ITN, insecticide-treated net.
[a]Results from adjusted models presented.

areas with low or moderate SP resistance, the IPTp strategy does not completely prevent PM and the protective effects depend on the timing of the first dose and the interval between treatments (Nosten and McGready 2015).

Alternatives to IPTp-SP

Dihydroartemisinin–Piperaquine

A comparison between three doses of IPTp-SP and three doses or monthly dihydroartemisinin–piperaquine (DP) was recently conducted in Uganda (Kakuru et al. 2016). Peripheral blood parasitemia detected by LAMP was significantly higher in the IPTp-SP group than three doses or monthly DP. Similarly, PM (combined active and past infection) was significantly higher among women who received IPTp-SP than women that received three doses or monthly treatment with DP. Although, among primigravid women, the rate of PM was similar between the three groups, the amount of pigment deposition was significantly higher in the IPTp-SP groups, which might indicate higher parasite densities in past infections. The risk of any poor pregnancy outcome (PTD, LBW, congenital anomaly, stillbirth, spontaneous abortion) was significantly lower among women receiving monthly DP than women who received three doses of DP or IPTp-SP.

Mefloquine

In a comparison of IPTp-SP and IPTp-mefloquine (MQ) (Briand et al. 2009), Beninese women received either two doses of IPTp-SP or two doses of MQ (15 mg/kg) during pregnancy. PM was significantly less frequent in the MQ group, but other endpoints including birth weight, LBW, and maternal anemia were similar (Briand et al. 2009). Adverse events were more common with MQ, and overall tolerability was lower (Briand et al. 2009). Another trial compared two doses of IPTp with SP or MQ in women who also received long-lasting insecticide-treated nets. MQ was given as a single 15 mg/kg dose or as a split dose (Gonzalez et al. 2014a). The rates of maternal parasitemia (by BS) at delivery,

mild anemia at delivery, and clinical malaria during pregnancy were significantly lower in the MQ group, while PM (by BS or histology), birth weight, and LBW rates were similar (Gonzalez et al. 2014a). As in Benin, tolerability was poor even in the group that received MQ as a split dose (Gonzalez et al. 2014a).

IPTp-SP is not recommended for HIV-infected women who take daily cotrimoxazole prophylaxis, owing to the potential adverse effects of taking two antifolate drugs with a common mechanism of action (reviewed in Peters et al. 2007). Two trials evaluated MQ as IPTp in women taking cotrimoxazole (Gonzalez et al. 2014b;). In a multicenter study conducted in East and Southeast Africa, peripheral and placental parasitemia (defined by BS, PCR, or histology) and nonobstetric admission were less frequent among women that received three doses of IPTp-MQ, while maternal anemia, birth weight, and gestational age at delivery were similar between groups (Gonzalez et al. 2014b). Notably, IPTp-MQ was associated with increased mother-to-child transmission of HIV, and again showed poor tolerability (Gonzalez et al. 2014b). In West Africa, IPTp with three MQ doses (15 mg/kg) was compared with cotrimoxazole alone and cotrimoxazole plus IPTp-MQ (Denoeud-Ndam et al. 2014). At delivery, PM was not detected by PCR in any of the 105 women in the cotrimoxazole + IPTp-MQ group compared with 5/103 women in the cotrimoxazole alone group. Maternal anemia, infection rate during pregnancy detected by PCR, and birth weight did not differ between groups. Again, adverse events were more common among women receiving MQ (Denoeud-Ndam et al. 2014). Although MQ can be effective to reduce infection, tolerability has been poor even when used at a split dose, and thus may result in low compliance if used for prevention.

Chloroquine–Azithromycin Combination

The CQ–azithromycin combination was compared with SP for use as IPTp in a trial that included six sites in Africa. However, interim analyses showed that the new combination was not superior to the existing intervention, and the study was terminated early (ClinicalTrials .gov Identifier: NCT01103063).

Intermittent Screening and Treatment

The Intermittent Screening and Treatment in pregnancy (ISTp) strategy entails screening women for malaria infection during antenatal clinic visits using an RDT and treating infection with an antimalarial drug. A multicenter trial comparing ISTp-AL (artemether–lumefantrine) with IPTp-SP was recently conducted in West Africa in sites with seasonal malaria and low SP resistance (Tagbor et al. 2015). PM, birth weight, and maternal hemoglobin were similar between ISTp-AL and IPTp-SP in the overall analysis and within individual sites (Tagbor et al. 2015). Malaria infections between scheduled visits were significantly more frequent in women randomized to the ISTp-AL (Tagbor et al. 2015). In an area of high malaria transmission and high SP resistance in Kenya, women were randomized to three interventions: ISTp with dihydroartemisinin–piperaquine (DP), IPTp with DP, and IPTp-SP (Desai et al. 2015). Malaria infection at delivery was diagnosed by detection of parasites with BS on peripheral or placental blood, or with RDT or PCR on peripheral blood. Risks of malaria infection, mild anemia (HGB < 11 g/dL), stillbirth, and early infant mortality were significantly reduced in women receiving IPTp-DP rather than IPTp-SP or ISTp-DP, while ISTp-DP and IPTp-SP groups did not differ (Desai et al. 2015). The failure of ISTp-DP to improve on IPTp with the failing drug SP echoes the early evaluation of IPTp-SP in 1992–1994 (Parise et al. 1998) in which case management was inferior to IPTp-SP.

Differences in ISTp efficacy between the two studies could result from different transmission patterns, being highly seasonal in West Africa versus perennial with seasonal peaks in Kenya. Peripheral parasite density at delivery in Kenya was much lower than the density at enrollment in West Africa. Although the different assessment times could influence BS results, lower parasite densities might explain the lower sensitivity of RDT to detect PM, potentially rendering the IST strategy ineffective in Kenya (Fried et al. 2012; Desai et al. 2015).

Treatment of Malaria during Pregnancy

Currently, artemisinin combination therapy (ACT) is the first-line treatment for malaria in nonpregnant individuals. Owing to safety concerns, WHO recommends that pregnant women be treated with quinine and clindamycin during the first trimester and with ACT in the second and third trimesters. A multicenter trial reported high cure rate with four different ACTs (artemether–lumefantrine, amodiaquine–artesunate, dihydroartemisinin–piperaquine, and mefloquine–artesunate), with artemether–lumefantrine showing the lowest cure rate of 94.8% (The PREGACT Study Group 2016). Pregnancy outcomes were similar between the four groups and both artemether–lumefantrine and dihydroartemisinin–piperaquine had fewer adverse events than amodiaquine–artesunate, and mefloquine–artesunate (The PREGACT Study Group 2016). Analyses of first-trimester antimalarial treatment records at Shoklo Malaria Research Unit in Thailand have shown that artesunate is as safe as choloroquine and quinine (McGready et al. 2012). In a similar study in Kenya, ACT treatment during the first-trimester (based on the review of treatment records) did not increase the risk of miscarriage, compared with women who did not receive any treatment or women who received quinine (Dellicour et al. 2015). However, community surveillance, which included cases without a treatment record, suggested that exposure to ACT may increase the risk of miscarriage compared with women that never received antimalarial drugs (Dellicour et al. 2015). Because both symptomatic and asymptomatic malaria infections (with *P. falciparum* or *P. vivax*) during the first trimester increase the risk of miscarriage (McGready et al. 2012), it might be difficult to assess the contribution attributable to ACT when the comparison group includes never-infected women. Both studies had a small number of women that received either ACT or quinine, and clinical trials to compare the safety of ACT to quinine during the first trimester are needed.

FUTURE PERSPECTIVES

Pregnant women are at increased risk of malaria, making this demographic group an important parasite reservoir in the community and a key target for interventions during elimination efforts (Fig. 1). However, pregnant women and women of childbearing age will require special considerations during any mass administration campaigns. Semi-immune women often carry *P. falciparum* PM with low peripheral parasite burdens and few acute symptoms, hindering diagnosis and complicating efforts to use targeted treatment as a strategy. Drugs currently used for malaria prevention during pregnancy have lost or are losing their efficacy, and finding new drugs is stymied by concerns for teratogenicity and embryotoxicity; dihydroartemisinin–piperaquine has shown promise as the monthly presumptive treatment to prevent poor pregnancy outcomes, although it may not reduce PM prevalence. Vaccines have been important tools for the elimination of other infectious pathogens, and women commonly receive vaccines such as tetanus toxoid during pregnancy. Vaccines could be particularly useful for the control of PM: *P. falciparum* parasites sequester in the human placenta by adhesion to CSA, and women acquire antibodies against CSA-binding parasites over successive pregnancies, rendering primigravidae most susceptible and suggesting a vaccine is feasible. Vaccines that control PM, prevent human infection, or block onward transmission to mosquitoes, will require testing to assess their ability to interrupt transmission through pregnant women. More effort must be made to address the safety of drugs, vaccines, and antivector measures among women of childbearing age, particularly during the first trimester of pregnancy when safety concerns are greatest.

CONCLUDING REMARKS

Tens of millions of pregnant women are at risk of malaria every year, but the management of malaria is particularly complex in this population. In areas of low transmission, women lacking immunity are at increased risk of acute severe disease and of death during *P. falciparum* infection, and therefore active surveillance and prompt treatment of malaria in these women is paramount. In areas of high stable transmission, acquired immunity can mask acute symptoms but leave women vulnerable to insidious effects such as severe maternal anemia and perinatal, neonatal, or postneonatal death for their offspring. Existing diagnostic tools are inadequate to detect malaria infection in semi-immune women, and the drugs CQ and SP used as preventive interventions have lost or are losing their benefits; a replacement drug has yet to be identified that is sufficiently safe, tolerable, and effective as prevention, although studies of dihydroartemisinin–piperaquine are encouraging. Naturally acquired resistance to malaria suggests that vaccines are feasible by inducing antibodies against the CSA-binding parasites that sequester in the human placenta. Passive or active immunization that provides women with a window of coverage throughout pregnancy is an appealing alternative to drug prevention strategies. The need for new preventive and diagnostic tools for this vulnerable population is urgent, but is often overlooked by policymakers and funding agencies. This dearth of safe and effective tools to control malaria in pregnant women will hinder future malaria elimination campaigns, because any woman of childbearing age will likely be excluded from participation if pregnancy status is unknown.

ACKNOWLEDGMENTS

The authors acknowledge J. Patrick Gorres (Laboratory of Malaria Immunology and Vaccinology, National Institutes of Health [NIH]) for proofreading and editing this review, and Alan Hoofring (NIH Medical Arts, NIH) for preparing the illustration. M.F. and P.E.D. are supported by the Intramural Research Program of the National Institute of Allergy and Infectious Diseases (NIAID), NIH.

REFERENCES

Abrams ET, Brown H, Chensue SW, Turner GD, Tadesse E, Lema VM, Molyneux ME, Rochford R, Meshnick SR,

 Cite this article as *Cold Spring Harb Perspect Med* doi: 10.1101/cshperspect.a025551

Rogerson SJ. 2003. Host response to malaria during pregnancy: Placental monocyte recruitment is associated with elevated β chemokine expression. *J Immunol* **170:** 2759–2764.

Achur RN, Valiyaveettil M, Alkhalil A, Ockenhouse CF, Gowda DC. 2000. Characterization of proteoglycans of human placenta and identification of unique chondroitin sulfate proteoglycans of the intervillous spaces that mediate the adherence of *Plasmodium falciparum*–infected erythrocytes to the placenta. *J Biol Chem* **275:** 40344–40356.

Aitken EH, Mbewe B, Luntamo M, Maleta K, Kulmala T, Friso MJ, Fowkes FJ, Beeson JG, Ashorn P, Rogerson SJ. 2010. Antibodies to chondroitin sulfate A-binding infected erythrocytes: Dynamics and protection during pregnancy in women receiving intermittent preventive treatment. *J Infect Dis* **201:** 1316–1325.

Alkhalil A, Achur RN, Valiyaveettil M, Ockenhouse CF, Gowda DC. 2000. Structural requirements for the adherence of *Plasmodium falciparum*–infected erythrocytes to chondroitin sulfate proteoglycans of human placenta. *J Biol Chem* **275:** 40357–40364.

Andrews KT, Klatt N, Adams Y, Mischnick P, Schwartz-Albiez R. 2005. Inhibition of chondroitin-4-sulfate-specific adhesion of *Plasmodium falciparum*–infected erythrocytes by sulfated polysaccharides. *Infect Immun* **73:** 4288–4294.

Arinaitwe E, Ades V, Walakira A, Ninsiima B, Mugagga O, Patil TS, Schwartz A, Kamya MR, Nasr S, Chang M, et al. 2013. Intermittent preventive therapy with sulfadoxine-pyrimethamine for malaria in pregnancy: A cross-sectional study from Tororo, Uganda. *PLoS ONE* **8:** e73073.

Ataide R, Hasang W, Wilson DW, Beeson JG, Mwapasa V, Molyneux ME, Meshnick SR, Rogerson SJ. 2010. Using an improved phagocytosis assay to evaluate the effect of HIV on specific antibodies to pregnancy-associated malaria. *PLoS ONE* **5:** e10807.

Ataide R, Mwapasa V, Molyneux ME, Meshnick SR, Rogerson SJ. 2011. Antibodies that induce phagocytosis of malaria infected erythrocytes: Effect of HIV infection and correlation with clinical outcomes. *PLoS ONE* **6:** e22491.

Awine T, Belko MM, Oduro AR, Oyakhirome S, Tagbor H, Chandramohan D, Milligan P, Cairns M, Greenwood B, Williams JE. 2016. The risk of malaria in Ghanaian infants born to women managed in pregnancy with intermittent screening and treatment for malaria or intermittent preventive treatment with sulfadoxine/pyrimethamine. *Malaria J* **15:** 46.

Babakhanyan A, Leke RG, Salanti A, Bobbili N, Gwanmesia P, Leke RJ, Quakyi IA, Chen JJ, Taylor DW. 2014. The antibody response of pregnant Cameroonian women to VAR2CSA ID1-ID2a, a small recombinant protein containing the CSA-binding site. *PLoS ONE* **9:** e88173.

Bardaji A, Sigauque B, Bruni L, Romagosa C, Sanz S, Mabunda S, Mandomando I, Aponte J, Sevene E, Alonso PL, et al. 2008. Clinical malaria in African pregnant women. *Malaria J* **7:** 27.

Beeson JG, Brown GV, Molyneux ME, Mhango C, Dzinjalamala F, Rogerson SJ. 1999. *Plasmodium falciparum* isolates from infected pregnant women and children are associated with distinct adhesive and antigenic properties. *J Infect Dis* **180:** 464–472.

Beeson JG, Mann EJ, Elliott SR, Lema VM, Tadesse E, Molyneux ME, Brown GV, Rogerson SJ. 2004. Antibodies to variant surface antigens of *Plasmodium falciparum*–infected erythrocytes and adhesion inhibitory antibodies are associated with placental malaria and have overlapping and distinct targets. *J Infect Dis* **189:** 540–551.

Brabin BJ. 1983. An analysis of malaria in pregnancy in Africa. *Bull World Health Org* **61:** 1005–1016.

Braun V, Rempis E, Schnack A, Decker S, Rubaihayo J, Tumwesigye NM, Theuring S, Harms G, Busingye P, Mockenhaupt FP. 2015. Lack of effect of intermittent preventive treatment for malaria in pregnancy and intense drug resistance in western Uganda. *Malaria J* **14:** 372.

Briand V, Bottero J, Noel H, Masse V, Cordel H, Guerra J, Kossou H, Fayomi B, Ayemonna P, Fievet N, et al. 2009. Intermittent treatment for the prevention of malaria during pregnancy in Benin: A randomized, open-label equivalence trial comparing sulfadoxine-pyrimethamine with mefloquine. *J Infect Dis* **200:** 991–1001.

Brolin KJ, Persson KE, Wahlgren M, Rogerson SJ, Chen Q. 2010. Differential recognition of *P. falciparum* VAR2CSA domains by naturally acquired antibodies in pregnant women from a malaria endemic area. *PLoS ONE* **5:** e9230.

Chaisavaneeyakorn S, Moore JM, Mirel L, Othoro C, Otieno J, Chaiyaroj SC, Shi YP, Nahlen BL, Lal AA, Udhayakumar V. 2003. Levels of macrophage inflammatory protein 1 α (MIP-1 α) and MIP-1 β in intervillous blood plasma samples from women with placental malaria and human immunodeficiency virus infection. *Clin Diagn Lab Immunol* **10:** 631–636.

Cisse M, Sangare I, Lougue G, Bamba S, Bayane D, Guiguemde RT. 2014. Prevalence and risk factors for *Plasmodium falciparum* malaria in pregnant women attending antenatal clinic in Bobo-Dioulasso (Burkina Faso). *BMC Infect Dis* **14:** 631.

Coulibaly SO, Kayentao K, Taylor S, Guirou EA, Khairallah C, Guindo N, Djimde M, Bationo R, Soulama A, Dabira E, et al. 2014. Parasite clearance following treatment with sulphadoxine-pyrimethamine for intermittent preventive treatment in Burkina-Faso and Mali: 42-day in vivo follow-up study. *Malaria J* **13:** 41.

Dechavanne S, Srivastava A, Gangnard S, Nunes-Silva S, Dechavanne C, Fievet N, Deloron P, Chene A, Gamain B. 2015. Parity-dependent recognition of DBL1X-3X suggests an important role of the VAR2CSA high-affinity CSA-binding region in the development of the humoral response against placental malaria. *Infect Immun* **83:** 2466–2474.

Denoeud-Ndam L, Zannou DM, Fourcade C, Taron-Brocard C, Porcher R, Atadokpede F, Komongui DG, Dossou-Gbete L, Afangnihoun A, Ndam NT, et al. 2014. Cotrimoxazole prophylaxis versus mefloquine intermittent preventive treatment to prevent malaria in HIV-infected pregnant women: Two randomized controlled trials. *J Acquir Immune Defic Syndr* **65:** 198–206.

Dellicour S, Tatem AJ, Guerra CA, Snow RW, ter Kuile FO. 2010. Quantifying the number of pregnancies at risk of malaria in 2007: A demographic study. *PLoS Med* **7:** e1000221.

Dellicour S, Desai M, Aol G, Oneko M, Ouma P, Bigogo G, Burton DC, Breiman RF, Hamel MJ, Slutsker L, et al. 2015. Risks of miscarriage and inadvertent exposure to artemisinin derivatives in the first trimester of pregnancy: A prospective cohort study in western Kenya. *Malaria J* **14:** 461.

Desai M, Gutman J, L'Lanziva A, Otieno K, Juma E, Kariuki S, Ouma P, Were V, Laserson K, Katana A, et al. 2015. Intermittent screening and treatment or intermittent preventive treatment with dihydroartemisinin–piperaquine versus intermittent preventive treatment with sulfadoxine-pyrimethamine for the control of malaria during pregnancy in western Kenya: An open-label, three-group, randomised controlled superiority trial. *Lancet* **386:** 2507–2519.

Diakite OS, Kayentao K, Traore BT, Djimde A, Traore B, Diallo M, Ongoiba A, Doumtabe D, Doumbo S, Traore MS, et al. 2011. Superiority of 3 over 2 doses of intermittent preventive treatment with sulfadoxine-pyrimethamine for the prevention of malaria during pregnancy in mali: A randomized controlled trial. *Clin Infect Dis* **53:** 215–223.

Dong S, Kurtis JD, Pond-Tor S, Kabyemela E, Duffy PE, Fried M. 2012. CXC ligand 9 response to malaria during pregnancy is associated with low-birth-weight deliveries. *Infect Immun* **80:** 3034–3038.

Duffy PE. 2001. Immunity to malaria: Different host, different parasite. In *Malaria in pregnancy: Deadly parasite, susceptible host* (ed. Duffy PE, Fried M), pp. 71–127. Taylor & Francis, New York.

Duffy PE, Desowitz RS. 2001. Pregnancy malaria throughout history: Dangerous labors. In *Malaria in pregnancy: Deadly parasite, susceptible host* (ed. Duffy PE, Fried M), pp. 1–25. Taylor & Francis, New York.

Duffy PE, Fried M. 2003. Antibodies that inhibit *Plasmodium falciparum* adhesion to chondroitin sulfate A are associated with increased birth weight and the gestational age of newborns. *Infect Immun* **71:** 6620–6623.

Duffy PE, Fried M. 2011. Pregnancy malaria: Cryptic disease, apparent solution. *Mem Inst Oswaldo Cruz* **106:** 64–69.

Eastman RT, Fidock DA. 2009. Artemisinin-based combination therapies: A vital tool in efforts to eliminate malaria. *Nat Rev Microbiol* **7:** 864–874.

Elliott SR, Brennan AK, Beeson JG, Tadesse E, Molyneux ME, Brown GV, Rogerson SJ. 2005. Placental malaria induces variant-specific antibodies of the cytophilic subtypes immunoglobulin G1 (IgG1) and IgG3 that correlate with adhesion inhibitory activity. *Infect Immun* **73:** 5903–5907.

Feng G, Aitken E, Yosaatmadja F, Kalilani L, Meshnick SR, Jaworowski A, Simpson JA, Rogerson SJ. 2009. Antibodies to variant surface antigens of *Plasmodium falciparum*–infected erythrocytes are associated with protection from treatment failure and the development of anemia in pregnancy. *J Infect Dis* **200:** 299–306.

Feng G, Simpson JA, Chaluluka E, Molyneux ME, Rogerson SJ. 2010. Decreasing burden of malaria in pregnancy in Malawian women and its relationship to use of intermittent preventive therapy or bed nets. *PLoS ONE* **5:** e12012.

Fievet N, Ringwald P, Bickii J, Dubois B, Maubert B, Le Hesran JY, Cot M, Deloron P. 1996. Malaria cellular immune responses in neonates from Cameroon. *Parasite Immunol* **18:** 483–490.

Fievet N, Le Hesran JY, Cottrell G, Doucoure S, Diouf I, Ndiaye JL, Bertin G, Gaye O, Sow S, Deloron P. 2006. Acquisition of antibodies to variant antigens on the surface of *Plasmodium falciparum*–infected erythrocytes during pregnancy. *Infect Genet Evol* **6:** 459–463.

Fried M, Duffy PE. 1996. Adherence of *Plasmodium falciparum* to chondroitin sulfate A in the human placenta. *Science* **272:** 1502–1504.

Fried M, Nosten F, Brockman A, Brabin BJ, Duffy PE. 1998a. Maternal antibodies block malaria. *Nature* **395:** 851–852.

Fried M, Muga RO, Misore AO, Duffy PE. 1998b. Malaria elicits type 1 cytokines in the human placenta: IFN-γ and TNF-α associated with pregnancy outcomes. *J Immunol* **160:** 2523–2530.

Fried M, Lauder RM, Duffy PE. 2000. *Plasmodium falciparum*: Adhesion of placental isolates modulated by the sulfation characteristics of the glycosaminoglycan receptor. *Exp Parasitol* **95:** 75–78.

Fried M, Domingo GJ, Gowda CD, Mutabingwa TK, Duffy PE. 2006. *Plasmodium falciparum*: Chondroitin sulfate A is the major receptor for adhesion of parasitized erythrocytes in the placenta. *Exp Parasitol* **113:** 36–42.

Fried M, Muehlenbachs A, Duffy PE. 2012. Diagnosing malaria in pregnancy: An update. *Expert Rev Anti Infect Ther* **10:** 1177–1187.

Garner P, Gulmezoglu AM. 2006. Drugs for preventing malaria in pregnant women. *Cochrane Database Syst Rev* doi: 10.1002/14651858.CD000169.pub2.

Garnham PCC. 1938. The placenta in malaria with special reference to reticulo-endothelial immunity. *Trans R Soc Trop Med Hyg* **32:** 13–34.

Gies S, Coulibaly SO, Ky C, Ouattara FT, Brabin BJ, D'Alessandro U. 2009. Community-based promotional campaign to improve uptake of intermittent preventive antimalarial treatment in pregnancy in Burkina Faso. *Am J Trop Med Hyg* **80:** 460–469.

Gnidehou S, Jessen L, Gangnard S, Ermont C, Triqui C, Quiviger M, Guitard J, Lund O, Deloron P, Ndam NT. 2010. Insight into antigenic diversity of VAR2CSA-DBL5ε domain from multiple *Plasmodium falciparum* placental isolates. *PLoS ONE* **5:** e13105.

Goncalves BP, Huang CY, Morrison R, Holte S, Kabyemela E, Prevots DR, Fried M, Duffy PE. 2014. Parasite burden and severity of malaria in Tanzanian children. *N Engl J Med* **370:** 1799–1808.

Gonzalez R, Mombo-Ngoma G, Ouedraogo S, Kakolwa MA, Abdulla S, Accrombessi M, Aponte JJ, Akerey-Diop D, Basra A, Briand V, et al. 2014a. Intermittent preventive treatment of malaria in pregnancy with mefloquine in HIV-negative women: A multicentre randomized controlled trial. *PLoS Med* **11:** e1001733.

Gonzalez R, Desai M, Macete E, Ouma P, Kakolwa MA, Abdulla S, Aponte JJ, Bulo H, Kabanywanyi AM, Katana A, et al. 2014b. Intermittent preventive treatment of malaria in pregnancy with mefloquine in HIV-infected women receiving cotrimoxazole prophylaxis: A multicenter randomized placebo-controlled trial. *PLoS Med* **11:** e1001735.

Greenwood BM, Greenwood AM, Snow RW, Byass P, Bennett S, Hatib-N'Jie AB. 1989. The effects of malaria chemoprophylaxis given by traditional birth attendants on the course and outcome of pregnancy. *Trans R Soc Trop Med Hyg* **83:** 589–594.

Greenwood AM, Armstrong JR, Byass P, Snow RW, Greenwood BM. 1992. Malaria chemoprophylaxis, birth weight and child survival. *Trans R Soc Trop Med Hyg* **86:** 483–485.

Gutman J, Mwandama D, Wiegand RE, Ali D, Mathanga DP, Skarbinski J. 2013. Effectiveness of intermittent preventive treatment with sulfadoxine-pyrimethamine during pregnancy on maternal and birth outcomes in Machinga district, Malawi. *J Infect Dis* **208:** 907–916.

Gutman J, Kalilani L, Taylor S, Zhou Z, Wiegand RE, Thwai KL, Mwandama D, Khairallah C, Madanitsa M, Chaluluka E, et al. 2015. The A581G mutation in the gene encoding *Plasmodium falciparum* dihydropteroate synthetase reduces the effectiveness of sulfadoxine-pyrimethamine preventive therapy in Malawian pregnant women. *J Infect Dis* **211:** 1997–2005.

Harrington WE, Mutabingwa TK, Muehlenbachs A, Sorensen B, Bolla MC, Fried M, Duffy PE. 2009. Competitive facilitation of drug-resistant *Plasmodium falciparum* malaria parasites in pregnant women who receive preventive treatment. *Proc Natl Acad Sci* **106:** 9027–9032.

Hommerich L, von Oertzen C, Bedu-Addo G, Holmberg V, Acquah PA, Eggelte TA, Bienzle U, Mockenhaupt FP. 2007. Decline of placental malaria in southern Ghana after the implementation of intermittent preventive treatment in pregnancy. *Malaria J* **6:** 144.

Ismail MR, Ordi J, Menendez C, Ventura PJ, Aponte JJ, Kahigwa E, Hirt R, Cardesa A, Alonso PL. 2000. Placental pathology in malaria: A histological, immunohistochemical, and quantitative study. *Hum Pathol* **31:** 85–93.

Jaworowski A, Fernandes LA, Yosaatmadja F, Feng G, Mwapasa V, Molyneux ME, Meshnick SR, Lewis J, Rogerson SJ. 2009. Relationship between human immunodeficiency virus type 1 coinfection, anemia, and levels and function of antibodies to variant surface antigens in pregnancy-associated malaria. *Clin Vaccine Immunol* **16:** 312–319.

Kabyemela ER, Fried M, Kurtis JD, Mutabingwa TK, Duffy PE. 2008. Fetal responses during placental malaria modify the risk of low birth weight. *Infect Immun* **76:** 1527–1534.

Kabyemela E, Goncalves BP, Prevots DR, Morrison R, Harrington W, Gwamaka M, Kurtis JD, Fried M, Duffy PE. 2013. Cytokine profiles at birth predict malaria severity during infancy. *PLoS ONE* **8:** e77214.

Kakuru A, Jagannathan P, Muhindo MK, Natureeba P, Awori P, Nakalembe M, Opira B, Olwoch P, Ategeka J, Nayebare P, et al. 2016. Dihydroartemisinin–piperaquine for the prevention of malaria in pregnancy. *N Engl J Med* **374:** 928–939.

Kattenberg JH, Tahita CM, Versteeg IA, Tinto H, Traore-Coulibaly M, Schallig HD, Mens PF. 2012. Antigen persistence of rapid diagnostic tests in pregnant women in Nanoro, Burkina Faso, and the implications for the diagnosis of malaria in pregnancy. *Trop Med Int Health* **17:** 550–557.

Keen J, Serghides L, Ayi K, Patel SN, Ayisi J, van Eijk A, Steketee R, Udhayakumar V, Kain KC. 2007. HIV impairs opsonic phagocytic clearance of pregnancy-associated malaria parasites. *PLoS Med* **4:** e181.

King CL, Malhotra I, Wamachi A, Kioko J, Mungai P, Wahab SA, Koech D, Zimmerman P, Ouma J, Kazura JW. 2002. Acquired immune responses to *Plasmodium falciparum* merozoite surface protein-1 in the human fetus. *J Immunol* **168:** 356–364.

Kublin JG, Dzinjalamala FK, Kamwendo DD, Malkin EM, Cortese JF, Martino LM, Mukadam RA, Rogerson SJ, Lescano AG, Molyneux ME, et al. 2002. Molecular markers for failure of sulfadoxine-pyrimethamine and chlorproguanil-dapsone treatment of *Plasmodium falciparum* malaria. *J Infect Dis* **185:** 380–388.

Leke RF, Djokam RR, Mbu R, Leke RJ, Fogako J, Megnekou R, Metenou S, Sama G, Zhou Y, Cadigan T, et al. 1999. Detection of the *Plasmodium falciparum* antigen histidine-rich protein 2 in blood of pregnant women: Implications for diagnosing placental malaria. *J Clin Microbiol* **37:** 2992–2996.

Mace KE, Chalwe V, Katalenich BL, Nambozi M, Mubikayi L, Mulele CK, Wiegand RE, Filler SJ, Kamuliwo M, Craig AS, et al. 2015. Evaluation of sulphadoxine-pyrimethamine for intermittent preventive treatment of malaria in pregnancy: A retrospective birth outcomes study in Mansa, Zambia. *Malaria J* **14:** 69.

Malhotra I, Mungai P, Muchiri E, Ouma J, Sharma S, Kazura JW, King CL. 2005. Distinct Th1- and Th2-Type prenatal cytokine responses to *Plasmodium falciparum* erythrocyte invasion ligands. *Infect Immun* **73:** 3462–3470.

Malhotra I, Dent A, Mungai P, Wamachi A, Ouma JH, Narum DL, Muchiri E, Tisch DJ, King CL. 2009. Can prenatal malaria exposure produce an immune tolerant phenotype? A–prospective birth cohort study in Kenya. *PLoS Med* **6:** e1000116.

Mankhambo L, Kanjala M, Rudman S, Lema VM, Rogerson SJ. 2002. Evaluation of the OptiMAL rapid antigen test and species-specific PCR to detect placental *Plasmodium falciparum* infection at delivery. *J Clin Microbiol* **40:** 155–158.

Maubert B, Fievet N, Tami G, Cot M, Boudin C, Deloron P. 1999. Development of antibodies against chondroitin sulfate A–adherent *Plasmodium falciparum* in pregnant women. *Infect Immun* **67:** 5367–5371.

Maubert B, Fievet N, Tami G, Boudin C, Deloron P. 2000. Cytoadherence of *Plasmodium falciparum*–infected erythrocytes in the human placenta. *Parasite Immunol* **22:** 191–199.

Mayor A, Rovira-Vallbona E, Machevo S, Bassat Q, Aguilar R, Quinto L, Jimenez A, Sigauque B, Dobano C, Kumar S, et al. 2011. Parity and placental infection affect antibody responses against *Plasmodium falciparum* during pregnancy. *Infect Immun* **79:** 1654–1659.

Mayor A, Moro L, Aguilar R, Bardaji A, Cistero P, Serra-Casas E, Sigauque B, Alonso PL, Ordi J, Menendez C. 2012. How hidden can malaria be in pregnant women? Diagnosis by microscopy, placental histology, polymerase chain reaction and detection of histidine-rich protein 2 in plasma. *Clin Infect Dis* doi: 10.1093/cid/cis236.

Mayor A, Kumar U, Bardaji A, Gupta P, Jimenez A, Hamad A, Sigauque B, Singh B, Quinto L, Kumar S, et al. 2013. Improved pregnancy outcomes in women exposed to malaria with high antibody levels against *Plasmodium falciparum*. *J Infect Dis* **207:** 1664–1674.

Mayor A, Bardaji A, Macete E, Nhampossa T, Fonseca AM, Gonzalez R, Maculuve S, Cistero P, Ruperez M, Campo J, et al. 2015. Changing trends in *P. falciparum* burden, immunity, and disease in pregnancy. *N Engl J Med*. **373:** 1607–1617.

Mayxay M, Pukrittayakamee S, Chotivanich K, Looareesuwan S, White NJ. 2001. Persistence of *Plasmodium falciparum* HRP-2 in successfully treated acute falciparum malaria. *Trans R Soc Trop Med Hyg* **95:** 179–182.

McGready R, Brockman A, Cho T, Levesque MA, Tkachuk AN, Meshnick SR, Nosten F. 2002. Haemozoin as a marker of placental parasitization. *Trans R Soc Trop Med Hyg* **96:** 644–646.

McGready R, Lee SJ, Wiladphaingern J, Ashley EA, Rijken MJ, Boel M, Simpson JA, Paw MK, Pimanpanarak M, Mu O, et al. 2012. Adverse effects of falciparum and vivax malaria and the safety of antimalarial treatment in early pregnancy: A population-based study. *Lancet Infect Dis* **12:** 388–396.

McGregor IA. 1984. Epidemiology, malaria and pregnancy. *Am J Trop Med Hyg* **33:** 517–525.

Megnekou R, Staalsoe T, Taylor DW, Leke R, Hviid L. 2005. Effects of pregnancy and intensity of *Plasmodium falciparum* transmission on immunoglobulin G subclass responses to variant surface antigens. *Infect Immun* **73:** 4112–4118.

Menendez C, Todd J, Alonso PL, Lulat S, Francis N, Greenwood BM. 1994. Malaria chemoprophylaxis, infection of the placenta and birth weight in Gambian primigravidae. *J Trop Med Hyg* **97:** 244–248.

Menendez C, Bardaji A, Sigauque B, Romagosa C, Sanz S, Serra-Casas E, Macete E, Berenguera A, David C, Dobano C, et al. 2008. A randomized placebo-controlled trial of intermittent preventive treatment in pregnant women in the context of insecticide treated nets delivered through the antenatal clinic. *PLoS ONE* **3:** e1934.

Mockenhaupt FP, Ulmen U, von Gaertner C, Bedu-Addo G, Bienzle U. 2002. Diagnosis of placental malaria. *J Clin Microbiol* **40:** 306–308.

Mockenhaupt FP, Bedu-Addo G, Junge C, Hommerich L, Eggelte TA, Bienzle U. 2007. Markers of sulfadoxine-pyrimethamine-resistant *Plasmodium falciparum* in placenta and circulation of pregnant women. *Antimicrob Agents Chemother* **51:** 332–334.

Moormann AM, Sullivan AD, Rochford RA, Chensue SW, Bock PJ, Nyirenda T, Meshnick SR. 1999. Malaria and pregnancy: Placental cytokine expression and its relationship to intrauterine growth retardation. *J Infect Dis* **180:** 1987–1993.

Mpogoro FJ, Matovelo D, Dosani A, Ngallaba S, Mugono M, Mazigo HD. 2014. Uptake of intermittent preventive treatment with sulphadoxine-pyrimethamine for malaria during pregnancy and pregnancy outcomes: A cross-sectional study in Geita district, North-Western Tanzania. *Malaria J* **13:** 455.

Muehlenbachs A, Fried M, Lachowitzer J, Mutabingwa TK, Duffy PE. 2007. Genome-wide expression analysis of placental malaria reveals features of lymphoid neogenesis during chronic infection. *J Immunol* **179:** 557–565.

Muehlenbachs A, Fried M, McGready R, Harrington WE, Mutabingwa TK, Nosten F, Duffy PE. 2010. A novel histological grading scheme for placental malaria applied in areas of high and low malaria transmission. *J Infect Dis* **202:** 1608–1616.

Muthusamy A, Achur RN, Valiyaveettil M, Botti JJ, Taylor DW, Leke RF, Gowda DC. 2007. Chondroitin sulfate proteoglycan but not hyaluronic acid is the receptor for the adherence of *Plasmodium falciparum*–infected erythrocytes in human placenta, and infected red blood cell adherence up-regulates the receptor expression. *Am J Pathol* **170:** 1989–2000.

Naidoo I, Roper C. 2013. Mapping "partially resistant," "fully resistant," and "super resistant" malaria. *Trends Parasitol* **29:** 505–515.

Ndam NT, Denoeud-Ndam L, Doritchamou J, Viwami F, Salanti A, Nielsen MA, Fievet N, Massougbodji A, Luty AJ, Deloron P. 2015. Protective antibodies against placental malaria and poor outcomes during pregnancy, Benin. *Emerg Infect Dis* **21:** 813–823.

Ndyomugyenyi R, Clarke SE, Hutchison CL, Hansen KS, Magnussen P. 2011. Efficacy of malaria prevention during pregnancy in an area of low and unstable transmission: An individually-randomised placebo-controlled trial using intermittent preventive treatment and insecticide-treated nets in the Kabale Highlands, southwestern Uganda. *Trans R Soc Trop Med Hyg* **105:** 607–616.

Nosten F, McGready R. 2015. Intermittent presumptive treatment in pregnancy with sulfadoxine-pyrimethamine: A counter perspective. *Malaria J* **14:** 248.

Nosten F, ter Kuile F, Maelankirri L, Decludt B, White NJ. 1991. Malaria during pregnancy in an area of unstable endemicity. *Trans R Soc Trop Med Hyg* **85:** 424–429.

Oleinikov AV, Rossnagle E, Francis S, Mutabingwa TK, Fried M, Duffy PE. 2007. Effects of sex, parity, and sequence variation on seroreactivity to candidate pregnancy malaria vaccine antigens. *J Infect Dis* **196:** 155–164.

O'Neil-Dunne I, Achur RN, Agbor-Enoh ST, Valiyaveettil M, Naik RS, Ockenhouse CF, Zhou A, Megnekou R, Leke R, Taylor DW, et al. 2001. Gravidity-dependent production of antibodies that inhibit binding of *Plasmodium falciparum*–infected erythrocytes to placental chondroitin sulfate proteoglycan during pregnancy. *Infect Immun* **69:** 7487–7492.

Ordi J, Ismail MR, Ventura PJ, Kahigwa E, Hirt R, Cardesa A, Alonso PL, Menendez C. 1998. Massive chronic intervillositis of the placenta associated with malaria infection. *Am J Surg Pathol* **22:** 1006–1011.

Parise ME, Ayisi JG, Nahlen BL, Schultz LJ, Roberts JM, Misore A, Muga R, Oloo AJ, Steketee RW. 1998. Efficacy of sulfadoxine-pyrimethamine for prevention of placental malaria in an area of Kenya with a high prevalence of malaria and human immunodeficiency virus infection. *Am J Trop Med Hyg* **59:** 813–822.

Peters PJ, Thigpen MC, Parise ME, Newman RD. 2007. Safety and toxicity of sulfadoxine/pyrimethamine: Implications for malaria prevention in pregnancy using intermittent preventive treatment. *Drug Saf* **30:** 481–501.

Radeva-Petrova D, Kayentao K, ter Kuile FO, Sinclair D, Garner P. 2014. Drugs for preventing malaria in pregnant women in endemic areas: Any drug regimen versus placebo or no treatment. *Cochrane Database Syst Rev* **10:** CD000169.

Rahman MM, Abe SK, Rahman MS, Kanda M, Narita S, Bilano V, Ota E, Gilmour S, Shibuya K. 2016. Maternal anemia and risk of adverse birth and health outcomes in low- and middle-income countries: Systematic review and meta-analysis. *Am J Clin Nutr* doi: 10.3945/ajcn.115.107896.

Ricke CH, Staalsoe T, Koram K, Akanmori BD, Riley EM, Theander TG, Hviid L. 2000. Plasma antibodies from malaria-exposed pregnant women recognize variant surface antigens on *Plasmodium falciparum*–infected erythrocytes in a parity-dependent manner and block parasite adhesion to chondroitin sulfate A. *J Immunol* **165:** 3309–3316.

Rogerson SJ, Brown HC, Pollina E, Abrams ET, Tadesse E, Lema VM, Molyneux ME. 2003. Placental tumor necrosis factor α but not γ interferon is associated with placental malaria and low birth weight in Malawian women. *Infect Immun* **71:** 267–270.

Salanti A, Staalsoe T, Lavstsen T, Jensen AT, Sowa MP, Arnot DE, Hviid L, Theander TG. 2003. Selective upregulation of a single distinctly structured var gene in chondroitin sulphate A-adhering *Plasmodium falciparum* involved in pregnancy-associated malaria. *Mol Microbiol* **49:** 179–191.

Salanti A, Dahlback M, Turner L, Nielsen MA, Barfod L, Magistrado P, Jensen AT, Lavstsen T, Ofori MF, Marsh K, et al. 2004. Evidence for the involvement of VAR2CSA in pregnancy-associated malaria. *J Exp Med* **200:** 1197–1203.

Schultz LJ, Steketee RW, Macheso A, Kazembe P, Chitsulo L, Wirima JJ. 1994. The efficacy of antimalarial regimens containing sulfadoxine-pyrimethamine and/or chloroquine in preventing peripheral and placental *Plasmodium falciparum* infection among pregnant women in Malawi. *Am J Trop Med Hyg* **51:** 515–522.

Schwarz NG, Adegnika AA, Breitling LP, Gabor J, Agnandji ST, Newman RD, Lell B, Issifou S, Yazdanbakhsh M, Luty AJ, et al. 2008. Placental malaria increases malaria risk in the first 30 months of life. *Clin Infect Dis* **47:** 1017–1025.

Serra-Casas E, Menendez C, Bardaji A, Quinto L, Dobano C, Sigauque B, Jimenez A, Mandomando I, Chauhan VS, Chitnis CE, et al. 2010. The effect of intermittent preventive treatment during pregnancy on malarial antibodies depends on HIV status and is not associated with poor delivery outcomes. *J Infect Dis* **201:** 123–131.

Shulman CE, Dorman EK, Cutts F, Kawuondo K, Bulmer JN, Peshu N, Marsh K. 1999. Intermittent sulphadoxine-pyrimethamine to prevent severe anaemia secondary to malaria in pregnancy: A randomised placebo-controlled trial. *Lancet* **353:** 632–636.

Shulman CE, Marshall T, Dorman EK, Bulmer JN, Cutts F, Peshu N, Marsh K. 2001. Malaria in pregnancy: Adverse effects on haemoglobin levels and birthweight in primigravidae and multigravidae. *Trop Med Int Health* **6:** 770–778.

Singer LM, Newman RD, Diarra A, Moran AC, Huber CS, Stennies G, Sirima SB, Konate A, Yameogo M, Sawadogo R, et al. 2004. Evaluation of a malaria rapid diagnostic test for assessing the burden of malaria during pregnancy. *Am J Trop Med Hyg* **70:** 481–485.

Staalsoe T, Megnekou R, Fievet N, Ricke CH, Zornig HD, Leke R, Taylor DW, Deloron P, Hviid L. 2001. Acquisition and decay of antibodies to pregnancy-associated variant antigens on the surface of *Plasmodium falciparum*–in-

fected erythrocytes that protect against placental parasitemia. *J Infect Dis* **184:** 618–626.

Staalsoe T, Shulman CE, Bulmer JN, Kawuondo K, Marsh K, Hviid L. 2004. Variant surface antigen-specific IgG and protection against clinical consequences of pregnancy-associated *Plasmodium falciparum* malaria. *Lancet* **363:** 283–289.

Suguitan AL Jr, Cadigan TJ, Nguyen TA, Zhou A, Leke RJ, Metenou S, Thuita L, Megnekou R, Fogako J, Leke RG, et al. 2003a. Malaria-associated cytokine changes in the placenta of women with pre-term deliveries in Yaounde, Cameroon. *Am J Trop Med Hyg* **69:** 574–581.

Suguitan AL Jr, Leke RG, Fouda G, Zhou A, Thuita L, Metenou S, Fogako J, Megnekou R, Taylor DW. 2003b. Changes in the levels of chemokines and cytokines in the placentas of women with *Plasmodium falciparum* malaria. *J Infect Dis* **188:** 1074–1082.

Tagbor H, Bruce J, Browne E, Greenwood B, Chandramohan D. 2008. Performance of the OptiMAL dipstick in the diagnosis of malaria infection in pregnancy. *Ther Clin Risk Manag* **4:** 631–636.

Tagbor H, Cairns M, Bojang K, Coulibaly SO, Kayentao K, Williams J, Abubakar I, Akor F, Mohammed K, Bationo R, et al. 2015. A non-inferiority, individually randomized trial of intermittent screening and treatment versus intermittent preventive treatment in the control of malaria in pregnancy. *PLoS ONE* **10:** e0132247.

The PREGACT Study Group; Pekyi D, Ampromfi AA, Tinto H, Traore-Coulibaly M, Tahita MC, Valea I, Mwapasa V, Kalilani-Phiri L, Kalanda G, et al. 2016. Four artemisinin-based treatments in African pregnant women with Malaria. *N Engl J Med* **374:** 913–927.

Tiono AB, Ouedraogo A, Bougouma EC, Diarra A, Konate AT, Nebie I, Sirima SB. 2009. Placental malaria and low birth weight in pregnant women living in a rural area of Burkina Faso following the use of three preventive treatment regimens. *Malaria J* **8:** 224.

Tjitra E, Suprianto S, McBroom J, Currie BJ, Anstey NM. 2001. Persistent ICT malaria P.f/P.v panmalarial and HRP-2 antigen reactivity after treatment of *Plasmodium falciparum* malaria is associated with gametocytemia and results in false-positive diagnoses of *Plasmodium vivax* in convalescence. *J Clin Microbiol* **39:** 1025–1031.

Tonga C, Kimbi HK, Anchang-Kimbi JK, Nyabeyeu HN, Bissemou ZB, Lehman LG. 2013. Malaria risk factors in women on intermittent preventive treatment at delivery and their effects on pregnancy outcome in Sanaga-Maritime, Cameroon. *PLoS ONE* **8:** e65876.

Tort J, Rozenberg P, Traore M, Fournier P, Dumont A. 2015. Factors associated with postpartum hemorrhage maternal death in referral hospitals in Senegal and Mali: A cross-sectional epidemiological survey. *BMC Pregnancy Childbirth* **15:** 235.

Toure OA, Kone PL, Coulibaly MA, Ako BA, Gbessi EA, Coulibaly B, LT NG, Koffi D, Beourou S, Soumahoro A, et al. 2014. Coverage and efficacy of intermittent preventive treatment with sulphadoxine pyrimethamine against malaria in pregnancy in Cote d'Ivoire five years after its implementation. *Parasit Vectors* **7:** 495.

Tuikue Ndam NG, Fievet N, Bertin G, Cottrell G, Gaye A, Deloron P. 2004. Variable adhesion abilities and overlapping antigenic properties in placental *Plasmodium falciparum* isolates. *J Infect Dis* **190:** 2001–2009.

Tuikue Ndam NG, Salanti A, Bertin G, Dahlback M, Fievet N, Turner L, Gaye A, Theander T, Deloron P. 2005. High level of var2csa transcription by *Plasmodium falciparum* isolated from the placenta. *J Infect Dis* **192:** 331–335.

Tuikue Ndam NG, Salanti A, Le-Hesran JY, Cottrell G, Fievet N, Turner L, Sow S, Dangou JM, Theander T, Deloron P. 2006. Dynamics of anti-VAR2CSA immunoglobulin G response in a cohort of Senegalese pregnant women. *J Infect Dis* **193:** 713–720.

Tutterrow YL, Avril M, Singh K, Long CA, Leke RJ, Sama G, Salanti A, Smith JD, Leke RG, Taylor DW. 2012a. High levels of antibodies to multiple domains and strains of VAR2CSA correlate with the absence of placental malaria in Cameroonian women living in an area of high *Plasmodium falciparum* transmission. *Infect Immun* **80:** 1479–1490.

Tutterrow YL, Salanti A, Avril M, Smith JD, Pagano IS, Ako S, Fogako J, Leke RG, Taylor DW. 2012b. High avidity antibodies to full-length VAR2CSA correlate with absence of placental malaria. *PLoS ONE* **7:** e40049.

Umbers AJ, Unger HW, Rosanas-Urgell A, Wangnapi RA, Kattenberg JH, Jally S, Silim S, Lufele E, Karl S, Ome-Kaius M, et al. 2015. Accuracy of an HRP-2/panLDH rapid diagnostic test to detect peripheral and placental *Plasmodium falciparum* infection in Papua New Guinean women with anaemia or suspected malaria. *Malaria J* **14:** 412.

VanderJagt TA, Ikeh EI, Ujah IO, Belmonte J, Glew RH, VanderJagt DJ. 2005. Comparison of the OptiMAL rapid test and microscopy for detection of malaria in pregnant women in Nigeria. *Trop Med Int Health* **10:** 39–41.

Vanga-Bosson HA, Coffie PA, Kanhon S, Sloan C, Kouakou F, Eholie SP, Kone M, Dabis F, Menan H, Ekouevi DK. 2011. Coverage of intermittent prevention treatment with sulphadoxine-pyrimethamine among pregnant women and congenital malaria in Cote d'Ivoire. *Malaria J* **10:** 105.

van Spronsen JH, Schneider TA, Atasige S. 2012. Placental malaria and the relationship to pregnancy outcome at Gushegu District Hospital, Northern Ghana. *Trop Doct* **42:** 80–84.

Verhoeff FH, Brabin BJ, Chimsuku L, Kazembe P, Russell WB, Broadhead RL. 1998. An evaluation of the effects of intermittent sulfadoxine-pyrimethamine treatment in pregnancy on parasite clearance and risk of low birthweight in rural Malawi. *Ann Trop Med Parasitol* **92:** 141–150.

Williams JE, Cairns M, Njie F, Laryea Quaye S, Awine T, Oduro A, Tagbor H, Bojang K, Magnussen P, Ter Kuile FO, et al. 2015. The performance of a rapid diagnostic test in detecting malaria infection in pregnant women and the impact of missed infections. *Clin Infect Dis* doi: 10.1093/cid/civ1198.

Williams J, Njie F, Cairns M, Bojang K, Coulibaly SO, Kayentao K, Abubakar I, Akor F, Mohammed K, Bationo R, et al. 2016. Non-falciparum malaria infections in pregnant women in West Africa. *Malaria J* **15:** 53.

Wilson NO, Ceesay FK, Obed SA, Adjei AA, Gyasi RK, Rodney P, Ndjakani Y, Anderson WA, Lucchi NW, Stiles JK. 2011. Intermittent preventive treatment with sulfadoxine-pyrimethamine against malaria and anemia in pregnant women. *Am J Trop Med Hyg* **85:** 12–21.

Wongsrichanalai C, Chuanak N, Tulyayon S, Thanoosingha N, Laboonchai A, Thimasarn K, Brewer TG, Heppner DG. 1999. Comparison of a rapid field immunochromatographic test to expert microscopy for the detection of *Plasmodium falciparum* asexual parasitemia in Thailand. *Acta Trop* **73:** 263–273.

Malaria Genomics in the Era of Eradication

Daniel E. Neafsey[1] and Sarah K. Volkman[2,3,4]

[1]Genome Sequencing and Analysis Program, Broad Institute of MIT and Harvard, Cambridge, Massachusetts 02142

[2]Department of Immunology and Infectious Disease, Harvard T.H. Chan School of Public Health, Boston, Massachusetts 02115

[3]Infectious Disease Initiative, Broad Institute of MIT and Harvard, Cambridge Massachusetts 02142

[4]School of Nursing and Health Sciences, Simmons College, Boston, MA 02115

Correspondence: neafsey@broadinstitute.org; svolkman@hsph.harvard.edu

The first reference genome assembly for the *Plasmodium falciparum* malaria parasite was completed over a decade ago, and the impact of this and other genomic resources on malaria research has been significant. Genomic resources for other malaria parasites are being established, even as *P. falciparum* continues to be the focus of development of new genomic methods and applications. Here we review the impact and applications of genomic data on malaria research, and discuss future needs and directions as genomic data generation becomes less expensive and more decentralized. Specifically, we focus on how population genomic strategies can be utilized to advance the malaria eradication agenda.

The past decade has been marked by tremendous cost reductions for generating genomic data, coupled with considerable knowledge increases required for analysis and interpretation of these genomic data. Consequently, thousands of parasite and vector genomes have been sequenced since the original *Plasmodium falciparum* reference genome assembly in 2002 (Gardner et al. 2002). The maturation of next-generation sequencing (NGS) technology has reduced the cost of sequencing a malaria parasite genome from millions to tens of dollars. The challenge now is how to interpret these genomic data to inform important biological or operational questions, and to prospectively generate genomic data in a strategic manner. Some of the ways genomic approaches can guide or advance the eradication agenda include addressing questions such as: Are intervention approaches working? Where are new infections coming from? Are intervention approaches like drugs and vaccines inducing resistance in parasite populations or only working on a subset of the population? In this review, we examine the application of genomic data toward understanding and eradicating malaria, and outline opportunities for extracting even more value from such data through defined sampling strategies and collection of relevant metadata and phenotypes.

AN ABUNDANCE OF GENOMIC DATA

To date, large genomic datasets have provided a framework for the forward-thinking work needed to apply malaria genomic information toward the goal of malaria eradication. Following the generation of reference genome assemblies, malaria investigators followed the path of other organisms in the postgenomic era and characterized genomic diversity through sequencing surveys (Jeffares et al. 2007; Mu et al. 2007; Volkman et al. 2007; Tan et al. 2011; Neafsey et al. 2012) and later genome-wide single nucleotide polymorphism (SNP) arrays (Neafsey et al. 2008, 2010; Mu et al. 2010; Tan et al. 2011; Van Tyne et al. 2011). Such work illuminated the recent demographic history of multiple parasite and vector species, defined sometimes complex gene flow boundaries, and revealed the impact of immune, drug, or insecticide selection on the genomes of malaria parasites and vectors. Subsequently, more comprehensive characterizations of genetic diversity have yielded thorough inventories of genomic diversity across many geographic regions (Amambua-Ngwa et al. 2012; Manske et al. 2012; Miotto et al. 2013, 2015; MalariaGEN *P. falciparum* Community Project 2016), refining our understanding of population boundaries and diversity differences between populations. Collectively, this deep genomic sequencing dataset, for example, represented in the open-access Pf3k collaboration and database (www.malariagen.net/projects/pf3k), facilitates informed development of markers for genotyping to analyze even larger sample collections. To ensure that sequencing data remain accessible and maximally useful to the malaria research community, it will be essential that prospective sequencing data generation efforts contribute sequencing data and a minimum increment of sample metadata (e.g., location and date of sample collection) to open repositories such as Pf3K and/or PlasmoDB in a timely manner with as few restrictions as possible. Strategies for how to accomplish this remain largely undetermined, but community-generated and -accessible databases are critical for leveraging genomic information to advance malaria elimination efforts.

DEVELOPING THE TOOLKIT

Although whole genome sequencing (WGS) efforts have provided a critical foundation for genomic tool development, WGS data may not be necessary to address some key considerations for malaria eradication. In fact, a major current limitation to the use of genomics for malaria eradication efforts is the limited availability of samples of sufficient quality or amount for WGS that have been collected with important clinical, epidemiological, or biological metadata. Although the cost of genome sequencing has fallen substantially, it can still be technically difficult and costly to sequence clinical samples heavily contaminated with host DNA. Two strategies have been developed to address this challenge: processes that enrich the parasite DNA either at the time of collection or from the already extracted nucleic acid material and use of genotyping tools that do not require removal of host DNA. Approaches, including hybrid selection (Melnikov et al. 2011; Bright et al. 2012) and selective whole genome amplification (Leichty and Brisson 2014), enable efficient sequencing by enriching for parasite over host genetic material. Filtration methods at the time of collection have also been employed to reduce host material, with variable success (Venkatesan et al. 2012). However, polymerase chain reaction (PCR)-based approaches that either genotype small collections of SNPs or a limited number of highly polymorphic regions (amplicons) are inexpensive ways of extracting genomic data from samples that are limited in amount or contaminated with large amounts of host DNA.

Several groups have explored the use of so-called SNP "barcodes" to distinguish unique versus clonal parasite lineages and track changes in disease transmission over time (Campino et al. 2011; Daniels et al. 2013, 2008, 2015; Echeverry et al. 2013; Nkhoma et al. 2013). Other groups have used amplification of highly polymorphic regions of the parasite genome to create haplotypes, which is the basis of merozoite surface protein type 1 (MSP) typing strate-

Cite this article as *Cold Spring Harb Perspect Med* doi: 10.1101/cshperspect.a025544

gies used to distinguish parasite reinfection (Tanabe et al. 1998). This latter strategy is particularly useful for polygenomic infections, where more than one parasite genome contributes to human infection. Both approaches (SNP barcodes and MSP typing) allow one to estimate the complexity of infection (COI) level across patient populations, or the mean number of genetically distinct parasite lineages infecting a person, which has been used to distinguish between high and low transmission levels. Statistical tools like COIL (complexity of infection using likelihood) can estimate the COI level of a malaria sample using only knowledge of SNP minor allele frequencies (MAFs) and a sample's genotype (Galinsky et al. 2015). SNP-based barcodes have also proven useful for distinguishing malaria parasites hailing from different geographic regions (Preston et al. 2014; Baniecki et al. 2015), suggesting they could be helpful in identifying the source of imported infections in pre-elimination settings. Amplicon-based sequencing approaches have also been useful in other intervention contexts, such as characterizing polymorphism in vaccine candidates (Juliano et al. 2010; Bailey et al. 2012; Gandhi et al. 2012, 2014; Aragam et al. 2013; Neafsey et al. 2015; Mideo et al. 2016).

One consideration important for obtaining value from large collections of SNP genotyping data will be some means of ensuring that data and findings are portable between studies conducted by different investigators. Numerous groups have put forth proposed collections of nuclear genetic markers for genotyping, while other groups have pursued whole mitochondrial sequencing to make demographic inferences about populations. Comparing findings between studies that employed nuclear and mitochondrial markers (Sutton 2013; Koepfli et al. 2015) can be challenging because of the different modes of inheritance, genetic effective population sizes, and mutation rates of those genomes. Use of markers that are neutral or potentially under selection (e.g., immune or drug) adds another level of consideration about which markers are most informative and/or appropriate for a given question. Within the nuclear genome, SNPs and microsatellite markers exhibit

extremely different modes and rates of mutation, requiring very different analysis strategies for interpretation. Microsatellites themselves exhibit highly variable mutation rates, related to the length of the repeat unit and the number of copies of the repeat, with greater repeat counts generally leading to a higher mutation rate.

Studies that simultaneously explore the signals of multiple marker sets, for example, nuclear SNPs and microsatellite markers, will be necessary to understand the transferability of findings employing a single class of markers. As methods to call microsatellite repeat length variation from NGS data improve, there will be an opportunity to use WGS data from parasites to explore the degree of concordance within and among different classes of markers from the same samples. The development and refinement of new tools to analyze genotype data for malaria applications will help to organize the field around specific sets of markers. Ultimately, the most powerful way to ensure comparability of findings from different genotyping studies will be community adoption of a common set of genotypic markers. Even if there is motivation to include population-specific genotype markers, for example, because of local questions relating to drug resistance or selection, analysis of a common core of genotype markers will contribute to building a collection of data that can be critically compared across disease elimination settings in a meta-analytical framework. Observing the behavior of a common set of markers in a range of elimination settings with disparate outcomes will be key to furthering our understanding of effective uses of genotyping tools.

DEPLOYMENT OF A GENOMICS TOOLKIT FOR THE ERADICATION AGENDA

Now that we have extensive catalogs of genomic variation data for *P. falciparum*, with efforts underway to produce comparable compendia of genomic variants for *Plasmodium vivax* and other parasite species, how do we apply these resources as effectively as possible to the goal of malaria eradication? Below we outline several ways we believe genomic data can continue to

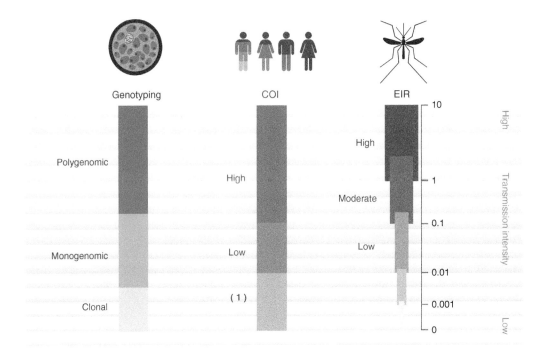

Figure 1. Range of transmission intensity. A schematic representing signals detected from mosquito, human, and parasite populations that are anticipated as transmission intensity declines. As the transmission intensity decreases from high to low levels, changes in mosquito (entomological inoculation rate [EIR]; human complexity of infection [COI]), and parasite (genotyping) indicators are anticipated to change. With relatively high transmission (e.g., EIR > 1), we see high COI levels and a predominance of polygenomic infections as assessed through genotyping methods. As transmission decreases to more moderate (e.g., EIR from 0.1 to 1) or lower levels (e.g., EIR from 0.01 to 0.1), we detect decreases in COI and increases in the proportion of individuals harboring monogenomic infections. Eventually as transmission intensity is very low (e.g., EIR from 0 to 0.01) we detect evidence of COI = 1 and clonal parasite populations among monogenomic infections detected using genotyping methods.

be a cost-effective and invaluable resource for understanding and controlling malaria and providing critical information about elimination activities. We focus this discussion on ways genomic information can be used to monitor changes in transmission intensity, evaluate of the impact of intervention methods, and track the movement of parasites between human populations. Critical for the success of these applications is the collection of samples with epidemiological, clinical, or biological metadata. Here we focus on study design and use of epidemiological and clinical metadata to inform changes in transmission or evaluate the impact of an intervention. However, genomic approaches for biological discovery, as are generally applied to understanding of mechanisms

of drug resistance or drug action, are also an important application of genomics that will be considered.

GENOMICS FOR STUDYING TRANSMISSION

The use of genomics to monitor changes in transmission intensity and evaluate intervention impact is grounded in basic population genetic principles (Fig. 1). As transmission intensity decreases there is a reduction in outcrossing during the mosquito stages of the lifecycle. This predicts that, over time, COI will decline among human infections, and parasites will become increasingly genetically similar because of inbreeding and recent common ancestry (Volkman et al. 2012). One can follow these signals over time to monitor increased parasite relatedness, as outward indicators of reduced transmission such as prevalence or incidence of malaria are detected using epidemiological or clinical measures. Such an approach has recently documented changing parasite population dynamics over time in Senegal, with modeling approaches employed to confirm sensitivity for detection of both transmission decrease and rebound patterns of malaria transmission (Daniels et al. 2015). There is tremendous value in samples collected over time, either across sequential transmission seasons, or in longitudinal or cohort design studies. To be useful for observing changes in transmission dynamics over time, longitudinal sample collections only need to be large enough to overcome a binomial sampling error within individual time points, and, often, signals indicating transmission changes can be detected by repeatedly sampling 100 samples or fewer. Thus, use of genomics has the potential to track transmission dynamics over time and monitor changes in these dynamics related to epidemiological and clinical variables.

Important for our understanding of transmission dynamics is determining the relative contributions of cotransmission and superinfection. Cotransmission occurs when multiple parasites enter the human host during a single mosquito-feeding event, whereas superinfection occurs when parasites enter the human host during multiple mosquito-feeding events. Cotransmission is expected to introduce parasites that are genetically more alike, perhaps coming from the same recombination events in the mosquito midgut. In contrast, depending on the genetic variation in the population, superinfection may introduce more highly diverse parasite types into the human host. Genomics, including single-cell genotyping and sequencing (Nkhoma et al. 2012; Nair et al. 2014), as well as population-based approaches, has the opportunity to help resolve distinct parasite types within either the human or mosquito host, and may be used to better estimate the contributions of these two different transmission patterns and their influence under various transmission settings to onward infection.

INTERVENTION IMPACT ASSESSMENT

Related to the concept of monitoring parasite population structure is the use of genomics to evaluate the impact of interventions (Fig. 2). Two main strategies are employed, using either drugs or vaccines, to reduce the clinical burden of malaria. Genomics has the potential to assess how such interventions are working, and provide an early warning system to potential failure of these strategies as resistant parasite populations emerge through natural selection. For example, application of drug pressure selects for drug-resistant variants that increasingly contribute to the overall parasite population infecting humans. At a certain point, these drug-resistant variants are sufficiently prevalent in the population that drug responses are compromised and these agents become limited or ineffective clinically. Genomics has the power to not only to discover drug-resistant variants by detecting genomic variants that increase in frequency over time, but also to monitor the consequences of drug pressure, such as under mass drug administration (MDA) projects that are being rolled out as part of the malaria eradication efforts. Application of MDA can boost frequency of drug-resistant parasites in the population by simultaneously compressing the parasite population while selecting for drug-resistant variants, and potentially compromise drug efficacy for future MDA projects.

To circumvent the emergence of drug resistance, specific genomic loci can be identified (e.g., *dhodh* [Ross et al. 2014] and *pfcrt* [Lukens et al. 2014]) that exist in two alternate allelic states (Fig. 3). In one allelic state, the locus is susceptible to the first drug while resistant to a second drug. In the alternate allelic state, the locus is resistant to the first drug, but susceptible to the second drug. Thus, one compound selects for genetic variants that are susceptible to the second compound, and vice versa. Such approaches provide promise for use of novel drug combinations where one drug selects for para-

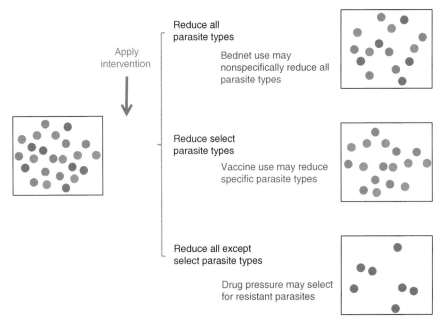

Figure 2. Intervention effect on parasite population. This schematic represents the potential impact of different interventions (e.g., bednets, vaccines, or drugs) on allele frequencies in the parasite population. The different colored circles represent a specific locus of interest such as an allele or haplotype that may be subject to selection by a vaccine (green circle) or drug (red circle). As a vaccine (e.g., a monovalent protein subunit vaccine like RTS,S) is applied, there may be reduction in specific parasite types that harbor the target locus (e.g., the circumsporozoite [CS] locus that matches the type found in the vaccine), thus reducing parasite types with that specific locus from the parasite population. As a drug is applied, there may be selection for a specific drug resistance locus resulting in an increase in the frequency of parasite types that harbor that specific drug-resistant variant. For comparison, use of a bednet might reduce the overall parasite types (represented by fewer circles that are proportionally reduced), but may not specifically select for or against any particular locus or allele within parasites in that population.

sites that are then susceptible to a second drug. The combined use of such paired compounds could offset emergence of resistance altogether, or, used sequentially, one drug could drive the emergence of parasite populations susceptible to the second drug, and vice versa. Thus, alternating drug pressure using a paired set of compounds could maintain the effectiveness of the compounds over time. Genomics can be used to identify genetic loci that have these alternate allelic states and facilitate identification of paired drugs that could prevent emergence of drug-resistant parasites. Surveillance of these critical allelic states can then be used to identify critical inflection points where drug strategies need to shift to remain effective.

Several malaria vaccine candidates have been associated with allele-specific protective responses (Takala et al. 2007, 2009; Takala and Plowe 2009; Thera et al. 2011; Neafsey et al. 2015). Allele-specific protective efficacy may compromise the overall efficacy of a vaccine, but can be characterized with PCR amplicon sequencing data. We recently demonstrated that the RTS,S/AS01 vaccine, which targets a highly polymorphic region of the circumsporozoite (CS) protein, exhibits significantly higher vaccine efficacy against infections matching the 3D7 vaccine strain compared with infections that do not match the vaccine strain (Neafsey et al. 2015) Thus, genomic information provides insight into vaccine effectiveness, and can perhaps contribute to improvements in vaccine efficacy for highly polymorphic vaccine targets, as well as helping predict the impact of a vaccine on a given target population.

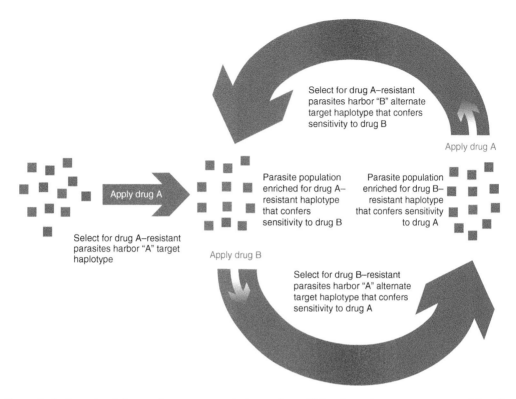

Figure 3. Anticorrelated drug resistance—an evolutionary loop. This schematic represents a potential evolutionary loop whereby two different drugs (A in red and B in blue) act on the same locus with each drug selecting a different variant or haplotype than the alternate drug. For example, as drug A (red) is applied to the parasite population, the haplotype conferring resistance to A will increase in frequency in the population. If the alternate drug (B, blue) is applied to this population, the alternate haplotype conferring resistance to B will increase in the population. This creates a population with increased resistance to B, but increased susceptibility to the alternate drug A. Application of drug A will now reverse the dynamics of the haplotype frequency such that the variant that confers resistance to A will again increase in frequency in the population. This alternating use of paired drugs with anticorrelated resistance will thus create an evolutionary loop.

TRACKING PARASITES

Genomics also has the potential to track transmission patterns, including detecting the movement of parasites and identifying new sources of infection. Genotyping approaches such as barcode methods or amplicon-sequencing approaches can identify specific parasite types, much like creating a "fingerprint" that identifies each kind of parasite within an infection. Such methods provide an opportunity to track specific parasite types in space and time. Human migration patterns, identified either from demographic or cell phone data, can be used to predict sources and sinks of malaria parasite

migration. If such patterns are present, targeting interventions to the source site could consequently reduce infections in the sink site. Genomic tools can test this "sink-source" hypothesis, by fingerprinting parasites and following them in space and time.

As we are better able to detect and track parasites, we still need to develop more sensitive methods for parasite identification, especially as we move toward malaria elimination and parasite density within human infections decreases. Specifically, sensitive molecular genetic approaches can identify parasite reservoirs, possibly among large numbers of asymptomatic individuals, and define whether these contribute to incident infection. One strategy is using case investigation or reactive case detection, where cases identified through passive case detection are then followed to determine whether other individuals in the household or neighborhood are also infected. Genomic tools have also been used for outbreak investigation (Obaldia et al. 2015) and may assist in identifying parasite types under "prevention of reintroduction" conditions in elimination settings. Genomic strategies not only provide a sensitive means of identifying who is infected, but also provide evidence for the spatial and temporal relationships among infected individuals. Such strategies can identify individuals who may not be treated as they are asymptomatic, yet may be a local source of new infection. Mapping of infected individuals may also identify pockets of infection that can then be investigated for mosquito breeding sites or other factors that contribute to maintaining these reservoirs of infection. For example, genomics can be coupled with strategies such as serology mapping in elimination phases to identify recent exposure history with serology, and then use molecular genetic approaches to determine who harbors infections and whether these contribute to new infections to map transmission networks and develop malaria risk maps.

Other useful information and strategies that might be obtained using genetic approaches include detection of gametocyte reservoirs, evaluating whether asymptomatic individuals harbor parasites that are infectious (i.e., determining the risk of seeding new infections), and understanding the intrahost dynamics between strains. As we move toward regional elimination, it is also critical to assess whether new cases are a result of rebound of autochthonous malaria, or whether it is a result of importation. In the context of "prevention of new infections" it will be important to be able to distinguish between local or external sources of these new infections to better define operational responses to distinct parasite sources. Some of the challenges we are likely to face as we move to elimination are the reduction of parasite types and increases in parasite relatedness. Thus, use of markers that differentiate between local and ex-

ternal populations will become increasingly challenging. Likely we will require use of a combination of markers including those that are rapidly evolving, such as microsatellites, and possibly the use of expression profiling such as can be obtained through RNAseq or Nanostring approaches.

FUTURE PERSPECTIVES FOR APPLICATION OF GENOMIC DATA

With a growing catalog of parasite population genomic information, we now need to develop strategies to apply these genomic data and approaches to promote malaria elimination. Although genomic sequencing provides a great deal of information about genetic variation within and between populations, key to application of these data to malaria eradication will involve population genetics strategies. Some of these approaches will involve use of changing parasite population genetics to monitor transmission dynamics and with modeling to inform best strategies and combinations of approaches to reduce the malaria burden. As drugs, vaccines, or other intervention measures impose selective pressures on the genomes of parasites and vectors, we can expect selected variants to measurably change in frequency within a few years, owing to the relatively short generation times. This method of detecting the targets of natural selection could identify the genomic basis of drug or insecticide resistance, as well as identify compensatory mutations that do not directly contribute to resistance but restore organismal fitness in the presence of resistance mutations.

To estimate changes in allele frequencies within a population over time, Figure 4 depicts the results of a binomial sampling-based simulation of changes in derived allele frequency (DAF) in a parasite population over time for neutral ($s = 0$; gray) and selected ($s = 0.01$; red) alleles, starting from a common DAF of 5% (assumes effective populations size (N_e) is constant and equal to 1000). Assuming that there are approximately 10 parasite generations per year, these simulations approximate the observable allele frequency changes in a clinical

Cite this article as *Cold Spring Harb Perspect Med* doi: 10.1101/cshperspect.a025544

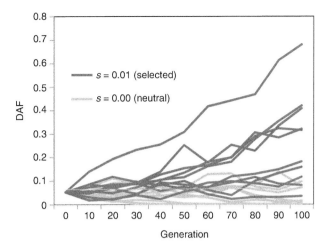

Figure 4. Expected changes in derived allele frequency. A simulation of expected changes in derived allele frequency (DAF) over time in a population with 1000 individuals for alleles that are selectively neutral (gray lines) or that confer a 1% fitness advantage (red lines). Time is measured in generations.

sample set collected over the span of a decade, the interval of time during which artemisinin resistance became widespread in Southeast Asia (Dondorp et al. 2009). Both neutral and selected alleles oscillate in frequency because of random genetic drift, but a significant fraction of selected alleles increase markedly in frequency over this relatively short time interval, with a conservatively low fitness advantage (1%). This suggests that careful analysis of longitudinally collected genomic datasets, taking into account factors such as population structure and demography, could be highly powered to detect and monitor the evolutionary impact of disease intervention efforts in both parasites and vectors. To produce such datasets in a practical and cost-effective manner, technical innovations will be necessary to ensure that clinical samples can be efficiently sequenced from an easily collectable source material (e.g., dried blood spots on filter paper), using such methods as hybrid selection, host DNA depletion, and/or selective whole genome amplification.

Whether future malaria genomic datasets are produced from longitudinal studies or focused on individual transmission seasons, these data must be analyzed and made public as quickly as possible to be truly useful. It will be of little practical value to understand the nature

of a pre-elimination outbreak from a genomic perspective 2 years after the fact; as a community we need tools to render actionable information from applied sequencing studies very quickly. Modeling genomic data in a manner that is integrated with epidemiological, clinical, serological, and other data types will be essential to distill the most informative signals about when and how to act in the context of elimination activities. In the future, easy-to-use tools like simple cell phone applications that display converted genomic signals into decision-making outputs for program officers in National Malaria Control Programs within the Ministry of Health would be ideal.

Malaria genomics is ready to move from a descriptive field to a practical tool informing elimination efforts, but, to successfully undergo that transition, the field will need to produce data and analyses closely tied to epidemiological and public health needs. Furthermore, the field will need new metrics and accepted modes of recognizing important contributions. A manuscript published in a prestigious journal years after samples have been collected and analyzed is of value to the investigators for future grant applications, but release of a dataset accompanied by a more cursory but actionable analysis in a forum like BioRxiv (bioRxiv.org) may be more useful for rapid dissemination of new molecular drug-resistance markers. Community engagement about how to create, support, and recognize contributions required for this timely generation, sharing, and interpretation of genomic data to inform operational activities is paramount.

CONCLUDING REMARKS

Recent developments in the field of nanopore sequencing point to new directions that malaria genomics may follow in the era of eradication. The prospect of inexpensive, disposable sequencing hardware, paired with largely automated analysis for common applications, will be powerful forces in the decentralization of genomic data generation. Although there are many reasons to celebrate increased access to the means of genomic data generation by investigators in malaria-endemic countries, that access will be of low value unless it is accompanied by training in the analysis, interpretation, and use of such data for operational activities. Thus, genomic data must become a local, interpretable, and actionable resource for the malaria community. The malaria research community needs to work hard to ensure that scientists from malaria-endemic countries are empowered to generate and analyze their own data, as the era of exporting both samples and intellectual ownership for the execution of malaria genomics studies to nonendemic countries is rapidly drawing to a close.

To avoid unnecessary and counterproductive duplication of efforts in an era of decentralized data production, the field should identify "best practice" methodologies for the generation and analysis of data, and repositories that can efficiently absorb data produced by a large number of contributors, as well as develop guidelines for use of these data. The malaria genomics field is fortunate to already have several central data repositories, including PlasmoDB (http://www.plasmodb.org) and the Pf3K project (www.malariagen.net/projects/parasite/pf3k) for parasite data, as well as VectorBase (vectorbase.org) and the Ag1000g project (www.malariagen.net/projects/vector/ag1000g) for vector data. It will be incumbent on the malaria research community, however, to ensure that the resources and tools provided by these repositories truly serve the goals of the malaria research community in the era of eradication. Care and attention to study design and sampling with connected metadata, including clinical, epidemiological, and biological information, will only enrich our ability to apply genomic strategies to increase our chances of reducing the malaria disease burden toward eradication.

ACKNOWLEDGMENTS

We thank Dyann F. Wirth, Daniel Hartl, and Bronwyn MacInnis for ongoing discussions about the ideas presented.

REFERENCES

Amambua-Ngwa A, Tetteh KK, Manske M, Gomez-Escobar N, Stewart LB, Deerhake ME, Cheeseman IH, Newbold CI, Holder AA, Knuepfer E, et al. 2012. Population genomic scan for candidate signatures of balancing selection to guide antigen characterization in malaria parasites. *PLoS Genet* **8:** e1002992.

Aragam NR, Thayer KM, Nge N, Hoffman I, Martinson F, Kamwendo D, Lin FC, Sutherland C, Bailey JA, Juliano JJ. 2013. Diversity of T cell epitopes in *Plasmodium falciparum* circumsporozoite protein likely due to protein–protein interactions. *PLoS ONE* **8:** e62427.

Bailey JA, Mvalo T, Aragam N, Weiser M, Congdon S, Kamwendo D, Martinson F, Hoffman I, Meshnick SR, Juliano JJ. 2012. Use of massively parallel pyrosequencing to evaluate the diversity of and selection on *Plasmodium falciparum csp* T-cell epitopes in Lilongwe, Malawi. *J Infect Dis* **206:** 580–587.

Baniecki ML, Faust AL, Schaffner SF, Park DJ, Galinsky K, Daniels RF, Hamilton E, Ferreira MU, Karunaweera ND, Serre D, et al. 2015. Development of a single nucleotide polymorphism barcode to genotype *Plasmodium vivax* infections. *PLoS Negl Trop Dis* **9:** e0003539.

Bright AT, Tewhey R, Abeles S, Chuquiyauri R, Llanos-Cuentas A, Ferreira MU, Schork NJ, Vinetz JM, Winzeler EA. 2012. Whole genome sequencing analysis of *Plasmodium vivax* using whole genome capture. *BMC Genomics* **13:** 262.

Campino S, Auburn S, Kivinen K, Zongo I, Ouedraogo JB, Mangano V, Djimde A, Doumbo OK, Kiara SM, Nzila A, et al. 2011. Population genetic analysis of *Plasmodium falciparum* parasites using a customized Illumina GoldenGate genotyping assay. *PLoS ONE* **6:** e20251.

Daniels R, Volkman SK, Milner DA, Mahesh N, Neafsey DE, Park DJ, Rosen D, Angelino E, Sabeti PC, Wirth DF, et al. 2008. A general SNP-based molecular barcode for *Plas-*

Cite this article as *Cold Spring Harb Perspect Med* doi: 10.1101/cshperspect.a025544

modium falciparum identification and tracking. *Malaria J* **7:** 223.

Daniels R, Chang HH, Sene PD, Park DC, Neafsey DE, Schaffner SF, Hamilton EJ, Lukens AK, Van Tyne D, Mboup S, et al. 2013. Genetic surveillance detects both clonal and epidemic transmission of malaria following enhanced intervention in Senegal. *PLoS ONE* **8:** e60780.

Daniels RF, Schaffner SF, Wenger EA, Proctor JL, Chang HH, Wong W, Baro N, Ndiaye D, Fall FB, Ndiop M, et al. 2015. Modeling malaria genomics reveals transmission decline and rebound in Senegal. *Proc Natl Acad Sci* **112:** 7067–7072.

Dondorp AM, Nosten F, Yi P, Das D, Phyo AP, Tarning J, Lwin KM, Ariey F, Hanpithakpong W, Lee SJ, et al. 2009. Artemisinin resistance in *Plasmodium falciparum* malaria. *N Engl J Med* **361:** 455–467.

Echeverry DF, Nair S, Osorio L, Menon S, Murillo C, Anderson TJ. 2013. Long term persistence of clonal malaria parasite *Plasmodium falciparum* lineages in the Colombian Pacific region. *BMC Genet* **14:** 2.

Galinsky K, Valim C, Salmier A, de Thoisy B, Musset L, Legrand E, Faust A, Baniecki ML, Ndiaye D, Daniels RF, et al. 2015. COIL: A methodology for evaluating malarial complexity of infection using likelihood from single nucleotide polymorphism data. *Malaria J* **14:** 4.

Gandhi K, Thera MA, Coulibaly D, Traore K, Guindo AB, Doumbo OK, Takala-Harrison S, Plowe CV. 2012. Next generation sequencing to detect variation in the *Plasmodium falciparum* circumsporozoite protein. *Am J Trop Med Hyg* **86:** 775–781.

Gandhi K, Thera MA, Coulibaly D, Traore K, Guindo AB, Ouattara A, Takala-Harrison S, Berry AA, Doumbo OK, Plowe CV. 2014. Variation in the circumsporozoite protein of *Plasmodium falciparum*: Vaccine development implications. *PLoS ONE* **9:** e101783.

Gardner MJ, Hall N, Fung E, White O, Berriman M, Hyman RW, Carlton JM, Pain A, Nelson KE, Bowman S, et al. 2002. Genome sequence of the human malaria parasite *Plasmodium falciparum. Nature* **419:** 498–511.

Jeffares DC, Pain A, Berry A, Cox AV, Stalker J, Ingle CE, Thomas A, Quail MA, Siebenthall K, Uhlemann AC, et al. 2007. Genome variation and evolution of the malaria parasite *Plasmodium falciparum. Nat Genet* **39:** 120–125.

Juliano JJ, Porter K, Mwapasa V, Sem R, Rogers WO, Ariey F, Wongsrichanalai C, Read A, Meshnick SR. 2010. Exposing malaria in-host diversity and estimating population diversity by capture-recapture using massively parallel pyrosequencing. *Proc Natl Acad Sci* **107:** 20138–20143.

Koepfli C, Rodrigues PT, Antao T, Orjuela-Sanchez P, Van den Eede P, Gamboa D, van Hong N, Bendezu J, Erhart A, Barnadas C, et al. 2015. *Plasmodium vivax* diversity and population structure across four continents. *PLoS Negl Trop Dis* **9:** e0003872.

Leichty AR, Brisson D. 2014. Selective whole genome amplification for resequencing target microbial species from complex natural samples. *Genetics* **198:** 473–481.

Lukens AK, Ross LS, Heidebrecht R, Javier Gamo F, Lafuente-Monasterio MJ, Booker ML, Hartl DL, Wiegand RC, Wirth DF. 2014. Harnessing evolutionary fitness in *Plasmodium falciparum* for drug discovery and suppressing resistance. *Proc Natl Acad Sci* **111:** 799–804.

MalariaGEN *Plasmodium falciparum* Community Project. 2016. Genomic epidemiology of artemisinin resistant malaria. *eLife* **5:** e08714.

Manske M, Miotto O, Campino S, Auburn S, Almagro-Garcia J, Maslen G, O'Brien J, Djimde A, Doumbo O, Zongo I, et al. 2012. Analysis of *Plasmodium falciparum* diversity in natural infections by deep sequencing. *Nature* **487:** 375–379.

Melnikov A, Galinsky K, Rogov P, Fennell T, Van Tyne D, Russ C, Daniels R, Barnes KG, Bochicchio J, Ndiaye D, et al. 2011. Hybrid selection for sequencing pathogen genomes from clinical samples. *Genome Biol* **12:** R73.

Mideo N, Bailey JA, Hathaway NJ, Ngasala B, Saunders DL, Lon C, Kharabora O, Jamnik A, Balasubramanian S, Bjorkman A, et al. 2016. A deep sequencing tool for partitioning clearance rates following antimalarial treatment in polyclonal infections. *Evol Med Public Health* **2016:** 21–36.

Miotto O, Almagro-Garcia J, Manske M, Macinnis B, Campino S, Rockett KA, Amaratunga C, Lim P, Suon S, Sreng S, et al. 2013. Multiple populations of artemisinin-resistant *Plasmodium falciparum* in Cambodia. *Nat Genet* **45:** 648–655.

Miotto O, Amato R, Ashley EA, MacInnis B, Almagro-Garcia J, Amaratunga C, Lim P, Mead D, Oyola SO, Dhorda M, et al. 2015. Genetic architecture of artemisinin-resistant *Plasmodium falciparum. Nat Genet* **47:** 226–234.

Mu J, Awadalla P, Duan J, McGee KM, Keebler J, Seydel K, McVean GA, Su XZ. 2007. Genome-wide variation and identification of vaccine targets in the *Plasmodium falciparum* genome. *Nat Genet* **39:** 126–130.

Mu J, Myers RA, Jiang H, Liu S, Ricklefs S, Waisberg M, Chotivanich K, Wilairatana P, Krudsood S, White NJ, et al. 2010. *Plasmodium falciparum* genome-wide scans for positive selection, recombination hot spots and resistance to antimalarial drugs. *Nat Genet* **42:** 268–271.

Nair S, Nkhoma SC, Serre D, Zimmerman PA, Gorena K, Daniel BJ, Nosten F, Anderson TJ, Cheeseman IH. 2014. Single-cell genomics for dissection of complex malaria infections. *Genome Res* **24:** 1028–1038.

Neafsey DE, Schaffner SF, Volkman SK, Park D, Montgomery P, Milner DA Jr, Lukens A, Rosen D, Daniels R, Houde N, et al. 2008. Genome-wide SNP genotyping highlights the role of natural selection in *Plasmodium falciparum* population divergence. *Genome Biol* **9:** R171.

Neafsey DE, Lawniczak MK, Park DJ, Redmond SN, Coulibaly MB, Traore SF, Sagnon N, Costantini C, Johnson C, Wiegand RC, et al. 2010. SNP genotyping defines complex gene-flow boundaries among African malaria vector mosquitoes. *Science* **330:** 514–517.

Neafsey DE, Galinsky K, Jiang RH, Young L, Sykes SM, Saif S, Gujja S, Goldberg JM, Young S, Zeng Q, et al. 2012. The malaria parasite *Plasmodium vivax* exhibits greater genetic diversity than *Plasmodium falciparum. Nat Genet* **44:** 1046–1050.

Neafsey DE, Juraska M, Bedford T, Benkeser D, Valim C, Griggs A, Lievens M, Abdulla S, Adjei S, Agbenyega T, et al. 2015. Genetic diversity and protective efficacy of the RTS,S/AS01 malaria vaccine. *N Engl J Med* **373:** 2025–2037.

Nkhoma SC, Nair S, Cheeseman IH, Rohr-Allegrini C, Singlam S, Nosten F, Anderson TJ. 2012. Close kinship within multiple-genotype malaria parasite infections. *Proc Biol Sci* **279:** 2589–2598.

Nkhoma SC, Nair S, Al-Saai S, Ashley E, McGready R, Phyo AP, Nosten F, Anderson TJ. 2013. Population genetic correlates of declining transmission in a human pathogen. *Mol Ecol* **22:** 273–285.

Obaldia N 3rd, Baro NK, Calzada JE, Santamaria AM, Daniels R, Wong W, Chang HH, Hamilton EJ, Arevalo-Herrera M, Herrera S, et al. 2015. Clonal outbreak of *Plasmodium falciparum* infection in eastern Panama. *J Infect Dis* **211:** 1087–1096.

Preston MD, Campino S, Assefa SA, Echeverry DF, Ocholla H, Amambua-Ngwa A, Stewart LB, Conway DJ, Borrmann S, Michon P, et al. 2014. A barcode of organellar genome polymorphisms identifies the geographic origin of *Plasmodium falciparum* strains. *Nat Commun* **5:** 4052.

Ross LS, Gamo FJ, Lafuente-Monasterio MJ, Singh OM, Rowland P, Wiegand RC, Wirth DF. 2014. In vitro resistance selections for *Plasmodium falciparum* dihydroorotate dehydrogenase inhibitors give mutants with multiple point mutations in the drug-binding site and altered growth. *J Biol Chem* **289:** 17980–17995.

Sutton PL. 2013. A call to arms: On refining *Plasmodium vivax* microsatellite marker panels for comparing global diversity. *Malaria J* **12:** 447.

Takala SL, Plowe CV. 2009. Genetic diversity and malaria vaccine design, testing and efficacy: Preventing and overcoming "vaccine resistant malaria." *Parasite Immunol* **31:** 560–573.

Takala SL, Coulibaly D, Thera MA, Dicko A, Smith DL, Guindo AB, Kone AK, Traore K, Ouattara A, Djimde AA, et al. 2007. Dynamics of polymorphism in a malaria vaccine antigen at a vaccine-testing site in Mali. *PLoS Med* **4:** e93.

Takala SL, Coulibaly D, Thera MA, Batchelor AH, Cummings MP, Escalante AA, Ouattara A, Traore K, Niangaly A, Djimde AA, et al. 2009. Extreme polymorphism in a vaccine antigen and risk of clinical malaria: Implications for vaccine development. *Sci Transl Med* **1:** 2ra5.

Tan JC, Miller BA, Tan A, Patel JJ, Cheeseman IH, Anderson TJ, Manske M, Maslen G, Kwiatkowski DP, Ferdig MT. 2011. An optimized microarray platform for assaying genomic variation in *Plasmodium falciparum* field populations. *Genome Biol* **12:** R35.

Tanabe K, Sakihama N, Kaneko O, Saito-Ito A, Kimura M. 1998. A PCR method for molecular epidemiology of *Plasmodium falciparum* Msp-1. *Tokai J Exp Clin Med* **23:** 375–381.

Thera MA, Doumbo OK, Coulibaly D, Laurens MB, Ouattara A, Kone AK, Guindo AB, Traore K, Traore I, Kouriba B, et al. 2011. A field trial to assess a blood-stage malaria vaccine. *N Engl J Med* **365:** 1004–1013.

Van Tyne D, Park DJ, Schaffner SF, Neafsey DE, Angelino E, Cortese JF, Barnes KG, Rosen DM, Lukens AK, Daniels RF, et al. 2011. Identification and functional validation of the novel antimalarial resistance locus PF10_0355 in *Plasmodium falciparum*. *PLoS Genet* **7:** e1001383.

Venkatesan M, Amaratunga C, Campino S, Auburn S, Koch O, Lim P, Uk S, Socheat D, Kwiatkowski DP, Fairhurst RM, et al. 2012. Using CF11 cellulose columns to inexpensively and effectively remove human DNA from *Plasmodium falciparum*–infected whole blood samples. *Malaria J* **11:** 41.

Volkman SK, Sabeti PC, DeCaprio D, Neafsey DE, Schaffner SF, Milner DA Jr, Daily JP, Sarr O, Ndiaye D, Ndir O, et al. 2007. A genome-wide map of diversity in *Plasmodium falciparum*. *Nat Genet* **39:** 113–119.

Volkman SK, Neafsey DE, Schaffner SF, Park DJ, Wirth DF. 2012. Harnessing genomics and genome biology to understand malaria biology. *Nat Rev Genet* **13:** 315–328.

Malaria Epigenetics

Alfred Cortés[1,2] and Kirk W. Deitsch[3]

[1]ISGlobal, Barcelona Centre for International Health Research (CRESIB), Hospital Clínic - Universitat de Barcelona, Barcelona, Catalonia 08036, Spain

[2]ICREA, Barcelona, Catalonia 08010, Spain

[3]Department of Microbiology and Immunology, Weill Medical College of Cornell University, New York, New York 10065

Correspondence: alfred.cortes@isglobal.org; kwd2001@med.cornell.edu

Organisms with identical genome sequences can show substantial differences in their phenotypes owing to epigenetic changes that result in different use of their genes. Epigenetic regulation of gene expression plays a key role in the control of several fundamental processes in the biology of malaria parasites, including antigenic variation and sexual differentiation. Some of the histone modifications and chromatin-modifying enzymes that control the epigenetic states of malaria genes have been characterized, and their functions are beginning to be unraveled. The fundamental principles of epigenetic regulation of gene expression appear to be conserved between malaria parasites and model eukaryotes, but important peculiarities exist. Here, we review the current knowledge of malaria epigenetics and discuss how it can be exploited for the development of new molecular markers and new types of drugs that may contribute to malaria eradication efforts.

Epigenetic regulation of gene expression refers to heritable changes in transcription that occur in the absence of alterations in the primary sequence of DNA. Numerous important biological pathways in eukaryotes involve epigenetic regulation, both in health and during disease. Chromatin is the main platform where epigenetic processes take place, such that epigenetic traits are typically mediated by DNA modifications (such as methylation) or by changes in chromatin structure such as histone posttranslational modifications or use of histone variants. In fact, there is an accepted "relaxed" use of the term epigenetics that includes all chromatin-based processes that affect transcription, regardless of whether or not information is transmitted through cell division.

In malaria parasites, epigenetic regulation of gene expression has been extensively studied only in *Plasmodium falciparum*. For many years, studying epigenetics in this parasite was almost synonymous to studying the regulation of *var* genes, which are important for antigenic variation and virulence (Kyes et al. 2001). However, recent findings have revealed a more general role for epigenetics in malaria parasite biology, including processes as diverse as erythrocyte invasion, solute transport, or formation of sexual forms necessary for human-to-mosquito transmission. The contribution of epigenetic regula-

Cite this article as *Cold Spring Harb Perspect Med* doi: 10.1101/cshperspect.a025528

tion of gene expression to these processes stems from the clonally variant expression of some of the genes involved. Silencing of clonally variant genes, which is a process truly controlled at the epigenetic level (Cortés et al. 2012), generally depends on histone modifications that result in reversible formation of repressive chromatin structures (heterochromatin), but several additional layers of regulation operate specifically on particular gene families such as *var* genes.

Genome-wide studies of heterochromatin marks or transcriptional variation identified many genes regulated at the epigenetic level that are not involved in the processes mentioned above, indicating that epigenetic regulation of gene expression plays a role in the control of other as-yet-uncharacterized biological processes (Flueck et al. 2009; Lopez-Rubio et al. 2009; Rovira-Graells et al. 2012). In the years to come, the biological significance of epigenetic regulation of these genes should be revealed. In all cases, epigenetic changes are likely to imply translating the same genome into alternative transcriptomes and phenotypes, increasing the plasticity of parasite populations and favoring their survival.

PROCESSES REGULATED AT THE EPIGENETIC LEVEL IN MALARIA PARASITES

Numerous *P. falciparum* genes involved in host–parasite interactions show clonally variant expression, such that they are expressed in some individual parasites, but not in others that are genetically identical (Table 1). The active or silenced states of these genes are clonally transmitted during asexual replication, with switches between the two states occurring at low frequencies. The predicted functions for clonally variant genes suggest that transcriptional variation results in both antigenic and functional differences at several stages along the parasite's life cycle (Fig. 1), but the phenotypic alterations associated with changes in the expression of specific clonally variant genes have been elucidated in only a few cases. In this section, we describe the known processes in which epigenetic changes determine alternative phenotypes. A common theme is that, for

processes in which the parasite requires alternative operational states to adapt to changes in its environment or to evade host immune responses, alternative epigenetic states exist for some of the genes linked to the process.

Antigenic Variation and Cytoadherence

Observations of both human and animal infections clearly show that malaria parasites are capable of maintaining persistent, chronic infections for extended periods of time, even in the presence of a robust antibody response of the infected host. In experimental human infections, parasites have been observed to persist for over a year, frequently displaying characteristic waves of parasites reminiscent of similar population dynamics displayed by other infectious organisms including African trypanosomes (Miller et al. 1994). Thus, it is clear that malaria parasites are capable of showing systematic antigenic variation that results in immune evasion, presumably through alterations made to proteins displayed on the surface of infected erythrocytes. In the case of *P. falciparum*, the formation of knobs on the infected erythrocyte membrane as well as the induction of cytoadherent properties of infected cells provided additional evidence for the placement of antigenically variant molecules on the infected cell surface (Miller et al. 2002). The variant surface properties of the infected erythrocytes were linked to epigenetic regulation of gene expression with the discovery and description in *P. falciparum* of the *var* multicopy gene family and the multitude of alternative forms of the *P. falciparum* erythrocyte membrane protein 1 (PfEMP1) that it encodes (Baruch et al. 1995; Smith et al. 1995; Su et al. 1995).

Individual parasites typically express only one *var* gene at a time, a pattern known as mutually exclusive expression that operates on top of a clonal variation and results in a single form of PfEMP1 on the erythrocyte surface. All variants of PfEMP1 include a single transmembrane domain that passes through the erythrocyte membrane, thus anchoring a long, hypervariable portion of the protein that binds to endothelial surface receptors and thereby

Cite this article as *Cold Spring Harb Perspect Med* doi: 10.1101/cshperspect.a025528

Table 1. Examples of genes or gene families that display clonally variant expression linked to the histone modification H3K9me3 (when transcriptionally silent) in *Plasmodium falciparum*

Gene ID (previous ID)	Protein name	Proposed function	Notes	References
PF3D7_1222600 (PFL1085w)	PfAP2-G	Transcription factor implicated in sexual differentiation	Protein contains an AP2 DNA-binding domain	Kafsack et al. 2014
PF3D7_1036300 (PF10_0355)	MSPDBL2	A likely merozoite surface protein, possibly involved in erythrocyte invasion	Gene under strong balancing selection Possible role in drug resistance	Amambua-Ngwa et al. 2012; Hodder et al. 2012; Van Tyne et al. 2013
PF3D7_1301600 (MAL13P1.60)	EBA140	Merozoite protein involved in erythrocyte invasion, binds to glycophorin C	Enables parasites to use alternative invasion pathways	Maier et al. 2003; Cortés et al. 2007; Crowley et al. 2011
PF3D7_0424200 (PFD1150c)	PfRH4	Merozoite protein involved in erythrocyte invasion, binds to complement receptor 1 (CR1)	Enables parasites to use alternative invasion pathways	Stubbs et al. 2005; Jiang et al. 2010
var gene family (approximately 60 members)	PfEMP1	Cytoadhesive protein displayed on the surface of the infected erythrocyte	Displays mutually exclusive expression, changes in expression enable antigenic variation	Chookajorn et al. 2007; Lopez-Rubio et al. 2007; Jiang et al. 2013
rif gene family (approximately 160 members)	RIFIN	Displayed on the surface of the infected erythrocyte, some members of the family have been linked to rosetting	Most members of the family silent at any given time, expression has also been reported in merozoites	Kyes et al 1999; Fernandez et al. 1999; Mwakalinga et al. 2012; Goel et al. 2015
stevor gene family (approximately 31 members)	STEVOR	Displayed on the surface of the infected erythrocyte; contribute to infected erythrocyte mechanical properties	Most members of the family silent at any given time, expression has also been reported in merozoites and gametocytes	Lavazec et al. 2007; Sanyal et al. 2012; Niang et al. 2014
Pfmc-2tm gene family (approximately 12 members)	PFMC-2TM	Displayed on the surface of the infected erythrocyte	Most members of the family silent at any given time	Sam-Yellowe et al. 2004; Lavazec et al. 2007
surfin gene family (approximately 10 members)	SURFIN	Unknown function	Several localizations reported including infected erythrocyte surface and merozoites	Winter et al. 2005; Mphande et al. 2008
clag gene family (five members)	CLAG	At least some members are implicated in the formation of the PSAC channel found in the infected erythrocyte membrane	*clag3.1* and *clag3.2* are expressed in a mutually exclusive fashion, whereas *clag2* shows independent clonally variant expression	Cortés et al. 2007; Comeaux et al. 2011; Crowley et al. 2011; Nguitragool et al. 2011

Continued

Table 1. *Continued*

Gene ID (previous ID)	Protein name	Proposed function	Notes	References
phist gene families (approximately 79 members)	PHIST-domain proteins	Cytoadherence/erythrocyte remodeling	Various families of exported proteins; at least some PHIST-domain proteins interact with PfEMP1 at knobs	Sargeant et al. 2006; Proellocks et al. 2014; Oberli et al. 2014
exported dnaj III gene family (approximately nine members)	DnaJ III/HSP40	Erythrocyte remodeling	Exported proteins with a J-domain; HSP40-type chaperones	Sargeant et al. 2006
hyp gene families (approximately 55 members)	HYP	Unknown function	Various families of exported proteins	Sargeant et al. 2006
fikk gene family (approximately 23 members)	FIKK	Erythrocyte remodeling	Exported kinases	Sargeant et al. 2006; Nunes et al. 2007; Kats et al. 2014
gbp gene family (three members)	Glycophorin binding protein (GBP)	Unknown	Exported proteins	(Sargeant et al. 2006)
acs gene family (approximately 13 members)	Acyl-CoA synthetase (ACS)	Lipid metabolism (synthesis and/or transport)	Gene family specifically amplified in *P. falciparum*	Bethke et al. 2006
acbp gene family (four members)	Acyl-coA binding protein (ACBP)	Lipid metabolism (synthesis and/or transport)	Not characterized	Bethke et al. 2006

Inclusion of a gene or gene family in this table is based on the direct observation of clonally variant expression (Rovira-Graells et al. 2012) and the presence of epigenetic marks of silencing (Flueck et al. 2009; Lopez-Rubio et al. 2009) in genome-wide studies, or in the specific references provided. Both current 3D7 ID numbers and previous ID numbers are provided, along with a brief, general description of the predicted function. The estimates of the number of genes in each family do not include pseudogenes.

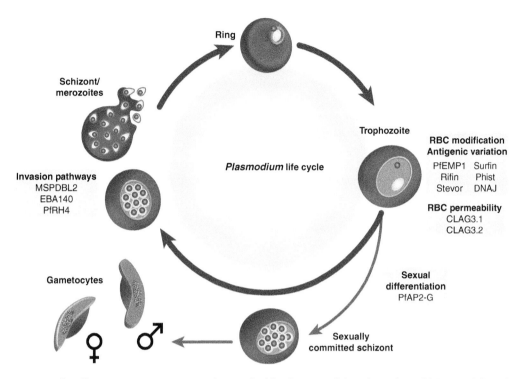

Figure 1. Clonally variant gene expression during the blood stages of the *Plasmodium falciparum* life cycle. Asexual replication occurs within human erythrocytes and progresses through different morphological stages, including rings, trophozoites, schizonts, and merozoites (cycle at *top* of figure). In trophozoites, several clonally variant proteins involved in erythrocyte modification, antigenic variation, and cell permeability are expressed. Similarly, in schizonts/merozoites, clonally variant proteins that determine alternative erythrocyte invasion pathways are expressed. In a small proportion of cells, the sexual differentiation process is initiated through the activation of PfAP2-G, leading to the production of male and female gametocytes (*bottom*).

mediates cytoadhesion. Cytoadhesion of infected erythrocytes effectively removes them from the peripheral circulation, a phenomenon referred to as sequestration, thereby enabling them to avoid passage through the spleen where they would be detected and destroyed. The different forms of PfEMP1 display different binding specificities, utilizing alternative host endothelial surface ligands for adhesion. This results in parasitized erythrocytes sequestering within different host tissues depending on which *var* gene (and the encoded form of PfEMP1) is expressed (Montgomery et al. 2007). Sequestration within the brain and the placenta has been directly linked to cerebral malaria and pregnancy-associated malaria, respectively, thus making PfEMP1 the best-characterized virulence factor of malaria caused by *P. falciparum*. PfEMP1 also

mediates rosetting, the binding of infected to noninfected erythrocytes that is also associated with virulence (Miller et al. 2002).

With the availability of complete genome sequences for several *Plasmodium* species infecting both primates and rodents, it has become possible to catalogue the many multicopy gene families found within these genomes. Gene families encoding variant surface proteins have been discovered in multiple *Plasmodium* species, suggesting that this is a universal characteristic of malaria parasites. Although some of these gene families are conserved throughout the *Plasmodium* lineage, others appear to be species-specific. In addition to the *var* gene family, which includes approximately 60 members per haploid genome, *P. falciparum* also possesses several other large, multicopy gene families likely involved in antigenic variation. These include the *rif/stevor/Pfmc-2tm* (approximately 200 copies) and the surfins (approximately 10 copies) (Weber 1988; Kyes et al. 1999; Sam-Yellowe et al. 2004; Winter et al. 2005). The largest multi-copy gene family in *P. vivax* is referred to as *vir* (approximately 350 copies) (del Portillo et al. 2001), which appears to have orthologous gene families in the primate parasite *P. knowlesi* (*kir*) and in the rodent parasites *P. berghei* (*bir*), *P. yoelii* (*yir*), and *P. chabaudi* (*cir*) (Fischer et al. 2003; Janssen et al. 2004) and is also likely a distant ortholog of the *rif* genes of *P. falciparum* (Janssen et al. 2004). *Plasmodium knowlesi* also possesses the *sica-var* family (approximately 100 copies), which encodes a protein linked to cy-toadherence similar to PfEMP1 (al-Khedery et al. 1999). In all cases, expression is limited to one or a limited subset of the members of each gene family at any given time. Activation and silencing of the genes of these families, as well as switching expression between members, are all thought to be regulated epigenetically.

Erythrocyte Invasion

Invasion of erythrocytes is an essential step of the asexual cycle of malaria parasites. After schizonts burst, merozoites are released into the bloodstream and quickly invade new ery-throcytes to start a new cycle of replication. Ery-throcyte invasion involves several differentiated steps, starting with initial contact, followed by merozoite reorientation and apical attachment that lead to the formation of a moving junction that progresses until the merozoite is internal-ized (Wright and Rayner 2014; Weiss et al. 2015). The small *eba* and *Pfrh* gene families, each including four to five members, encode adhesins that are released from apical organelles and interact with erythrocyte receptors to me-diate merozoite reorientation/apical attach-ment. Of note, merozoites can use alternative pathways for this step of invasion, each involv-ing a different set of erythrocyte receptors. With the exception of *Pfrh5*, the genes of the *eba* and *Pfrh* families are nonessential and appear to be functionally redundant (Reed et al. 2000; Du-raisingh et al. 2003; Maier et al. 2003; Stubbs

et al. 2005; Wright and Rayner 2014). As expect-ed from the existence of alternative invasion pathways and the nonessentiality of these genes, several *eba* and *Pfrh* genes are spontaneously silenced in some parasite lines, and clonally var-iant expression mediated by epigenetic mecha-nisms has been directly shown in some cases (Taylor et al. 2002; Duraisingh et al. 2003; Cortés et al. 2007; Jiang et al. 2010; Crowley et al. 2011). Importantly, variant expression of invasion ad-hesins has also been observed in field isolates (Cortés 2008; Gomez-Escobar et al. 2010). Al-though the relation between *eba* and *Pfrh* ex-pression patterns and the use of specific inva-sion pathways is complex and not completely understood, it is generally accepted that changes in the expression of these genes lead to pheno-typic variation in the process of invasion (Du-raisingh et al. 2003; Cortés 2008; Wright and Rayner 2014).

Understanding what selective advantage the clonally variant expression of invasion adhesins confers to parasites is an unresolved question. Although flexibility in front of genetic variabil-ity in host erythrocytes is an appealing possibil-ity, mutations in the majority of erythrocyte receptors that *P. falciparum* uses for invasion are rare, especially in Africa. Immune evasion provides an alternative explanation for the po-tential advantage that variant expression of invasion ligands may confer to the parasites. The number of genes in the *eba* or *Pfrh* families is small for "classic" antigenic variation, but variant expression may act synergistically with genetic polymorphism among different isolates to evade acquired immune responses (Cortés 2008; Wright and Rayner 2014).

The proteins encoded by some members of the variantly expressed large multigene families *rif, stevor,* and *surfin* discussed above also appear to be expressed in merozoites (Chan et al. 2014), although their function in the merozoite re-mains unknown and may be unrelated to inva-sion. Another gene encoding a protein ex-pressed in merozoites that shows clonally variant expression is *mspdbl2*, a member of the small *msp3-like* family. MSPDBL2 is located at the merozoite surface, where it may play a role in the initial steps of erythrocyte invasion. This

Cite this article as *Cold Spring Harb Perspect Med* doi: 10.1101/cshperspect.a025528

intriguing gene, which carries the epigenetic marks of silencing associated with clonally variant gene expression (Flueck et al. 2009; Lopez-Rubio et al. 2009), appears to be silenced in the vast majority of parasites and activated in only small subpopulations (~1% of parasites in most lines) (Amambua-Ngwa et al. 2012). However, the phenotypic differences resulting from the alternative transcriptional states of *mspdbl2* remain unknown.

Infected Erythrocyte Permeability

The transport of many solutes across the infected erythrocyte membranes is mediated by the plasmodial surface anion channel (PSAC), a broad selectivity channel with several unusual transport properties (Desai 2014). Recent research has established that the product of the parasite genes *clag3.1* or *clag3.2* is required for the formation of functional PSAC and efficient nutrient acquisition (Nguitragool et al. 2011; Pillai et al. 2012). This was an unexpected finding because these genes were previously thought to participate in either cytoadherence or erythrocyte invasion (Gupta et al. 2015).

The link between solute uptake and epigenetics comes from studies demonstrating that *clag3* genes show clonally variant expression regulated at the epigenetic level (Cortés et al. 2007; Comeaux et al. 2011; Crowley et al. 2011). Interestingly, *clag3* genes generally show mutually exclusive expression, such that individual parasites express either *clag3.1* or *clag3.2* (Cortés et al. 2007). However, it appears to not be strict, with occasional parasites escaping mutual exclusion (Rovira-Graells et al. 2015). Although the driving force for the epigenetic regulation of the expression of *clag3* genes remains unclear, it is reasonable to hypothesize that expression of alternative *clag3* genes may result in different solute transport phenotypes, which may play a role in the adaptation of the parasite to varying concentrations of nutrients and other solutes in the host plasma. This might explain why mutually exclusive expression need not be strict because silencing or expressing both genes simultaneously could provide additional phenotypic plasticity to parasite populations. In support of

this view, challenging *P. falciparum* cultures with the toxic compound blasticidin S, which requires the PSAC for transport across the infected erythrocyte membrane, results in the selection of parasites with dramatic switches in *clag3* expression (Mira-Martínez et al. 2013; Sharma et al. 2013). This is indicative of a role for *clag3* epigenetic regulation in the trade-off between excluding toxic compounds from infected erythrocytes and allowing the entrance of nutrients necessary for normal growth. These results also show that switches in *clag3* expression constitute a novel antimalarial drug resistance mechanism controlled at the epigenetic level. Finally, CLAG3 proteins are exposed on the erythrocyte surface (Nguitragool et al. 2011), so in addition to influencing solute transport, switches in the expression of *clag3* genes may also play a role in antigenic variation and immune evasion.

Sexual Conversion

The complex life cycle of malaria parasites includes multiple well-differentiated stages through which the parasite progresses in an ordered manner. The single developmental decision for the parasite occurs during asexual growth in the bloodstream: at each cycle of replication, the parasite makes a choice between continuing asexual multiplication, as the majority of parasites do, and irreversibly converting into male or female gametocytes, which are the sexual forms of the parasite necessary for transmission to another host via a mosquito vector (Fig. 1).

Genome-wide studies on transcriptional variation and epigenomic studies identified a member of the ApiAP2 family of transcriptional regulators that shows clonally variant expression (Rovira-Graells et al. 2012) and carries epigenetic marks of silencing (Flueck et al. 2009; Lopez-Rubio et al. 2009). The characterization of this transcriptional regulator, termed PfAP2-G, revealed that it plays an essential role in triggering sexual differentiation, such that the gene is by default silenced by heterochromatin-based epigenetic mechanisms, and only the few parasites in which the gene is stochastically activated convert into gametocytes (Kafsack et al. 2014). These results raised the idea that sexual conversion is regulated at the epigenetic level, a view that was later corroborated by studies in which specific epigenetic factors were depleted (Brancucci et al. 2014; Coleman et al. 2014). The ortholog of *pfap2-g* in the distantly related murine malaria parasite *P. berghei*, *pbap2-g*, also plays a key role in gametocyte formation (Sinha et al. 2014). This observation suggests that *ap2-g* is a conserved regulator of sexual conversion in malaria parasites; whether or not epigenetic control of the process is a conserved feature in all *Plasmodium* species awaits experimental confirmation.

The proportion of parasites that convert into sexual forms varies among isogenic parasite subclones (Kafsack et al. 2014). Spontaneous sexual conversion rates in these subclones are stable, indicating that as-yet-uncharacterized epigenetic mechanisms transmit the probability of *pfap2-g* activation and subsequent sexual conversion. Additionally, sexual conversion rates are affected by some environmental conditions (Bousema and Drakeley 2011), which opens up exciting perspectives about the possibility that environmental cues influence *pfap2-g* epigenetic states. This would provide one of the first examples in malaria of the parasite sensing the state of its host and producing a directed transcriptional response.

Epigenetic Variation and Adaptation to Environmental Changes: Bet-Hedging

Clonally variant expression is an intrinsic property of many *P. falciparum* gene families involved in disparate cellular processes (Rovira-Graells et al. 2012). This implies that isogenic parasite populations spontaneously become transcriptionally heterogeneous during normal growth, such that different individual parasites have different combinations of active and epigenetically silenced genes. This diversity confers plasticity to parasite populations because it provides the grounds for dynamic natural selection of parasites with highest fitness as changes in the environment occur. Adaptive strategies based on the stochastic generation of phenotypic di-

versity within populations before any challenge occurs, as opposed to directed adaptive responses, are commonly referred to as bet-hedging (Veening et al. 2008; Simons 2011).

The high level of spontaneous transcriptional diversity observed within isogenic parasite populations and the apparently stochastic nature of expression switches in clonally variant genes support the view that malaria parasites commonly use bet-hedging adaptive strategies (Rovira-Graells et al. 2012). This idea is also supported by the proposed limited ability of *P. falciparum* to adapt via directed transcriptional responses (Ganesan et al. 2008; Le Roch et al. 2008), although this remains controversial (Deitsch et al. 2007). In addition to the processes described above, in which epigenetic changes can be ascribed to alterations in specific phenotypes, the predicted functions of some of the clonally variant genes identified (Table 1) make it tempting to speculate that they modulate fitness in front of the majority of conditions that commonly fluctuate in the human blood, which is the environment where *P. falciparum* asexual stages reside. However, altogether there are few examples of well-defined adaptive pathways to specific challenges via bet-hedging in malaria, so it is still unclear whether epigenetic variation and bet-hedging play a general role in the adaptation of malaria parasite populations to changes in their environment. More experimental insight into the association between epigenetic diversity and long-term fitness in natural environments, and the identification of the clonally variant genes that mediate adaptation to specific changes in the parasite environment, are clearly needed to determine the actual contribution of bet-hedging to malarial adaptation.

EPIGENETIC MECHANISMS IN *Plasmodium falciparum*

Given the important role that epigenetic regulation of gene expression plays in the biology of malaria parasites, considerable work has focused on determining the molecular mechanisms that underlie these processes. The lion's share of this work has been performed with *P. falciparum*, although additional work has also been performed in the rodent models of malaria. In this section, we summarize recent studies that shed light on the molecular basis for epigenetic regulation in *P. falciparum*.

Chromatin Structure across the Life Cycle

As mentioned briefly above, epigenetic regulation of gene expression involves heritable modifications to the way the genome is packaged, which influence gene activation and silencing. Many of these modifications occur on histones, the protein subunits that comprise the nucleosomes around which the DNA strands of the chromosomes are wrapped. Modifications that increase the affinity of the histones to the DNA, thereby resulting in a more condensed chromatin structure that is less accessible to transcription complexes (called heterochromatin), lead to silencing of gene expression, whereas those that result in more open chromatin (called euchromatin) are associated with active regions of the genome. Typical nucleosome modifications include the incorporation of histone variants or posttranslational modifications (most often acetylation or methylation) to the amino-terminal "tails" of histones H3 and H4. Many of the enzymes that catalyze the addition or removal of these modifications have been identified encoded in the *P. falciparum* genome and some have been experimentally characterized (Table 2). Once formed, heterochromatin and euchromatin are separated within the nucleus, with heterochromatin generally found segregated to the nuclear periphery. In *P. falciparum*, as in other eukaryotes, many regions of the genome are found in either a euchromatic or a constitutively heterochromatic state that is the same in all cells, indicating that the chromatin state in such regions is likely dictated by the underlying primary DNA sequence. Although constitutive heterochromatin is, in general, transcriptionally silent, some long noncoding RNAs (lncRNAs) are expressed from subtelomeric repeats heterochromatin (Sierra-Miranda et al. 2012; Broadbent et al. 2015). However, other regions of the genome can be found in alternative chromatin states in different individual cells (Fig. 2). In such regions, known as facultative heterochromatin or bistable chromatin, once one or the other state is established, the resulting gene expression patterns are heritable through multiple cell generations, a phenomenon frequently referred to as epigenetic memory. However, these states are reversible, thus a gene that is silenced for many generations can once again revert to the active state, and vice versa. Herein lies the mechanistic basis for clonally variant expression and the biological phenomena described above.

Progression through the different stages of the asexual cycle of *P. falciparum* requires a tightly regulated cascade of gene expression in which most of the 5300 genes display a narrowly defined timing of activation (Bozdech et al. 2003; Le Roch et al. 2003). The general chromatin structure of the genome as a whole similarly displays cyclical, dynamic changes. The density of nucleosomes along the length of the chromosomes, called nucleosome occupancy, is somewhat depleted as cells enter S phase in the trophozoite stage, then becomes maximal in schizonts (Bunnik et al. 2014). Nucleosomes also appear to be clearly positioned around transcriptional landmark sites, including transcription start sites, regulatory elements, and splice donor and acceptor sites (Kensche et al. 2016). Euchromatic upstream regulatory regions of most genes are typically associated with the presence of the histone variants H2A.Z and H2B.Z, acetylation of histone H3 on the lysine in the ninth position (H3K9ac) and methylation of the lysine in the fourth position (H3K4me3). The presence of both of these histone modifications shows dynamic changes over the course of the asexual cycle, such that H3K9ac levels directly correlate with temporal patterns of gene expression, whereas H3K4me3 increases throughout the genome from low levels in rings to highly enriched levels late in the cycle (Lopez-Rubio et al. 2009; Salcedo-Amaya et al. 2009; Bartfai et al. 2010; Hoeijmakers et al. 2013). Other histone modifications similarly correlate with transcript levels, and their incorporation into the chromatin at specific regions of the genome appears to depend on the underlying DNA sequence (Gupta et al. 2013). All of these dynamic chromatin changes that occur over the course of the asexual cycle

Table 2. List of putative epigenetic factors involved in controlling chromatin structure and epigenetic regulation in *P. falciparum*

Protein name	Gene ID (previous ID)	Proposed function	References
Histone methyltransferases			
PfSET1	PF3D7_0629700 (PFF1440w)	Involved in the deposition of the epigenetic mark H3K4me3	Cui et al. 2008a
PfSET2 (also called PfSETvs)	PF3D7_1322100 (MAL13P1.122)	Involved in the deposition of the epigenetic mark H3K36me2/3, participates in *var* regulation	Cui et al. 2008a; Kishore et al. 2013; Jiang et al. 2013; Ukaegbu et al. 2014
PfSET3 (also called PfKMT1)	PF3D7_0827800 (PF08_0012)	Involved in the deposition of the epigenetic mark H3K9me2/3	Cui et al. 2008a; Lopez-Rubio et al. 2009; Volz et al. 2010
PfSET4	PF3D7_0910000 (PFI0485c)	Involved in the deposition of epigenetic marks on H3K4	Cui et al. 2008a; Volz et al. 2010; Jiang et al. 2013
PfSET5	PF3D7_1214200 (PFL0690c)	Involved in the deposition of unknown epigenetic marks; mitochondrial localization also reported	Cui et al. 2008a; Volz et al. 2010; Jiang et al. 2013
PfSET6	PF3D7_1355300 (PF13_0293)	Involved in the deposition of epigenetic marks on H3K4	Cui et al. 2008a; Volz et al. 2010
PfSET7	PF3D7_1115200 (PF11_0160)	In vitro data suggest methylation of H3K4 and H3K9	Cui et al. 2008a; Chen et al. 2016
PfSET8	PF3D7_0403900 (PFD0190w)	Involved in the deposition of the epigenetic mark H4K20me1/2/3	Cui et al. 2008a; Kishore et al. 2013; Jiang et al. 2013
PfSET9	PF3D7_0508100 (PFE0400w)	Involved in the deposition of unknown epigenetic marks	Cui et al. 2008a
PfSET10	PF3D7_1221000 (PFL1010c)	Involved in the deposition of the epigenetic mark H3K4me3, localized to the *var* expression site	Volz et al. 2012
Histone demethylases			
JmjC1	PF3D7_0809900 (MAL8P1.111)	Involved in the removal of epigenetic marks from H3K9 and H3K36	Cui et al. 2008a; Jiang et al. 2013
JmjC2	PF3D7_0602800 (PFF0135w)	Involved in the removal of unknown epigenetic marks	Cui et al. 2008a; Jiang et al. 2013
LSD1	PF3D7_1211600 (PFL0575w)	Involved in the removal of unknown epigenetic marks	Iyer et al. 2008; Volz et al. 2010; Jiang et al. 2013
Histone acetyltransferases			
PfGCN5	PF3D7_0823300 (PF08_0034)	Involved in the deposition of the epigenetic marks H3K9ac and H3K14ac	Fan et al. 2004; Cui et al. 2007
PfHAT1	PF3D7_0416400 (PFD0795w)	Probable ortholog to HAT1 in higher eukaryotes	
PfMYST	PF3D7_1118600 (PF11_0192)	Member of the MYST family of acetyltransferases, proposed to acetylate H4K5, K8, K12, and K16	Miao et al. 2010
Histone deacetylases			
PfSIR2A PfSIR2B	PF3D7_1328800 (PF13_0152) PF3D7_1451400 (PF14_0489)	Involved in telomere maintenance and regulation of *var* gene expression	Duraisingh et al. 2005; Freitas-Junior et al. 2005; Tonkin et al. 2009; Merrick et al. 2015

Continued

Cite this article as *Cold Spring Harb Perspect Med* doi: 10.1101/cshperspect.a025528

Table 2. *Continued*

Protein name	Gene ID (previous ID)	Proposed function	References
PfHDAC1	PF3D7_0925700 (PFI1260c)	Putative class I histone deacetylase, probable ortholog of Rpd3 from yeast	Joshi et al. 1999; Andrews et al. 2012b
PfHDAC2	PF3D7_1472200 (PF14_0690)	Putative class II histone deacetylase	Andrews et al. 2012b
PfHDAC3 (also called PfHda2)	PF3D7_1008000 (PF10_0078)	Putative class II histone deacetylase, linked to *var* gene silencing and sexual differentiation	Andrews et al. 2012b; Coleman et al. 2014
Other			
PfBDP1	PF3D7_1033700 (PF10_0328)	Bromodomain protein 1, involved in the regulation of genes linked to erythrocyte invasion	Josling et al. 2015
PfHP1	PF3D7_1220900 (PFL1005c)	Heterochromatin protein 1, involved in the maintenance of silenced regions of the genome, linked to *var* gene silencing and sexual differentiation	Perez-Toledo et al. 2009; Flueck et al. 2009; Brancucci et al. 2014

Both current 3D7 ID numbers and previous numbers are provided, along with a brief, general description of the predicted function. Many of the listed functions are predicted based on computational analysis and have not been experimentally verified. Several additional uncharacterized putative epigenetic factors have been predicted by in silico analysis (Bischoff and Vaquero 2010).

within constitutively euchromatic regions of the genome are unlikely to carry heritable information (Cortés et al. 2012), but together they contribute to the cascade of gene activation that enables the parasites to faithfully complete each round of schizogony. Special chromatin also forms at centromeres, including the incorporation of the variant histone cenH3. The centromeres from the different chromosomes cluster together within the nucleus during mitosis and cytokinesis, but dissociate after the merozoites reinvade erythrocytes and reinitiate a new cycle (Hoeijmakers et al. 2012). Additionally, DNA methylation has also been detected and proposed to contribute to transcriptional regulation (Ponts et al. 2013).

General Mechanisms Regulating Clonally Variant Gene Expression

As mentioned above, genes that display clonally variant expression are associated with bistable chromatin, which can be found as either euchromatin or facultative heterochromatin, resulting in either activation or silencing, respec-

tively. This chromatin state is heritable and, thus, must be faithfully reproduced as the genome transitions through multiple rounds of replication and division during schizogony. Only relatively rarely does a gene switch transcriptional states; however, the ability to switch is key for parasites to be able to display clonally variant expression and is indispensable for processes like antigenic variation that depend on generating variability over time, and for bet-hedging strategies that enable parasite populations to respond to changes in their environment. In addition to switching transcriptional states, some genes also belong to gene families in which only one or a small number of genes are active at a time (frequently referred to as mutually exclusive expression). Thus, activation of one gene necessitates the simultaneous silencing of the previously active member of the family, therefore requiring a mechanism of coordination within the family.

Significant progress has been made in recent years in identifying and characterizing the epigenetic components associated with activation and silencing of individual genes. Much less is

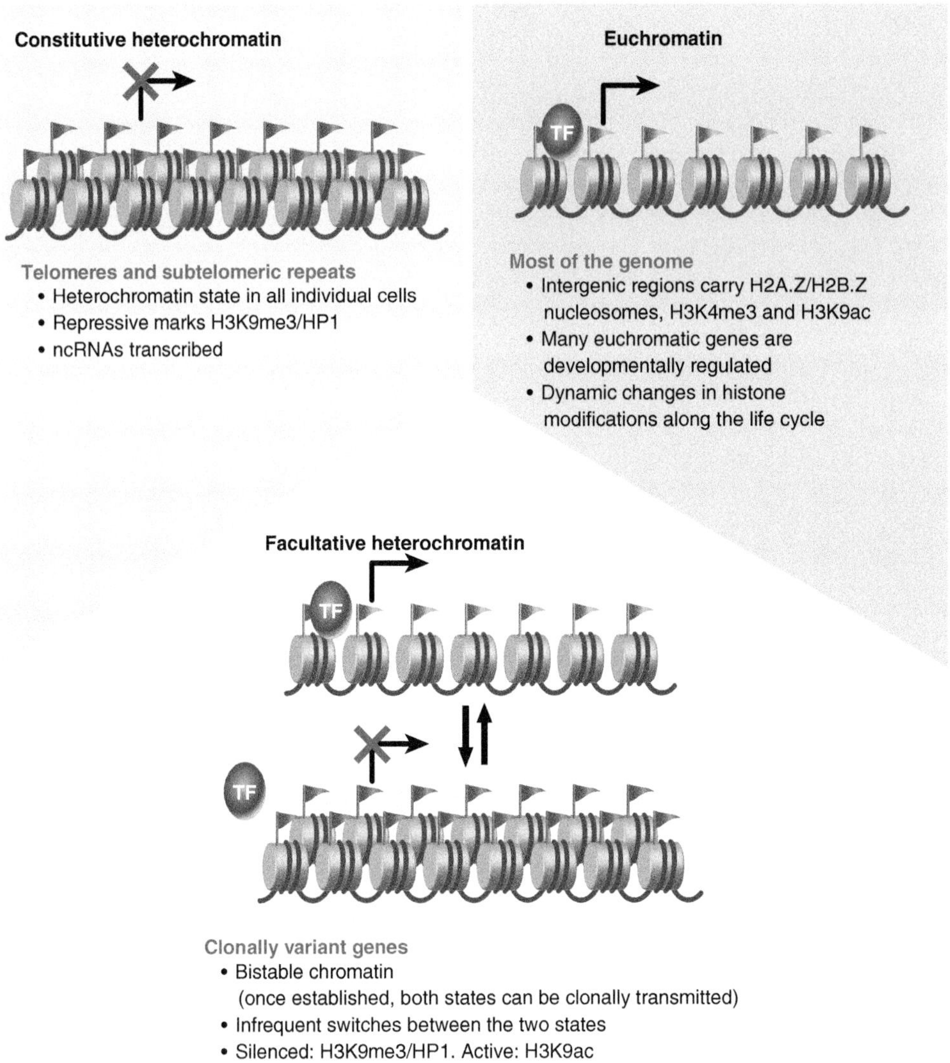

Figure 2. Chromatin compartments in *Plasmodium falciparum*. As in other eukaryotes, the chromatin of malaria parasites can be roughly divided into three separate compartments with very distinct properties. Green and red flags represent histone marks generally associated with transcriptional activation or silencing, respectively. *P. falciparum* constitutive heterochromatin (*upper left*) is generally transcriptionally silent but allows transcription of some noncoding RNAs (ncRNAs). Euchromatic regions (*upper right*) are typified by the incorporation of the variant histones H2A.Z and H2B.Z as well as the histone modifications H3K4me3 and H3K9ac. Stage-specific transcription largely depends on the presence of specific transcription factors (TFs), whereas in facultative heterochromatin (*bottom*) transcription depends on both the presence of the relevant transcription factor(s) and chromatin accessibility. The latter is determined by which of the possible chromatin states has been assembled at a specific locus in a given cell. Typically, chromatin at silent loci incorporates the histone modification H3K9me3 and is bound by HP1, whereas active genes are associated with the histone modification H3K9ac.

understood regarding what controls switching between transcriptional states, and the molecular basis for mutually exclusive expression within gene families remains entirely mysterious. The clonally variant genes involved in antigenic variation (*var*, *rifin*, *stevor*, *Pfmc-2tm*), alternative erythrocyte invasion pathways (*eba* and *Pfrh*), infected erythrocyte permeability (*clag3.1* and *clag3.2*), and sexual conversion (*pfap2-g*) all share certain epigenetic characteristics. When they are transcriptionally silent, they are bound by nucleosomes that incorporate the silent mark H3K9me3, in particular surrounding the transcriptional start site (Chookajorn et al. 2007; Lopez-Rubio et al. 2009; Jiang et al. 2010; Crowley et al. 2011; Kafsack et al. 2014). When individual genes are activated, H3K9me3 is replaced by H3K9ac, and this appears to be a key step in switching the transcriptional state of the gene (Lopez-Rubio et al. 2007; Crowley et al. 2011). Once in place, the activating or silencing histone marks are maintained throughout the remainder of the asexual cycle, even at points in the cycle when the genes are inactive. Furthermore, these marks are faithfully reproduced as the genome replicates through schizogony, resulting in epigenetic memory. Changes in these histone modifications occur at low frequencies, resulting in clonal variation. The H3K9me3 modification is recognized by heterochromatin protein 1 (HP1) that begins the chromatin condensation process that results in segregation into the nuclear periphery and prevents transcription (Flueck et al. 2009; Perez-Toledo et al. 2009). The importance of HP1 in this process is shown by experiments in which its expression is disrupted. In the absence of HP1, all clonally variant genes become transcriptionally active simultaneously, leading to disruption of antigenic variation and rapid differentiation into the sexual conversion pathway (Brancucci et al. 2014). A similar phenotype results from disruption of the histone deacetylase PfHda2 (Coleman et al. 2014), further demonstrating the shared epigenetic mechanisms controlling expression of clonally variant gene families. These profound phenotypes reveal the importance of proper regulation of heterochromatin for parasite biology.

Specific Mechanisms Regulating *var* Gene Expression

Of the genes that undergo clonally variant expression, the most work has focused on the *var* gene family that encodes the variant surface protein PfEMP1. The haploid genome of any given parasite includes approximately 60 *var* genes, which are expressed in a mutually exclusive manner. As described above, the active gene is associated with chromatin that incorporates the H3K9ac modification, whereas the remaining, silent members of the family are marked by histones carrying H3K9me3. As expected, the silent genes are bound by HP1 and incorporated into heterochromatin that is segregated into the nuclear periphery, in which they group together into five to seven clusters (Freitas-Junior et al. 2000). Interestingly, the active member of the family is also found at the nuclear periphery, but it is separated from the silent genes into a subnuclear position that also includes the histone methyltransferase PfSET10 (Duraisingh et al. 2005; Ralph et al. 2005; Volz et al. 2012). It is postulated that this methyltransferase is responsible for the H3K4me3 modification found at the active *var* gene (Volz et al. 2012). An additional histone mark that appears to be important for *var* gene regulation is H3K36me3, a modification incorporated by the methyltransferase PfSET2 (Cui et al. 2008a) that in model eukaryotes is typically associated with transcriptional elongation. Surprisingly, disruption of the gene encoding PfSET2 completely disrupts mutually exclusive expression, leading to simultaneous expression of all members of the family and suggesting that H3K36me3 might be required for *var* gene silencing (Jiang et al. 2013). However, H3K36me3 is found within the body of both active and silent *var* genes, suggesting an alternative model in which this histone mark is required for the recognition of *var* genes as members of the *var* gene family. This hypothesis has implications for coordination of gene expression and mutually exclusive expression.

In addition to specific histone modifications associated with active and silent *var* genes, incorporation of variant histones into the nucleosomes found at specific regions of the genome also appears to contribute to *var* gene regulation. The variant histone H2A.Z is found within nucleosomes throughout the genome wherever H3K9ac and H3K4me3 are found (Bartfai et al. 2010; Petter et al. 2011), consistent with a role in maintaining euchromatin. Although at most genes incorporation of H2A.Z is stable throughout the asexual cycle, at the single active *var* gene H2A.Z incorporation into nucleosomes at the promoter appears to be temporally regulated and is observed only at the point in the cycle when the *var* gene is actively transcribed (Petter et al. 2011), thus nucleosome exchange could play a role in *var* gene activation. In contrast, silent *var* genes are devoid of this histone variant. More recent work has identified double-variant histones that incorporate both H2A.Z and H2B.Z at transcriptionally active genomic regions, including the active *var* gene promoter (Hoeijmakers et al. 2013; Petter et al. 2013). The amount of double-variant histones found within intergenic regions correlates with the strength of the nearby promoters as well as the base composition of the underlying DNA, suggesting a model in which double-variant histones help to demarcate transcriptionally active and silent regions of the genome.

Although the histone marks associated with active or silent *var* genes have now been identified, it is not yet clear how the histone modifiers are selectively targeted to specific genes to properly mark them for activation or silencing. DNA regulatory elements have been identified both within individual *var* genes (Avraham et al. 2012; Brancucci et al. 2012) and separating genes within *var* tandem arrays (Wei et al. 2015), but their possible role in recruiting epigenetic factors remains uncharacterized. ncRNAs have been implicated in this process in many model eukaryotic systems, and similar mechanisms are likely to be at play with *var* genes. ncRNAs were first identified associated with *var* genes when this gene family was initially discovered, although their function was not understood (Su et al. 1995). These RNAs are transcribed from an RNA pol II promoter found within the conserved intron located within all *var* genes (Kyes et al. 2007). The intron is re-

quired for the recognition of *var* genes for mutually exclusive expression (Deitsch et al. 2001; Dzikowski et al. 2007), and it has been shown to transcribe an antisense ncRNA from the single active gene while producing sense ncRNAs from all members of the family (Jiang et al. 2013; Amit-Avraham et al. 2015). The role of the ncRNAs themselves is not known; however, targeting the antisense transcripts for degradation or overexpression greatly alters *var* gene expression patterns (Amit-Avraham et al. 2015), and an RNA exosome was recently identified that appears to be important for controlling antisense ncRNA levels (Zhang et al. 2014). Disruption of the RNAse activity of this exosome strongly affects *var* gene expression patterns. In addition to the ncRNAs themselves, the RNA pol II complex that transcribes them might also play a direct role in recruiting histone modifiers to *var* loci. PfSET2, the histone methyltransferase that deposits the H3K36me3 mark at *var* genes, binds to the carboxy-terminal domain of RNA pol II and, thus, could be recruited by the polymerase while it is transcribing the sense ncRNAs (Ukaegbu et al. 2014). This would explain why both active and silent genes are marked by H3K36me3, and is consistent with the hypothesis that this mark is responsible for genes to be recognized as members of the *var* gene family. Additional work will begin to decipher how these different aspects of *var* gene regulation integrate into an overall mechanism of control, and further how mutually exclusive expression and switching are coordinated. Work in the field will also help to determine how *var* gene switching integrates with selection by the human immune system (Abdi et al. 2016), a topic that has not been extensively studied, and also how transmission through the mosquito potentially "resets" the expression patterns of clonally variant gene families (Spence et al. 2015).

IMPORTANCE OF RESEARCH ON MALARIA EPIGENETICS IN THE CONTEXT OF ERADICATION

The new paradigm in the fight against malaria is eradication. An agenda has been developed to guide the steps that need to be undertaken to achieve this ambitious aim (Alonso et al. 2011). Considering the low expectations of having a highly effective vaccine available in the next few years, elimination efforts will have to rely mainly on vector control strategies and antimalarial drugs that could be used in mass drug administration schemes. Monitoring and diagnostic tools will also play important roles in elimination campaigns. Research on malaria epigenetics can contribute to the development of new public health tools that could facilitate elimination.

Monitoring Malaria Phenotypes: Genes under Epigenetic Regulation as Markers for Virulence and Transmission Potential

Malaria elimination campaigns will represent an extremely strong selective pressure for malaria parasites, which makes it reasonable to fear that such interventions may result in accelerated parasite evolution. There is a risk that elimination efforts may select for "super-parasites" with undesirable traits, such as increased virulence, more efficient transmission, increased resilience in front of low vector availability, increased resistance to multiple drugs, or even an increased ability to generate resistance to new drugs reminiscent of the "accelerated resistance to multiple drugs" (ARMD) phenotype (Rathod et al. 1997). Monitoring how parasite traits evolve during elimination campaigns is essential to avoid potentially disastrous consequences of the attempts to eradicate the disease. Monitoring will be necessary at the epidemiological level, but also at the genetic, phenotypic, and epigenetic levels. Strong pressures can obviously result in the selection of genetic variants that confer increased fitness in front of the new challenges, but it is also possible that there is a selection of parasites with epigenetic patterns that have an analogous effect. As described above, some parasite traits are associated with the expression of specific clonally variant genes: for example, expression of some *var* genes is associated with increased risk of severe disease (Jensen et al. 2004; Rottmann et al. 2006; Avril et al. 2012; Claessens et al. 2012; Lavstsen et al. 2012), and *pfap2-g* expression levels could be

used as a proxy for parasite investment into sexual conversion and transmission. Expression of these genes and several others should be characterized in parasites that persist in settings in which elimination efforts are not completely successful and a residual parasite population survives, albeit with altered epidemiology. This could help to understand the adaptive pathways of surviving parasites, as well as to appreciate the potential risks associated with the evolved parasites (e.g., increased virulence), or to identify their Achilles' heels.

Epigenetic Regulation of Gene Expression as a Target for Therapeutic Intervention: "Epidrugs"

It is unclear whether existing drugs, used wisely, are sufficient to achieve success in malaria elimination campaigns. In any case, new antimalarial drugs with desirable properties, such as being effective against all parasite stages or requiring a single dose, if available, would certainly facilitate the task. In this regard, epigenetic regulators are considered a promising new class of drug targets, with some attractive characteristics described below.

Epigenetic regulation of gene expression is a highly dynamic process, implying that it is possible to alter normal epigenetic states through modulation of the enzymes involved in the process. Interfering pharmacologically with the delicate balance between the alternative epigenetic states of clonally variant genes could compromise parasite survival in several ways (Fig. 3). First, inhibiting the epigenetic factors that are necessary for *var* silencing could result in parasites that simultaneously express multiple forms of PfEMP1, inducing the development of broadly reactive immune responses that eliminate the current infection and additionally confer protection against future infections. An analogous strategy to disrupt normal antigenic variation has been successfully applied to induce protective immunity against *Giardia lamblia* in rodent models of disease (Rivero et al. 2010). Second, altering the balance between the active and silenced states of *pfap2-g* could result in either massive sexual conversion or no pro-

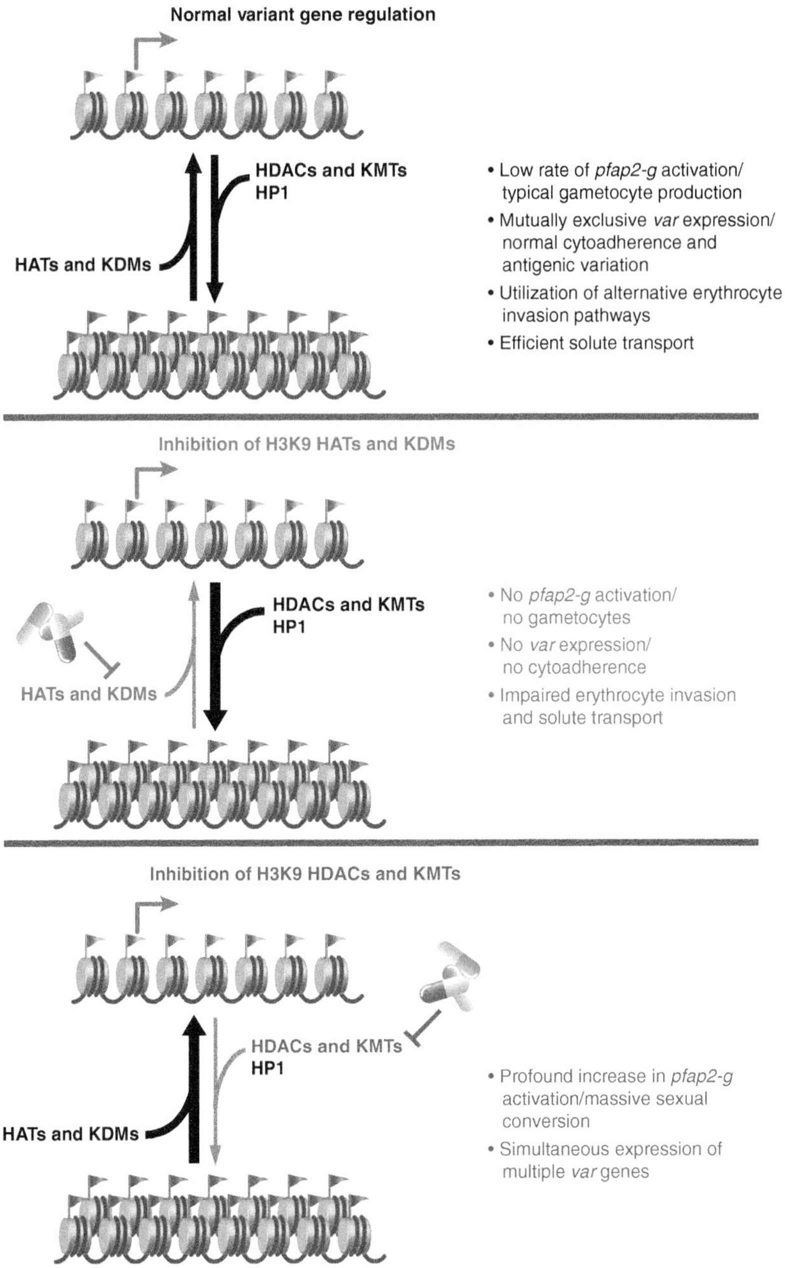

Figure 3. Epigenetic factors as targets for drug development. The normal balance between the euchromatic (active) and heterochromatic (silenced) states of clonally variant genes (*top* panel) can be altered pharmacologically. Drugs that inhibit the factors that catalyze the transition to or the maintenance of the active state are expected to shift the balance toward the silenced state (*middle* panel). In contrast, drugs that inhibit the factors that catalyze the transition to or the maintenance of the silenced state are expected to shift the balance toward the active state (*bottom* panel). The predicted effects of chemical inhibition of enzymes that participate in the regulation of clonally variant genes in general are listed. As examples, enzymes that operate on H3K9 are shown, but inhibition of enzymes that regulate the deposition or removal of other histone modifications (e.g., H4K20me3) may have similar effects. Inhibitors of epigenetic factors that participate in the regulation of only some clonally variant gene families (e.g., *var* genes) are expected to have family-specific effects. The predicted histone acetyltransferases (HATs), lysine demethylases (KDMs), histone deacetylases (HDACs), and lysine methyltransferases (KMTs) that operate on H3K9 are described in Table 2.

Cite this article as *Cold Spring Harb Perspect Med* doi: 10.1101/cshperspect.a025528

duction of sexual forms, both with catastrophic consequences for the parasite. It is important to note that malaria elimination efforts would tremendously benefit from drugs that kill gametocytes and consequently prevent transmission, but gametocytes are highly resilient to chemical attack and most current antimalarial drugs are not efficient against them (malERA Consultative Group on Drugs 2011). Thus, inhibiting the epigenetic mechanisms that drive the conversion of parasites into sexual forms arguably provides an attractive alternative to directly targeting gametocytes. Third, inhibiting malaria chromatin modifiers that do not specifically regulate clonally variant genes but participate in normal cell cycle progression could directly kill the parasites.

Orthologs of many known chromatin modifiers have been identified in the *P. falciparum* genome (Cui et al. 2008a; Bischoff and Vaquero 2010). The first obvious targets for antimalarial "epidrug" development are the enzymes that add or remove acetyl or methyl groups from histone tails (Table 2). Importantly, inhibitors of this type of enzymes have been developed for the fight against other diseases such as cancer, providing a large number of chemical starting points and a wealth of knowledge that could be used for the development of malaria-specific epigenetic inhibitors (Arrowsmith et al. 2012). Several compounds that were identified as inhibitors of histone deacetylases (HDACs) or acetyltransferases (HATs) in other eukaryotes inhibit *P. falciparum* growth, and some of them have a more potent effect on malaria parasites than on human cells (Merrick and Duraisingh 2007; Cui et al. 2008b; Andrews et al. 2012a,b; Duffy et al. 2014). Inhibitors of *P. falciparum* lysine methyltransferases (KMTs) have also been identified and shown to effectively kill malaria parasites of different species and at different stages of development (Malmquist et al. 2012, 2015). Furthermore, a sublethal concentration of one such compound, chaetocin, was recently shown to alter the epigenetic regulation of *var* gene expression by increasing the frequency of expression switches in this gene family (Ukaegbu et al. 2015). Interestingly, another KMT inhibitor was shown to activate dormant liver forms called hypnozoites (Dembele et al. 2014), which are produced by some malaria parasite species including *P. vivax* and are considered one of the less accessible malaria infection reservoirs. This observation raises the intriguing possibility that hypnozoite activation may be regulated at the epigenetic level. If this is the case, it may be possible to target these highly resilient forms with epigenetic drugs.

FUTURE PERSPECTIVES

Epigenetics continues to be a vibrant field of investigation in all eukaryotic systems, from animals to plants to protozoans. Given their somewhat "stripped down" repertoire of transcription factors, it is likely to play an even bigger role in the biology of malaria parasites. With the development of drugs that target epigenetic factors as therapies for human diseases like autoimmune disorders or cancer, this rapidly evolving technology can be applied to the development of antimalarial compounds that kill parasites, reduce virulence, and disrupt transmission, all key components of any elimination/eradication campaign. Along the way, these compounds will also serve as tools for investigating the basic biology of these evolutionarily distant and fascinating organisms. The recent development of new technologies for genetic manipulation of the parasites, including powerful methods for genome editing, will also contribute to addressing some of the burning questions in the malaria epigenetics field described in this chapter. Considering that epigenetics often studies properties that vary from one cell to another, it will be important to also develop improved technologies for analysis at the single-cell level, which could bring enormous progress to the field.

CONCLUDING REMARKS

It is exciting to once again consider the prospects of malaria elimination and eradication after such plans were previously abandoned decades ago. Recent gains in reducing the global malaria burden provide tantalizing hope that elimination is indeed possible. Nonetheless, for progress against the disease to be sustained, new intervention strategies will be required as drug and insecticide resistance inevitably arise. As funds and resources are devoted to disease reduction in the field, it will be important not to neglect basic research into the fundamental biology of the parasite and its mosquito vector. It is this discovery process that will yield the drugs, vaccines, and intervention strategies of the future that will be required for the ultimate eradication of malaria. Epigenetics is one such field that is rapidly developing and likely to be a rich source of novel targets for antimalaria strategies.

ACKNOWLEDGMENTS

We apologize for important work that could not be cited owing to space restrictions. A.C. is supported by Spanish Ministry of Economy and Competitiveness (MINECO; Grant SAF2013-43601-R), co-funded by the European Regional Development Fund (ERDF, European Union), and Grant 2014 SGR 485 from the Secretary for Universities and Research under the Department of Economy and Knowledge of the Government of Catalonia. K.W.D. is supported by Grants AI052390 and AI099327 from the National Institutes of Health.

REFERENCES

Abdi AI, Warimwe GM, Muthui MK, Kivisi CA, Kiragu EW, Fegan GW, Bull PC. 2016. Global selection of *Plasmodium falciparum* virulence antigen expression by host antibodies. *Sci Rep* 6: 19882.

al-Khedery B, Barnwell JW, Galinski MR. 1999. Antigenic variation in malaria: A 3' genomic alteration associated with the expression of a *P. knowlesi* variant antigen. *Mol Cell* 3: 131–141.

Alonso PL, Brown G, Arevalo-Herrera M, Binka F, Chitnis C, Collins F, Doumbo OK, Greenwood B, Hall BF, Levine MM, et al. 2011. A research agenda to underpin malaria eradication. *PLoS Med* 8: e1000406.

Amambua-Ngwa A, Tetteh KK, Manske M, Gomez-Escobar N, Stewart LB, Deerhake ME, Cheeseman IH, Newbold CI, Holder AA, Knuepfer E, et al. 2012. Population genomic scan for candidate signatures of balancing selection to guide antigen characterization in malaria parasites. *PLoS Genet* 8: e1002992.

Amit-Avraham I, Pozner G, Eshar S, Fastman Y, Kolevzon N, Yavin E, Dzikowski R. 2015. Antisense long noncoding RNAs regulate *var* gene activation in the malaria parasite *Plasmodium falciparum*. *Proc Natl Acad Sci* 112: E982–E991.

Andrews KT, Gupta AP, Tran TN, Fairlie DP, Gobert GN, Bozdech Z. 2012a. Comparative gene expression profiling of *P. falciparum* malaria parasites exposed to three different histone deacetylase inhibitors. *PLoS ONE* 7: e31847.

Andrews KT, Haque A, Jones MK. 2012b. HDAC inhibitors in parasitic diseases. *Immunol Cell Biol* 90: 66–77.

Arrowsmith CH, Bountra C, Fish PV, Lee K, Schapira M. 2012. Epigenetic protein families: A new frontier for drug discovery. *Nat Rev Drug Discov* 11: 384–400.

Avraham I, Schreier J, Dzikowski R. 2012. Insulator-like pairing elements regulate silencing and mutually exclusive expression in the malaria parasite *Plasmodium falciparum*. *Proc Natl Acad Sci* 109: E3678–E3686.

Avril M, Tripathi AK, Brazier AJ, Andisi C, Janes JH, Soma VL, Sullivan DJ Jr, Bull PC, Stins MF, Smith JD. 2012. A restricted subset of *var* genes mediates adherence of *Plasmodium falciparum*–infected erythrocytes to brain endothelial cells. *Proc Natl Acad Sci* 109: E1782–E1790.

Bartfai R, Hoeijmakers WA, Salcedo-Amaya AM, Smits AH, Janssen-Megens E, Kaan A, Treeck M, Gilberger TW, Francoijs KJ, Stunnenberg HG. 2010. H2A.Z demarcates intergenic regions of the *Plasmodium falciparum* epigenome that are dynamically marked by H3K9ac and H3K4me3. *PLoS Pathog* 6: e1001223.

Baruch DI, Pasloske BL, Singh HB, Bi X, Ma XC, Feldman M, Taraschi TF, Howard RJ. 1995. Cloning the *P. falciparum* gene encoding PfEMP1, a malarial variant antigen and adherence receptor on the surface of parasitized human erythrocytes. *Cell* 82: 77–87.

Bethke LL, Zilversmit M, Nielsen K, Daily J, Volkman SK, Ndiaye D, Lozovsky ER, Hartl DL, Wirth DF. 2006. Duplication, gene conversion, and genetic diversity in the species-specific acyl-CoA synthetase gene family of *Plasmodium falciparum*. *Mol Biochem Parasitol* 150: 10–24.

Bischoff E, Vaquero C. 2010. *In silico* and biological survey of transcription-associated proteins implicated in the transcriptional machinery during the erythrocytic development of *Plasmodium falciparum*. *BMC Genomics* 11: 34.

Bousema T, Drakeley C. 2011. Epidemiology and infectivity of *Plasmodium falciparum* and *Plasmodium vivax* gametocytes in relation to malaria control and elimination. *Clin Microbiol Rev* 24: 377–410.

Bozdech Z, Llinas M, Pulliam BL, Wong ED, Zhu J, DeRisi JL. 2003. The transcriptome of the intraerythrocytic developmental cycle of *Plasmodium falciparum*. *PLoS Biol* 1: E5.

Brancucci NM, Witmer K, Schmid CD, Flueck C, Voss TS. 2012. Identification of a cis-acting DNA-protein interaction implicated in singular *var* gene choice in *Plasmodium falciparum*. *Cell Microbiol* 14: 1836–1848.

Brancucci NM, Bertschi NL, Zhu L, Niederwieser I, Chin WH, Wampfler R, Freymond C, Rottmann M, Felger I, Bozdech Z, et al. 2014. Heterochromatin protein 1 secures survival and transmission of malaria parasites. *Cell Host Microbe* 16: 165–176.

Broadbent KM, Broadbent JC, Ribacke U, Wirth D, Rinn JL, Sabeti PC. 2015. Strand-specific RNA sequencing in *Plasmodium falciparum* malaria identifies developmentally regulated long non-coding RNA and circular RNA. *BMC Genomics* **16**: 454.

Bunnik EM, Polishko A, Prudhomme J, Ponts N, Gill SS, Lonardi S, Le Roch KG. 2014. DNA-encoded nucleosome occupancy is associated with transcription levels in the human malaria parasite *Plasmodium falciparum*. *BMC Genomics* **15**: 347.

Chan JA, Fowkes FJ, Beeson JG. 2014. Surface antigens of *Plasmodium falciparum*–infected erythrocytes as immune targets and malaria vaccine candidates. *Cell Mol Life Sci* **71**: 3633–3657.

Chen PB, Ding S, Zanghi G, Soulard V, DiMaggio PA, Fuchter MJ, Mecheri S, Mazier D, Scherf A, Malmquist NA. 2016. *Plasmodium falciparum* PfSET7: Enzymatic characterization and cellular localization of a novel protein methyltransferase in sporozoite, liver and erythrocytic stage parasites. *Sci Rep* **6**: 21802.

Chookajorn T, Dzikowski R, Frank M, Li F, Jiwani AZ, Hartl DL, Deitsch KW. 2007. Epigenetic memory at malaria virulence genes. *Proc Natl Acad Sci* **104**: 899–902.

Claessens A, Adams Y, Ghumra A, Lindergard G, Buchan CC, Andisi C, Bull PC, Mok S, Gupta AP, Wang CW, et al. 2012. A subset of group A-like *var* genes encodes the malaria parasite ligands for binding to human brain endothelial cells. *Proc Natl Acad Sci* **109**: E1772–E1781.

Coleman BI, Skillman KM, Jiang RH, Childs LM, Altenhofen LM, Ganter M, Leung Y, Goldowitz I, Kafsack BF, Marti M, et al. 2014. A *Plasmodium falciparum* histone deacetylase regulates antigenic variation and gametocyte conversion. *Cell Host Microbe* **16**: 177–186.

Comeaux CA, Coleman BI, Bei AK, Whitehurst N, Duraisingh MT. 2011. Functional analysis of epigenetic regulation of tandem *RhopH1/clag* genes reveals a role in *Plasmodium falciparum* growth. *Mol Microbiol* **80**: 378–390.

Cortés A. 2008. Switching *Plasmodium falciparum* genes on and off for erythrocyte invasion. *Trends Parasitol* **24**: 517–524.

Cortés A, Carret C, Kaneko O, Yim Lim BY, Ivens A, Holder AA. 2007. Epigenetic silencing of *Plasmodium falciparum* genes linked to erythrocyte invasion. *PLoS Pathog* **3**: e107.

Cortés A, Crowley VM, Vaquero A, Voss TS. 2012. A view on the role of epigenetics in the biology of malaria parasites. *PLoS Pathog* **8**: e1002943.

Crowley VM, Rovira-Graells N, de Pouplana LR, Cortés A. 2011. Heterochromatin formation in bistable chromatin domains controls the epigenetic repression of clonally variant *Plasmodium falciparum* genes linked to erythrocyte invasion. *Mol Microbiol* **80**: 391–406.

Cui L, Miao J, Furuya T, Li X, Su XZ, Cui L. 2007. PfGCN5-mediated histone H3 acetylation plays a key role in gene expression in *Plasmodium falciparum*. *Eukaryot Cell* **6**: 1219–1227.

Cui L, Fan Q, Cui L, Miao J. 2008a. Histone lysine methyltransferases and demethylases in *Plasmodium falciparum*. *Int J Parasitol* **38**: 1083–1097.

Cui L, Miao J, Furuya T, Fan Q, Li X, Rathod PK, Su XZ, Cui L. 2008b. Histone acetyltransferase inhibitor anacardic acid causes changes in global gene expression during in vitro *Plasmodium falciparum* development. *Eukaryot Cell* **7**: 1200–1210.

Deitsch KW, Calderwood MS, Wellems TE. 2001. Malaria. Cooperative silencing elements in *var* genes. *Nature* **412**: 875–876.

Deitsch K, Duraisingh M, Dzikowski R, Gunasekera A, Khan S, Le Roch K, Llinas M, Mair G, McGovern V, Roos D, et al. 2007. Mechanisms of gene regulation in *Plasmodium*. *Am J Trop Med Hyg* **77**: 201–208.

del Portillo HA, Fernandez-Becerra C, Bowman S, Oliver K, Preuss M, Sanchez CP, Schneider NK, Villalobos JM, Rajandream MA, Harris D, et al. 2001. A superfamily of variant genes encoded in the subtelomeric region of *Plasmodium vivax*. *Nature* **410**: 839–842.

Dembele L, Franetich JF, Lorthiois A, Gego A, Zeeman AM, Kocken CH, Le Grand R, Dereuddre-Bosquet N, van Gemert GJ, Sauerwein R, et al. 2014. Persistence and activation of malaria hypnozoites in long-term primary hepatocyte cultures. *Nat Med* **20**: 307–312.

Desai SA. 2014. Why do malaria parasites increase host erythrocyte permeability? *Trends Parasitol* **30**: 151–159.

Duffy MF, Selvarajah SA, Josling GA, Petter M. 2014. Epigenetic regulation of the *Plasmodium falciparum* genome. *Brief Funct Genomics* **13**: 203–216.

Duraisingh MT, Triglia T, Ralph SA, Rayner JC, Barnwell JW, McFadden GI, Cowman AF. 2003. Phenotypic variation of *Plasmodium falciparum* merozoite proteins directs receptor targeting for invasion of human erythrocytes. *EMBO J* **22**: 1047–1057.

Duraisingh MT, Voss TS, Marty AJ, Duffy MF, Good RT, Thompson JK, Freitas-Junior LH, Scherf A, Crabb BS, Cowman AF. 2005. Heterochromatin silencing and locus repositioning linked to regulation of virulence genes in *Plasmodium falciparum*. *Cell* **121**: 13–24.

Dzikowski R, Li F, Amulic B, Eisberg A, Frank M, Patel S, Wellems TE, Deitsch KW. 2007. Mechanisms underlying mutually exclusive expression of virulence genes by malaria parasites. *EMBO Rep* **8**: 959–965.

Fan Q, An L, Cui L. 2004. *Plasmodium falciparum* histone acetyltransferase, a yeast GCN5 homologue involved in chromatin remodeling. *Eukaryot Cell* **3**: 264–276.

Fernandez V, Hommel M, Chen Q, Hagblom P, Wahlgren M. 1999. Small, clonally variant antigens expressed on the surface of the *Plasmodium falciparum*–infected erythrocyte are encoded by the *rif* gene family and are the target of human immune responses. *J Exp Med* **190**: 1393–1404.

Fischer K, Chavchich M, Huestis R, Wilson DW, Kemp DJ, Saul A. 2003. Ten families of variant genes encoded in subtelomeric regions of multiple chromosomes of *Plasmodium chabaudi*, a malaria species that undergoes antigenic variation in the laboratory mouse. *Mol Microbiol* **48**: 1209–1223.

Flueck C, Bartfai R, Volz J, Niederwieser I, Salcedo-Amaya AM, Alako BT, Ehlgen F, Ralph SA, Cowman AF, Bozdech Z, et al. 2009. *Plasmodium falciparum* heterochromatin protein 1 marks genomic loci linked to phenotypic variation of exported virulence factors. *PLoS Pathog* **5**: e1000569.

Freitas-Junior LH, Bottius E, Pirrit LA, Deitsch KW, Scheidig C, Guinet F, Nehrbass U, Wellems TE, Scherf A. 2000. Frequent ectopic recombination of virulence factor genes in telomeric chromosome clusters of *P. falciparum*. *Nature* **407**: 1018–1022.

Freitas-Junior LH, Hernandez-Rivas R, Ralph SA, Montiel-Condado D, Ruvalcaba-Salazar OK, Rojas-Meza AP, Mancio-Silva L, Leal-Silvestre RJ, Gontijo AM, Shorte S, et al. 2005. Telomeric heterochromatin propagation and histone acetylation control mutually exclusive expression of antigenic variation genes in malaria parasites. *Cell* 121: 25–36.

Ganesan K, Ponmee N, Jiang L, Fowble JW, White J, Kamchonwongpaisan S, Yuthavong Y, Wilairat P, Rathod PK. 2008. A genetically hard-wired metabolic transcriptome in *Plasmodium falciparum* fails to mount protective responses to lethal antifolates. *PLoS Pathog* 4: e1000214.

Goel S, Palmkvist M, Moll K, Joannin N, Lara P, Akhouri RR, Moradi N, Ojemalm K, Westman M, Angeletti D, et al. 2015. RIFINs are adhesins implicated in severe *Plasmodium falciparum* malaria. *Nat Med* 21: 314–317.

Gomez-Escobar N, Amambua-Ngwa A, Walther M, Okebe J, Ebonyi A, Conway DJ. 2010. Erythrocyte invasion and merozoite ligand gene expression in severe and mild *Plasmodium falciparum* malaria. *J Infect Dis* 201: 444–452.

Gupta AP, Chin WH, Zhu L, Mok S, Luah YH, Lim EH, Bozdech Z. 2013. Dynamic epigenetic regulation of gene expression during the life cycle of malaria parasite *Plasmodium falciparum*. *PLoS Pathog* 9: e1003170.

Gupta A, Thiruvengadam G, Desai SA. 2015. The conserved *clag* multigene family of malaria parasites: Essential roles in host-pathogen interaction. *Drug Resist Updat* 18: 47–54.

Hodder AN, Czabotar PE, Uboldi AD, Clarke OB, Lin CS, Healer J, Smith BJ, Cowman AF. 2012. Insights into Duffy binding-like domains through the crystal structure and function of the merozoite surface protein MSPDBL2 from *Plasmodium falciparum*. *J Biol Chem* 287: 32922–32939.

Hoeijmakers WA, Flueck C, Francoijs KJ, Smits AH, Wetzel J, Volz JC, Cowman AF, Voss T, Stunnenberg HG, Bartfai R. 2012. *Plasmodium falciparum* centromeres display a unique epigenetic makeup and cluster prior to and during schizogony. *Cell Microbiol* 14: 1391–1401.

Hoeijmakers WA, Salcedo-Amaya AM, Smits AH, Francoijs KJ, Treeck M, Gilberger TW, Stunnenberg HG, Bartfai R. 2013. H2A.Z/H2B.Z double-variant nucleosomes inhabit the AT-rich promoter regions of the *Plasmodium falciparum* genome. *Mol Microbiol* 87: 1061–1073.

Iyer LM, Anantharaman V, Wolf MY, Aravind L. 2008. Comparative genomics of transcription factors and chromatin proteins in parasitic protists and other eukaryotes. *Int J Parasitol* 38: 1–31.

Janssen CS, Phillips RS, Turner CM, Barrett MP. 2004. *Plasmodium* interspersed repeats: the major multigene superfamily of malaria parasites. *Nucleic Acids Res* 32: 5712–5720.

Jensen AT, Magistrado P, Sharp S, Joergensen L, Lavstsen T, Chiucchiuini A, Salanti A, Vestergaard LS, Lusingu JP, Hermsen R, et al. 2004. *Plasmodium falciparum* associated with severe childhood malaria preferentially expresses PfEMP1 encoded by group A *var* genes. *J Exp Med* 199: 1179–1190.

Jiang L, Lopez-Barragan MJ, Jiang H, Mu J, Gaur D, Zhao K, Felsenfeld G, Miller LH. 2010. Epigenetic control of the variable expression of a *Plasmodium falciparum* receptor protein for erythrocyte invasion. *Proc Natl Acad Sci* 107: 2224–2229.

Jiang L, Mu J, Zhang Q, Ni T, Srinivasan P, Rayavara K, Yang W, Turner L, Lavstsen T, Theander TG, et al. 2013. PfSETvs methylation of histone H3K36 represses virulence genes in *Plasmodium falciparum*. *Nature* 499: 223–227.

Joshi MB, Lin DT, Chiang PH, Goldman ND, Fujioka H, Aikawa M, Syin C. 1999. Molecular cloning and nuclear localization of a histone deacetylase homologue in *Plasmodium falciparum*. *Mol Biochem Parasitol* 99: 11–19.

Josling GA, Petter M, Oehring SC, Gupta AP, Dietz O, Wilson DW, Schubert T, Langst G, Gilson PR, Crabb BS, et al. 2015. A *Plasmodium falciparum* bromodomain protein regulates invasion gene expression. *Cell Host Microbe* 17: 741–751.

Kafsack BF, Rovira-Graells N, Clark TG, Bancells C, Crowley VM, Campino SG, Williams AE, Drought LG, Kwiatkowski DP, Baker DA, et al. 2014. A transcriptional switch underlies commitment to sexual development in malaria parasites. *Nature* 507: 248–252.

Kats LM, Fernandez KM, Glenister FK, Herrmann S, Buckingham DW, Siddiqui G, Sharma L, Bamert R, Lucet I, Guillotte M, et al. 2014. An exported kinase (FIKK4.2) that mediates virulence-associated changes in *Plasmodium falciparum*–infected red blood cells. *Int J Parasitol* 44: 319–328.

Kensche PR, Hoeijmakers WA, Toenhake CG, Bras M, Chappell L, Berriman M, Bartfai R. 2016. The nucleosome landscape of *Plasmodium falciparum* reveals chromatin architecture and dynamics of regulatory sequences. *Nucleic Acids Res* 44: 2110–2124.

Kishore SP, Stiller JW, Deitsch KW. 2013. Horizontal gene transfer of epigenetic machinery and evolution of parasitism in the malaria parasite *Plasmodium falciparum* and other apicomplexans. *BMC Evol Biol* 13: 37.

Kyes SA, Rowe JA, Kriek N, Newbold CI. 1999. Rifins: A second family of clonally variant proteins expressed on the surface of red cells infected with *Plasmodium falciparum*. *Proc Natl Acad Sci* 96: 9333–9338.

Kyes S, Horrocks P, Newbold C. 2001. Antigenic variation at the infected red cell surface in malaria. *Annu Rev Microbiol* 55: 673–707.

Kyes S, Christodoulou Z, Pinches R, Kriek N, Horrocks P, Newbold C. 2007. *Plasmodium falciparum var* gene expression is developmentally controlled at the level of RNA polymerase II–mediated transcription initiation. *Mol Microbiol* 63: 1237–1247.

Lavazec C, Sanyal S, Templeton TJ. 2007. Expression switching in the *stevor* and *Pfmc-2TM* superfamilies in *Plasmodium falciparum*. *Mol Microbiol* 64: 1621–1634.

Lavstsen T, Turner L, Saguti F, Magistrado P, Rask TS, Jespersen JS, Wang CW, Berger SS, Baraka V, Marquard AM, et al. 2012. *Plasmodium falciparum* erythrocyte membrane protein 1 domain cassettes 8 and 13 are associated with severe malaria in children. *Proc Natl Acad Sci* 109: E1791–E1800.

Le Roch KG, Zhou Y, Blair PL, Grainger M, Moch JK, Haynes JD, De La Vega P, Holder AA, Batalov S, Carucci DJ, et al. 2003. Discovery of gene function by expression profiling of the malaria parasite life cycle. *Science* 301: 1503–1508.

Cite this article as *Cold Spring Harb Perspect Med* doi: 10.1101/cshperspect.a025528

Le Roch KG, Johnson JR, Ahiboh H, Chung DW, Prud-homme J, Plouffe D, Henson K, Zhou Y, Witola W, Yates JR, et al. 2008. A systematic approach to understand the mechanism of action of the bisthiazolium compound T4 on the human malaria parasite, *Plasmodium falciparum*. *BMC Genomics* **9**: 513.

Lopez-Rubio JJ, Gontijo AM, Nunes MC, Issar N, Hernan-dez Rivas R, Scherf A. 2007. 5′ flanking region of *var* genes nucleate histone modification patterns linked to phenotypic inheritance of virulence traits in malaria parasites. *Mol Microbiol* **66**: 1296–1305.

Lopez-Rubio JJ, Mancio-Silva L, Scherf A. 2009. Genome-wide analysis of heterochromatin associates clonally variant gene regulation with perinuclear repressive centers in malaria parasites. *Cell Host Microbe* **5**: 179–190.

Maier AG, Duraisingh MT, Reeder JC, Patel SS, Kazura JW, Zimmerman PA, Cowman AF. 2003. *Plasmodium falciparum* erythrocyte invasion through glycophorin C and selection for Gerbich negativity in human populations. *Nat Med* **9**: 87–92.

malERA Consultative Group on Drugs. 2011. A research agenda for malaria eradication: Drugs. *PLoS Med* **8**: e1000402.

Malmquist NA, Moss TA, Mecheri S, Scherf A, Fuchter MJ. 2012. Small-molecule histone methyltransferase inhibitors display rapid antimalarial activity against all blood stage forms in *Plasmodium falciparum*. *Proc Natl Acad Sci* **109**: 16708–16713.

Malmquist NA, Sundriyal S, Caron J, Chen P, Witkowski B, Menard D, Suwanarusk R, Renia L, Nosten F, Jimenez-Diaz MB, et al. 2015. Histone methyltransferase inhibitors are orally bioavailable, fast-acting molecules with activity against different species causing malaria in humans. *Antimicrob Agents Chemother* **59**: 950–959.

Merrick CJ, Duraisingh MT. 2007. *Plasmodium falciparum* Sir2: An unusual sirtuin with dual histone deacetylase and ADP-ribosyltransferase activity. *Eukaryot Cell* **6**: 2081–2091.

Merrick CJ, Jiang RH, Skillman KM, Samarakoon U, Moore RM, Dzikowski R, Ferdig MT, Duraisingh MT. 2015. Functional analysis of sirtuin genes in multiple *Plasmodium falciparum* strains. *PLoS ONE* **10**: e0118865.

Miao J, Fan Q, Cui L, Li X, Wang H, Ning G, Reese JC. 2010. The MYST family histone acetyltransferase regulates gene expression and cell cycle in malaria parasite *Plasmodium falciparum*. *Mol Microbiol* **78**: 883–902.

Miller LH, Good MF, Milon G. 1994. Malaria pathogenesis. *Science* **264**: 1878–1883.

Miller LH, Baruch DI, Marsh K, Doumbo OK. 2002. The pathogenic basis of malaria. *Nature* **415**: 673–679.

Mira-Martínez S, Rovira-Graells N, Crowley VM, Altenho-fen LM, Llinás M, Cortés A. 2013. Epigenetic switches in *clag3* genes mediate blasticidin S resistance in malaria parasites. *Cell Microbiol* **15**: 1913–1923.

Montgomery J, Mphande FA, Berriman M, Pain A, Roger-son SJ, Taylor TE, Molyneux ME, Craig A. 2007. Differential *var* gene expression in the organs of patients dying of falciparum malaria. *Mol Microbiol* **65**: 959–967.

Mphande FA, Ribacke U, Kaneko O, Kironde F, Winter G, Wahlgren M. 2008. SURFIN4.1, a schizont-merozoite associated protein in the SURFIN family of *Plasmodium falciparum*. *Malar J* **7**: 116.

Mwakalinga SB, Wang CW, Bengtsson DC, Turner L, Dinko B, Lusingu JP, Arnot DE, Sutherland CJ, Theander TG, Lavstsen T. 2012. Expression of a type B RIFIN in *Plasmodium falciparum* merozoites and gametes. *Malar J* **11**: 429.

Nguitragool W, Bokhari AA, Pillai AD, Rayavara K, Sharma P, Turpin B, Aravind L, Desai SA. 2011. Malaria parasite *clag3* genes determine channel-mediated nutrient uptake by infected red blood cells. *Cell* **145**: 665–677.

Niang M, Bei AK, Madnani KG, Pelly S, Dankwa S, Kanjee U, Gunalan K, Amaladoss A, Yeo KP, Bob NS, et al. 2014. STEVOR is a *Plasmodium falciparum* erythrocyte binding protein that mediates merozoite invasion and rosetting. *Cell Host Microbe* **16**: 81–93.

Nunes MC, Goldring JP, Doerig C, Scherf A. 2007. A novel protein kinase family in *Plasmodium falciparum* is differentially transcribed and secreted to various cellular compartments of the host cell. *Mol Microbiol* **63**: 391–403.

Oberli A, Slater LM, Cutts E, Brand F, Mundwiler-Pachlatko E, Rusch S, Masik MF, Erat MC, Beck HP, Vakonakis I. 2014. A *Plasmodium falciparum* PHIST protein binds the virulence factor PfEMP1 and comigrates to knobs on the host cell surface. *FASEB J* **28**: 4420–4433.

Perez-Toledo K, Rojas-Meza AP, Mancio-Silva L, Hernan-dez-Cuevas NA, Delgadillo DM, Vargas M, Martinez-Calvillo S, Scherf A, Hernandez-Rivas R. 2009. *Plasmodium falciparum* heterochromatin protein 1 binds to tri-methylated histone 3 lysine 9 and is linked to mutually exclusive expression of *var* genes. *Nucleic Acids Res* **37**: 2596–2606.

Petter M, Lee CC, Byrne TJ, Boysen KE, Volz J, Ralph SA, Cowman AF, Brown GV, Duffy MF. 2011. Expression of *P. falciparum var* genes involves exchange of the histone variant H2A.Z at the promoter. *PLoS Pathog* **7**: e1001292.

Petter M, Selvarajah SA, Lee CC, Chin WH, Gupta AP, Boz-dech Z, Brown GV, Duffy MF. 2013. H2A.Z and H2B.Z double-variant nucleosomes define intergenic regions and dynamically occupy *var* gene promoters in the malaria parasite *Plasmodium falciparum*. *Mol Microbiol* **87**: 1167–1182.

Pillai AD, Nguitragool W, Lyko B, Dolinta K, Butler MM, Nguyen ST, Peet NP, Bowlin TL, Desai SA. 2012. Solute restriction reveals an essential role for *clag3*-associated channels in malaria parasite nutrient acquisition. *Mol Pharmacol* **82**: 1104–1114.

Ponts N, Fu L, Harris EY, Zhang J, Chung DW, Cervantes MC, Prudhomme J, Atanasova-Penichon V, Zehraoui E, Bunnik EM, et al. 2013. Genome-wide mapping of DNA methylation in the human malaria parasite *Plasmodium falciparum*. *Cell Host Microbe* **14**: 696–706.

Proellocks NI, Herrmann S, Buckingham DW, Hanssen E, Hodges EK, Elsworth B, Morahan BJ, Coppel RL, Cooke BM. 2014. A lysine-rich membrane-associated PHISTb protein involved in alteration of the cytoadhesive properties of *Plasmodium falciparum*–infected red blood cells. *FASEB J* **28**: 3103–3113.

Ralph SA, Scheidig-Benatar C, Scherf A. 2005. Antigenic variation in *Plasmodium falciparum* is associated with movement of *var* loci between subnuclear locations. *Proc Natl Acad Sci* **102**: 5414–5419.

Rathod PK, McErlean T, Lee PC. 1997. Variations in frequencies of drug resistance in *Plasmodium falciparum*. *Proc Natl Acad Sci* **94:** 9389–9393.

Reed MB, Caruana SR, Batchelor AH, Thompson JK, Crabb BS, Cowman AF. 2000. Targeted disruption of an erythrocyte binding antigen in *Plasmodium falciparum* is associated with a switch toward a sialic acid-independent pathway of invasion. *Proc Natl Acad Sci* **97:** 7509–7514.

Rivero FD, Saura A, Prucca CG, Carranza PG, Torri A, Lujan HD. 2010. Disruption of antigenic variation is crucial for effective parasite vaccine. *Nat Med* **16:** 551–557.

Rottmann M, Lavstsen T, Mugasa JP, Kaestli M, Jensen AT, Muller D, Theander T, Beck HP. 2006. Differential expression of *var* gene groups is associated with morbidity caused by *Plasmodium falciparum* infection in Tanzanian children. *Infect Immun* **74:** 3904–3911.

Rovira-Graells N, Gupta AP, Planet E, Crowley VM, Mok S, Ribas de Pouplana L, Preiser PR, Bozdech Z, Cortés A. 2012. Transcriptional variation in the malaria parasite *Plasmodium falciparum*. *Genome Res* **22:** 925–938.

Rovira-Graells N, Crowley VM, Bancells C, Mira-Martínez S, Ribas de Pouplana L, Cortés A. 2015. Deciphering the principles that govern mutually exclusive expression of *Plasmodium falciparum clag3* genes. *Nucleic Acids Res* **43:** 8243–8257.

Salcedo-Amaya AM, van Driel MA, Alako BT, Trelle MB, van den Elzen AM, Cohen AM, Janssen-Megens EM, van de Vegte-Bolmer M, Selzer RR, Iniguez AL, et al. 2009. Dynamic histone H3 epigenome marking during the intra-erythrocytic cycle of *Plasmodium falciparum*. *Proc Natl Acad Sci* **106:** 9655–9660.

Sam-Yellowe TY, Florens L, Johnson JR, Wang T, Drazba JA, Le Roch KG, Zhou Y, Batalov S, Carucci DJ, Winzeler EA, et al. 2004. A *Plasmodium* gene family encoding Maurer's cleft membrane proteins: Structural properties and expression profiling. *Genome Res* **14:** 1052–1059.

Sanyal S, Egee S, Bouyer G, Perrot S, Safeukui I, Bischoff E, Buffet P, Deitsch KW, Mercereau-Puijalon O, David PH, et al. 2012. *Plasmodium falciparum* STEVOR proteins impact erythrocyte mechanical properties. *Blood* **119:** e1–e8.

Sargeant TJ, Marti M, Caler E, Carlton JM, Simpson K, Speed TP, Cowman AF. 2006. Lineage-specific expansion of proteins exported to erythrocytes in malaria parasites. *Genome Biol* **7:** R12.

Sharma P, Wollenberg K, Sellers M, Zainabadi K, Galinsky K, Moss E, Nguitragool W, Neafsey D, Desai SA. 2013. An epigenetic antimalarial resistance mechanism involving parasite genes linked to nutrient uptake. *J Biol Chem* **288:** 19429–19440.

Sierra-Miranda M, Delgadillo DM, Mancio-Silva L, Vargas M, Villegas-Sepulveda N, Martinez-Calvillo S, Scherf A, Hernandez-Rivas R. 2012. Two long non-coding RNAs generated from subtelomeric regions accumulate in a novel perinuclear compartment in *Plasmodium falciparum*. *Mol Biochem Parasitol* **185:** 36–47.

Simons AM. 2011. Modes of response to environmental change and the elusive empirical evidence for bet hedging. *Proc Biol Sci* **278:** 1601–1609.

Sinha A, Hughes KR, Modrzynska KK, Otto TD, Pfander C, Dickens NJ, Religa AA, Bushell E, Graham AL, Cameron R, et al. 2014. A cascade of DNA-binding proteins for sexual commitment and development in *Plasmodium*. *Nature* **507:** 253–257.

Smith JD, Chitnis CE, Craig AG, Roberts DJ, Hudson-Taylor DE, Peterson DS, Pinches R, Newbold CI, Miller LH. 1995. Switches in expression of *Plasmodium falciparum var* genes correlate with changes in antigenic and cytoadherent phenotypes of infected erythrocytes. *Cell* **82:** 101–110.

Spence PJ, Brugat T, Langhorne J. 2015. Mosquitoes reset malaria parasites. *PLoS Pathog* **11:** e1004987.

Stubbs J, Simpson KM, Triglia T, Plouffe D, Tonkin CJ, Duraisingh MT, Maier AG, Winzeler EA, Cowman AF. 2005. Molecular mechanism for switching of *P. falciparum* invasion pathways into human erythrocytes. *Science* **309:** 1384–1387.

Su XZ, Heatwole VM, Wertheimer SP, Guinet F, Herrfeldt JA, Peterson DS, Ravetch JA, Wellems TE. 1995. The large diverse gene family *var* encodes proteins involved in cytoadherence and antigenic variation of *Plasmodium falciparum*–infected erythrocytes. *Cell* **82:** 89–100.

Taylor HM, Grainger M, Holder AA. 2002. Variation in the expression of a *Plasmodium falciparum* protein family implicated in erythrocyte invasion. *Infect Immun* **70:** 5779–5789.

Tonkin CJ, Carret CK, Duraisingh MT, Voss TS, Ralph SA, Hommel M, Duffy MF, Silva LM, Scherf A, Ivens A, et al. 2009. Sir2 paralogues cooperate to regulate virulence genes and antigenic variation in *Plasmodium falciparum*. *PLoS Biol* **7:** e1000084.

Ukaegbu UE, Kishore SP, Kwiatkowski DL, Pandarinath C, Dahan-Pasternak N, Dzikowski R, Deitsch KW. 2014. Recruitment of PfSET2 by RNA polymerase II to variant antigen encoding loci contributes to antigenic variation in *P. falciparum*. *PLoS Pathog* **10:** e1003854.

Ukaegbu UE, Zhang X, Heinberg AR, Wele M, Chen Q, Deitsch KW. 2015. A unique virulence gene occupies a principal position in immune evasion by the malaria parasite *Plasmodium falciparum*. *PLoS Genet* **11:** e1005234.

Van Tyne D, Uboldi AD, Healer J, Cowman AF, Wirth DF. 2013. Modulation of PF10_0355 (MSPDBL2) alters *Plasmodium falciparum* response to antimalarial drugs. *Antimicrob Agents Chemother* **57:** 2937–2941.

Veening JW, Smits WK, Kuipers OP. 2008. Bistability, epigenetics, and bet-hedging in bacteria. *Annu Rev Microbiol* **62:** 193–210.

Volz J, Carvalho TG, Ralph SA, Gilson P, Thompson J, Tonkin CJ, Langer C, Crabb BS, Cowman AF. 2010. Potential epigenetic regulatory proteins localise to distinct nuclear sub-compartments in *Plasmodium falciparum*. *Int J Parasitol* **40:** 109–121.

Volz JC, Bartfai R, Petter M, Langer C, Josling GA, Tsuboi T, Schwach F, Baum J, Rayner JC, Stunnenberg HG, et al. 2012. PfSET10, a *Plasmodium falciparum* methyltransferase, maintains the active *var* gene in a poised state during parasite division. *Cell Host Microbe* **11:** 7–18.

Weber JL. 1988. Interspersed repetitive DNA from *Plasmodium falciparum*. *Mol Biochem Parasitol* **29:** 117–124.

Wei G, Zhao Y, Zhang Q, Pan W. 2015. Dual regulatory effects of non-coding GC-rich elements on the expression of virulence genes in malaria parasites. *Infect Genet Evol* **36:** 490–499.

Weiss GE, Gilson PR, Taechalertpaisarn T, Tham WH, de Jong NW, Harvey KL, Fowkes FJ, Barlow PN, Rayner JC, Wright GJ, et al. 2015. Revealing the sequence and resulting cellular morphology of receptor-ligand interactions during *Plasmodium falciparum* invasion of erythrocytes. *PLoS Pathog* **11:** e1004670.

Winter G, Kawai S, Haeggstrom M, Kaneko O, von Euler A, Kawazu S, Palm D, Fernandez V, Wahlgren M. 2005. SURFIN is a polymorphic antigen expressed on *Plasmodium falciparum* merozoites and infected erythrocytes. *J Exp Med* **201:** 1853–1863.

Wright GJ, Rayner JC. 2014. *Plasmodium falciparum* erythrocyte invasion: Combining function with immune evasion. *PLoS Pathog* **10:** e1003943.

Zhang Q, Siegel TN, Martins RM, Wang F, Cao J, Gao Q, Cheng X, Jiang L, Hon CC, Scheidig-Benatar C, et al. 2014. Exonuclease-mediated degradation of nascent RNA silences genes linked to severe malaria. *Nature* **513:** 431–435.

Antimalarial Drug Resistance: A Threat to Malaria Elimination

Didier Menard[1] and Arjen Dondorp[2]

[1]Malaria Molecular Epidemiology Unit, Institut Pasteur in Cambodia, Phnom Penh 12201, Cambodia

[2]Mahidol-Oxford Tropical Medicine Research Unit, Faculty of Tropical Medicine, Mahidol University, Bangkok 73170, Thailand

Correspondence: arjen@tropmedres.ac

Increasing antimalarial drug resistance once again threatens effective antimalarial drug treatment, malaria control, and elimination. Artemisinin combination therapies (ACTs) are first-line treatment for uncomplicated falciparum malaria in all endemic countries, yet partial resistance to artemisinins has emerged in the Greater Mekong Subregion. Concomitant emergence of partner drug resistance is now causing high ACT treatment failure rates in several areas. Genetic markers for artemisinin resistance and several of the partner drugs have been established, greatly facilitating surveillance. Single point mutations in the gene coding for the Kelch propeller domain of the K13 protein strongly correlate with artemisinin resistance. Novel regimens and strategies using existing antimalarial drugs will be needed until novel compounds can be deployed. Elimination of artemisinin resistance will imply elimination of all falciparum malaria from the same areas. In vivax malaria, chloroquine resistance is an increasing problem.

The two main pillars for malaria control and beyond remain targeting the anopheline mosquito vector and effective case management, which is crucially dependent on the efficacy of the deployed antimalarial drugs (Bhatt et al. 2015). Antimalarial drug resistance in *Plasmodium falciparum* tends to emerge in low-transmission settings, in particular in Southeast Asia or South America, before expanding to high-transmission settings in sub-Saharan Africa (White 2004). Resistance to chloroquine and later to sulfadoxine–pyrimethamine have followed this route and have contributed to millions of excess malaria attributable mortality in African children (Trape et al. 1998; Trape 2001;

Korenromp et al. 2003). At the end of the last century, introduction of the artemisinin combination therapies (ACTs) provided a much needed, highly efficacious antimalarial treatment, which became the first-line treatment for uncomplicated falciparum malaria in all endemic countries (WHO 2001, 2015a). Parenteral artesunate became the first-line treatment for severe malaria. However, partial artemisinin resistance characterized by much slower clearance of parasitemia in the first 3 days of treatment following artemisinin monotherapy or ACT was identified in western Cambodia in 2008–2009 (Noedl et al. 2008; Dondorp et al. 2009), and subsequently in all countries of the Greater

Mekong Subregion (Amaratunga et al. 2012; Hien et al. 2012; Phyo et al. 2012; Ashley et al. 2014; Huang et al. 2015). Artemisinin resistance has selected for concomitant resistance to ACT partner drugs, resulting in high late treatment failure rates with dihydroartemisinin–piperaquine in Cambodia (Leang et al. 2013, 2015; Lon et al. 2014; Saunders et al. 2014; Duru et al. 2015; Spring et al. 2015; Amaratunga et al. 2016) and with artesunate–mefloquine on the Thai–Myanmar border (Carrara et al. 2013). Close surveillance of the emergence and the distribution of artemisinin and partner drugs resistance are important to guide public health measures. This will require drug efficacy studies in sentinel sites, but can be greatly facilitated by the increasing availability of genetic markers for antimalarial drug resistance. New antimalarial treatments are urgently needed. It is expected that new compounds will not be ready for deployment before 2020 (Wells et al. 2015). Until then, novel strategies and regimes using existing antimalarial drugs will have to be implemented to ensure effective treatment. Elimination of artemisinin resistance will imply elimination of all falciparum malaria from the same areas before falciparum malaria becomes untreatable (Maude et al. 2009). This paradigm has contributed to the adoption of a malaria elimination agenda for the Greater Mekong Subregion, which also includes vivax malaria (WHO 2015b). In this respect, increasing resistance to *Plasmodium vivax* to chloroquine in Indonesia and beyond is an important notice.

This article discusses driving forces of antimalarial drug resistance, the global antimalarial drug resistance situation for *P. falciparum* and *P. vivax*, current insights in the molecular markers and mechanisms of antimalarial drug resistance with a focus on the artemisinins, and possible strategies for the treatment of artemisinin and multiple drug-resistant malaria in the context of malaria elimination.

ORIGINS OF ANTIMALARIAL DRUG RESISTANCE

De novo emergence of antimalarial drug resistance requires the spontaneous arising of mutations or gene duplications conferring reduced drug susceptibility, which is then selected in the individual by the presence of antimalarial drug concentrations sufficient to kill or inhibit the growth of sensitive parasites, but allowing expansion of the resistant clone. For the resistant parasite to be successful, the gene alterations conferring resistance should not affect parasite fitness to a large extent (White 2004; Barnes and White 2005). Drug-resistant mutations can arise in the sexual parasite stages in the mosquito (where diploidy and meiosis occur), in the preerythrocytic liver stages or in the asexual erythrocytic parasite stages, and there has been much debate on the most likely source (Pongtavornpinyo et al. 2009). It seems that resistant parasites are most likely to emerge during high levels of asexual-stage parasitemia in patients with subtherapeutic drug levels and, less likely, in the liver stages (Pongtavornpinyo et al. 2009; White et al. 2009). Antimalarial drugs will be more prone to resistance when requiring a limited number of genetic events conferring a considerable level of resistance (such as atovaquone or mefloquine), and when its pharmacokinetic properties include a long terminal half-life translating into a long period of subtherapeutic drug levels (such as piperaquine). Once resistance starts emerging, its transmission and, thus, spread are facilitated by the increased production of gametocytes in partial resistant strains, as shown, for instance, for sulfadoxine–pyrimethamine (Barnes et al. 2008).

Although the total number of circulating *P. falciparum* parasites and, thus, the number of spontaneous genetic events is much higher in high transmission settings in sub-Saharan Africa, history shows that antimalarial drug resistance is much more likely to emerge successfully in low transmission settings. In particular, Southeast Asia has in the last decades been the cradle for the emergence of *P. falciparum* resistance to chloroquine (Eyles et al. 1963; Young et al. 1963), sulfadoxine–pyrimethamine (Hofler 1980; Hurwitz et al. 1981), mefloquine (Boudreau et al. 1982; Smithuis et al. 1993), and more recently to artemisinins (Noedl et al. 2008; Dondorp et al. 2009) and piperaquine (Leang et al. 2013; Saunders et al.

Cite this article as *Cold Spring Harb Perspect Med* doi: 10.1101/cshperspect.a025619

2014). An important reason for this apparent brake on resistance emergence in regions with high stable transmission is host immunity, which can contribute substantially to parasite clearance of partial resistant parasite and also makes that older children and adults can carry substantial numbers of parasites without causing illness (Sarda et al. 2009; Lopera-Mesa et al. 2013). Because these individuals will not seek treatment, the associated large asymptomatic reservoir dilutes the selective pressure provided by antimalarial drugs at the population level (White 2004). In addition, in high transmission areas, patients have multiple strain infections transmitted to the mosquito vector. Crossing over of genes during meiosis in the mosquito can then break up resistance and compensatory mutations, and this greater opportunity for recombination will result in increased parasite diversity and direct competition between different parasite strains, with less opportunity for resistant alleles to become fixed (Jiang et al. 2011; Takala-Harrison and Laufer 2015). This is not the case in low transmission areas where multiple infections are much less common, infected individuals are less preimmune, usually more prone to be symptomatic, and, as a consequence, to be treated with possible poor-quality antimalarial drugs, incomplete treatment courses, or (artemisinin) monotherapies. *P. falciparum* parasite populations in Southeast Asia are highly structured with high rates of parasite inbreeding; particular genetic background alleles seem to predispose to the development of resistance-causing mutations through multistage processes in natural parasite populations (Miotto et al. 2013). Moreover, hemoglobinopathies (mainly HbAE or HbEE) and glucose-6-phosphate dehydrogenase deficiency, which are highly prevalent in Southeast Asian human populations, may have selected parasites less susceptible to oxidative stress while most antimalarial drugs currently in clinical use exert their activities, at least in part, by increasing oxidative stress in the parasitized erythrocyte (Becker et al. 2004).

Poor drug stewardship has been an important driver of antimalarial drug resistance, and in particular the emergence of artemisinin resistance in Southeast Asia. In the early 1960s, pyrimethamine and later chloroquine were added to salt for consumption as a measure of population malaria prophylaxis in Cambodia (Verdrager 1986). Although the artemisinins have been deployed as combination therapies in ACTs, unregulated artemisinin or artesunate monotherapy has been available since the mid-1970s in the region. In most countries, including Cambodia where artemisinin resistance was first recognized, the majority of patients obtain their antimalarial treatment through the private sector, which consisted until recent years mainly of artesunate monotherapy (Yeung et al. 2008). A ban on artemisinin monotherapies and deployment of fixed dose combinations for the majority of ACTs have been an important step forward. Counterfeited or substandard drugs that contain less active ingredients than stated are additional sources of subtherapeutic dosing of artemisinins, which may also have contributed to the selection of resistant parasite strains (Newton et al. 2003). Moreover, it is possible that the different pharmacokinetic properties of artemisinins in subgroups of the population, such as pregnant women and children, have resulted in underdosing (Kloprogge et al. 2015). It is thought that an important driver of the rapid spread of resistance to sulfadoxine–pyrimethamine in Africa has been underdosing of the drug in children with falciparum malaria (Barnes et al. 2006).

CURRENT MAP OF ANTIMALARIAL DRUG RESISTANCE IN *P. falciparum* AND *P. vivax*

The emergence and spread of antimalarial drug resistance is a dynamic process that can change by year. Figure 1 provides an overview of the current situation of falciparum artemisinin resistance (Fig. 1A) and vivax chloroquine resistance (Fig. 1B). For updated information, there are several sources intending to provide information in real time on the global antimalarial drug-resistance situation. The World Health Organization (WHO) maintains a network of sentinel sites in malaria-endemic countries performing therapeutic efficacy studies of first- and second-line antimalarial drugs using a

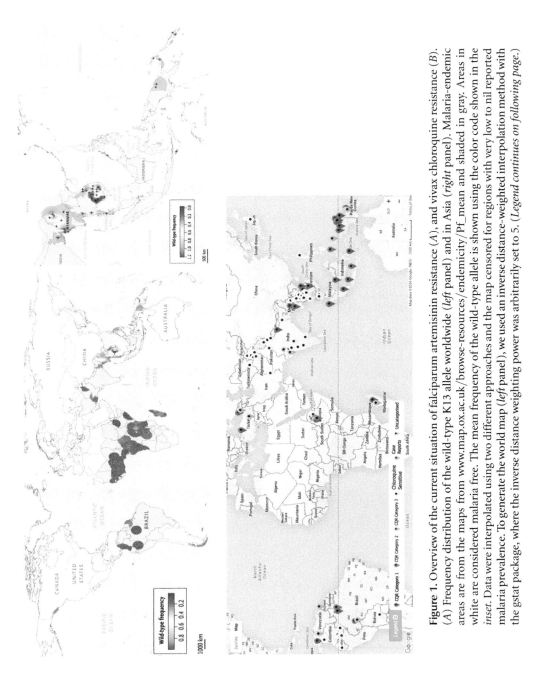

Figure 1. Overview of the current situation of falciparum artemisinin resistance (*A*), and vivax chloroquine resistance (*B*). (*A*) Frequency distribution of the wild-type K13 allele worldwide (*left* panel) and in Asia (*right* panel). Malaria-endemic areas are from the maps from www.map.ox.ac.uk/browse-resources/endemicity/Pf_mean and shaded in gray. Areas in white are considered malaria free. The mean frequency of the wild-type allele is shown using the color code shown in the *inset*. Data were interpolated using two different approaches and the map censored for regions with very low to nil reported malaria prevalence. To generate the world map (*left* panel), we used an inverse distance-weighted interpolation method with the gstat package, where the inverse distance weighting power was arbitrarily set to 5. (*Legend continues on following page.*)

standard protocol. Combined with information from national malaria control programs, the findings are regularly updated on the WHO website (www.who.int/topics/malaria/en). The WorldWide Antimalarial Resistance Network (WWARN) provides updated maps on antimalarial drug resistance from clinical and laboratory studies, including molecular markers, with a focus on academic and other research groups (www.wwarn.org). The KARMA international consortium (K13 Artemisinin Resistance Multicenter Assessment) launched in 2014 and led by the Institut Pasteur and the WHO provides a worldwide map of the polymorphism in the propeller domain of the *P. falciparum* K13 gene (see below) (Menard et al. 2016). The International Centers of Excellence for Malaria Research also established a network for monitoring of antimalarial drug efficacy (Cui et al. 2015). A number of research groups monitor drug efficacy through clinical and laboratory studies, which are published in peer-reviewed journals. Close cooperation between academic and research groups, and national malaria control programs is important for quick incorporation of results into drug policy.

ASSESSING ANTIMALARIAL DRUG EFFICACY

Sources of information on antimalarial drug efficacy include clinical drug efficacy studies, ex vivo and in vitro assessments of drug sensitivity, and molecular markers. Regarding clinical studies, it is important that follow-up of patients is sufficiently long to assess appropriate parasitological and clinical cure, in particular when trialing antimalarial drugs with long terminal half-lives, such as mefloquine or piperaquine. Short follow-up will miss up to 90% (at 14 d) or 50% (at 28 d) of late recrudescence infections, which can occur up to 63 d after the start of therapy (Stepniewska and White 2006). In trials on drug efficacy in falciparum malaria, it is important to distinguish between reinfection and recrudescence as the source of recurrent infection, using genotyping methods of parasite strains (WHO 2007). This is a major issue in vivax malaria, as genotyping cannot reliably classify recurrent infection into a relapsing infection (parasites released from liver hypnozoites) or recrudescent infection (resistant parasites), because parasites from relapse infection can be issued from a similar or a different hypnozoite clone than the initial clone (Chen et al. 2007; Imwong et al. 2007).

In vitro assays assessing the sensitivity of *P. falciparum* malaria parasites to antimalarial drugs is a research tool, which is frequently used to complement data from clinical studies and for providing data on the epidemiology of drug-resistant malaria. In vitro sensitivity testing can contribute to the early detection of emergence of drug resistance, changing trends in parasite drug susceptibility over time and space, or changes in the in vitro responses of indiv-

Figure 1. (*Continued*) A 100-km radius surrounding the coordinate sampling site(s) was used. To generate the Asia map (*right* panel), we used the well-established spatial statistical interpolation of ordinary kriging using a 50-km radius for the area surrounding the coordinate sampling site(s). The individual sites of sample collection are indicated with a cross (reproduced, with permission). (*B*) Chloroquine resistance in *Plasmodium vivax* infections. The map summarizes evidence from published and unpublished data from 1980 to 2015 compiled by the WWARN, available at www.wwarn.org. Category 1: >10% recurrent infections by day 28 (with a lower 95% CI of >5%), irrespective of confirmation of adequacy of blood chloroquine concentrations at the moment of recurrence. The presence of >10% recurrent infections is highly suggestive of chloroquine resistance. Category 2: parasitological confirmed recurrent infection within 28 d, in the presence of adequate whole-blood chloroquine concentrations (>100 nM) at the moment of recurrence. This confirms chloroquine resistance. Category 3: >5% recurrent infections by day 28 (lower 95%, CI of <5%), irrespective of confirmation of adequacy of blood chloroquine concentrations at the moment of recurrence. In this category, the contribution of other factors than drug resistance, such as poor drug absorption or drug quality, cannot be ruled out. Category 4: chloroquine-sensitive *P. vivax* infections, concluded from studies reporting on ≥10 symptomatic patients with symptomatic malaria, treated with chloroquine monotherapy (without early primaquine treatment), showing fewer than 5% recurrent infections within 28 d. (Reproduced, with permission, from WWARN.)

idual drugs currently deployed in combination therapies) (Guiguemde et al. 1994; Philipps et al. 1998; Ringwald et al. 2000; Menard et al. 2013). In vitro assessments are also useful for drug development (drug screening, isobologram studies for drug combinations, cross-resistance studies, in vitro phenotype comparisons of pre- and posttreatment isolates, baseline parasite susceptibility to a new drug before country implementation) and for validating candidate molecular markers associated with drug resistance. However, a limited number of laboratories in malaria-endemic countries have the capacity to perform in vitro assays, which requires sophisticated equipment, extensive resources, training, and expertise. There is no universally accepted, standardized protocol for in vitro drug sensitivity assays available, yet, but most protocols are based on the assessment of the 48-h *P. falciparum* in vitro development of isolates freshly collected in the field (ex vivo) or of short-/long-term culture-adapted parasite strains (in vitro), in the presence of increasing concentrations of antimalarial drugs (Basco 2007). The procedures for the parasite culture are those defined by Trager and Jensen (1976). The readout of the ex vivo or in vitro tests is parasite growth (at 48 h or later), evaluated by various methods including microscopy (Rieckmann et al. 1978), radioisotopic activity (isotopic test) (Desjardins et al. 1979), colorimetry (ELISA based on HRP2 and pLDH detection) (Makler and Hinrichs 1993; Brasseur et al. 2001; Noedl et al. 2002), fluorescence (Pico Green or Sybr Green dyes) (Smilkstein et al. 2004; Bacon et al. 2007; Rason et al. 2008), or flow cytometry (Pattanapanyasat et al. 1997; Contreras et al. 2004). In vitro susceptibility parameters of *P. falciparum* isolates are expressed as the 50% inhibitory concentration (IC_{50}) or the 90% inhibitory concentration (IC_{90}) defined as the minimal concentration of antimalarial drug that inhibits parasite growth by 50% or 90% compared with the development in drug-free control wells. IC_{50} and IC_{90} estimations can be calculated by a variety of means, including algorithms within software packages or freely available tools based on log-probit (Grab and Wernsdorfer 1983), polynomial (Noedl et al. 2002),

and sigmoid inhibition (Le Nagard et al. 2011) models. Easy-to-use online tools, such as ICEstimator 1.2 (www.antimalarial-icestimator.net) or IVART (www.wwarn.org/tools-resources/toolkit/analyse/ivart), are available for free.

The main advantage of in vitro susceptibility testing is that inhibitory constants calculated from the parasite growth are an inherent trait of the parasite and are not affected by host factors, such as acquired immunity, bioavailability, or pharmacokinetics of antimalarial drugs (e.g., low drug absorption or metabolic alterations) (Woodrow et al. 2013). However, for some drugs, classical in vitro assays have limited sensitivity for detecting resistant parasites. This is, in particular, the case for artemisinin derivatives. Most of the initial studies investigating in vitro susceptibility to artemisinin showed that the delayed parasite clearance phenotype does not correspond to increased artemisinin 50% inhibitory concentration (IC_{50}) values. Slightly increased IC_{50} values for dihydroartemisinin (the active metabolite of all artemisinins) were reported for slow-clearing parasites (Noedl et al. 2008), but they substantially overlap with those for fast-clearing parasites (Dondorp et al. 2009; Amaratunga et al. 2012). Studies with culture-adapted resistant parasite lines showed that artemisinin resistance was associated with decreased susceptibility of ring stages (Witkowski et al. 2010, 2013a,b; Cui et al. 2012; Klonis et al. 2013) and in some lines to mature stages (Cui et al. 2012; Teuscher et al. 2012). A novel in vitro assay (ring-stage survival assay [RSA]) that measures susceptibility of 0–3 h postinvasion *P. falciparum* ring stages to a pharmacologically relevant, short exposure (700 nM for 6 h) to dihydroartemisinin developed by Witkowski and colleagues demonstrated significant higher survival rates of culture-adapted parasites (in vitro $RSA^{0-3\,h}$) or fresh isolates (ex vivo RSA) in slow-clearing *P. falciparum* infections (threshold >1%) compared with isolates collected from fast-clearing infections (Witkowski et al. 2013a). In contrast, late rings and trophozoites from slow- and fast-clearing infections showed no difference in their susceptibility to dihydroartemisinin. Parasite survival rates in the RSA also significantly correlated with parasite clearance half-life, including in areas where artemisinin-resistant parasites had not yet been described, designating this assay as the current reference platform to detect in vitro artemisinin resistance.

Molecular markers associated with antimalarial drug resistance, when they are validated, are highly relevant to detect and monitor in real time the geospatial distribution of resistant parasites. To date, known molecular signatures are mutations in genes or changes in the copy number of genes encoding to the drug's parasite target or to transport proteins involved in intraparasitic influx/efflux of the drugs. Markers represent useful surveillance tools as their prevalence in a parasite population is often a good indicator of the level of clinical resistance. Different methods, including classical polymerase chain reaction (PCR), followed by direct sequencing, allele-specific PCR, PCR-RFLP, PCR-SSOP, FRET-MCA, PCR with molecular beacons, SNPE, PCR-LDR-FMA, and real-time PCR can be used depending on resources (Wilson et al. 2005; Barnadas et al. 2011). Their main advantage is that they allow us to test thousands of small volumes of blood samples (capillary blood collected by finger prick, spotted into filter paper, and stored at ambient temperature) at a wide scale by high-throughput automated approaches (Menard and Ariey 2015). Validated or candidate genetic markers are available for a limited number of antimalarial drugs, as described in Tables 1 and 2. Current molecular markers associated with antimalarial drug resistance are summarized in Table 1. These include markers for resistance to chloroquine (*Pfcrt*, *Pfmdr-1*), sulfonamides, and sulfones, including sulfadoxine (*Pfdhps*), pyrimethamine, cycloguanil and chlorcycloguanil (*Pfdhfr*), atovaquone (*Pfcytb*), mefloquine and halofantrine (*Pfmdr-1* amplification), amodiaquine (*Pfcrt*, *Pfmdr-1*), quinine (*Pfcrt*, *Pfmdr-1*, *Pfnhe-1*), and, most recently, artemisinins (*PfK13*).

Located on chromosome 13 (*PfK13* gene, PF3D7_1343700, previous ID: PF13_0238), *PfK13* is a single exon gene, which encodes a 726 amino acid protein that constitutes three domains, including a *Plasmodium*-specific/ Apicomplexa-specific domain, a BTB/POZ domain, and a six-blade β-propeller Kelch domain. Seminal studies performed by Ariey et al. (2014) demonstrated that a single mutation in the β-propeller domain of the K13 gene was a major determinant of resistance to artemisinin derivatives (see paragraph below). The identification of K13 mutant-allele parasites in patients with a slow parasite clearance rate and site-specific genome-editing experiments using zinc-finger nucleases (Straimer et al. 2015) or the CRISPR-Cas9 system (Ghorbal et al. 2014) provided final evidence that this molecular marker was a major determinant of resistance to artemisinin derivatives. However, because this is a laborious process, to date only four mutant alleles have been validated by genome editing (580C → Y, 539R → T, 543I → T, and 493Y → H) among the 173 nonsynonymous mutations described to date (Straimer et al. 2015; Menard et al. 2016). The discovery of K13 polymorphism as the major determinant of *P. falciparum* artemisinin resistance opened unprecedented opportunities for resistance monitoring and soon after this discovery several molecular epidemiology studies were conducted to map the extended artemisinin resistance (Ashley et al. 2014; Takala-Harrison et al. 2015; Tun et al. 2015). The KARMA project is the largest study, yet, and provides critical information for drug policymakers in the following years, by clarifying the roadmap for future surveillance activities involving samples collected across 59 malaria-endemic countries (Menard et al. 2016).

CURRENT INSIGHTS IN ARTEMISININ RESISTANCE

The clinical phenotype of artemisinin resistance is characterized by delayed parasite clearance after treatment with artemisinin monotherapy or an ACT. Delayed clearance can be assessed as an increased parasite half-life assessed from the log-linear part of the peripheral blood parasite clearance curve or as persistence of parasitemia at 72 h after the start of treatment (Flegg et al. 2011; White et al. 2015). In addition to resistance of the parasite to the artemisinins, para-

Table 1. Catalogue of the current molecular markers associated with antimalarial drug resistance

Plasmodium falciparum chloroquine resistance transporter (PfCRT)

Located on chromosome 7 (*Pfcrt* gene, PF3D7_0709000, previous ID: MAL7P1.27), *Pfcrt* encodes a food vacuole membrane transporter protein, member of the drug/metabolite transporter superfamily (Tran and Saier 2004). The mutation at codon 76 (K → T) always associated with other nonsynonymous mutations (at codons 72, 74, or 75) (Warhurst 2001; Sidhu et al. 2002) is the primary mediator of chloroquine resistance, by increasing the export of chloroquine from the food vacuole, away from its target (Sanchez et al. 2007). Laboratory experiments have shown that *Pfcrt* is also involved in decreasing parasites' susceptibility to monodesethylamodiaquine (SVMNT, 7G8 allele) and quinine (Cooper et al. 2007; Tinto et al. 2008) and mediates increased susceptibility to mefloquine and artemisinins. In areas where *Pfcrt* mutant-type alleles are not fixed, like Africa, an increase in the frequency of the wild-type allele has been observed after the discontinuation of chloroquine (Laufer et al. 2006; Noranate et al. 2007). In South America, where SVMNT alleles are almost fixed, emergence of a mutation at codon 350 (C → R) mediates both increase susceptibility to chloroquine and resistance to piperaquine (Pelleau et al. 2015).

P. falciparum multidrug resistance protein 1 (PfMDR1)

Located on chromosome 5 (*Pfmdr-1* gene, PF3D7_0523000, previous ID: MAL5P1.230, PFE1150w), *Pfmdr-1* encodes an ABC transporter (ATP-binding cassette, P-glycoprotein homolog). MDR1, located in the membrane of the food vacuole, is involved in the modulation of the susceptibility to several antimalarial drugs and, more particularly, in the hydrophobic antimalarial efflux (Duraisingh and Cowman 2005). Resistance mechanisms are associated to (1) increased copy number of *Pfmdr-1* leading to an increase in the expression of the protein (Nishiyama et al. 2004) and resistance to mefloquine, lumefantrine, quinine, and artemisinins (Cowman et al. 1994; Pickard et al. 2003; Price et al. 2004; Sidhu et al. 2006), and (2) mutations at codons 86N → Y and 1246D → Y (found in Africa) mediating decreased susceptibility to chloroquine and amodiaquine, but increased sensitivity to lumefantrine, mefloquine, and artemisinins (Duraisingh et al. 2000; Reed et al. 2000; Mwai et al. 2009) or at codons 1034C → S and 1042N → D (observed outside Africa), which have been associated with altered sensitivity to lumefantrine, mefloquine, and artemisinins (Reed et al. 2000; Pickard et al. 2003; Sidhu et al. 2005, 2006). Opposite effects on different drugs have been reported between chloroquine and mefloquine: the 86N → Y mutation decreases the parasite susceptibility to chloroquine, but increases mefloquine sensibility (Duraisingh and Cowman 2005). Similarly, increased copy number of *Pfmdr-1* increases resistance to mefloquine, but conversely increases the sensitivity to chloroquine and to piperaquine (Leang et al. 2013, 2015; Duru et al. 2015; Lim et al. 2015; Amaratunga et al. 2016)

P. falciparum bifunctional dihydrofolate reductase-thymidylate synthase (PfDHFR-TS)

Located on chromosome 4 (*Pfdhfr-ts* gene, PF3D7_0417200, previous ID: MAL4P1.161, PFD0830w), *Pfdhfr-ts* encodes an enzyme involved in the pathway of the folate synthesis (Foote and Cowman 1994; Gregson and Plowe 2005). DHFR-TS is the target of the antifolate drugs such as pyrimethamine and proguanil (metabolized in vivo to the active form cycloguanil). Antifolate drugs act by inhibiting DHFR-TS activity, blocking the pyrimidine synthesis, and the replication of the parasite DNA (Hankins et al. 2001; Sibley et al. 2001). The accumulation of several specific nonsynonymous mutations in *Pfdhfr-ts* mediates high clinical treatment failure rates and increase in vitro susceptibility to pyrimethamine (codons 51N → I, 59C → R, 108 S → N, and 164I → L) and to cycloguanil (codons 16A → V, 108S → T).

P. falciparum hydroxymethyl–dihydropterin pyrophosphokinase–dihydropteroate synthase (PfPPK-DHPS)

Located on chromosome 8 (*Pfhppk-dhps* gene, PF3D7_0810800, previous ID: PF08_0095), *Pfpppk-dhps*, this gene encodes another parasite-specific enzyme involved in the de novo synthesis of essential folate coenzymes. Resistance to sulfa drugs (sulfonamide, sulfadoxine, sulfone, and dapsone), most commonly involves the changes at codons 436S → A, 437K → G, 540K → E, 581A → G, and 613A → S/T (Hyde 2002; Gregson and Plowe 2005). Accumulation of mutations in *Pfdhfr-ts* and *Pfhppk-dhps* genes is strongly associated to clinical failure rates in patients treated with sulfadoxine–pyrimethaminecombination, widely used in Africa in pregnant women or in children in the intermittent preventive treatment strategy (Kublin et al. 2002). The most frequent resistant combination in HPPK-DHPS and DHFR-TS (quintuple mutant for which frequencies of 70% or higher in some areas of East Africa is currently

Continued

Table 1. *Continued*

observed) is the double-mutant form 437A → G, 540K → E with the triple-mutant form of DHFR (51N → I, 59C → R, 108 S → N) (Pearce et al. 2009; Naidoo and Roper 2010).

P. falciparum multidrug resistance-associated protein 1 (PfMRP1)

Located on chromosome 1 (*Pfmrp1* gene, PF3D7_0112200, previous ID: MAL1P3.03, PFA0590w), PfMRP1 is an ABC transporter (Koenderink et al. 2010). The *Pfmrp1* gene knockout in culture-adapted parasite lines causes a reduction in parasite growth and increased susceptibility to chloroquine, suggesting that MRP1 is involved in the efflux of antimalarial drugs from the parasite and is important for parasite fitness (Raj et al. 2009). Polymorphisms in *Pfmrp1* have been associated to decreased sensitivity to chloroquine and quinine (Mu et al. 2003) in in vitro susceptibility assays of culture-adapted cloned isolates and mefloquine, pyronaridine, and lumefantrine from Southeast Asian field isolates (Gupta et al. 2014).

P. falciparum cytochrome *b* (PfCYTB)

Located on the mitochondrial genome (*Pfcytb* gene, mal_mito_3), the *Pfcytb* gene encodes the mitochondrial cytochrome *bc1* complex involved in the electron transport and ATP synthesis, and is the target of atovaquone (Fry and Pudney 1992; Birth et al. 2014; Siregar et al. 2015). A single mutation at codon 268 (Y → N/S/C) highly decreases sensitivity to atovaquone (Korsinczky et al. 2000; Fivelman 2002; Farnert 2003), in combination with proguanil (Malarone) currently widely used for malaria chemoprophylaxis in travelers (Kain et al. 2001). Mutations at codon 268 are rarely detected in field isolates, and are mostly intrahost selected following atovaquone–proguanil treatment in patients experiencing clinical failure (Musset et al. 2007; Nuralitha et al. 2015).

P. falciparum sodium–hydrogen exchanger gene Na^+, H^+ antiporter (PfNHE)

Located on chromosome 13 (*Pfnhe-1* gene, PF3D7_1303500, previous ID: PF13_0019), *Pfnhe-1* encodes a putative sodium–hydrogen exchanger protein involved in parasite homeostasis by increasing the cytosolic pH (pH_{cyt}) and compensating acidosis caused by anaerobic glycolysis (Bosia et al. 1993; Nkrumah et al. 2009). Using quantitative trait loci analysis of the genetic cross of the HB3 and Dd2 clones, it has been demonstrated that three genes including *Pfnhe-1* were associated with quinine-reduced susceptibility (Ferdig et al. 2004). Sequencing analysis of *P. falciparum* culture-adapted isolates and reference lines from Southeast Asia, Africa, and South America revealed significant associations between variations in ms4760 intragenic microsatellite (alleles with >2 DNNND repeat motifs in block II, such as ms4760–1), and in vitro quinine response. However, the reliability of polymorphisms in the *Pfnhe-1* gene as molecular markers of quinine resistance appeared restricted to endemic areas from Southeast Asia or possibly east African countries and needs to be confirmed (Menard et al. 2013a).

P. falciparum non-SERCA-type Ca^{2+}-transporting P-ATPase (PfATP4)

Located on chromosome 12 (*Pfatp4*, PF3D7_1211900, previous ID: 2277.t00119, MAL12P1.118, PFL0590c), *Pfatp4* encodes a plasma membrane protein involved in the sodium efflux (Spillman et al. 2013). Recent laboratory investigations demonstrated that nonsynonymous mutations in this gene were associated to the resistance of new antimalarial compounds, including the spiroindolones, the pyrazoles, and the dihydroisoquinolones (Rottmann et al. 2010; Jimenez-Diaz et al. 2014; Vaidya et al. 2014; Spillman and Kirk 2015).

site clearance dynamics are also, to some extent, affected by the differences in host immunity (causing a variance of 0.5–1 h in parasite half-life), partner drug efficacy, splenic function, and other factors (Dondorp et al. 2010). Persistence of parasitemia at 72 h as a measure of artemisinin resistance is much dependent on the initial parasitemia and on the sensitivity of the method assessing parasitemia at 72 h (White et al. 2015). Because *P. falciparum* parasites in the second half of their asexual-stage development sequester in the microcirculation, delayed clearance suggests that ring-stage sensitivity is affected by artemisinin resistance. Artemisinins are the only class of antimalarial drugs with potent and rapid parasiticidal action against ring-stage parasites translating to a 10,000-fold decrease in parasitemia 48 h after the start of treatment

Table 2. Recommended antimalarial drugs: epidemiological, biological, and molecular characteristics

Artemisinin derivatives (artesunate, artemether, dihydroartemisinin)

Chemical structure	Sesquiterpene lactone endoperoxide
Introduced in	1980s (monotherapy), 2000s (combined with a partner drug in ACT)
First report of resistance in	2008 (partial resistance)
Half-life	0.5–2.0 h (artesunate, dihydroartemisinin) 5–7 h (artemether)
Mode of action	Not fully understood. Active against blood-stage parasites, from the ring stages to early schizonts as well as young gametocytes, involving cation-mediated generation of reactive intermediates and reduction of the peroxide bridge.
Molecular signatures of resistance	
Validated	$PfK13$ gene at codons 580 (C $\rightarrow$ Y), 539 (R $\rightarrow$ T), 543 (I $\rightarrow$ T), 493 (Y $\rightarrow$ H), 561 (R $\rightarrow$ H)
Associated	$PfK13$ gene at codons 441 (P $\rightarrow$ L), F446 $\rightarrow$ I, G449 $\rightarrow$ A, N458 $\rightarrow$ Y, M476 $\rightarrow$ I, N537 $\rightarrow$ D, P553 $\rightarrow$ L, V568 $\rightarrow$ G, P574 $\rightarrow$ L, M579 $\rightarrow$ I, D584 $\rightarrow$ V, A675 $\rightarrow$ V, H719 $\rightarrow$ N
In vitro susceptibility threshold value for resistance	Survival rate >1% in the $RSA^{0-3\ h}$
In vitro cross-resistance (IC_{50} correlation)	—
Spatial distribution of confirmed resistance	Southeast Asia

Quinine

Chemical structure	Aryl-amino alcohol
Introduced in	1632 (cinchona), 1820 (quinine)
First report of resistance in	1908
Half-life	3–36 h
Mode of action	Active against large rings and trophozoites by inhibiting intraparasitic haem detoxification in the parasite's digestive vacuole. Active against gametocytes (except for *Plasmodium falciparum*).
Molecular signatures of resistance	
Validated	None
Associated	$Pfcrt$ at codon 76 (K $\rightarrow$ T) Pfmdr-1 at codons 1042 (N $\rightarrow$ D), 1034 (S $\rightarrow$ C) or 1246 (D $\rightarrow$ Y) ms4760 variation in Pfnhe1 gene (increase in DNNND repeats in block II) (in Asian parasite populations)
In vitro susceptibility threshold value for resistance	IC50 > 500–800 nM
In vitro cross-resistance (IC_{50} correlation)	Positively correlated with chloroquine, lumefantrine, mefloquine, halofantrine

Cite this article as *Cold Spring Harb Perspect Med* doi: 10.1101/cshperspect.a025619

Spatial distribution of confirmed resistance	Sporadic worldwide cases (but mainly in Southeast Asia)
Chloroquine	
Chemical structure	4-Aminoquinoline
Introduced in	1945
First reports of resistance in	1957
Half-life	5–12 d (chloroquine and monodesthylchloroquine)
Mode of action	Active by inhibiting intraparasitic haem detoxification in the parasite's digestive vacuole. Chloroquine may also act on the biosynthesis of nucleic acids.
Molecular signatures of resistance	
Validated	*Pfcrt* at codon 76 (K $\rightarrow$ T) with other mutations: Dd2 Southeast Asian allele (74 M $\rightarrow$ I, 75 N $\rightarrow$ E) or 7G8 South American allele (72 C $\rightarrow$ S)
Associated	*Pfmdr-1* a codons 86 (N $\rightarrow$ Y), 1034 (S $\rightarrow$ C), 1042 (N $\rightarrow$ D), and 1246 (D $\rightarrow$ Y)
In vitro susceptibility threshold value for resistance	IC50 >100 nM
In vitro cross-resistance (IC_{50} correlation)	Positively correlated with quinine, monodesethylamodiaquine, piperaquine. Negatively correlated with mefloquine.
Spatial distribution of confirmed resistance	Worldwide
Amodiaquine	
Chemical structure	4-Aminoquinoline
Introduced in	1945
First reports of resistance in	1990s
Half-life	3–12 h (amodiaquine) 4–10 d (monodesethylamodiaquine)
Mode of action	Active by accumulation in the parasite's digestive vacuole and inhibition of the haem detoxification
Molecular signatures of resistance	
Validated	*Pfcrt* at codons 72 (C $\rightarrow$ S) and 76 (K $\rightarrow$ T) (7G8 South American allele SVMNT)
Associated	*Pfmdr-1* at codons 86 (N $\rightarrow$ Y) and 1246 (D $\rightarrow$ Y) (on the Pfcrt CVIET allele genetic background)
In vitro susceptibility threshold value for resistance	Amodiaquine > 80 nM monodesethylamodiaquine IC_{50} > 60 nM
In vitro cross-resistance (IC_{50} correlation)	Positively correlated with chloroquine and quinine
Spatial distribution of confirmed resistance	South America, Asia, and East Africa

Continued

Table 2. *Continued*

Mefloquine

Chemical structure	4-methanolquinoline
Introduced in	1984
First reports of resistance in	1991
Half-life	8–15 d
Mode of action	Active by inhibiting intraparasitic haem detoxification in the parasite's digestive vacuole and endocytosis of the cytosol by the parasite
Molecular signatures of resistance	
Validated	Increase expression of the amplified ($\geq$ 2 wild-type *Pfmdr-1* gene copy) *Pfmdr-1* gene
Associated	—
In vitro susceptibility threshold value for resistance	$IC_{50} > 30$ nM
In vitro cross-resistance (IC_{50} correlation)	Positively correlated with halofantrine and lumefantrine and negatively correlated with chloroquine and piperaquine
Spatial distribution of confirmed resistance	Southeast Asia, and sporadically in South America, India, Africa

Lumefantrine

Chemical structure	Aryl-amino alcohol
Introduced in	2000s (combined with artemether)
First reports of resistance in	—
Half-life	2–11 d
Mode of action	Active by inhibiting intraparasitic haem detoxification in the parasite's digestive vacuole and endocytosis of the cytosol by the parasite
Molecular signatures of resistance	
Validated	—
Associated	*Pfmdr-1* at codons 184 (Y $\rightarrow$ F), 1034 (S $\rightarrow$ C) and 1042 (N $\rightarrow$ D) (on the *Pfcrt* CVIET allele genetic background)
In vitro susceptibility threshold value for resistance	—
In vitro cross-resistance (IC_{50} correlation)	Positively correlated with mefloquine and halofantrine and negatively correlated with chloroquine and piperaquine
Spatial distribution of confirmed resistance	—

Piperaquine

Chemical structure	Bis-4-aminoquinolin
Introduced in	1960s (monotherapy), 2008 (combined with dihydroartemisinin)
First reports of resistance in	1970s

Cite this article as *Cold Spring Harb Perspect Med* doi: 10.1101/cshperspect.a025619

Half-life	13–28 d
Mode of action	Not fully understood. Active by inhibiting intraparasitic haem detoxification in the parasite's digestive vacuole. Chloroquine may also act on the biosynthesis of nucleic acids.
Molecular signatures of resistance	
Validated	—
Associated	*Pfcrt* at codon 350 (C → R). Deamplification of an 82-kb region of chromosome 5 (including *Pfmdr-1* gene) and amplification of an adjacent 63-kb region of chromosome 5.
In vitro susceptibility threshold value for resistance	Survival rate >10% in the PSA (piperaquine survival assay)
In vitro cross-resistance (IC$_{50}$ correlation)	Positively correlated with chloroquine and negatively correlated with mefloquine
Spatial distribution of confirmed resistance	Southeast Asia, China
Primaquine	
Chemical structure	8-Aminoquinoline
Introduced in	1950
First reports of resistance in	—
Half-life	4–9 h
Mode of action	Active by disrupting the metabolic processes of *Plasmodium* mitochondria and by interferencing with the function of ubiquinone as an electron carrier in the respiratory chain and by producing highly reactive metabolites generating toxic intracellular oxidative potentials
Molecular signatures of resistance	
Validated	—
Associated	—
In vitro susceptibility threshold value for resistance	—
In vitro cross-resistance (IC$_{50}$ correlation)	—
Spatial distribution of confirmed resistance	—
Sulfadoxine	
Chemical structure	Sulfonamide
Introduced in	1937
First reports of resistance in	1970s (in association with pyrimethamine)
Half-life	4–11 d

Continued

Table 2. *Continued*

Mode of action	Active by inhibiting the enzyme dihydropteroate synthase (DHPS), a component of the folate biosynthetic pathway and the replication of the parasite DNA
Molecular signatures of resistance	
Validated	*Pfdhps* at codons 436 (S → A), 437 (K → G), 540 (K → E), 581 (A → G), and 613 (A → S/T)
Associated	—
In vitro susceptibility threshold value for resistance	—
In vitro cross-resistance (IC_{50} correlation)	—
Spatial distribution of confirmed resistance	Worldwide
Pyrimethamine	
Chemical structure	Diaminopyrimidine derivative
Available since	1940s
First report of resistance in	1952 and 1970s (in association with sulfadoxine)
Half-life	2–19 d
Mode of action	Active by inhibiting the bifunctional dihydrofolate reductase–thymidylate synthase activity, blocking the pyrimidine synthesis and the replication of the parasite DNA
Molecular signatures of resistance	
Validated	*Pfdhfr* at codons 51 (N → I), 59 (C → R), 108 (S → N), and 164 (I → L). In South America, mutation at codon 50 C → R instead of 59 (C → R).
Associated	—
In vitro susceptibility threshold value for resistance	IC_{50} >100 nM
In vitro cross-resistance (IC_{50} correlation)	—
Spatial distribution of confirmed resistance	Worldwide
Proguanil	
Chemical structure	Biguanide
Available since	1940s

Cite this article as *Cold Spring Harb Perspect Med* doi: 10.1101/cshperspect.a025619

First report of resistance in	1949
Half-life	Proguanil (8–18 h); cycloguanil (16–23 h)
Mode of action	Active through its active triazine metabolite (cycloguanil) by inhibiting the bifunctional dihydrofolate reductase–thymidylate synthase activity, blocking the pyrimidine synthesis and the replication of the parasite DNA
Molecular signatures of resistance	
Validated	$Pfdhfr$ at codons 16 (A → V) and 108 (S → T)
Associated	–
In vitro susceptibility threshold value for resistance	$IC_{50} > 15$ nM
In vitro cross-resistance (IC_{50} correlation)	–
Spatial distribution of confirmed resistance	Sporadic worldwide cases
Atovaquone	
Chemical structure	Hydroxynaphthoquinone
Available since	1996
First report of resistance in	1996
Half-life	1–6 d
Mode of action	Active by inhibiting the transport of several parasite enzymes and by interfering with the cytochrome electron transport system, resulting in the collapse of the mitochondrial membrane potential
Molecular signatures of resistance	
Validated	$Pfcytb$ at codon 268 (Y → N/S/C)
Associated	–
In vitro susceptibility threshold value for resistance	$IC50 > 10$ nM
In vitro cross-resistance (IC_{50} correlation)	–
Spatial distribution of confirmed resistance	Sporadic worldwide cases

(White 2008). This sensitivity of ring-stage *P. falciparum* parasites seems what is primarily affected in artemisinin resistance as suggested by the clinical observations and later confirmed by ring-stage-specific sensitivity tests described above (Dondorp et al. 2009; Flegg et al. 2011; Saralamba et al. 2011; Ariey et al. 2014). The ring-stage survival assay performed on early ring parasites (0–3 h postinvasion, $RSA^{0-3\ h}$) showed a strong correlation between clinical data (parasite clearance half-life) and in vitro parasite survival rates (Witkowski et al. 2013a; Amaratunga et al. 2014). Transcriptomic and cell biological studies suggest that the important contributors to reduced ring-stage sensitivity are a deceleration in ring-stage development (early ring forms are intrinsically less susceptible) and an up-regulation of the "unfolded protein" stress response (UPR) (Dogovski et al. 2015; Mok et al. 2015). This was confirmed by additional population transcriptional studies (Mok et al. 2015; Shaw et al. 2015), which showed an increased expression of the UPR pathways involving the major PROSC and TRiC chaperone complexes to mitigate protein damage caused by artemisinin.

As discussed above, mutations in the K13 gene coding for the propeller region of the *P. falciparum* Kelch protein are a cause of artemisinin resistance. The Kelch protein has a wide range of biological functions, one of which is facilitating polyubiquination leading to protein degradation in the proteosome (Dogovski et al. 2015; Mbengue et al. 2015). In Kelch-mutated parasites, lower levels of ubiquitinated proteins can be observed, which is in accordance with UPR up-regulation (Dogovski et al. 2015). In addition, it was recently shown that artemisinins target *P. falciparum* phosphatidylinositol-3-kinase (PfPI3K) and Kelch-mutated parasites, through reduced ubiquitination, have increased levels of PfPI3K and its lipid product phosphatidylinositol-3-phosphate (PI3P), conferring reduced artemisinin sensitivity (Mbengue et al. 2015).

Following the discovery of the K13 genetic marker, additional genomewide studies suggested a specific genetic background in Southeast Asia parasite populations associated to ar-temisinin resistance (Miotto et al. 2015). This genetic background on which *kelch13* mutations are particularly likely to arise includes several nonsynonymous mutations: 193D → Y in PF3D7_1318100 (ferredoxin putative gene), 127V → M in PF3D7_1460900 (apicoplast ribosomal protein S10 precursor gene), 484T → I in PF3D7_1447900 (multidrug resistance protein 2 gene), and 356I → T in PF3D7_0709000 (chloroquine resistance transporter gene). Further research on defining this genetic backbone is ongoing.

Genetic studies also showed that two different foci of resistance originated in Asia, with virtually no overlap between the sets of mutations and haplotypes in Thailand–Myanmar–China and Cambodia–Vietnam–Lao PDR, confirming recent observations (Takala-Harrison et al. 2015; Menard et al. 2016). In Cambodia where artemisinin-resistant mutants in western provinces are almost fixed, haplotyping of K13 neighboring loci revealed multiple independent origins of common mutations alongside numerous sporadic localized mutational events, creating a large repertoire of mutants (Menard et al. 2016). The independent emergence of various K13 mutations will have to be reconciled with the observation that the area in Southeast Asia harboring the artemisinin-resistant phenotype is expanding over time.

South America, Oceania, Philippines, and Central/South Asia are currently areas free of K13 mutant parasites. In Africa, highly diverse and low-frequent K13 mutant alleles have been observed, with no evidence of selection, and none of these were associated with clinical artemisinin resistance assessed by the presence of parasites on day 3 following artesunate mono-therapy or a 3-d ACT course. It is thought that artemisinin resistance has not been established in Africa, supported by the additional absence of evidence of invasion by Asian K13 alleles validated as molecular marker of artemisinin resistance (C580Y, R539T, I543T, Y493H), confirming previous smaller-sized studies (Conrad et al. 2014; Torrentino-Madamet et al. 2014; Cooper et al. 2015; Escobar et al. 2015; Hawkes et al. 2015; Isozumi et al. 2015; Kamau et al. 2015; Taylor et al. 2015). Haplotyping studies on the most common African mutant 578A → S does not show evidence of selection of the mutation in the African parasite population. In addition, the 578A → S mutation seems phenotypically neutral, because genome editing of the Dd2 line indicated that this mutation did not affect artemisinin susceptibility in in vitro sensitivity testing with the $RSA^{0-3 \text{ h}}$ assay, whereas this was clearly the case for other Kelch mutations (Straimer et al. 2015; Menard et al. 2016). Figure 2 summarizes current insights in artemisinin resistance from the molecular to the public health level.

P. vivax ANTIMALARIAL DRUG RESISTANCE

Vivax malaria is treated with antimalarial drugs highly effective against blood-stage parasites. For radical cure, which includes sterilization of liver hypnozoites, primaquine has to be added to the drug regimen. To date, in vivax malaria resistance has only emerged against chloroquine, a drug used worldwide for decades. Chloroquine resistance was first recognized in the late 1980s in New Guinea, 30 years after the emergence of *P. falciparum* chloroquine resistance (Rieckmann et al. 1989) and later in Eastern Indonesia, and nowadays in many countries in which vivax malaria is endemic (Price et al. 2014). Until now, the detection of chloroquine resistance is challenging, as recurrence after treatment may be a recrudescence (true resistance), a relapse or a reinfection (false resistance). As no reliable genotyping method is available, caution is required to conclude arrival of resistance. A consensus definition of resistance is the capability of a parasite strain to grow in the presence of an adequate drug blood concentration (100 ng/mL in whole blood). Unfortunately, this information is often missing in clinical studies, because of technical constraints. In vitro drug sensitivity testing is an alternative option to assess drug resistance for *P. vivax*, but only "one-shot" ex vivo drug sensitivity assays can be performed yet, because continuous culturing is not possible for *P. vivax* (Russell et al. 2012). Such assays are difficult to implement (the assay needs to be conducted within few hours of blood collection) and to

interpret, because isolates from patients generally contain a mixture of parasite stages ranging from early ring stages to mature trophozoites and sensitivity of *P. vivax* to chloroquine depends on its parasite stage: ring forms are highly sensitive, whereas trophozoites are more resistant (Kerlin et al. 2012). To date, no validated molecular marker associated with chloroquine resistance in vivax malaria has been identified, and the mechanisms of parasite resistance to this drug remain unknown. However, current ACTs remain fully effective to kill blood-stage *P. vivax* parasites and through their posttreatment prophylactic effect protect against relapses for weeks after treatment (Gogtay et al. 2013). Thus, in chloroquine-resistance areas, ACTs provide an effective alternative treatment, decreasing the risk of chloroquine resistance spreading.

FUTURE PERSPECTIVES: TOWARD THE ELIMINATION OF ARTEMISININ AND MULTIPLE DRUG-RESISTANT FALCIPARUM MALARIA IN SOUTHEAST ASIA

Because the artemisinins have much shorter plasma half-lives (∼1 h) compared with the ACT partner drugs (days to weeks), the reduction in artemisinin sensitivity has left partner drugs exposed to a larger biomass of parasites after the usual 3-d ACT course. For this reason, artemisinin resistance contributes to the selection for partner drug resistance (Dondorp et al. 2010). Indeed, an increase in concomitant partner drug resistance has been observed in recent years and, as a consequence, treatment failures after ACTs are becoming more widespread in Southeast Asia. Late failure rates (within 21–28 d after the initial treatment) of >30% for dihydroartemisinin–piperaquine and mefloquine–artesunate have been documented in western Cambodia (Leang et al. 2013, 2015; Lon et al. 2014; Saunders et al. 2014; Duru et al. 2015; Spring et al. 2015; Amaratunga et al. 2016) and the western Thailand border areas (Carrara et al. 2013), respectively. Failure of first-line ACTs will damage current control and elimination efforts and accelerate the emergence and spread of resistance. Although

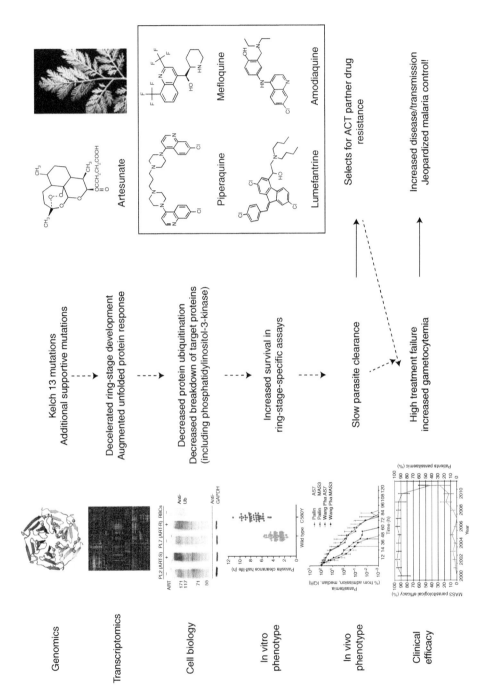

Figure 2. Current insights in artemisinin resistance from the molecular to the public health level.

Cite this article as *Cold Spring Harb Perspect Med* doi: 10.1101/cshperspect.a025619

promising new compounds are currently in phase II and phase III trials, their deployment is not expected before 2020. Promising new drug classes include ozonides, spiroindolones, and imidozole piperazines (Wells et al. 2015). There is an urgent need to evaluate alternative treatments where standard courses of ACTs are failing, and to develop combinations of existing drugs that will not fall rapidly to resistance and can be deployed immediately. Possible strategies include drug rotation between different ACTs, in particular DHA–piperaquine and artesunate–mefloquine. It has been shown that withdrawal of mefloquine as antimalarial treatment is followed by the recovery of mefloquine sensitivity in *P. falciparum*, resulting from the quick loss of *mdr-1* gene amplification, which exerts an important fitness cost in the absence of drug pressure (Preechapornkul et al. 2009; Leang et al. 2013, 2015; Duru et al. 2015; Lim et al. 2015; Amaratunga et al. 2016). This strategy is currently implemented in large parts of Cambodia suffering from high failure rates with DHA–piperaquine. Another possibility is extension of the usual 3-d ACT course to 5 or 7 d, for instance, using artemether-lumefantrine. A 5-d course of the latter drug combination is currently (2015) being trialed. A novel ACT, artesunate–pyronaridine, was recently trialed in western Cambodia, but showed suboptimal efficacy in an area of artemisinin and piperaquine resistance (Leang et al. 2016). A synthetic endoperoxide trioxane, arterolane, which is marketed in India in combination with piperaquine, might be efficacious in areas with high ACT failure, but cross-resistance with the artemisinins cannot be excluded. Sequential deployment of two alternative full ACT courses could likely restore cure rates. Adherence to the longer treatment course might hinder adherence, and interaction of the long half-life partner drugs will need to be assessed. It should also be noted that a total cumulative dose >20 mg/kg of artesunate has been associated with bone marrow toxicity (Bethell et al. 2010; Das et al. 2013). Finally, a promising approach is the combination of artemisinin derivatives with two slowly eliminated partner drugs in a 3-d triple ACT. The principle of combining three antimicrobial drugs is a standard approach for the treatment of HIV and tuberculosis. Several groups have advocated for the same approach as the new paradigm for the treatment of falciparum malaria (Shanks et al. 2015). There is a fortuitous inverse correlation between susceptibility to amodiaquine and lumefantrine and between piperaquine and mefloquine, which in addition have reasonably well-matching pharmacokinetic profiles. The combinations artemether–lumefantrine–amodiaquine and DHA–piperaquine–mefloquine are currently studied for their efficacy and safety in the treatment of uncomplicated falciparum malaria in areas of artemisinin and partner drug resistance.

CONCLUDING REMARKS

Artemisinin and partner drug resistance in *P. falciparum* are an increasing problem in Southeast Asia, causing high failure rates with ACTs in several countries of the Greater Mekong subregion. This jeopardizes the malaria elimination agenda of the region. Arrival in sub-Saharan Africa of these very difficult-to-treat parasite strains can have a huge impact on malaria morbidity and mortality, and intense surveillance is indicated. Monitoring of the genetic marker for artemisinin resistance, K13, has greatly facilitated surveillance, supplementing the more labor-intensive clinical studies identifying the slow clearance phenotype. The ring-stage-specific assay, $RSA^{0-3\,h}$, has become the reference in vitro sensitivity test, which has helped to uncover the important aspects of the underlying biological mechanisms conferring artemisinin resistance. Until new antimalarials become available, creative deployment of existing drugs will be essential, which could include triple combination therapies. Accelerated elimination of all falciparum malaria in the Greater Mekong subregion will be needed to counter the threat of artemisinin and partner drug resistance. In vivax malaria, increasing chloroquine resistance is an increasing problem. Its surveillance is hampered by the absence of validated molecular markers or easy deployable in vitro sensitivity assays. ACTs are an effective alternative treatment for *P. vivax*, with the addition of primaquine for radical cure of the infection.

ACKNOWLEDGMENTS

A.D. is funded by the Wellcome Trust of Great Britain and D. M. by the Institut Pasteur and the Institut Pasteur International Network. D.M. is deeply grateful to the staff of the Molecular Epidemiology Unit at Institut Pasteur in Cambodia, especially to Valentine Duru and Jean Popovici for having provided critical thinking and to his main collaborators in Cambodia and beyond.

REFERENCES

Amaratunga C, Sreng S, Suon S, Phelps ES, Stepniewska K, Lim P, Zhou C, Mao S, Anderson JM, Lindegardh N, et al. 2012. Artemisinin-resistant *Plasmodium falciparum* in Pursat province, western Cambodia: A parasite clearance rate study. *Lancet Infect Dis* **12:** 851–858.

Amaratunga C, Witkowski B, Khim N, Menard D, Fairhurst RM. 2014. Artemisinin resistance in *Plasmodium falciparum*. *Lancet Infect Dis* **14:** 449–450.

Amaratunga C, Lim P, Suon S, Sreng S, Mao S, Sopha C, Sam B, Dek D, Try V, Amato R, et al. 2016. Dihydroartemisinin–piperaquine resistance in *Plasmodium falciparum* malaria in Cambodia: A multisite prospective cohort study. *Lancet Infect Dis* **16:** 357–365.

Ariey F, Witkowski B, Amaratunga C, Beghain J, Langlois AC, Khim N, Kim S, Duru V, Bouchier C, Ma L, et al. 2014. A molecular marker of artemisinin-resistant *Plasmodium falciparum* malaria. *Nature* **505:** 50–55.

Ashley EA, Dhorda M, Fairhurst RM, Amaratunga C, Lim P, Suon S, Sreng S, Anderson JM, Mao S, Sam B, et al. 2014. Spread of artemisinin resistance in *Plasmodium falciparum* malaria. *N Engl J Med* **371:** 411–423.

Bacon DJ, Latour C, Lucas C, Colina O, Ringwald P, Picot S. 2007. Comparison of a SYBR green I-based assay with a histidine-rich protein II enzyme-linked immunosorbent assay for in vitro antimalarial drug efficacy testing and application to clinical isolates. *Antimicrob Agents Chemother* **51:** 1172–1178.

Barnadas C, Kent D, Timinao L, Iga J, Gray LR, Siba P, Mueller I, Thomas PJ, Zimmerman PA. 2011. A new high-throughput method for simultaneous detection of drug resistance associated mutations in *Plasmodium vivax* dhfr, dhps and mdr1 genes. *Malaria J* **10:** 282.

Barnes KI, White NJ. 2005. Population biology and antimalarial resistance: The transmission of antimalarial drug resistance in *Plasmodium falciparum*. *Acta Tropica* **94:** 230–240.

Barnes KI, Little F, Smith PJ, Evans A, Watkins WM, White NJ. 2006. Sulfadoxine-pyrimethamine pharmacokinetics in malaria: Pediatric dosing implications. *Clin Pharmacol Ther* **80:** 582–596.

Barnes KI, Little F, Mabuza A, Mngomezulu N, Govere J, Durrheim D, Roper C, Watkins B, White NJ. 2008. Increased gametocytemia after treatment: An early parasitological indicator of emerging sulfadoxine-pyrimethamine resistance in falciparum malaria. *J Infect Dis* **197:** 1605–1613.

Basco LK. 2007. *Field application of in vitro assays for the sensitivity of human malaria parasites to antimalarial drugs*. WHO Press, Geneva.

Becker K, Tilley L, Vennerstrom JL, Roberts D, Rogerson S, Ginsburg H. 2004. Oxidative stress in malaria parasite-infected erythrocytes: Host-parasite interactions. *Int J Parasitol* **34:** 163–189.

Bethell D, Se Y, Lon C, Socheat D, Saunders D, Teja-Isavadharm P, Khemawoot P, Darapiseth S, Lin J, Sriwichai S, et al. 2010. Dose-dependent risk of neutropenia after 7-day courses of artesunate monotherapy in Cambodian patients with acute *Plasmodium falciparum* malaria. *Clin Infect Dis* **51:** e105–e114.

Bhatt S, Weiss DJ, Cameron E, Bisanzio D, Mappin B, Dalrymple U, Battle KE, Moyes CL, Henry A, Eckhoff PA, et al. 2015. The effect of malaria control on *Plasmodium falciparum* in Africa between 2000 and 2015. *Nature* **526:** 207–211.

Birth D, Kao WC, Hunte C. 2014. Structural analysis of atovaquone-inhibited cytochrome *bc*1 complex reveals the molecular basis of antimalarial drug action. *Nat Commun* **5:** 4029.

Bosia A, Ghigo D, Turrini F, Nissani E, Pescarmona GP, Ginsburg H. 1993. Kinetic characterization of Na^+/H^+ antiport of *Plasmodium falciparum* membrane. *J Cell Physiol* **154:** 527–534.

Boudreau EF, Webster HK, Pavanand K, Thosingha L. 1982. Type II mefloquine resistance in Thailand. *Lancet* **2:** 1335.

Brasseur P, Agnamey P, Moreno A, Druilhe P. 2001. Evaluation of in vitro drug sensitivity of antimalarials for *Plasmodium falciparum* using a colorimetric assay (DELI-microtest). *Med Trop* **61:** 545–547.

Carrara VI, Lwin KM, Phyo AP, Ashley E, Wiladphaingern J, Sriprawat K, Rijken M, Boel M, McGready R, Proux S, et al. 2013. Malaria burden and artemisinin resistance in the mobile and migrant population on the Thai–Myanmar border, 1999–2011: An observational study. *PLoS Med* **10:** e1001398.

Chen N, Auliff A, Rieckmann K, Gatton M, Cheng Q. 2007. Relapses of *Plasmodium vivax* infection result from clonal hypnozoites activated at predetermined intervals. *J Infect Dis* **195:** 934–941.

Conrad MD, Bigira V, Kapisi J, Muhindo M, Kamya MR, Havlir DV, Dorsey G, Rosenthal PJ. 2014. Polymorphisms in K13 and falcipain-2 associated with artemisinin resistance are not prevalent in *Plasmodium falciparum* isolated from Ugandan children. *PloS ONE* **9:** e105690.

Contreras CE, Rivas MA, Dominguez J, Charris J, Palacios M, Bianco NE, Blanca I. 2004. Stage-specific activity of potential antimalarial compounds measured in vitro by flow cytometry in comparison to optical microscopy and hypoxanthine uptake. *Mem Inst Oswaldo Cruz* **99:** 179–184.

Cooper RA, Conrad MD, Watson QD, Huezo SJ, Ninsiima H, Tumwebaze P, Nsobya SL, Rosenthal PJ. 2015. Lack of artemisinin resistance in *Plasmodium falciparum* in

Uganda based on parasitological and molecular assays. *Antimicrob Agents Chemother* **59:** 5061–5064.

Cui L, Wang Z, Miao J, Miao M, Chandra R, Jiang H, Su XZ, Cui L. 2012. Mechanisms of in vitro resistance to dihydroartemisinin in *Plasmodium falciparum. Mol Microbiol* **86:** 111–128.

Cui L, Mharakurwa S, Ndiaye D, Rathod PK, Rosenthal PJ. 2015. Antimalarial drug resistance: Literature review and activities and findings of the ICEMR network. *Am J Trop Med Hyg* **93:** 57–68.

Das D, Tripura R, Phyo AP, Lwin KM, Tarning J, Lee SJ, Hanpithakpong W, Stepniewska K, Menard D, Ringwald P, et al. 2013. Effect of high-dose or split-dose artesunate on parasite clearance in artemisinin-resistant falciparum malaria. *Clinical Infect Dis* **56:** e48–58.

Desjardins RE, Canfield CJ, Haynes JD, Chulay JD. 1979. Quantitative assessment of antimalarial activity in vitro by a semiautomated microdilution technique. *Antimicrob Agents Chemother* **16:** 710–718.

Dogovski C, Xie SC, Burgio G, Bridgford J, Mok S, McCaw JM, Chotivanich K, Kenny S, Gnadig N, Straimer J, et al. 2015. Targeting the cell stress response of *Plasmodium falciparum* to overcome artemisinin resistance. *PLoS Biol* **13:** e1002132.

Dondorp AM, Nosten F, Yi P, Das D, Phyo AP, Tarning J, Lwin KM, Ariey F, Hanpithakpong W, Lee SJ, et al. 2009. Artemisinin resistance in *Plasmodium falciparum* malaria. *N Engl J Med* **361:** 455–467.

Dondorp AM, Yeung S, White L, Nguon C, Day NP, Socheat D, von Seidlein L. 2010. Artemisinin resistance: Current status and scenarios for containment. *Nat Rev Microbiol* **8:** 272–280.

Duru V, Khim N, Leang R, Kim S, Domergue A, Kloeung N, Ke S, Chy S, Eam R, Khean C, et al. 2015. *Plasmodium falciparum* dihydroartemisinin–piperaquine failures in Cambodia are associated with mutant K13 parasites presenting high survival rates in novel piperaquine in vitro assays: Retrospective and prospective investigations. *BMC Med* **13:** 305.

Escobar C, Pateira S, Lobo E, Lobo L, Teodosio R, Dias F, Fernandes N, Arez AP, Varandas L, Nogueira F. 2015. Polymorphisms in *Plasmodium falciparum* K13-propeller in Angola and Mozambique after the introduction of the ACTs. *PLoS ONE* **10:** e0119215.

Eyles DE, Hoo CC, Warren M, Sandosham AA. 1963. *Plasmodium falciparum* resistant to chloroquine in Cambodia. *Am J Trop Med Hyg* **12:** 840–843.

Farnert A, Lindberg J, Gil P, Swedberg G, Berqvist Y, Thapar MM, Lindegardh N, Berezcky S, Bjorkman A. 2003. Evidence of *Plasmodium falciparum* malaria resistant to atovaquone and proguanil hydrochloride: Case reports. *BMJ* **326:** 628–629.

Ferdig MT, Cooper RA, Mu J, Deng B, Joy DA, Su XZ, Wellems TE. 2004. Dissecting the loci of low-level quinine resistance in malaria parasites. *Mol Microbiol* **52:** 985–997.

Fivelman QL, Butcher GA, Adagu IS, Warhurst DC, Pasvol G. 2002. Malarone treatment failure and in vitro confirmation of resistance of *Plasmodium falciparum* isolate from Lagos, Nigeria. *Malaria J* **1:** 1.

Flegg JA, Guerin PJ, White NJ, Stepniewska K. 2011. Standardizing the measurement of parasite clearance in falciparum malaria: The parasite clearance estimator. *Malaria J* **10:** 339.

Fry M, Pudney M. 1992. Site of action of the antimalarial hydroxynaphthoquinone, 2-[trans-4-(4′-chlorophenyl) cyclohexyl]-3-hydroxy-1,4-naphthoquinone (566C80). *Biochem Pharmacol* **43:** 1545–1553.

Ghorbal M, Gorman M, Macpherson CR, Martins RM, Scherf A, Lopez-Rubio JJ. 2014. Genome editing in the human malaria parasite *Plasmodium falciparum* using the CRISPR-Cas9 system. *Nat Biotechnol* **32:** 819–821.

Gogtay N, Kannan S, Thatte UM, Olliaro PL, Sinclair D. 2013. Artemisinin-based combination therapy for treating uncomplicated *Plasmodium vivax* malaria. *Cochrane Database Syst Rev* **10:** CD008492.

Grab B, Wernsdorfer WH. 1983. Evaluation of in vitro tests for drug sensitivity in *Plasmodium falciparum*: Probit analysis of logdose/response test from 3–8 points assay (see more at apps.who.int/iris/handle/10665/65879#sthash.hw4wohyT.dpuf). WHO Press, Geneva.

Guiguemde TR, Aouba A, Ouedraogo JB, Lamizana L. 1994. Ten-year surveillance of drug-resistant malaria in Burkina Faso (1982–1991). *Am J Trop Med Hyg* **50:** 699–704.

Gupta B, Xu S, Wang Z, Sun L, Miao J, Cui L, Yang Z. 2014. *Plasmodium falciparum* multidrug resistance protein 1 (*pfmrp1*) gene and its association with in vitro drug susceptibility of parasite isolates from north-east Myanmar. *J Antimicrob Chemother* **69:** 2110–2117.

Hawkes M, Conroy AL, Opoka RO, Namasopo S, Zhong K, Liles WC, John CC, Kain KC. 2015. Slow clearance of *Plasmodium falciparum* in severe pediatric malaria, Uganda, 2011–2013. *Emerg Infect Dis* **21:** 1237–1239.

Hien TT, Thuy-Nhien NT, Phu NH, Boni MF, Thanh NV, Nha-Ca NT, Thai le H, Thai CQ, Toi PV, Thuan PD, et al. 2012. In vivo susceptibility of *Plasmodium falciparum* to artesunate in Binh Phuoc Province, Vietnam. *Malaria J* **11:** 355.

Hofler W. 1980. Sulfadoxine-pyrimethamine resistant falciparum malaria from Cambodia. *Dtsch Med Wochenschr* **105:** 350–351.

Huang F, Takala-Harrison S, Jacob CG, Liu H, Sun X, Yang H, Nyunt MM, Adams M, Zhou S, Xia Z, et al. 2015. A single mutation in K13 predominates in Southern China and is associated with delayed clearance of *Plasmodium falciparum* following artemisinin treatment. *J Infect Dis* **212:** 1629–1635.

Hurwitz ES, Johnson D, Campbell CC. 1981. Resistance of *Plasmodium falciparum* malaria to sulfadoxine-pyrimethamine ("Fansidar") in a refugee camp in Thailand. *Lancet* **1:** 1068–1070.

Imwong M, Snounou G, Pukrittayakamee S, Tanomsing N, Kim JR, Nandy A, Guthmann JP, Nosten F, Carlton J, Looareesuwan S, et al. 2007. Relapses of *Plasmodium vivax* infection usually result from activation of heterologous hypnozoites. *J Infect Dis* **195:** 927–933.

Isozumi R, Uemura H, Kimata I, Ichinose Y, Logedi J, Omar AH, Kaneko A. 2015. Novel mutations in K13 propeller gene of artemisinin-resistant *Plasmodium falciparum*. *Emerg Infect Dis* **21:** 490–492.

Jiang H, Li N, Gopalan V, Zilversmit MM, Varma S, Nagarajan V, Li J, Mu J, Hayton K, Henschen B, et al. 2011. High recombination rates and hotspots in a *Plasmodium falciparum* genetic cross. *Genome Biol* **12:** pR33.

Jimenez-Diaz MB, Ebert D, Salinas Y, Pradhan A, Lehane AM, Myrand-Lapierre ME, O'Loughlin KG, Shackleford DM, Justino de Almeida M, Carrillo AK, et al. 2014. (+)-SJ733, a clinical candidate for malaria that acts through ATP4 to induce rapid host-mediated clearance of *Plasmodium*. *Proc Natl Acad Sci* 111: E5455-E5462.

Kamau E, Campino S, Amenga-Etego L, Drury E, Ishengoma D, Johnson K, Mumba D, Kekre M, Yavo W, Mead D, et al. 2015. K13-propeller polymorphisms in *Plasmodium falciparum* parasites from sub-Saharan Africa. *J Infect Dis* 211: 1352-1355.

Kerlin DH, Boyce K, Marfurt J, Simpson JA, Kenangalem E, Cheng Q, Price RN, Gatton ML. 2012. An analytical method for assessing stage-specific drug activity in *Plasmodium vivax* malaria: Implications for ex vivo drug susceptibility testing. *PLoS Negl Trop Dis* 6: e1772.

Klonis N, Xie SC, McCaw JM, Crespo-Ortiz MP, Zaloumis SG, Simpson JA, Tilley L. 2013. Altered temporal response of malaria parasites determines differential sensitivity to artemisinin. *Proc Natl Acad Sci* 110: 5157-5162.

Kloprogge F, McGready R, Phyo AP, Rijken MJ, Hanpithakpon W, Than HH, Hlaing N, Zin NT, Day NP, White NJ, et al. 2015. Opposite malaria and pregnancy effect on oral bioavailability of artesunate—A population pharmacokinetic evaluation. *Br J Clin Pharmacol* 80: 642-653.

Korenromp EL, Williams BG, Gouws E, Dye C, Snow RW. 2003. Measurement of trends in childhood malaria mortality in Africa: An assessment of progress toward targets based on verbal autopsy. *Lancet Infect Dis* 3: 349-358.

Le Nagard H, Vincent C, Mentre F, Le Bras J. 2011. Online analysis of in vitro resistance to antimalarial drugs through nonlinear regression. *Comput Methods Programs Biomed* 104: 10-18.

Leang R, Barrette A, Bouth DM, Menard D, Abdur R, Duong S, Ringwald P. 2013. Efficacy of dihydroartemisinin–piperaquine for treatment of uncomplicated *Plasmodium falciparum* and *Plasmodium vivax* in Cambodia, 2008 to 2010. *Antimicrob Agents Chemother* 57: 818-826.

Leang R, Taylor WR, Bouth DM, Song L, Tarning J, Char MC, Kim S, Witkowski B, Duru V, Domergue A, et al. 2015. Evidence of *Plasmodium falciparum* malaria multidrug resistance to artemisinin and piperaquine in western Cambodia: Dihydroartemisinin–piperaquine open-label multicenter clinical assessment. *Antimicrob Agents Chemother* 59: 4719-4726.

Leang R, Canavati SE, Khim N, Vestergaard LS, Borghini Fuhrer I, Kim S, Denis MB, Heng P, Tol B, Huy R, et al. 2016. Efficacy and safety of pyronaridine–artesunate for the treatment of uncomplicated *Plasmodium falciparum* malaria in western Cambodia. *Antimicrob Agents Chemother* 60: 3884-3890.

Lim P, Dek D, Try V, Sreng S, Suon S, Fairhurst RM. 2015. Decreasing pfmdr1 copy number suggests that *Plasmodium falciparum* in western Cambodia is regaining in vitro susceptibility to mefloquine. *Antimicrob Agents Chemother* 59: 2934-2937.

Lon C, Manning JE, Vanachayangkul P, So M, Sea D, Se Y, Gosi P, Lanteri C, Chaorattanakawee S, Sriwichai S, et al. 2014. Efficacy of two versus three-day regimens of dihydroartemisinin–piperaquine for uncomplicated malaria in military personnel in northern Cambodia: An open-label randomized trial. *PloS ONE* 9: e93138.

Lopera-Mesa TM, Doumbia S, Chiang S, Zeituni AE, Konate DS, Doumbouya M, Keita AS, Stepniewska K, Traore K, Diakite SA, et al. 2013. *Plasmodium falciparum* clearance rates in response to artesunate in Malian children with malaria: Effect of acquired immunity. *J Infect Dis* 207: 1655-1663.

Makler MT, Hinrichs DJ. 1993. Measurement of the lactate dehydrogenase activity of *Plasmodium falciparum* as an assessment of parasitemia. *Am J Trop Med Hyg* 48: 205-210.

Maude RJ, Pontavornpinyo W, Saralamba S, Aguas R, Yeung S, Dondorp AM, Day NP, White NJ, White LJ. 2009. The last man standing is the most resistant: Eliminating artemisinin-resistant malaria in Cambodia. *Malaria J* 8: 31.

Mbengue A, Bhattacharjee S, Pandharkar T, Liu H, Estiu G, Stahelin RV, Rizk SS, Njimoh DL, Ryan Y, Chotivanich K, et al. 2015. A molecular mechanism of artemisinin resistance in *Plasmodium falciparum* malaria. *Nature* 520: 683-687.

Menard D, Ariey F. 2015. Towards real-time monitoring of artemisinin resistance. *Lancet Infect Dis* 15: 367-368.

Menard D, Ariey F, Mercereau-Puijalon O. 2013. *Plasmodium falciparum* susceptibility to antimalarial drugs: Global data issued from the Pasteur Institutes international network. *Med Sci (Paris)* 29: 647-655.

Menard D, Khim N, Beghain J, Adegnika AA, Shafiul-Alam M, Amodu O, Rahim-Awab G, Barnadas C, Berry A, Boum Y, et al. 2016. A worldwide map of *Plasmodium falciparum* K13-propeller polymorphisms. *N Eng J Med* 374: 2453-2464.

Miotto O, Almagro-Garcia J, Manske M, Macinnis B, Campino S, Rockett KA, Amaratunga C, Lim P, Suon S, Sreng S, et al. 2013. Multiple populations of artemisinin-resistant *Plasmodium falciparum* in Cambodia. *Nat Genet* 45: 648-655.

Miotto O, Amato R, Ashley EA, MacInnis B, Almagro-Garcia J, Amaratunga C, Lim P, Mead D, Oyola SO, Dhorda M, et al. 2015. Genetic architecture of artemisinin-resistant *Plasmodium falciparum*. *Nat Genet* 47: 226-234.

Mok S, Ashley EA, Ferreira PE, Zhu L, Lin Z, Yeo T, Chotivanich K, Imwong M, Pukrittayakamee S, Dhorda M, et al. 2015. Drug resistance. Population transcriptomics of human malaria parasites reveals the mechanism of artemisinin resistance. *Science* 347: 431-435.

Mu J, Ferdig MT, Feng X, Joy DA, Duan J, Furuya T, Subramanian G, Aravind L, Cooper RA, Wootton JC, et al. 2003. Multiple transporters associated with malaria parasite responses to chloroquine and quinine. *Mol Microbiol* 49: 977-989.

Musset L, Le Bras J, Clain J. 2007. Parallel evolution of adaptive mutations in *Plasmodium falciparum* mitochondrial DNA during atovaquone–proguanil treatment. *Mol Biol Evol* 24: 1582-1585.

Newton PN, Dondorp A, Green M, Mayxay M, White NJ. 2003. Counterfeit artesunate antimalarials in Southeast Asia. *Lancet* 362: 169.

Nkrumah LJ, Riegelhaupt PM, Moura P, Johnson DJ, Patel J, Hayton K, Ferdig MT, Wellems TE, Akabas MH, Fidock DA. 2009. Probing the multifactorial basis of *Plasmodium falciparum* quinine resistance: Evidence for a strain-specific contribution of the sodium-proton exchanger PfNHE. *Mol Biochem Parasitol* 165: 122-131.

Cite this article as *Cold Spring Harb Perspect Med* doi: 10.1101/cshperspect.a025619

Noedl H, Wernsdorfer WH, Miller RS, Wongsrichanalai C. 2002. Histidine-rich protein. II: A novel approach to malaria drug sensitivity testing. *Antimicrob Agents Chemother* **46:** 1658–1664.

Noedl H, Se Y, Schaecher K, Smith BL, Socheat D, Fukuda MM. 2008. Artemisinin Resistance in Cambodia, 1 Study C. Evidence of artemisinin-resistant malaria in western Cambodia. *N Engl J Med* **359:** 2619–2620.

Nuralitha S, Siregar JE, Syafruddin D, Roelands J, Verhoef J, Hoepelman AI, Marzuki S. 2015. Within-host selection of drug resistance in a mouse model of repeated incomplete malaria treatment: Comparison between atovaquone and pyrimethamine. *Antimicrob Agents Chemother* **60:** 258–263.

Pattanapanyasat K, Thaithong S, Kyle DE, Udomsangpetch R, Yongvanitchit K, Hider RC, Webster HK. 1997. Flow cytometric assessment of hydroxypyridinone iron chelators on in vitro growth of drug-resistant malaria. *Cytometry* **27:** 84–91.

Philipps J, Radloff PD, Wernsdorfer W, Kremsner PG. 1998. Follow-up of the susceptibility of *Plasmodium falciparum* to antimalarials in Gabon. *Am J Trop Med Hyg* **58:** 612–618.

Phyo AP, Nkhoma S, Stepniewska K, Ashley EA, Nair S, McGready R, ler Moo C, Al-Saai S, Dondorp AM, Lwin KM, et al. 2012. Emergence of artemisinin-resistant malaria on the western border of Thailand: A longitudinal study. *Lancet* **379:** 1960–1966.

Pongtavornpinyo W, Hastings IM, Dondorp A, White LJ, Maude RJ, Saralamba S, Day NP, White NJ, Boni MF. 2009. Probability of emergence of antimalarial resistance in different stages of the parasite life cycle. *Evol Appl* **2:** 52–61.

Preechapornkul P, Imwong M, Chotivanich K, Pongtavornpinyo W, Dondorp AM, Day NP, White NJ, Pukrittayakamee S. 2009. *Plasmodium falciparum pfmdr1* amplification, mefloquine resistance, and parasite fitness. *Antimicrob Agents Chemother* **53:** 1509–1515.

Price RN, von Seidlein L, Valecha N, Nosten F, Baird JK, White NJ. 2014. Global extent of chloroquine-resistant *Plasmodium vivax*: A systematic review and meta-analysis. *Lancet Infect Dis* **14:** 982–991.

Raj DK, Mu J, Jiang H, Kabat J, Singh S, Sullivan M, Fay MP, McCutchan TF, Su XZ. 2009. Disruption of a *Plasmodium falciparum* multidrug resistance–associated protein (PfMRP) alters its fitness and transport of antimalarial drugs and glutathione. *J Biol Chem* **284:** 7687–7696.

Rason MA, Randriantsoa T, Andrianantenaina H, Ratsimbasoa A, Menard D. 2008. Performance and reliability of the SYBR Green I based assay for the routine monitoring of susceptibility of *Plasmodium falciparum* clinical isolates. *Trans R Soc Trop Med Hyg* **102:** 346–351.

Rieckmann KH, Campbell GH, Sax LJ, Mrema JE. 1978. Drug sensitivity of *Plasmodium falciparum*. An in vitro microtechnique. *Lancet* **1:** 22–23.

Rieckmann KH, Davis DR, Hutton DC. 1989. *Plasmodium vivax* resistance to chloroquine? *Lancet* **2:** 1183–1184.

Ringwald P, Same Ekobo A, Keundjian A, Kedy Mangamba D, Basco LK. 2000. Chemoresistance of *P. falciparum* in urban areas of Yaounde, Cameroon. Part 1: Surveillance of in vitro and in vivo resistance of *Plasmodium falciparum* to chloroquine from 1994 to 1999 in Yaounde, Cameroon. *Trop Med Int Health* **5:** 612–619.

Rottmann M, McNamara C, Yeung BK, Lee MC, Zou B, Russell B, Seitz P, Plouffe DM, Dharia NV, Tan J, et al. 2010. Spiroindolones, a potent compound class for the treatment of malaria. *Science* **329:** 1175–1180.

Russell B, Suwanarusk R, Malleret B, Costa FT, Snounou G, Kevin Baird J, Nosten F, Renia L. 2012. Human ex vivo studies on asexual *Plasmodium vivax*: The best way forward. *Int J Parasitol* **42:** 1063–1070.

Saralamba S, Pan-Ngum W, Maude RJ, Lee SJ, Tarning J, Lindegardh N, Chotivanich K, Nosten F, Day NP, Socheat D, et al. 2011. Intrahost modeling of artemisinin resistance in *Plasmodium falciparum*. *Proc Natl Acad Sci* **108:** 397–402.

Sarda V, Kaslow DC, Williamson KC. 2009. Approaches to malaria vaccine development using the retrospectroscope. *Infect Immun* **77:** 3130–3140.

Saunders DL, Vanachayangkul P, Lon C. 2014. Dihydroartemisinin–piperaquine failure in Cambodia. *N Engl J Med* **371:** 484–485.

Shanks GD, Edstein MD, Jacobus D. 2015. Evolution from double to triple-antimalarial drug combinations. *Trans R Soc Trop Med Hyg* **109:** 182–188.

Shaw PJ, Chaotheing S, Kaewprommal P, Piriyapongsa J, Wongsombat C, Suwannakitti N, Koonyosying P, Uthaipibull C, Yuthavong Y, Kamchonwongpaisan S. 2015. Plasmodium parasites mount an arrest response to dihydroartemisinin, as revealed by whole transcriptome shotgun sequencing (RNA-seq) and microarray study. *BMC Genomics* **16:** 830.

Siregar JE, Kurisu G, Kobayashi T, Matsuzaki M, Sakamoto K, Mi-ichi F, Watanabe Y, Hirai M, Matsuoka H, Syafruddin D, et al. 2015. Direct evidence for the atovaquone action on the *Plasmodium* cytochrome *bc*1 complex. *Parasitol Int* **64:** 295–300.

Smilkstein M, Sriwilaijaroen N, Kelly JX, Wilairat P, Riscoe M. 2004. Simple and inexpensive fluorescence-based technique for high-throughput antimalarial drug screening. *Antimicrob Agents Chemother* **48:** 1803–1806.

Smithuis FM, van Woensel JB, Nordlander E, Vantha WS, ter Kuile FO. 1993. Comparison of two mefloquine regimens for treatment of *Plasmodium falciparum* malaria on the northeastern Thai–Cambodian border. *Antimicrob Agents Chemother* **37:** 1977–1981.

Spillman NJ, Kirk K. 2015. The malaria parasite cation ATPase PfATP4 and its role in the mechanism of action of a new arsenal of antimalarial drugs. *Int J Parasitol Drugs Drug Resist* **5:** 149–162.

Spring MD, Lin JT, Manning JE, Vanachayangkul P, Somethy S, Bun R, Se Y, Chann S, Ittiverakul M, Sia-ngam P, et al. 2015. Dihydroartemisinin–piperaquine failure associated with a triple mutant including *kelch13 C580Y* in Cambodia: An observational cohort study. *Lancet Infect Dis* **15:** 683–691.

Stepniewska K, White NJ. 2006. Some considerations in the design and interpretation of antimalarial drug trials in uncomplicated falciparum malaria. *Malaria J* **5:** 127.

Straimer J, Gnadig NF, Witkowski B, Amaratunga C, Duru V, Ramadani AP, Dacheux M, Khim N, Zhang L, Lam S, et al. 2015. Drug resistance. K13-propeller mutations confer artemisinin resistance in *Plasmodium falciparum* clinical isolates. *Science* **347**: 428–431.

Takala-Harrison S, Laufer MK. 2015. Antimalarial drug resistance in Africa: Key lessons for the future. *Ann NY Acad Sci* **1342**: 62–67.

Takala-Harrison S, Jacob CG, Arze C, Cummings MP, Silva JC, Dondorp AM, Fukuda MM, Hien TT, Mayxay M, Noedl H, et al. 2015. Independent emergence of artemisinin resistance mutations among *Plasmodium falciparum* in Southeast Asia. *J Infect Dis* **211**: 670–679.

Taylor SM, Parobek CM, DeConti DK, Kayentao K, Coulibaly SO, Greenwood BM, Tagbor H, Williams J, Bojang K, Njie F, et al. 2015. Absence of putative artemisinin resistance mutations among *Plasmodium falciparum* in sub-Saharan Africa: A molecular epidemiologic study. *J Infect Dis* **211**: 680–688.

Teuscher F, Chen N, Kyle DE, Gatton ML, Cheng Q. 2012. Phenotypic changes in artemisinin-resistant *Plasmodium falciparum* lines in vitro: Evidence for decreased sensitivity to dormancy and growth inhibition. *Antimicrob Agents Chemother* **56**: 428–431.

Torrentino-Madamet M, Fall B, Benoit N, Camara C, Amalvict R, Fall M, Dionne P, Ba Fall K, Nakoulima A, Diatta B, et al. 2014. Limited polymorphisms in k13 gene in *Plasmodium falciparum* isolates from Dakar, Senegal in 2012–2013. *Malaria J* **13**: 472.

Trager W, Jensen JB. 1976. Human malaria parasites in continuous culture. *Science* **193**: 673–675.

Trape JF. 2001. The public health impact of chloroquine resistance in Africa. *Am J Trop Med Hyg* **64**: 12–17.

Trape JF, Pison G, Preziosi MP, Enel C, Desgrees du Lou A, Delaunay V, Samb B, Lagarde E, Molez JF, Simondon F. 1998. Impact of chloroquine resistance on malaria mortality. *C R Acad Sci III* **321**: 689–697.

Tun KM, Imwong M, Lwin KM, Win AA, Hlaing TM, Hlaing T, Lin K, Kyaw MP, Plewes K, Faiz MA, et al. 2015. Spread of artemisinin-resistant *Plasmodium falciparum* in Myanmar: A cross-sectional survey of the K13 molecular marker. *Lancet Infect Dis* **15**: 415–421.

Vaidya AB, Morrisey JM, Zhang Z, Das S, Daly TM, Otto TD, Spillman NJ, Wyvratt M, Siegl P, Marfurt J, et al. 2014. Pyrazoleamide compounds are potent antimalarials that target Na$^+$ homeostasis in intraerythrocytic *Plasmodium falciparum*. *Nat Commun* **5**: 5521.

Verdrager J. 1986. Epidemiology of the emergence and spread of drug-resistant falciparum malaria in South-East Asia and Australasia. *J Trop Med Hyg* **89**: 277–289.

Wells TN, Hooft van Huijsduijnen R, Van Voorhis WC. 2015. Malaria medicines: A glass half full? *Nat Rev Drug Discov* **14**: 424–442.

White NJ. 2004. Antimalarial drug resistance. *J Clin Invest* **113**: 1084–1092.

White NJ. 2008. Qinghaosu (artemisinin): The price of success. *Science* **320**: 330–334.

White NJ, Pongtavornpinyo W, Maude RJ, Saralamba S, Aguas R, Stepniewska K, Lee SJ, Dondorp AM, White LJ, Day NP. 2009. Hyperparasitaemia and low dosing are an important source of anti-malarial drug resistance. *Malaria J* **8**: 253.

WHO. 2001. *Antimalarial drug combination therapy*. WHO Press, Geneva.

WHO. 2007. *Methods and techniques for clinical trials on antimalarial drug efficacy: Genotyping to identify parasite populations*. WHO Press, Geneva.

WHO. 2015a. *Guidelines for the treatment of malaria*, 3rd ed. WHO Press, Geneva

WHO. 2015b. *Strategy for malaria elimination in the Greater Mekong subregion (2015–2030)*. WHO Press, Geneva.

Wilson PE, Alker AP, Meshnick SR. 2005. Real-time PCR methods for monitoring antimalarial drug resistance. *Trends Parasitol* **21**: 278–283.

Witkowski B, Lelievre J, Barragan MJ, Laurent V, Su XZ, Berry A, Benoit-Vical F. 2010. Increased tolerance to artemisinin in *Plasmodium falciparum* is mediated by a quiescence mechanism. *Antimicrob Agents Chemother* **54**: 1872–1877.

Witkowski B, Amaratunga C, Khim N, Sreng S, Chim P, Kim S, Lim P, Mao S, Sopha C, Sam B, et al. 2013a. Novel phenotypic assays for the detection of artemisinin-resistant *Plasmodium falciparum* malaria in Cambodia: In-vitro and ex-vivo drug-response studies. *Lancet Infect Dis* **13**: 1043–1049.

Witkowski B, Khim N, Chim P, Kim S, Ke S, Kloeung N, Chy S, Duong S, Leang R, Ringwald P, et al. 2013b. Reduced artemisinin susceptibility of *Plasmodium falciparum* ring stages in western Cambodia. *Antimicrob Agents Chemother* **57**: 914–923.

Witkowski B, Lelievre J, Barragan MJ, Laurent V, Su XZ, Berry A, Benoit-Vical F. 2010. Increased tolerance to artemisinin in *Plasmodium falciparum* is mediated by a quiescence mechanism. *Antimicrob Agents Chemother* **54**: 1872–1877.

Woodrow CJ, Dahlstrom S, Cooksey R, Flegg JA, Le Nagard H, Mentre F, Murillo C, Menard D, Nosten F, Sriprawat K, et al. 2013. High-throughput analysis of antimalarial susceptibility data by the WorldWide Antimalarial Resistance Network (WWARN) in vitro analysis and reporting tool. *Antimicrob Agents Chemother* **57**: 3121–3130.

Yeung S, Van Damme W, Socheat D, White NJ, Mills A. 2008. Access to artemisinin combination therapy for malaria in remote areas of Cambodia. *Malaria J* **7**: 96.

Young MD, Contacos PG, Stitcher JE, Millar JW. 1963. Drug resistance in *Plasmodium falciparum* from Thailand. *Am J Trop Med Hyg* **12**: 305–314.

Cite this article as *Cold Spring Harb Perspect Med* doi: 10.1101/cshperspect.a025619

Vaccines to Accelerate Malaria Elimination and Eventual Eradication

Julie Healer,[1] Alan F. Cowman,[1] David C. Kaslow,[2] and Ashley J. Birkett[3]

[1]Walter & Eliza Hall Institute of Medical Research, Melbourne, Victoria 3052, Australia

[2]PATH, Seattle, Washington 98121

[3]PATH Malaria Vaccine Initiative, Washington, D.C. 20001

Correspondence: healer@wehi.edu.au

Remarkable progress has been made in coordinated malaria control efforts with substantial reductions in malaria-associated deaths and morbidity achieved through mass administration of drugs and vector control measures including distribution of long-lasting insecticide-impregnated bednets and indoor residual spraying. However, emerging resistance poses a significant threat to the sustainability of these interventions. In this light, the malaria research community has been charged with the development of a highly efficacious vaccine to complement existing malaria elimination measures. As the past 40 years of investment in this goal attests, this is no small feat. The malaria parasite is a highly complex organism, exquisitely adapted for survival under hostile conditions within human and mosquito hosts. Here we review current vaccine strategies to accelerate elimination and the potential for novel and innovative approaches to vaccine design through a better understanding of the host–parasite interaction.

Following the reinstatement in 2007 of global malaria eradication as a long-term goal, the malaria eradication research agenda initiative was conceived as a scientific consultative process between funding groups, researchers, and interest groups to identify key knowledge gaps and new tools required to move toward elimination and the eventual eradication of malaria. The crux of this strategy was enabling development of strategies and mechanisms to interrupt transmission of malaria, without which eradication would not be achievable. In 2011, a comprehensive R&D agenda was published (www.ploscollections.org/malERA2011; a new updated version will be available soon) in which vaccine development was recognized as a key component, complementing other malaria interventions with the objective of interrupting transmission to bring about the eventual eradication of the parasite species responsible for causing malaria in humans. The MalERA agenda introduced the concept of vaccines to interrupt malaria (parasite) transmission (VIMT), which could potentially incorporate the classical transmission-blocking targets, the sexual/mosquito stages (transmission-blocking vaccine [TBV]); preerythrocytic vaccines that markedly reduce asexual- and transmission-stage prevalence rates; erythrocytic-stage vaccines that reduce asexual parasite and gameto-

Cite this article as *Cold Spring Harb Perspect Med* doi: 10.1101/cshperspect.a025627

cyte densities to impact malaria transmission; and mosquito antigens to disrupt development in the vector. Although the main target product profile (TPP) of a VIMT is to interrupt transmission, an important additional benefit would be to provide protection against malaria symptoms and, ideally, to prevent epidemic spread following reintroduction after elimination.

A fundamental principle that underpins the current strategic agenda of VIMT development is that population bottlenecks (i.e., points in the life cycle where parasite numbers are low) constitute weak points where targeted approaches have a greater potential for success. As shown in Figure 1, there are two main opportunities for targeting parasite density bottlenecks: during the early exoerythrocytic phase with sporozoite injection and intrahepatocyte infection and development within the mosquito midgut following uptake of gametocytes. The fewer parasites infecting the host tissues, the reasoning goes, the greater the likelihood that induced immune mediators can prevent onward development. This is conceptually attractive as a vaccine strategy to prevent infection. Immunity in this vaccine-induced scenario differs from that of naturally acquired immunity to malaria, which occurs only after several exposures, largely to asexual targets, and acts to suppress parasite density and thereby prevent malaria symptoms. Another key advantage of a VIMT approach is a smaller population of parasites subjected to immune selection, reducing the probability of vaccine escape mutants. Naturally acquired immunity does not prevent infection or effect complete destruction of parasites in the host (Hoffman et al. 1987; Doolan et al. 2009). Thus, vaccine strategies focused on recapitulating naturally acquired immunity, via the targeting of asexual-stage antigens, are poorly aligned with the VIMT concept.

IMPORTANT CONSIDERATIONS FOR PRODUCT DEVELOPMENT OF A VACCINE TO ACCELERATE GLOBAL MALARIA ELIMINATION

What Does a Malaria Vaccine Need to Do?

The outputs from the MalERA processes, which informed the subsequent updates to the Malaria Vaccine Technology Roadmap (who .int/immunization/topics/malaria/vaccine_ roadmap/TRM_update_nov13.pdf), have contributed to the establishment of clear community goals for development of a vaccine to interrupt malaria transmission. The 2013 updated Roadmap acknowledges the need for specific measures to tackle the burden of malaria caused by *Plasmodium vivax*, considered to be even more intractable than *Plasmodium falciparum* in some regions. The points below, generally presented in the context of *P. falciparum*, apply to *P. vivax* also.

In high-intensity transmission areas where malaria is not yet under control, a VIMT would synergize with existing or introduced control programs to move these regions toward elimination.

In areas where elimination has previously been achieved, such a vaccine would prevent reestablishment of transmission; and in the event of malaria resurgence (e.g., where previous control efforts have broken down [Cohen et al. 2012]), it would provide a safety net to prevent disease and death where naturally acquired immunity has waned (White 2014).

This issue is particularly relevant in the light of the spread of anopheline resistance to insecticides and the potential time bomb of resistance to artemisinin combination therapies (ACTs) crossing into Africa (Ashley et al. 2014; Mnzava et al. 2015).

Toward ensuring that such a vaccine meets requirements, the World Health Organiza-

---

Figure 1. Points of intervention of a malaria vaccine to accelerate toward elimination. (*A*) Within-host malaria parasite population dynamics showing bottlenecks post−mosquito injection and after uptake of the blood meal where the parasite is vulnerable to vaccine-induced immune mechanisms. (*B*) Vaccine-targetable processes within the *Plasmodium* life cycle. Areas susceptible to antibody-mediated mechanisms are shown in yellow and cell-mediated mechanisms in blue. This schematic does not account for the exoerythrocytic hypnozoite stage causing relapsing blood-stage *Plasmodium vivax* infections. RBC, Red blood cell; SPZ, sporozoite.

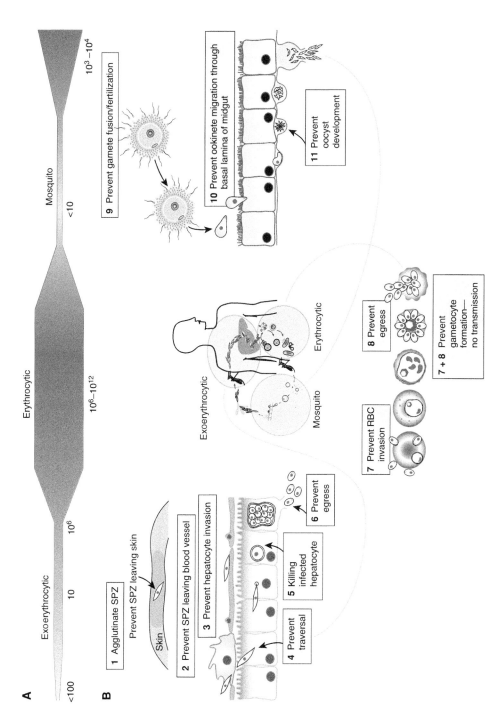

Figure 1. (*Legend on facing page.*)

tion (WHO) published a set of preferred product characteristics (PPCs) that describe the parameters for the vaccine (apps.who.int/iris/bitstream/10665/149822/1/WHO_IVB_14.09_eng.pdf). These include indications, target groups, and the clinical data required to assess safety and efficacy.

A critical knowledge gap in the PPC guidelines currently is the target protective efficacy and coverage required to confer population immunity and impact malaria transmission, in particular transmission settings. Currently, mathematical modeling using clinical trial data is our only tool to advise on these parameters and to predict how vaccine efficacy will impact malaria transmission. The controlled human malaria infection (CHMI) model offers a practical way to obtain initial efficacy estimates of a candidate vaccine in naïve volunteers. Vaccine efficacy is generally measured by evaluating the proportion of vaccinated individuals who are protected following malaria exposure. In clinical field trials, a number of endpoints may be considered including *Plasmodium* infection, number of clinical episodes, time to infection, and the number of severe malaria cases (White et al. 2015). A critical measure of vaccine efficacy, and one that has proven particularly difficult to achieve to date, is duration of protection; models can provide insight into how waning immune responses will potentially impact on malaria transmission over time. For transmission-blocking vaccines, in which the definitive measure of efficacy will be via cluster-randomized studies (either pre- or postlicensure), preclinical and early clinical studies currently place a heavy reliance on the standard membrane feeding assay (SMFA) to measure transmission reducing and/or blocking activity. Although significant progress has been made in qualifying this assay, additional work is needed to better correlate outcomes with natural transmission measures (i.e., via direct skin feeding), as well as to translate "individual level" outcomes to anticipated impact on populations. Mathematical models of malaria transmission provide a rational approach to estimating the public health impact of these interventions (White et al. 2009); however, it is important that such

models are maximally informed by biological data, an example being the nonclinical population transmission model, which has yielded unexpected findings regarding the potential impact of relatively low efficacy interventions on sustained parasite transmission (Blagborough et al. 2013).

APPROACHES TO DEVELOPMENT OF VIMT

Attacking the Exoerythrocytic Cycle— Preventing Mosquito-to-Human Transmission

To enter the liver, intradermally deposited sporozoites must leave the skin by encountering and penetrating blood vessels (Sinnis and Zavala 2012). Mutant sporozoites with decreased migratory behavior and motility speed show dramatic reductions in invasion and infectivity, indicating that migration from the inoculation site poses a significant barrier and thus an ideal opportunity for intervention (Hopp et al. 2015). Available data indicate that fewer than 100 sporozoites result in hepatocytic infection following the bite of a mosquito (Fig. 1B-1) (Kebaier et al. 2009).

Following inoculation, sporozoites migrate around CD31$^+$ endothelial junction cells before penetration of a blood vessel. Circumsporozoite protein (CSP) and thrombospondin-related adhesive protein (TRAP) have important roles in dermal emigration (Fig. 1B-1,2) (Coppi et al. 2011; Ejigiri et al. 2012). Sporozoites injected into the skin display a folded CSP conformation such that the amino-terminal region masks the carboxy-terminal thrombospondin repeat (TSR) domain. Although a number of sporozoites enter lymphatic vessels and do not contribute to hepatic invasion (Amino et al. 2006), these are crucial in priming CD8$^+$ T-cell immunity that targets intrahepatocytic infection (Fig. 1B-5) (Radtke et al. 2015). How sporozoites recognize liver proximity and by what mechanisms they exit the blood vessel and initiate liver cell entry are unknown, but an understanding of these processes would provide insights for targeted vaccine development (Fig. 1B-3).

On reaching the liver, the amino-terminal region of CSP is proteolytically cleaved, exposing the TSR that is crucial for hepatocyte adhesion and invasion (Coppi et al. 2005, 2011). Antibody-mediated prevention of this processing event inhibits sporozoite invasion in vitro (Espinosa et al. 2015), indicating that incorporating amino-terminal CSP targets may improve the efficacy of a CSP-based vaccine. Because the proteolytic cleavage site (region I) appears to be genetically conserved across species, it represents a promising target for induction of cross-species protection.

The liver vasculature, or sinusoids, is comprised of two cell types, the endothelial and macrophage-like Kupffer cells (Widmann et al. 1972). Kupffer cells are the main route of entry for sporozoites into the liver parenchyma (Meis et al. 1983; Frevert et al. 2005; Baer et al. 2007), although endothelial cells have also been observed as a route of sporozoite entry into the liver (Fig. 1B-3,4) (Tavares et al. 2013). Sporozoite traversal occurs via active penetration rather than phagocytosis (Vanderberg and Stewart 1990; Frevert et al. 2005) and CD68 is a receptor for Kupffer cell invasion, although the sporozoite ligand is not yet known (Cha et al. 2015). This would be a prime target for vaccination. How the sporozoite escapes triggering the respiratory burst is not completely understood, but involves CSP binding (Usynin et al. 2007); thus, antibodies bound to CSP may act to reverse this respiratory burst inhibition or provide an opsonization signal for phagocytic activity by Kupffer cells.

Once the process of traversal is complete and a suitable hepatocyte is identified, the process of active invasion occurs, leading to the establishment of the parasite inside a parasitophorous vacuole (PV) (Sibley 2011). The molecular determinants of this process are poorly understood but involve interactions between sporozoites and specific surface receptors on hepatocytes. These cells are recognized and bound by the amino-terminal region of CSP, mediating a signal for hepatocyte invasion (Coppi et al. 2007). Hepatocyte membrane-bound CD81 is one important receptor for sporozoites (Silvie et al. 2003), and EphA2, which associates with sporozoite proteins P52 and P36, is another (Kaushansky et al. 2015). Intra-

hepatocytic replication commences inside the PV. This provides a protective niche and prevents fusion with endosomal compartments. Once a liver schizont completes development, merozoites are released, initiating the self-replicating, pathogenic blood-stage cycle of malaria.

A fully effective vaccine that prevents sporozoite invasion of hepatocytes would also prevent emergence of blood-stage parasites, including gametocytes, and thus parasite transmission (inducing so-called sterile immunity).

Proof-of-principle evidence that sterile protection is achievable by vaccination comes from studies of irradiated sporozoites in humans and animal models (Nussenzweig et al. 1967; Clyde et al. 1973; McCarthy and Clyde 1977; Rieckmann et al. 1979). Complete protection against a sporozoite challenge can be induced when subjects are immunized with adequate numbers of attenuated parasites. Radiation-attenuated sporozoites undergo random DNA damage and arrest early in intrahepatocytic development, before DNA replication. What is not yet clear is the exact gene expression attenuation profile required to inactivate parasite development while still inducing protective immunity; nor is it clear what immune profile confers protection in protected individuals, although associations have been shown with CD8[+] T-cell responses targeting liver-stage antigens (Epstein et al. 2011; Seder et al. 2013). Answers to these questions will provide direct routes to targeted vaccine development, including development of genetically attenuated sporozoite vaccines, which are potentially safer in terms of quality control than irradiated vaccines, because identical clonal parasite lines are used in which the exact gene attenuation profile is known (Vaughan et al. 2010). These approaches benefit, at least in early-stage development, from the absence of a requirement to define specific protective antigens (a critical requirement for subunit vaccine development) and have the potential to enable identification of immune correlates of protection that could inform subunit vaccine development. The most advanced whole-parasite vaccine effort involves radiation-attenuated P. falciparum sporozoites, administered by the intravenous route. This approach, being developed by Sanaria (Rockville, MD), protected six out of six volunteers in the highest dose group from infection in CHMI studies (Richie et al. 2015). Studies are ongoing to replicate these initial findings in larger numbers of volunteers, and to generate evidence for sustained protection (via delayed challenge) and cross-strain protection (via heterologous challenge). Initial results from a field study in Mali have revealed a more modest level of efficacy (approximately 50% protection over 6 months of follow-up) (ECTMIH Special Issue 2015, http://www.ectmihbasel2015.ch/ectmih2015/home). Further, in view of the manufacturing substrate (sterile mosquitoes) reservations remain as to the feasibility of producing adequate material for global mass vaccination campaigns, as well as lack of alignment with current WHO PPCs for next-generation malaria vaccines, specifically with respect to need for intravenous delivery and a liquid nitrogen cold chain (apps.who.int/iris/bitstream/10665/149822/1/WHO_IVB_14.09_eng.pdf).

It has been postulated that the former issue, the numbers of irradiated sporozoites required, may be circumvented by adopting a similar strategy, known as ChemoProphylaxis with Sporozoites (CPS), where complete protection is induced by a fraction of the dose required in the *Plasmodium falciparum* sporozoite (PfSPZ) vaccine (Roestenberg et al. 2009). However, recent enthusiasm for the potential impact of this approach has been tempered by the report of disappointing levels of heterologous protection (Schats et al. 2015); further, challenges with ensuring safe and effective delivery of such a vaccine approach remain to be resolved.

Late liver-stage parasites show an overlapping transcriptomic profile with blood-stage parasites (Tarun et al. 2008) suggesting at least some of these antigens are expressed in both stages. Indeed, immunization with a late-arresting genetically attenuated parasite (GAP) did provide some protection against a low-dose blood-stage challenge, by a cell-mediated mechanism; however, in a CPS human challenge model, no protection was observed against direct blood challenge (Bijker et al. 2013). It has been determined that generation of preery-

throcytic immunity is dependent on sporozoite numbers (Bijker et al. 2014; Nahrendorf et al. 2015). This is consistent with the assertion that naturally acquired preerythrocytic immunity is absent in malaria-endemic situations (Tran et al. 2014). Protection against challenge in a rodent study model was only apparent after several cycles of replication in the bloodstream and indicates that lack of protection against blood-stage challenge in human volunteers may have resulted from the necessarily early treatment with chloroquine (CQ), before the onset of symptoms. Attenuation by other means, either chemical (Good et al. 2013) or genetic (Aly et al. 2011), could potentially provide protection against homologous and heterologous blood-stage challenge. Complete sterilizing immunity against sporozoite challenge in a late-arresting GAP liver infection model is conferred by only two, rather than three, immunizations in other GAP/RAS models, suggesting that late schizont/merozoite antigen expression may be important. This is supported by evidence that MSP1 can induce a multistage immune response with partial protection against liver stages (Draper et al. 2009).

The malaria vaccine candidate most advanced in development is RTS,S, comprising Hepatitis B surface antigen (HBsAg) and an HBsAg-circumsporozoite (CS) fusion protein, which are produced in yeast and form a particulate structure. It is formulated with the proprietary AS01 adjuvant system of GlaxoSmithKline (GSK). Results after a year of follow-up in a phase III efficacy (clinical malaria endpoint) and safety trial, involving more than 15,000 infants and young children, at 11 sites in seven African countries, showed that three doses of RTS,S reduced clinical malaria by approximately half in children 5–17 months of age at first vaccination (Agnandji et al. 2011). The final study results analyzed vaccine efficacy (VE), immunogenicity, safety, and impact of RTS,S/AS01 over a median of 38 and 48 months of follow-up (postdose 1) in infants and young children, respectively, including the effect of a fourth dose of vaccine (Greenwood 2015). These final results showed that vaccination with the three-dose primary series reduced clinical malaria cases by 28% (95% CI: 23.3; 32.9) in young children and 18% (95% CI: 11.7; 24.4) in infants to the end of the study. Adding a fourth dose of RTS,S, administered 18 months after the primary series, reduced the number of cases of clinical malaria in young children by 36% (95% CI: 31.8; 40.5) and in infants by 26% (95% CI: 19.9; 31.5) over the entire study period. Therefore, although the VE waned over time, the fourth dose contributed to enhancing VE, but not to the level observed following the first three doses. These results were achieved within the context of existing malaria interventions, such as insecticide-treated nets (ITNs), which were used by approximately 80% of the trial participants during the follow-up period.

In June 2014, GSK submitted an application for a scientific opinion on the RTS,S/AS01 candidate vaccine to the European Medicines Agency (EMA) under its Article 58 procedure. The EMA's Committee for Medicinal Products for Human Use (CHMP) evaluated data on the quality, safety, and efficacy of the RTS,S/AS01 vaccine candidate. In July 2015, CHMP adopted a positive scientific opinion for RTS,S/AS01, stating that the quality of the vaccine and the benefit-risk balance are considered favorable from a regulatory perspective. However, the EMA also requested that additional information needs be addressed in future studies, specifically with respect to (1) the timing of the fourth dose and evaluation of the safety and efficacy of an earlier fourth dose; (2) the efficacy and safety of multiple yearly doses and whether the vaccine predisposes to some degree of hyporesponsiveness to sequential doses; and (3) the potential utility of a delayed and fractionated third dose schedule in the target age group. Subsequent to the Article 58 process (WHO issued formal recommendations in January 2016 calling for large-scale pilot implementations of RTS,S; www.who.int/immunization/research/development/malaria_vaccine_qa/en).

The recommendations include that the pilot implementations use the four-dose schedule of the RTS,S/AS01 vaccine in three to five distinct epidemiological settings in sub-Saharan Africa, at the subnational level, covering moderate-to-high transmission settings, with three doses administered to children between 5 and 9 months of age, followed by a fourth dose 15–18 months later. Further recommendations for the pilot implementations are outlined in the WHO position paper.

Concurrent with the activities associated with the conduct and regulatory submission of the phase 3 RTS,S/AS01 clinical trial, PATH's (Program for Appropriate Technology in Health) malaria vaccine initiative (MVI) and GSK have continued to investigate opportunities to increase the efficacy and duration of protection against malaria infection toward development of a vaccine that could contribute to malaria elimination and eradication. An important milestone was achieved in 2014–2015, when an alternative regimen of RTS,S/AS01—in which the third dose is delayed by 6 months and fractionated to one-fifth of the standard dose (thus the term "FxRTS,S")—achieved 87% protection (95% CI: 67–95), compared to 63% (95% CI: 20–80) for the standard full-dose regimen, in a CHMI study. The fractional regimen increased antibody somatic hypermutation and avidity. Rechallenge showed waning efficacy in both groups, but fractional dose boosting maintained high protection (manuscript in preparation). These results were remarkably similar to findings reported in 1997, where six of seven volunteers were protected with a similar regimen of RTS,S/AS02 (Stoute et al. 1997); this regimen was not pursued at that time, as the results were generally viewed as being a "chance" finding in view of later studies (where the fractional booster dose was not implemented), and the nonalignment with the accepted expanded program on immunization (EPI) schedules, for which the vaccine was intended. The GSK/PATH partnership are proceeding to a phase 2b field study in young African children (aged 5 to 17 months at first vaccination) to evaluate the potential of FxRTS,S to prevent naturally acquired *P. falciparum* infection.

PREVENTION OF HUMAN–MOSQUITO TRANSMISSION—ATTACKING THE ERYTHROCYTIC STAGES

Early malaria vaccine development efforts focused on induction of an immune response that would clear or restrict fulminating parasitemia, thus preventing severe disease and death. The rationale for this approach came from resolution of malaria symptoms following clinical interventions involving passive transfer of hyperimmune adult sera to children experiencing severe malaria symptoms with high parasitemia (Cohen et al. 1961; Sabchaeron et al. 1991). The prospective targets for conferring such immunity were antigens expressed in the blood stages, many of which were correlated with immune protection in endemic regions or were identified by screening expression libraries with hyperimmune sera. Thus, there was a clear correspondence between induction of vaccine-induced protection and naturally acquired immunity to malaria. Despite a pressing medical need for a vaccine to prevent clinical malaria, as well as a strong rationale for vaccine-induced immunity against blood stages to provide a safety net in regions of waning naturally acquired immunity because of reductions in parasite transmission achieved by other measures, blood-stage vaccine research has been deprioritized in favor of targeting preerythrocytic- and mosquito-stage parasites. Reasons for deprioritizing blood-stage vaccines in an elimination agenda include the bottleneck phenomenon (Fig. 1): the perception that large numbers of circulating parasites, and genetic diversity of many, but not all potential asexual blood-stage target antigens, present an insurmountable hurdle to the vaccine-induced immunity. The disappointing clinical efficacy of AMA1- and MSP1-based vaccines have no doubt contributed to the idea that blood-stage parasitemia is intractable to control by vaccination (Spring et al. 2009; Sheehy et al. 2012; Payne et al. 2016). These unsuccessful clinical trials have highlighted the importance of judicious antigen choice, with conserved antigens preferable to polymorphic ones and prioritization of antigens capable of evoking protective responses at relatively low antibody concentrations.

These trials highlighted the benefit of early clinical testing of prospective approaches in CHMI models, toward determining whether induced responses reduce parasite replication in vivo, and CHMI is increasingly serving as a stage gate before endemic field testing (Duncan et al. 2011; Duncan and Draper 2012).

It still remains possible that a highly effective blood-stage immune response could form an integral part of a VIMT strategy if it successfully reduced death, disease, and transmission by limiting the asexual parasite density below a threshold required for infectious gametocyte production. How these factors are related is not well understood, however, and more research is required to address this particular knowledge gap.

The leading blood-stage vaccine candidate today is PfRh5, a conserved merozoite protein essential to erythrocyte invasion (Fig. 1B-7) (Baum et al. 2009; Douglas et al. 2011, 2015; Chen et al. 2014; Wright et al. 2014). Other merozoite protein clinical candidates remaining in the vaccine pipeline from the pre-eradication era are SERA5, MSP3, MSP1, GLURP, AMA1, and EBA-175 (Birkett 2015). Promising early clinical trial data support further investigation into MSP3 (Sirima et al. 2011) and SERA5 (Palacpac et al. 2013) as possible components in a next-generation malaria vaccine. Another antigen showing preclinical promise is schizont egress antigen-1 (SEA-1). This protein plays an essential role during schizont rupture during the blood stage (Fig. 1B-8) and carriage of antibodies to this protein was associated with reduced incidence of severe malaria (Raj et al. 2014). Whether antibodies to SEA-1 can also block liver schizont egress (Fig. 1B-6) is not known, but an essential process that could be blocked in multiple stages with a single vaccine antigen should be considered as a high priority for further investigation.

Antigens present on the surface of the parasitized erythrocyte membrane are associated with natural immunity to malaria; however, their high diversity presents a major roadblock for vaccine design. A vaccine aimed to prevent pregnancy-associated malaria, based on the relatively conserved PfEMP1 protein VAR2CSA, is close to clinical transition (Birkett 2015).

During a blood-stage infection, a proportion of parasites will divert to a sexual course of development, dependent on the uptake of mature gametocytes by a feeding mosquito. Conversion to gametocyte development is a poorly understood process (see Meibalan and Marti

2016 for details) that is constitutive in *Plasmodium*, but is also inducible by certain environmental conditions, indicating that parasites sense changes in their environment and respond to these cues. In *P. falciparum*, intracellular gametocytes develop through five distinct stages, and sequester in the bone marrow and spleen for 9–12 days until mature forms emerge into the peripheral circulation and are transmissible. Many sexual stage–specific antigens are expressed in the developing gametocyte, but do not play a role in nutrient acquisition or cytoadherence, and thus are not revealed to the immune system by presentation on the erythrocyte surface.

Until recently, it was widely held that circulating gametocytes were immunologically silent. The proteins exposed on the surface of gametocyte-infected erythrocytes are potentially involved in cytoadherence, conferring the ability of maturing stages to sequester until maturity, are poorly characterized but may include variant proteins such as STEVOR (McRobert et al. 2004), RIFIN (Sharp et al. 2006) or others yet to be identified (Saeed et al. 2008). This as-yet-unexplored area could present new opportunities for gametocyte-specific immune targeting to reduce transmission and move toward malaria elimination.

PREVENTION OF HUMAN–MOSQUITO TRANSMISSION—ATTACKING THE MOSQUITO STAGES

Once inside the midgut of the mosquito, the changed environment signals the gametocytes to break down the erythrocyte membrane and emerge as male and female gametes that can undergo fertilization. At this point, well-characterized antigens (clinical vaccine candidates Pfs230 and Pfs48/45) are exposed and are targetable by antibodies and complement (Table 1) (Sauerwein and Bousema 2015).

Mosquito midgut invasion by *Plasmodium* ookinetes is considered a promising target for transmission-blocking intervention, as parasite numbers undergo a major bottleneck at this stage (Sinden 2010). After the mosquito ingests an infected blood meal, male and female gametes fuse in the midgut lumen, giving rise to zygotes that differentiate into motile ookinetes.

After crossing the peritrophic matrix aided by chitinase secretion (Tsai et al. 2001), the ookinete establishes specific molecular interactions with the midgut epithelial cells, followed by their invasion and traversal. Several proteins from the ookinete, including the most advanced TBV candidate Pfs25 and the mosquito aminopeptidase 1 (AnAPN1), may be involved in this process (see Bousema and Drakeley 2016 for more details). AnAPN1 presents a conceptually attractive candidate because it potentially targets multiple *Plasmodium–Anopheles* species combinations, although preclinical studies have yet to confirm this. The only molecular interactions between the ookinete and the midgut characterized thus far are the in vitro interaction between parasite Pvs25 and mosquito calreticulin (Rodriguez Mdel et al. 2007) and between the ookinete enolase and the mosquito midgut enolase-binding protein (Vega-Rodriguez et al. 2014).

Table 1. Malaria vaccine candidates in clinical trials

Exoerythrocytic antigens	Erythrocytic-stage antigens	Transmission blocking	Multistage
RTS,S (CSP)	PfAMA1 (3)	Pfs25 + Pfs230-EPA	PfCSP + AMA1
PfME-TRAP	PfAMA1 + MSP1		PfTRAP + MSP1
PfSPZ (RAS, CPS)	PfGLURP + MSP3		PfTRAP + RH5 + Pfs25
PfCSP (3)	EBA-175		
PfCelTOS	PfRH5		
PvCSP	SERA5		
PfGAP (2)	PvDBP		

For up-to-date information, see the WHO rainbow tables at: www.who.int/immunization/research/development/Rainbow_tables/en.

The classical TBV candidates are antigens expressed on the surface membrane of gamete, zygote, and ookinete forms. The best characterized of these, Pfs25, is the lead TBV in clinical development. However, challenges in the induction of high titer antibody responses have been recently reported, with poor immunoreactivity in humans with this antigen, despite good preclinical results in nonhuman primates. For an in-depth recent review of the TBV candidate development status see Nikolaeva et al. (2015).

Two of the main challenges in TBV development have been: (1) producing immunogens with three-dimensional structures that mimic their native counterparts, and (2) inducing in humans the levels of functional antibodies observed in preclinical models. Although progress has been made in qualifying the SMFA (Miura et al. 2013), there remains a need to better understand the correlation between the readout of assays used to report the impact of TBVs and the longitudinal impact on malaria transmission (Blagborough et al. 2013; Kapulu et al. 2015). A rapid pipeline of proof-of-principle human trials for testing lead candidates would improve prioritization of new TBV candidates (Sauerwein and Bousema 2015). Target identification efforts that leverage available sera with high levels of naturally induced transmission-blocking activity have recently been initiated.

INNOVATION FOR DISCOVERY OF NEW TARGETS AND BIOMARKERS

Publication of the *P. falciparum* (Gardner et al. 2002) and *P. vivax* (Carlton et al. 2008) genomes revealed many novel potential candidate antigens. Transcriptome (Le Roch et al. 2003; Silvestrini et al. 2005; Xu et al. 2005; Young et al. 2005) and proteomic (Lasonder et al. 2002; Hall et al. 2005; Khan et al. 2005; Lal et al. 2009) studies have since confirmed expression of hundreds of *Plasmodium* proteins. Potentially, all of these could be investigated for their suitability as vaccine antigens and their roles in parasite development. However, only a few have been the subject of preclinical studies. Advances in other postgenomic areas such as metabolomics,

lipidomics, and functional genomics, particularly with CRISPR/Cas9 technology to expedite large screening projects, are also poised to yield exciting leads in vaccine R&D.

Conventional screening approaches used for antigen identification to date have included expression cloning of putative candidates followed by immunoreactivity testing of plasma by ELISA or western blot; elution and mass spectrometry sequencing of MHC-bound peptides; and in vitro testing of pools of overlapping peptides and reverse immunogenetics (Doolan et al. 2008). However, these methods are not applicable to high-throughput analysis of genomic data. Screening of protein microarray (Doolan et al. 2008; Felgner et al. 2013) or expression libraries (Richards et al. 2013; Arumugam et al. 2014; Osier et al. 2014) can be a useful alternative for identifying immunodominant antigens and immunoreactivity profiles from donors with defined malaria immune status. Antibody profiles from naturally immune individuals and those from CPS- or radiation-attenuated immunized, protected individuals have distinctly different profiles (Felgner et al. 2013), with a strong blood-stage bias in protective immunity from natural infection compared with largely preerythrocytic or mixed-stage targets via CPS vaccination, which is perhaps unsurprising given that CQ treatment is highly effective in preventing establishment of a blood-stage infection.

A key knowledge gap is what constitutes a protective immune response. This is used to inform which particular antigens or epitopes are likely to comprise the best targets, whether adjuvants will be required to optimize the induction of immune effectors, and which platforms may be best suited for durability and longevity of the protective response. Rational design of malaria vaccines can be facilitated by progress in the understanding of the host–parasite relationship, particularly, mechanisms of host protective immunity and molecular mechanisms of pathogen–host interactions, particularly those that are essential to parasites' survival and reproduction, and also those used to evade host immunity. To investigate protective immunity a combination of systems biology, -omics technologies, interrogation of the B-cell repertoire, cell-based assays, and epidemiological studies are all relevant.

The relative importance of different immune responses in endemic settings is difficult to gauge, inconsistent between studies and varies with seasonality and parasite density. Despite extensive use as surrogate markers of immunity, neither antibody levels nor interferon γ (IFN-γ) responses correlate consistently with protection between studies (Dunachie et al. 2015). Of particular note is the failure of the parasite growth-inhibition assay (GIA) to predict clinical outcomes from trials of blood-stage vaccines to date.

The availability of highly characterized parasites for challenge via CHMI offers significant advantages over the study of natural infections for gaining insight into protective mechanisms of antimalarial immunity following vaccination or exposure (reviewed in Sauerwein et al. 2011). In a CHMI study, participants are infected with parasites delivered via three alternative routes: with sporozoites via mosquito bite (Chulay et al. 1986; Roestenberg et al. 2012); via needle-based inoculation of cryopreserved sporozoites (Epstein 2013); or via thawed cryopreserved, infected red blood cells (Lawrence et al. 2000; Pombo et al. 2002; Duncan et al. 2011). CHMI by mosquito bite challenge has been the most widely adopted, and provides a cost-effective, highly reproducible assessment of vaccine candidates for their efficacy against infection. Two groups have reported successful challenge with *P. vivax*–infected mosquitoes opening up the potential for much-needed research on *P. vivax* vaccines (Herrera et al. 2009; Bennett et al. 2016).

Vaccine approaches designed to interrupt transmission of *P. vivax* parasites must account for two unique features that are distinct from *P. falciparum* parasites: (1) the relapse potential of liver-resident hypnozoites; and (2) accelerated transmissibility associated with direct emergence of gametocytes from the liver at the initiation of the asexual blood-stage infection. A highly efficacious preerythrocytic vaccine that prevents initial infections, and thereby preventing relapsing hypnozoites, has significant po-

tential in accelerating *P. vivax* elimination. Although relatively few *P. vivax* vaccine approaches have been tested in human clinical trials, a chimeric PvCSP protein (VMP001), developed by Walter Reed Army Institute of Research (WRAIR) and incorporating a truncated repeat region containing sequences from both the VK210 (type 1) and the VK247 (type 2) parasites has been evaluated in a single CHMI study. Although all volunteers immunized with VMP001/AS01 progressed to blood-stage parasitemia following challenge by infected mosquitoes, a significant delay in the median prepatency period was noted as compared to the infectivity controls (Bennett et al. 2016). These results suggest that induced immune responses partially blocked hepatocyte invasion by sporozoites and/or emergence of merozoites from infected hepatocytes. The development and testing of a particulate CS-based immunogen, and application of the delayed fractional booster dosing regimen, successfully applied to RTS,S/AS01, would appear to be logical next steps.

SPECIAL CONSIDERATIONS FOR A TBV

Classical TBVs, also known as SSM-VIMT (for sexual, sporogonic, and/or mosquito-stage vaccines interrupting malaria [parasite] transmission), target the mosquito stages of the life cycle by inducing antibodies within the human host that prevent onward transmission and, therefore, provide no direct and immediate clinical benefit to the vaccine recipient. Delayed individual benefit would be realized at the population level, when transmission is decreased or ceased. Despite the absence of direct and immediate benefit to the vaccine recipient, the United States Food and Drug Administration (FDA) has asserted that there is no legal bar to prevent a vaccine such as an SSM-TBV from being considered for licensure in the context of their review process. This is consistent with the continued implementation of pertussis vaccine, which from a public health standpoint primarily benefits the unborn children of pregnant women. Further, tetanus and influenza vaccines (along with pertussis) are recommended during pregnancy, and vaccine development efforts for respiratory syncytial virus (RSV) and group B streptococcus (GBS) are increasingly targeting maternal immunization as an approach to benefit newborns (Lindsey et al. 2013).

Another key consideration is how to monitor the efficacy and secure licensure of such a vaccine via clinical trials. Two approaches have been proposed: (1) a large-scale, phase 3 efficacy trial, which, in the case of an SSM-VIMT, has been proposed by regulators to be a cluster-randomized trial (CRT) to show vaccine impact on incidence of infection in the community; and (2) an accelerated approval pathway in which the vaccine would receive approval for use based on an analytically and biologically, but not clinically, validated surrogate of efficacy (which does not yet exist), with impact on transmission confirmed during postapproval studies (Nunes et al. 2014; Delrieu et al. 2015). The accelerated approval strategy would likely involve feeding mosquitoes directly on malaria-exposed trial participants or via drawn blood in membrane feeders. However, there are likely to be significant differences in transmission between humans and mosquitoes (e.g., age of volunteer, immune status, parasite and mosquito genotypes) (Smith et al. 2010; Tusting et al. 2014; Reiner et al. 2015); thus, trial size, as well as design, will be major considerations in ensuring statistical confidence in the results.

Further challenges are how to predict the public health impact from reducing transmission, and what criteria to apply regarding the minimal efficacy required to ensure that the significant financial and logistical investment required of such a vaccine is warranted.

TARGET POPULATION FOR A VACCINE TO ELIMINATE MALARIA

All individuals with the potential to become infected, including those who are asymptomatic and whose parasitemia is below detectable levels, should be considered capable of transmitting malaria parasites; therefore, everyone in the area of transmission would likely need to be immunized with a VIMT. This contrasts with

vaccine approaches intended to protect only those at greatest risk from the severe consequences of malaria, primarily young African children, who are targeted via the EPI schedule. Distinct implementation strategies, and other key considerations that need to be considered in development of these two classes of vaccine, have been the focus of increased recent attention (Nunes et al. 2014; Birkett 2015).

CONCLUDING REMARKS

The first 15 years of the 21st century have witnessed remarkable reductions in mortality attributable to malaria, in alignment with the coordinated implementation of a range of interventions. Approximately six million lives, mostly of young African children, have been spared during this period (www.who.int/malaria/media/world-malaria-report-2015/en). Emerging threats to the effectiveness of these interventions highlights the need for new and innovative approaches. The potential for a vaccine to contribute to maintaining the gains and potentially contributing to further reductions in disease and death has become closer to realization over the past 2 years with RTS,S/AS01, the most advanced vaccine candidate in development globally, completing phase 3 testing and receiving a positive opinion from the EMA. The future impact of RTS,S/AS01 will be defined by its performance in pilot implementations recommended by WHO to generate the supplemental evidence needed to support possible wide-scale implementation.

In the face of these advancements, the vaccine development community has been challenged to apply the proven attributes of this powerful intervention to contribute to reduced transmission, toward accelerating elimination and eventual eradication of the parasites responsible for causing malaria in humans. This has led to an increased focus on research to better understand the biological process associated with parasite invasion, particularly at the interface of the two obligate hosts, humans and female anopheline mosquitoes, critical for maintaining parasite transmission. Further understanding these invasion mechanisms could reveal potent new vaccine targets.

Vaccine development efforts, utilizing an array of subunit and whole parasite vaccine approaches, are increasingly focused on infection and transmission endpoints. Short-term protection levels (from infection) approaching 100% have recently been reported for two distinct vaccine approaches, RTS,S/AS01 and PfSPZ, in CHMI studies, resulting in significant optimism. For these leading approaches, efforts are underway to improve the durability of protective responses and ease implementation challenges. As these approaches transition to endemic field testing for assessment under conditions of natural transmission, clear "lines of sight" for development, regulatory approval, implementation, and financing will become increasingly important.

REFERENCES

*Reference is also in this collection.

Agnandji ST, Lell B, Soulanoudjingar SS, Fernandes JF, Abossolo BP, Conzelmann C, Methogo BG, Doucka Y, Flamen A, Mordmuller B, et al. 2011. First results of phase 3 trial of RTS,S/AS01 malaria vaccine in African children. *N Engl J Med* **365:** 1863–1875.

Aly AS, Lindner SE, MacKellar DC, Peng X, Kappe SH. 2011. SAP1 is a critical post-transcriptional regulator of infectivity in malaria parasite sporozoite stages. *Mol Microbiol* **79:** 929–939.

Amino R, Thiberge S, Shorte S, Frischknecht F, Menard R. 2006. Quantitative imaging of Plasmodium sporozoites in the mammalian host. *C R Biol* **329:** 858–862.

Arumugam TU, Ito D, Takashima E, Tachibana M, Ishino T, Torii M, Tsuboi T. 2014. Application of wheat germ cell-free protein expression system for novel malaria vaccine candidate discovery. *Expert Rev Vaccines* **13:** 75–85.

Ashley EA, Dhorda M, Fairhurst RM, Amaratunga C, Lim P, Suon S, Sreng S, Anderson JM, Mao S, Sam B, et al. 2014. Spread of artemisinin resistance in *Plasmodium falciparum* malaria. *N Engl J Med* **371:** 411–423.

Baer K, Roosevelt M, Clarkson AB Jr, van Rooijen N, Schnieder T, Frevert U. 2007. Kupffer cells are obligatory for *Plasmodium yoelii* sporozoite infection of the liver. *Cell Microbiol* **9:** 397–412.

Baum J, Chen L, Healer J, Lopaticki S, Boyle M, Triglia T, Ehlgen F, Ralph SA, Beeson JG, Cowman AF. 2009. Reticulocyte-binding protein homologue 5—An essential adhesin involved in invasion of human erythrocytes by *Plasmodium falciparum*. *Int J Parasitol* **39:** 371–380.

Bennett JW, Yadava A, Tosh D, Sattabongkot J, Komisar J, Ware LA, McCarthy WF, Cowden JJ, Regules J, Spring MD, et al. 2016. Phase 1/2a trial of *Plasmodium vivax*

malaria vaccine candidate VMP001/AS01B in malaria-naive adults: Safety, immunogenicity, and efficacy. *PLoS Negl Trop Dis* **10:** e0004423.

Bijker EM, Bastiaens GJ, Teirlinck AC, van Gemert GJ, Graumans W, van de Vegte-Bolmer M, Siebelink-Stoter R, Arens T, Teelen K, Nahrendorf W, et al. 2013. Protection against malaria after immunization by chloroquine prophylaxis and sporozoites is mediated by preerythrocytic immunity. *Proc Natl Acad Sci* **110:** 7862–7867.

Bijker EM, Teirlinck AC, Schats R, van Gemert GJ, van de Vegte-Bolmer M, van Lieshout L, IntHout J, Hermsen CC, Scholzen A, Visser LG, et al. 2014. Cytotoxic markers associate with protection against malaria in human volunteers immunized with *Plasmodium falciparum* sporozoites. *J Infect Dis* **210:** 1605–1615.

Birkett AJ. 2015. Building an effective malaria vaccine pipeline to address global needs. *Vaccine* **33:** 7538–7543.

Blagborough AM, Churcher TS, Upton LM, Ghani AC, Gething PW, Sinden RE. 2013. Transmission-blocking interventions eliminate malaria from laboratory populations. *Nat Commun* **4:** 1812.

* Bousema T, Drakeley C. 2016. Determinants of malaria transmission at the population level. *Cold Spring Harb Perspect Med* doi: 10.1101/cshperspect.a025510.

Carlton JM, Adams JH, Silva JC, Bidwell SL, Lorenzi H, Caler E, Crabtree J, Angiuoli SV, Merino EF, Amedeo P, et al. 2008. Comparative genomics of the neglected human malaria parasite *Plasmodium vivax*. *Nature* **455:** 757–763.

Cha SJ, Park K, Srinivasan P, Schindler CW, van Rooijen N, Stins M, Jacobs-Lorena M. 2015. CD68 acts as a major gateway for malaria sporozoite liver infection. *J Exp Med* **212:** 1391–1403.

Chen L, Xu Y, Healer J, Thompson JK, Smith BJ, Lawrence MC, Cowman AF. 2014. Crystal structure of PfRh5, an essential *P. falciparum* ligand for invasion of human erythrocytes. *eLife* **3:** e04187.

Chulay JD, Schneider I, Cosgriff TM, Hoffman SL, Ballou WR, Quakyi IA, Carter R, Trosper JH, Hockmeyer WT. 1986. Malaria transmitted to humans by mosquitoes infected from cultured *Plasmodium falciparum*. *Am J Trop Med Hyg* **35:** 66–68.

Clyde DF, Most H, McCarthy VC, Vanderberg JP. 1973. Immunization of man against sporozoite-induced falciparum malaria. *Am J Med Sci* **266:** 169–177.

Cohen S, McGregor IA, Carrington SC. 1961. γ-Globulin and acquired immunity to human malaria. *Nature* **192:** 733–737.

Cohen JM, Smith DL, Cotter C, Ward A, Yamey G, Sabot OJ, Moonen B. 2012. Malaria resurgence: A systematic review and assessment of its causes. *Malaria J* **11:** 122.

Coppi A, Pinzon-Ortiz C, Hutter C, Sinnis P. 2005. The Plasmodium circumsporozoite protein is proteolytically processed during cell invasion. *J Exp Med* **201:** 27–33.

Coppi A, Tewari R, Bishop JR, Bennett BL, Lawrence R, Esko JD, Billker O, Sinnis P. 2007. Heparan sulfate proteoglycans provide a signal to Plasmodium sporozoites to stop migrating and productively invade host cells. *Cell Host Microbe* **2:** 316–327.

Coppi A, Natarajan R, Pradel G, Bennett BL, James ER, Roggero MA, Corradin G, Persson C, Tewari R, Sinnis

P. 2011. The malaria circumsporozoite protein has two functional domains, each with distinct roles as sporozoites journey from mosquito to mammalian host. *J Exp Med* **208:** 341–356.

Delrieu I, Leboulleux D, Ivinson K, Gessner BD; Malaria Transmission Blocking Vaccine Technical Consultation. 2015. Design of a phase III cluster randomized trial to assess the efficacy and safety of a malaria transmission blocking vaccine. *Vaccine* **33:** 1518–1526.

Doolan DL, Mu Y, Unal B, Sundaresh S, Hirst S, Valdez C, Randall A, Molina D, Liang X, Freilich DA, et al. 2008. Profiling humoral immune responses to *P. falciparum* infection with protein microarrays. *Proteomics* **8:** 4680–4694.

Doolan DL, Dobano C, Baird JK. 2009. Acquired immunity to malaria. *Clin Microbiol Rev* **22:** 13–36.

Douglas AD, Williams AR, Illingworth JJ, Kamuyu G, Biswas S, Goodman AL, Wyllie DH, Crosnier C, Miura K, Wright GJ, et al. 2011. The blood-stage malaria antigen PfRH5 is susceptible to vaccine-inducible cross-strain neutralizing antibody. *Nat Commun* **2:** 601.

Douglas AD, Baldeviano GC, Lucas CM, Lugo-Roman LA, Crosnier C, Bartholdson SJ, Diouf A, Miura K, Lambert LE, Ventocilla JA, et al. 2015. A PfRH5-based vaccine is efficacious against heterologous strain blood-stage *Plasmodium falciparum* infection in Aotus monkeys. *Cell Host Microbe* **17:** 130–139.

Draper SJ, Goodman AL, Biswas S, Forbes EK, Moore AC, Gilbert SC, Hill AV. 2009. Recombinant viral vaccines expressing merozoite surface protein-1 induce antibody- and T cell-mediated multistage protection against malaria. *Cell Host Microbe* **5:** 95–105.

Dunachie S, Hill AV, Fletcher HA. 2015. Profiling the host response to malaria vaccination and malaria challenge. *Vaccine* **33:** 5316–5320.

Duncan CJ, Draper SJ. 2012. Controlled human blood stage malaria infection: Current status and potential applications. *Am J Trop Med Hyg* **86:** 561–565.

Duncan CJ, Sheehy SH, Ewer KJ, Douglas AD, Collins KA, Halstead FD, Elias SC, Lillie PJ, Rausch K, Aebig J, et al. 2011. Impact on malaria parasite multiplication rates in infected volunteers of the protein-in-adjuvant vaccine AMA1-C1/Alhydrogel+CPG 7909. *PLoS ONE* **6:** e22271.

Ejigiri I, Ragheb DR, Pino P, Coppi A, Bennett BL, Soldati-Favre D, Sinnis P. 2012. Shedding of TRAP by a rhomboid protease from the malaria sporozoite surface is essential for gliding motility and sporozoite infectivity. *PLoS Pathog* **8:** e1002725.

Epstein JE. 2013. Taking a bite out of malaria: Controlled human malaria infection by needle and syringe. *Am J Trop Med Hyg* **88:** 3–4.

Epstein JE, Tewari K, Lyke KE, Sim BK, Billingsley PF, Laurens MB, Gunasekera A, Chakravarty S, James ER, Sedegah M, et al. 2011. Live attenuated malaria vaccine designed to protect through hepatic CD8$^+$ T cell immunity. *Science* **334:** 475–480.

Espinosa DA, Gutierrez GM, Rojas-Lopez M, Noe AR, Shi L, Tse SW, Sinnis P, Zavala F. 2015. Proteolytic cleavage of the *Plasmodium falciparum* circumsporozoite protein is a target of protective antibodies. *J Infect Dis* **212:** 1111–1119.

Felgner PL, Roestenberg M, Liang L, Hung C, Jain A, Pablo J, Nakajima-Sasaki R, Molina D, Teelen K, Hermsen CC, et al. 2013. Pre-erythrocytic antibody profiles induced by controlled human malaria infections in healthy volunteers under chloroquine prophylaxis. *Sci Rep* **3:** 3549.

Frevert U, Engelmann S, Zougbede S, Stange J, Ng B, Matuschewski K, Liebes L, Yee H. 2005. Intravital observation of *Plasmodium berghei* sporozoite infection of the liver. *PLoS Biol* **3:** e192.

Gardner MJ, Hall N, Fung E, White O, Berriman M, Hyman RW, Carlton JM, Pain A, Nelson KE, Bowman S, et al. 2002. Genome sequence of the human malaria parasite *Plasmodium falciparum*. *Nature* **419:** 498–511.

Good MF, Reiman JM, Rodriguez IB, Ito K, Yanow SK, El-Deeb IM, Batzloff MR, Stanisic DI, Engwerda C, Spithill T, et al. 2013. Cross-species malaria immunity induced by chemically attenuated parasites. *J Clin Invest* doi: 10.1172/JCI66634.

Greenwood BR, S Clinical Trials Partnership. 2015. Efficacy and safety of RTS,S/AS01 malaria vaccine with or without a booster dose in infants and children in Africa: Final results of a phase 3, individually randomised, controlled trial. *Lancet* **386:** 60721–60728.

Hall N, Karras M, Raine JD, Carlton JM, Kooij TW, Berriman M, Florens L, Janssen CS, Pain A, Christophides GK, et al. 2005. A comprehensive survey of the *Plasmodium* life cycle by genomic, transcriptomic, and proteomic analyses. *Science* **307:** 82–86.

Herrera S, Fernandez O, Manzano MR, Murrain B, Vergara J, Blanco P, Palacios R, Velez JD, Epstein JE, Chen-Mok M, et al. 2009. Successful sporozoite challenge model in human volunteers with *Plasmodium vivax* strain derived from human donors. *Am J Trop Med Hyg* **81:** 740–746.

Hoffman SL, Oster CN, Plowe CV, Woollett GR, Beier JC, Chulay JD, Wirtz RA, Hollingdale MR, Mugambi M. 1987. Naturally acquired antibodies to sporozoites do not prevent malaria: Vaccine development implications. *Science* **237:** 639–642.

Hopp CS, Chiou K, Ragheb DR, Salman A, Khan SM, Liu AJ, Sinnis P. 2015. Longitudinal analysis of Plasmodium sporozoite motility in the dermis reveals component of blood vessel recognition. *eLife* **4.**

Kapulu MC, Da DF, Miura K, Li Y, Blagborough AM, Churcher TS, Nikolaeva D, Williams AR, Goodman AL, Sangare I, et al. 2015. Comparative assessment of transmission-blocking vaccine candidates against *Plasmodium falciparum*. *Sci Rep* **5:** 11193.

Kaushansky A, Douglass AN, Arang N, Vigdorovich V, Dambrauskas N, Kain HS, Austin LS, Sather DN, Kappe SH. 2015. Malaria parasites target the hepatocyte receptor EphA2 for successful host infection. *Science* **350:** 1089–1092.

Kebaier C, Voza T, Vanderberg J. 2009. Kinetics of mosquito-injected Plasmodium sporozoites in mice: Fewer sporozoites are injected into sporozoite-immunized mice. *PLoS Pathog* **5:** e1000399.

Khan SM, Franke-Fayard B, Mair GR, Lasonder E, Janse CJ, Mann M, Waters AP. 2005. Proteome analysis of separated male and female gametocytes reveals novel sex-specific *Plasmodium* biology. *Cell* **121:** 675–687.

Lal K, Prieto JH, Bromley E, Sanderson SJ, Yates JR III, Wastling JM, Tomley FM, Sinden RE. 2009. Characterisation of *Plasmodium* invasive organelles; an ookinete microneme proteome. *Proteomics* **9:** 1142–1151.

Lasonder E, Ishihama Y, Andersen JS, Vermunt AM, Pain A, Sauerwein RW, Eling WM, Hall N, Waters AP, Stunnenberg HG, et al. 2002. Analysis of the *Plasmodium falciparum* proteome by high-accuracy mass spectrometry. *Nature* **419:** 537–542.

Lawrence G, Cheng QQ, Reed C, Taylor D, Stowers A, Cloonan N, Rzepczyk C, Smillie A, Anderson K, Pombo D, et al. 2000. Effect of vaccination with three recombinant asexual-stage malaria antigens on initial growth rates of *Plasmodium falciparum* in non-immune volunteers. *Vaccine* **18:** 1925–1931.

Le Roch KG, Zhou Y, Blair PL, Grainger M, Moch JK, Haynes JD, De La Vega P, Holder AA, Batalov S, Carucci DJ, et al. 2003. Discovery of gene function by expression profiling of the malaria parasite life cycle. *Science* **301:** 1503–1508.

Lindsey B, Kampmann B, Jones C. 2013. Maternal immunization as a strategy to decrease susceptibility to infection in newborn infants. *Curr Opin Infect Dis* **26:** 248–253.

McCarthy VC, Clyde DF. 1977. *Plasmodium vivax*: Correlation of circumsporozoite precipitation (CSP) reaction with sporozoite-induced protective immunity in man. *Exp Parasitol* **41:** 167–171.

McRobert L, Preiser P, Sharp S, Jarra W, Kaviratne M, Taylor MC, Renia L, Sutherland CJ. 2004. Distinct trafficking and localization of STEVOR proteins in three stages of the *Plasmodium falciparum* life cycle. *Infect Immun* **72:** 6597–6602.

* Meibalan E, Marti M. 2016. Biology of malaria transmission. *Cold Spring Harb Perspect Med* doi: 10.1101/cshperspect.a025452.

Meis JF, Verhave JP, Jap PH, Meuwissen JH. 1983. An ultrastructural study on the role of Kupffer cells in the process of infection by *Plasmodium berghei* sporozoites in rats. *Parasitology* **86:** 231–242.

Miura K, Deng B, Tullo G, Diouf A, Moretz SE, Locke E, Morin M, Fay MP, Long CA. 2013. Qualification of standard membrane-feeding assay with *Plasmodium falciparum* malaria and potential improvements for future assays. *PLoS ONE* **8:** e57909.

Mnzava AP, Knox TB, Temu EA, Trett A, Fornadel C, Hemingway J, Renshaw M. 2015. Implementation of the global plan for insecticide resistance management in malaria vectors: Progress, challenges and the way forward. *Malaria J* **14:** 173.

Nahrendorf W, Spence PJ, Tumwine I, Levy P, Jarra W, Sauerwein RW, Langhorne J. 2015. Blood-stage immunity to *Plasmodium chabaudi* malaria following chemoprophylaxis and sporozoite immunization. *eLife* **4:** e05165.

Nikolaeva D, Draper SJ, Biswas S. 2015. Toward the development of effective transmission-blocking vaccines for malaria. *Exp Rev Vaccines* **14:** 653–680.

Nunes JK, Woods C, Carter T, Raphael T, Morin MJ, Diallo D, Leboulleux D, Jain S, Loucq C, Kaslow DC, et al. 2014. Development of a transmission-blocking malaria vaccine: Progress, challenges, and the path forward. *Vaccine* **32:** 5531–5539.

Nussenzweig RS, Vanderberg J, Most H, Orton C. 1967. Protective immunity produced by the injection of X-ir-

radiated sporozoites of *plasmodium berghei*. *Nature* **216:** 160–162.

Osier FH, Mackinnon MJ, Crosnier C, Fegan G, Kamuyu G, Wanaguru M, Ogada E, McDade B, Rayner JC, Wright GJ, et al. 2014. New antigens for a multicomponent blood-stage malaria vaccine. *Sci Transl Med* **6:** p247ra102.

Palacpac NM, Ntege E, Yeka A, Balikagala B, Suzuki N, Shirai H, Yagi M, Ito K, Fukushima W, Hirota Y, et al. 2013. Phase 1b randomized trial and follow-up study in Uganda of the blood-stage malaria vaccine candidate BK-SE36. *PLoS ONE* **8:** e64073.

Payne RO, Milne KH, Elias SC, Edwards NJ, Douglas AD, Brown RE, Silk SE, Biswas S, Miura K, Roberts R, et al. 2016. Demonstration of the blood-stage controlled human malaria infection model to assess efficacy of the *Plasmodium falciparum* AMA1 vaccine FMP2.1/AS01. *J Infect Dis* **213:** 1743–1751.

Pombo DJ, Lawrence G, Hirunpetcharat C, Rzepczyk C, Bryden M, Cloonan N, Anderson K, Mahakunkijcharoen Y, Martin LB, Wilson D, et al. 2002. Immunity to malaria after administration of ultra-low doses of red cells infected with *Plasmodium falciparum*. *Lancet* **360:** 610–617.

Radtke AJ, Kastenmuller W, Espinosa DA, Gerner MY, Tse SW, Sinnis P, Germain RN, Zavala FP, Cockburn IA. 2015. Lymph-node resident CD8α^+ dendritic cells capture antigens from migratory malaria sporozoites and induce CD8$^+$ T cell responses. *PLoS Pathog* **11:** e1004637.

Raj DK, Nixon CP, Nixon CE, Dvorin JD, DiPetrillo CG, Pond-Tor S, Wu HW, Jolly G, Pischel L, Lu A, et al. 2014. Antibodies to PfSEA-1 block parasite egress from RBCs and protect against malaria infection. *Science* **344:** 871–877.

Reiner RC Jr, Guerra C, Donnelly MJ, Bousema T, Drakeley C, Smith DL. 2015. Estimating malaria transmission from humans to mosquitoes in a noisy landscape. *J R Soc Interface* **12:** 20150478.

Richards JS, Arumugam TU, Reiling L, Healer J, Hodder AN, Fowkes FJ, Cross N, Langer C, Takeo S, Uboldi AD, et al. 2013. Identification and prioritization of merozoite antigens as targets of protective human immunity to *Plasmodium falciparum* malaria for vaccine and biomarker development. *J Immunol* **191:** 795–809.

Richie TL, Billingsley PF, Sim BK, James ER, Chakravarty S, Epstein JE, Lyke KE, Mordmuller B, Alonso P, Duffy PE, et al. 2015. Progress with *Plasmodium falciparum* sporozoite (PfSPZ)-based malaria vaccines. *Vaccine* **33:** 7452–7461.

Rieckmann KH, Beaudoin RL, Cassells JS, Sell KW. 1979. Use of attenuated sporozoites in the immunization of human volunteers against falciparum malaria. *Bull World Health Organ* **57:** 261–265.

Rodriguez Mdel C, Martinez-Barnetche J, Alvarado-Delgado A, Batista C, Argotte-Ramos RS, Hernandez-Martinez S, Gonzalez Ceron L, Torres JA, Margos G, Rodriguez MH. 2007. The surface protein Pvs25 of *Plasmodium vivax* ookinetes interacts with calreticulin on the midgut apical surface of the malaria vector *Anopheles albimanus*. *Mol Biochem Parasitol* **153:** 167–177.

Roestenberg M, McCall M, Hopman J, Wiersma J, Luty AJ, van Gemert GJ, van de Vegte-Bolmer M, van Schaijk B,

Teelen K, Arens T, et al. 2009. Protection against a malaria challenge by sporozoite inoculation. *N Engl J Med* **361:** 468–477.

Roestenberg M, de Vlas SJ, Nieman AE, Sauerwein RW, Hermsen CC. 2012. Efficacy of preerythrocytic and blood-stage malaria vaccines can be assessed in small sporozoite challenge trials in human volunteers. *J Infect Dis* **206:** 319–323.

Sabchaeron A, Burnouf T, Ouattara D, Attanath P, Bouharoun-Tayoun H, Chantavanich P, Foucault C, Chongsuphajaisiddhi T, Druilhe P. 1991. Parasitologic and clinical human response to immunoglobulin administration in falciparum malaria. *Am J Trop Med Hyg* **45:** 297–308.

Saeed M, Roeffen W, Alexander N, Drakeley CJ, Targett GA, Sutherland CJ. 2008. *Plasmodium falciparum* antigens on the surface of the gametocyte-infected erythrocyte. *PLoS ONE* **3:** e2280.

Sauerwein RW, Bousema T. 2015. Transmission blocking malaria vaccines: Assays and candidates in clinical development. *Vaccine* **33:** 7476–7482.

Sauerwein RW, Roestenberg M, Moorthy VS. 2011. Experimental human challenge infections can accelerate clinical malaria vaccine development. *Nat Rev Immunol* **11:** 57–64.

Schats R, Bijker EM, van Gemert GJ, Graumans W, van de Vegte-Bolmer M, van Lieshout L, Haks MC, Hermsen CC, Scholzen A, Visser LG, et al. 2015. Heterologous protection against malaria after immunization with *Plasmodium falciparum* sporozoites. *PLoS ONE* **10:** e0124243.

Seder RA, Chang LJ, Enama ME, Zephir KL, Sarwar UN, Gordon IJ, Holman LA, James ER, Billingsley PF, Gunasekera A, et al. 2013. Protection against malaria by intravenous immunization with a nonreplicating sporozoite vaccine. *Science* **341:** 1359–1365.

Sharp S, Lavstsen T, Fivelman QL, Saeed M, McRobert L, Templeton TJ, Jensen AT, Baker DA, Theander TG, Sutherland CJ. 2006. Programmed transcription of the *var* gene family, but not of *stevor*, in *Plasmodium falciparum* gametocytes. *Eukaryot Cell* **5:** 1206–1214.

Sheehy SH, Duncan CJ, Elias SC, Choudhary P, Biswas S, Halstead FD, Collins KA, Edwards NJ, Douglas AD, Anagnostou NA, et al. 2012. ChAd63-MVA-vectored blood-stage malaria vaccines targeting MSP1 and AMA1: Assessment of efficacy against mosquito bite challenge in humans. *Mol Ther* **20:** 2355–2368.

Sibley LD. 2011. Invasion and intracellular survival by protozoan parasites. *Immunol Rev* **240:** 72–91.

Silvestrini F, Bozdech Z, Lanfrancotti A, Di Giulio E, Bultrini E, Picci L, Derisi JL, Pizzi E, Alano P. 2005. Genome-wide identification of genes upregulated at the onset of gametocytogenesis in *Plasmodium falciparum*. *Mol Biochem Parasitol* **143:** 100–110.

Silvie O, Rubinstein E, Franetich JF, Prenant M, Belnoue E, Renia L, Hannoun L, Eling W, Levy S, Boucheix C, et al. 2003. Hepatocyte CD81 is required for *Plasmodium falciparum* and *Plasmodium yoelii* sporozoite infectivity. *Nat Med* **9:** 93–96.

Sinden RE. 2010. A biologist's perspective on malaria vaccine development. *Hum Vaccin* **6:** 3–11.

Sinnis P, Zavala F. 2012. The skin: Where malaria infection and the host immune response begin. *Semin Immunopathol* **34:** 787–792.

Sirima SB, Cousens S, Druilhe P. 2011. Protection against malaria by MSP3 candidate vaccine. *N Engl J Med* **365:** 1062–1064.

Smith DL, Drakeley CJ, Chiyaka C, Hay SI. 2010. A quantitative analysis of transmission efficiency versus intensity for malaria. *Nat Commun* **1:** 108.

Spring MD, Cummings JF, Ockenhouse CF, Dutta S, Reidler R, Angov E, Bergmann-Leitner E, Stewart VA, Bittner S, Juompan L, et al. 2009. Phase 1/2a study of the malaria vaccine candidate apical membrane antigen-1 (AMA-1) administered in adjuvant system AS01B or AS02A. *PLoS ONE* **4:** e5254.

Stoute JA, Slaoui M, Heppner DG, Momin P, Kester KE, Desmons P, Wellde BT, Garcon N, Krzych U, Marchand M, et al. 1997. A preliminary evaluation of a recombinant circumsporozoite protein vaccine against *Plasmodium falciparum*. *N Engl J Med* **336:** 86–91.

Tarun AS, Peng X, Dumpit RF, Ogata Y, Silva-Rivera H, Camargo N, Daly TM, Bergman LW, Kappe SH. 2008. A combined transcriptome and proteome survey of malaria parasite liver stages. *Proc Natl Acad Sci* **105:** 305–310.

Tavares J, Formaglio P, Thiberge S, Mordelet E, Van Rooijen N, Medvinsky A, Menard R, Amino R. 2013. Role of host cell traversal by the malaria sporozoite during liver infection. *J Exp Med* **210:** 905–915.

Tran TM, Ongoiba A, Coursen J, Crosnier C, Diouf A, Huang CY, Li S, Doumbo S, Doumtabe D, Kone Y, et al. 2014. Naturally acquired antibodies specific for *Plasmodium falciparum* reticulocyte-binding protein homologue 5 inhibit parasite growth and predict protection from malaria. *J Infect Dis* **209:** 789–798.

Tsai YL, Hayward RE, Langer RC, Fidock DA, Vinetz JM. 2001. Disruption of *Plasmodium falciparum* chitinase markedly impairs parasite invasion of mosquito midgut. *Infect Immun* **69:** 4048–4054.

Tusting LS, Bousema T, Smith DL, Drakeley C. 2014. Measuring changes in *Plasmodium falciparum* transmission: Precision, accuracy and costs of metrics. *Adv Parasitol* **84:** 151–208.

Usynin I, Klotz C, Frevert U. 2007. Malaria circumsporozoite protein inhibits the respiratory burst in Kupffer cells. *Cell Microbiol* **9:** 2610–2628.

Vanderberg JP, Stewart MJ. 1990. *Plasmodium* sporozoite-host cell interactions during sporozoite invasion. *Bull World Health Organ* **68:** 74–79.

Vaughan AM, Wang R, Kappe SH. 2010. Genetically engineered, attenuated whole-cell vaccine approaches for malaria. *Hum Vaccin* **6:** 107–113.

Vega-Rodriguez J, Ghosh AK, Kanzok SM, Dinglasan RR, Wang S, Bongio NJ, Kalume DE, Miura K, Long CA, Pandey A, et al. 2014. Multiple pathways for *Plasmodium* ookinete invasion of the mosquito midgut. *Proc Natl Acad Sci* **111:** E492–E500.

White NJ. 2014. Malaria: A molecular marker of artemisinin resistance. *Lancet* **383:** 1439–1440.

White LJ, Maude RJ, Pongtavornpinyo W, Saralamba S, Aguas R, Van Effelterre T, Day NP, White NJ. 2009. The role of simple mathematical models in malaria elimination strategy design. *Malaria J* **8:** 212.

White MT, Verity R, Churcher TS, Ghani AC. 2015. Vaccine approaches to malaria control and elimination: Insights from mathematical models. *Vaccine* **33:** 7544–7550.

Widmann JJ, Cotran RS, Fahimi HD. 1972. Mononuclear phagocytes (Kupffer cells) and endothelial cells. Identification of two functional cell types in rat liver sinusoids by endogenous peroxidase activity. *J Cell Biol* **52:** 159–170.

Wright KE, Hjerrild KA, Bartlett J, Douglas AD, Jin J, Brown RE, Illingworth JJ, Ashfield R, Clemmensen SB, de Jongh WA, et al. 2014. Structure of malaria invasion protein RH5 with erythrocyte basigin and blocking antibodies. *Nature* **515:** 427–430.

Xu X, Dong Y, Abraham EG, Kocan A, Srinivasan P, Ghosh AK, Sinden RE, Ribeiro JM, Jacobs-Lorena M, Kafatos FC, et al. 2005. Transcriptome analysis of *Anopheles stephensi*–*Plasmodium berghei* interactions. *Mol Biochem Parasitol* **142:** 76–87.

Young JA, Fivelman QL, Blair PL, de la Vega P, Le Roch KG, Zhou Y, Carucci DJ, Baker DA, Winzeler EA. 2005. The *Plasmodium falciparum* sexual development transcriptome: A microarray analysis using ontology-based pattern identification. *Mol Biochem Parasitol* **143:** 67–79.

Malaria Modeling in the Era of Eradication

Thomas A. Smith, Nakul Chitnis, Melissa Penny, and Marcel Tanner

Department of Epidemiology and Public Health, Swiss Tropical and Public Health Institute, Basel CH 4002, Switzerland; and University of Basel, Basel CH 4001, Switzerland

Correspondence: thomas-a.smith@unibas.ch

Mathematical models provide the essential basis of rational research and development strategies in malaria, informing the choice of which technologies to target, which deployment strategies to consider, and which populations to focus on. The Internet and remote sensing technologies also enable assembly of ever more relevant field data. Together with supercomputing technology, this has made available timely descriptions of the geography of malaria transmission and disease across the world and made it possible for policy and planning to be informed by detailed simulations of the potential impact of intervention programs. These information technology advances do not replace the basic understanding of the dynamics of malaria transmission that should be embedded in the thinking of anyone planning malaria interventions. The appropriate use of modeling may determine whether we are living in an era of hubris or indeed in an age of eradication.

The quantitative understanding of malaria dynamics that is essential for rational planning of intervention programs needs to be supported by mathematical models. These models must address considerably more challenges and factors than is generally the case for directly transmitted pathogens or for noncommunicable diseases. The malaria life cycle is complicated, as are host immune responses to the parasite and the consequent pathogenesis. The diversity of *Anopheles* vectors, with their own complex life cycles and distinct ecologies also complicate malaria dynamics, resulting in an enormous variety of situations and of potential intervention strategies. Evaluating all of these empirically in field trials is simply impossible, especially because effects can occur over long timescales. Malaria is, thus, an archetypical example of a complex system, in which mathematical modeling is needed for studying the magnitude of effects of different components and for explaining their interactions and for making predictions about their behavior and how this depends on multiple drivers.

The need for mathematical models that simultaneously consider the effects of these different factors was recognized by Ross (1911), not long after he elucidated the transmission cycle, making malaria one of the first infectious diseases to be analyzed mathematically. Ross showed that attacking the *Anopheles* mosquito could be effective in controlling malaria but that it was not necessary to completely eliminate the vector to eliminate the infection: This motivated substantial efforts in larval control in the early 20th century. The development of indoor residual spraying (IRS) using DDT in the mid-20th century as mainstream of the World Health

Organization (WHO) Global Malaria Eradication Program (GMEP) stimulated further development of mathematical models of malaria interventions, mainly led by George Macdonald (1956). The central insight of these models is that, despite the complexity of malaria transmission, many of the factors affecting it can be quantified in a single equation for R_0, the basic reproductive number (Fig. 1). This measures how many infectious humans could be expected to arise from a single infectious human, assuming all other humans and mosquitoes are susceptible. Using this equation, it is straightforward to compare impact of intervention at different stages of the malaria cycle and show that, assuming all other things being equal, killing adult female mosquitoes has a much greater transmission effect than an equivalent attack on any other stage in the life cycle of the parasite or vector considered in the model (Fig. 1). IRS with DDT provided an effective way of achieving exactly that, and armies of malaria workers were trained to implement what was perceived of as a one-size-fits-all campaign with well-defined activities and timelines (Pampana 1963). Although these efforts were successful in many parts of the world, they did not lead to interruption of transmission in every setting. A lesson of this was that malaria control and elimination require additional interventions, especially in Africa, where transmission is most intense.

BEYOND ROSS–MACDONALD

Much malaria modeling has been built on the Ross–Macdonald model (Smith et al. 2014) but the key insight remains valid: The most traction will generally be achieved in reducing transmission by targeting the adult female vector. This is borne out by the tremendous success of scale-up of insecticide-treated nets (ITNs) in reducing transmission across Africa in the last decade (Bhatt et al. 2015). In general, interventions that target malaria in humans need to achieve very high efficacy, coverage, and long duration if they are to be comparable with vector control in their impacts on transmission. So far, we do not have any such interventions.

At the same time, the basic Ross–Macdonald framework does not consider all elements even of the life cycle of the *Anopheles* mosquito or how best to reduce adult mosquito survival. The R_0 concept, elegant in its simplicity, is more complicated when heterogeneities in space and time (e.g., seasonality) need to be considered (Diekmann et al. 1990; Heffernan et al. 2005), and the aspects of malaria dynamics considered by Macdonald are only a subset of those that need modeling. Although computer technology continually increases the computational possibilities, modeling malaria in a complex, dynamic, rapidly changing world finds ever more challenges. Some of them are discussed below.

Surveillance Response

The models available did not address all the challenges of malaria programs recognized in the mid-20th century. In general, the impact on transmission of a malaria intervention program is maximal shortly after scale-up (Smith and Schapira 2012), so IRS programs were originally intended to be time-limited to achieve very rapid interruption of transmission (Pampana 1963; Macdonald and Göckel 1964). Once malaria transmission is very low or has been interrupted, an effective surveillance system is essential, and if significant residual vectorial capacity remains then the surveillance must have a reactive component consisting of well-tailored (to a given epidemiological setting) and validated integrated response packages that is effective in preventing transmission from imported cases. This can be very expensive and difficult to operate in tropical areas. Just as with transmission reduction, models are needed to identify the critical elements of surveillance-response approaches. This remains an underdeveloped area of modeling.

Temporal Dynamics

The timelines for elimination programs established for in the mid-20th century (Macdonald and Göckel 1964) no longer seem realistic. This is partly a consequence of the fact that recent intervention programs generally do not achieve maximal coverage at the start, and transmission-

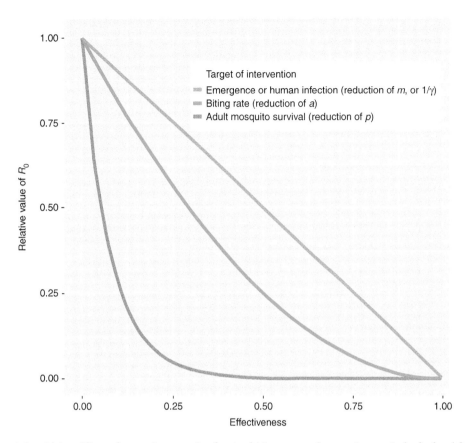

Figure 1. Sensitivity of R_0 to changes in mosquito density, biting rate, and mosquito survival calculated for the Ross–Macdonald model (based on Koella 1991). Macdonald's formula for R_0 is

$$R_0 = \frac{ma^2 \, bc \, p^\tau}{-\gamma \log(p)},$$

where the different parameters are m = the number of female mosquitoes per human host, a = the number of bites per mosquito per day, b = the probability of transmitting infection from an infectious mosquito to a human (per bite), c = the probability of transmission of infection from an infectious human to a mosquito (per bite), γ = rate of recovery of humans from infectiousness (equivalently, $1/\gamma$, duration of human infectiousness), p = the daily survival of adult mosquitoes, and τ = the period required for development of sporozoites from infection of the mosquito. Changes in parameter values are represented as the efficacy of shown factors relating to the original setting (e.g., an efficacy of 50% corresponds to a multiplication of m, or $1/\gamma$ by 0.5; m or $1/\gamma$ enter the equation for the basic reproductive number linearly); therefore, this efficacy corresponds to a 50% decrease in reproductive number. Biting rate, a, enters the reproductive number quadratically, so that an efficacy of 50% in reducing this leads to reduction in R_0 to $0.5^2 = 0.25$ times its original value. Efficacy in adulticiding of 50% corresponds to a 50% reduction in survival per unit time. This enters the formula for R_0 as a power function so decreases in this lead to the largest changes in R_0.

reducing interventions are consequently applied for long periods. The reasons are many: R_0 for *Plasmodium falciparum* can be extremely high (Smith et al. 2007), characteristics of the mosquitoes (such as exophily) limiting the effective-

ness of vector control measures; the populations needing coverage may be large, and therefore likely to encompass heterogeneities in transmission and in the health system leading to potentially reduced impact of interventions; and more gradual scale-up of impact is likely to be achieved with ITNs as the main transmission-reducing intervention rather than IRS. As malaria transmission is brought down, it is essential for the control and elimination program to reorient mainly toward intensified surveillance-response approaches as immunity in the population is gradually reduced.

Understanding of the temporal dynamics induced by long-term programs and optimizing decision rules for program adjustments require consideration of the time dimension of the different interventions. This depends on the technical characteristics of the intervention, on the induced effects on natural immunity, and on external drivers of seasonal and interannual variations in malaria transmission such as rainfall and temperature. Population models of malaria incorporating natural immunity are thus needed to predict these dynamics. There is a substantial mathematical literature on malaria immunity based around susceptible–exposed–infectious–recovered dynamics (Ngwa and Shu 2000; Mandal et al. 2011; Reiner et al. 2013), but these fail to capture fundamental aspects of what is known about superinfection in both *P. falciparum* and *Plasmodium vivax*. Other relatively simple compartment models (Dietz et al. 1974; Anderson and May 1991; Gupta and Day 1994) also failed to capture key aspects of malaria immunity, leading more recently to the use of a new generation of relatively complex compartment models and microsimulations (see below) (Smith et al. 2006, 2012; Griffin et al. 2010; Eckhoff 2011).

Spatial Variation and Movement

Because underlying transmission potential is everywhere highly heterogeneous and programs rarely achieve synchronous scale-up of vector control, transmission persists in pockets or foci. This reduces the impact of untargeted interventions but makes them more effective if they can target highly exposed hosts (Woolhouse et al. 1997). There is a substantial literature on extensions of models of vector-borne disease to take into account transmission heterogeneity following on from key publications

three decades ago (Dye and Hasibeder 1986). Heterogeneity in transmission potential is, however, not the only kind of heterogeneity needing to be considered in models of public health outcomes of malaria interventions (Ross and Smith 2010). It is particularly important to consider all such heterogeneities in predicting the outcome of programs that aim to eliminate the infection. Models of average outcomes (such as, e.g., Tatem et al. 2010) generally provide optimistic predictions because it is the challenging foci, not the average, that determine whether the infection is eliminated.

Other models consider the impact of movements of both humans and vector populations. These models have ranged from general theoretical models that have been used to show that human movement can lead to persistence of malaria where it would not have otherwise persisted (Cosner et al. 2009) to more detailed models that can provide estimates of numbers of imported cases in particular locations (Tatem et al. 2009; Le Menach et al. 2011) or help to plan spatial targeting of vector control interventions (Lutambi et al. 2013).

Stochasticity

Until the last decade, most widely used mathematical models for malaria transmission, including Macdonald's formulation and later models incorporating immunity (Dietz et al. 1974), have been deterministic continuous state models that consider average status in an undefined size of population. Such models cannot capture chance or stochastic phenomena that are particularly important when transmission rates are low. In particular, a deterministic system can achieve a stable state with very low transmission, although a stochastic simulation (or the real world) will sooner or later achieve extinction if average transmission is very low, irrespective of the estimated basic reproduction number.

Population size is critical for stochastic loss but has so far not been adequately addressed in malaria modeling. Even stochastic implementations of models that allow unlimited superinfection, such as those of Smith et al. (2006) and

Walker et al. (2015), cannot capture what happens in small foci. When parasite populations are small, a large proportion of inoculations represent recurrent exposure to the same parasite genotypes, and malaria therapy data show that this is less likely to result in infection than is inoculation with heterologous parasites (Molineaux et al. 2002; Collins et al. 2004). Because reduction of transmission leads to progressive fragmentation of parasite (or vector) populations into discrete foci, this in turn will lead to collapse of local genetic diversity. This is likely to be a key stage in interrupting transmission, but modeling of this is still poorly developed. We have, for instance, no good estimates of the minimum population size for endemic malaria (either *P. falciparum* or *P. vivax*).

Within-Host Dynamics

Just as there are variations in the vulnerability of the parasite at different stages in the transmission cycle between the mosquito vector and the human, there are also variations between stages within the human and within the mosquito in suitability as intervention targets. One driver of this is the enormous variation in biomass between different parasite stages (Sinden et al. 2007), which provides an indication of which stages might be most vulnerable within the host, because they represent a bottleneck in the parasite life cycle. This is potentially key information for choice of drug and vaccine targets. To understand how this translates into potential impacts of interventions needs models of the various density-dependent regulation processes, including the effects of the immune system (e.g., the within-host model of Molineaux et al. 2001).

New Interventions

The new era initiated by the 2007 Gates Malaria Forum (Roberts and Enserink 2007) is not just a time of appeals for disease eradication, it is also a time of technological change at an unprecedented rate. There is consensus that eradication is impossible without a new generation of tools and strategies (Alonso et al. 2011), therefore, at present, the only rational global eradication strategy is to focus on identifying and developing the transformative technologies that are needed. Some of these technologies will be improved versions of existing interventions, such as ITNs, drugs, and insecticides. Others will be novel deployment strategies, tools for more efficient dissemination of information (such as mHealth tools), and ways of integrating these such as new strategies for surveillance response.

Modeling should be an essential component of establishing target product profiles (TPPs) for vaccine, drugs, and diagnostics in the research and development process aiming at malaria elimination and eradication. Before product developers lock themselves into inappropriate development pathways, models need to be applied to address the questions of which deployment strategies to consider and how interventions, including both new and established ones, might best be combined with each other in integrated packages. Models should be used to evaluate the potential of deployment strategies before deciding whether to embark on full-scale field trials. For instance, modeling of vaccine combinations suggests that duration of protection, the choice of target group, the timing, and the deployment strategy are as important as antigen selection. Multiple components targeting the same parasite stage are likely to have more impact than multistage vaccines if they can achieve higher efficacy and longer duration of protection, and this needs to be considered in trial design. Transmission reduction could theoretically be achieved with vaccines targeting any parasite stage, but to substantially reduce transmission or achieve elimination they will need to reach very large proportions of the population (Penny et al. 2008). Vaccines with profiles similar to the recently evaluated RTS,S might be an important component of intervention packages designed for elimination in low-transmission settings if deployed across a wide age range.

Mosquito Ecology

Because of the importance of killing adult mosquitoes indicated by Macdonald's analysis, novel vector control interventions represent a particularly promising avenue, but there is an implicit assumption in Macdonald's analysis that the emergence of the next generation of mosquitoes will not be affected by adulticiding interventions. Different models are thus needed in planning interventions that hope to eliminate the mosquitoes. Such technologies are urgently needed because elimination of malaria from much of the world will require technologies that target outdoor biting and resting mosquitoes that are refractory to ITNs and IRS. These include models of larval competition (White et al. 2011; Smith et al. 2013) and of the systems needed to drive through the population interventions based on genetically modified mosquitoes (Boete and Koella 2002) or entomopathogens (Hancock et al. 2008) and of various kinds of insecticidal baits (Okumu et al. 2010).

Resistance and Evolutionary Models

A basic principle in evolutionary ecology is that interventions against an organism will increase the frequency of genetic variants that evade them. This applies to all malaria interventions, most obviously (but not exclusively) leading to drug (Escalante et al. 2009) and insecticide resistance. The best strategies for managing this are not always obvious (Hastings 2010). Evolutionary changes to evade interventions are not always harmful, and evolutionary models can help identify interventions that may push the evolution of vectors or parasites in directions that make them less harmful. For instance, by increasing the relative fitness of high fecundity, short lifespan mosquitoes (Ferguson et al. 2012) and increasing the relative fitness of zoophilic vectors, ITNs may select not only insecticide-resistant mosquitoes but also ones that are less competent malaria vectors. However, some studies have also shown that resistance to insecticide in mosquitoes could increase their susceptibility to *Plasmodium* infection (Ndiath et al. 2014) and further increase malaria transmission. Well-calibrated population genetics models of the evolution of resistance of both parasites (to drugs) and mosquitoes (to insecticides) are needed that can capture both

the drivers of the evolution of resistance and its impact on malaria transmission.

Prediction and Microsimulation Models

At the same time as modeling new interventions, there is a need to reduce disease burden as efficiently as possible using existing tools. This requires guidance on the likely impact in particular places of integrated programs consisting of an array of specific intervention deployments. Global resources allocated for malaria programs remain far below what is required to achieve universal coverage of all recommended interventions (WHO 2015b), making it essential to carry out economic evaluations for optimizing budget allocations, as well as epidemiological ones. Economic evaluations of health interventions have generally used rather simple static models of disease dynamics, but the recognition that the dynamic processes of feedback effects can radically modify cost-effectiveness has motivated linking of costing data with quantitative results from dynamic models of epidemiology. Economic evaluation of improvements in case management and in health systems in general remains a challenge.

At the policy level, modeling is again seen as a necessary step in the rollout of a new intervention strategy. This has motivated the development of complex simulation models that aim to capture as many factors as possible that might influence quantitative outcomes of intervention programs (Smith et al. 2006, 2012; Griffin et al. 2010; Eckhoff 2011). The recent publication of results from the Phase III trial of the RTS,S vaccine (RTS,S Clinical Trials Partnership 2015) has been accompanied by a major exercise to apply a multimodel ensemble to predict the impact of specific intervention strategies (Penny et al. 2015b). This provided an unprecedented opportunity to evaluate the degree of consensus among simulation models. Despite differences in assumptions and model structures the models included are in broad agreement on the strategies and settings in which RTS,S would have the greatest public health impact and cost-effectiveness and hence on recommendations on use of the vaccine.

Cite this article as *Cold Spring Harb Perspect Med* doi: 10.1101/cshperspect.a025460

Quantitative predictions of impact and cost-effectiveness make it possible to compare both between malaria interventions and with comparable interventions against other diseases. For instance, RTS,S is predicted to be relatively cost-effective compared with vaccines against other diseases, but may not be the most cost-effective way to reduce malaria burden. However, different interventions may be synergistic: RTS,S may be best used to reduce childhood malaria burden when implemented with existing high coverage of ITNs.

GEOGRAPHICAL SPECIFICITY

High-resolution open-access geographical databases of relevant data on human population distribution (Tatem et al. 2012), human and pathogen movement (Tatem 2014), and remote-sensed risk factors are becoming much more available (Bhatt et al. 2015). The malaria community now has particularly rich databases of geolocated parasitological survey data (Gething et al. 2011), which make it possible to use largely empirical sources to estimate disease burden. Mathematical models are still needed for assessing the feasibility of an elimination in a given setting as well as for projections of how interventions and specific intervention mixes will impact public health in the future. Finally, appropriate combination of mathematical and statistical approaches are providing a continually improving understand of how patterns of malaria and of interventions evolved in the recent past (Bhatt et al. 2015).

The availability of massive amounts of geolocation data means that modeling of the likely impacts of specific intervention programs (like RTS,S vaccination) in specific places and times has become feasible (Penny et al. 2015a), and these profuse data are available for calibration and validation of models. This sets a high bar for malaria modeling: Fitting complex models to multiple types of data is challenging, and model predictions are always likely to be unreliable at very high spatial resolution. The twin objectives of understanding the dynamics and making quantitative predictions can also be in conflict, because the push to include all relevant factors in a locally calibrated predictive model rapidly leads to complex behavior that can no longer be explained.

FUTURE PERSPECTIVES

The volume of data from remote sensing, available for parameterizing models of malaria in specific areas, will no doubt continue to grow massively. Electronic communications and data capture mean that disease surveillance systems will soon be accessing close to real-time data in cyberspace, enabling such models to propose optimized intervention responses tailored to particular places, at the appropriate level of spatial and temporal disaggregation.

If malaria is to be eradicated, modeling will need to contribute much more than datamining applications. Computers will not circumvent the need for humans to apply an understanding of the dynamics of malaria in considering which novel interventions to develop, in product development, and in designing and costing rational surveillance and intervention plans within national and regional strategies.

CONCLUDING REMARKS

Models are invaluable to support understanding of the impacts of interventions on malaria dynamics and represent a cornerstone for the implementation of the global technical strategy (WHO 2015a) at the global and national level. Some of these models can be built on the Ross–Macdonald framework. Just as an understanding of aerodynamics was needed by the astronauts who flew to the moon, the planners of malaria eradication need to understand these basic dynamics. However, rocket science based on physical laws is simple compared with disease eradication in complex biological systems. Multifarious phenomena need to be considered in malaria models.

All too often, models are seen as black boxes, and a considerable effort is required to understand them. Mathematical modeling is barely regulated, unlike most of the activities in pharmaceutical development and clinical trials, and the onus is on the modelers to communicate the basic structure of their models and how they are fitted to data and validated and at the same time be clear about where there is consensus and where there are major uncertainties in their predictions. Sensitivity analyses and analysis of uncertainty and understanding its implications are essential components of any responsible prediction exercise. Modeling of the RTS,S vaccine represents one example in which there has been considerable attention to critical evaluation and validation of models, including documentation, quality control, and comprehensive review. Evaluation of the structural uncertainties in model predictions via multimodel ensembles (Smith et al. 2012; Cameron et al. 2015) or assessment of the consequences of uncertainties in parameter values are generally much more time-consuming and challenging than the modeling itself. It is especially difficult to convey this message to decision-makers who struggle to know what to do about uncertainty. So, to paraphrase the much-abused words of George Box, it is challenging for a nonspecialist to distinguish modeling that is useful from poor-quality modeling that may support misguided policies.

The science of complex systems, not least, systems biology, warns us that there are limits to the predictability of the events we are interested in. Elimination and eradication are extreme events, and extreme events are the most difficult to reliably predict. All those planning intervention strategies and making policy need not only heed projections of mostly likely or preferred scenarios but also understand that they are embarking on a road that is not, and cannot be, mapped out with a great deal of confidence and to be prepared if the best predictions of the route prove either greatly optimistic or unduly pessimistic.

Not all the unknowns make eradication harder. We also live in an era of mass extinction: another process full of uncertainties. Eradication is deliberate extinction, so models of ecological catastrophe hold lessons for disease eradication. The system of *P. falciparum* malaria transmitted by Afrotropical vectors is exquisitely adapted to the ecology of African subsistence agriculture, with people living in mud and thatch houses in intimate contact with an environment rich in *Anopheles* breeding sites. *P. vivax* also has a specific ecology, which facilitated its disappearance from the industrialized world. As the lifestyles supporting it disappear, both major species of human malaria may retreat from the rest of the world. Intelligent deployment of interventions could end the disease sooner.

ACKNOWLEDGMENTS

The authors have received support from the Bill and Melinda Gates Foundation, Grant OPP1032350, and acknowledge the contributions of their colleagues Katya Galactionova, Amanda Ross, Peter Pemberton-Ross, Diggory Hardy, Tobias Thüring, Flavia Camponovo, and Olivier Briet to the Swiss Tropical and Public Health (TPH) malaria-modeling program.

REFERENCES

Alonso PL, Brown G, Arevalo-Herrera M, Binka F, Chitnis C, Collins F, Doumbo OK, Greenwood B, Hall BF, Levine MM, et al. 2011. A research agenda to underpin malaria eradication. *PLoS Med* **8:** e1000406.

Anderson RM, May RM. 1991. *Infectious diseases of humans: Dynamics and control.* Oxford University Press, Oxford.

Bhatt S, Weiss DJ, Cameron E, Bisanzio D, Mappin B, Dalrymple U, Battle KE, Moyes CL, Henry A, Eckhoff PA, et al. 2015. The effect of malaria control on *Plasmodium falciparum* in Africa between 2000 and 2015. *Nature* **526:** 207–211.

Boete C, Koella JC. 2002. A theoretical approach to predicting the success of genetic manipulation of malaria mosquitoes in malaria control. *Malaria J* **1:** 3.

Cameron E, Battle KE, Bhatt S, Weiss DJ, Bisanzio D, Mappin B, Dalrymple U, Hay SI, Smith DL, Griffin JT, et al. 2015. Defining the relationship between infection prevalence and clinical incidence of *Plasmodium falciparum* malaria: An ensemble model. *Nat Commun* **6:** 8170.

Collins WE, Jeffery GM, Roberts JM. 2004. A retrospective examination of reinfection of humans with *Plasmodium vivax*. *Am J Trop Med Hyg* **70:** 642–644.

Cosner C, Beier JC, Cantrell RS, Impoinvil D, Kapitanski L, Potts MD, Troyo A, Ruan S. 2009. The effects of human movement on the persistence of vector-borne diseases. *J Theor Biol* **258:** 550–560.

Diekmann O, Heesterbeek JA, Metz JA. 1990. On the definition and the computation of the basic reproduction ratio R_0 in models for infectious diseases in heterogeneous populations. *J Math Biol* **28:** 365–382.

Dietz K, Molineaux L, Thomas A. 1974. A malaria model tested in the African savannah. *Bull World Health Org* **50:** 347–357.

Cite this article as *Cold Spring Harb Perspect Med* doi: 10.1101/cshperspect.a025460

Dye C, Hasibeder G. 1986. Population dynamics of mosquito-borne disease: Effects of flies which bite some people more frequently than others. *Trans R Soc Trop Med Hyg* **80:** 69–77.

Eckhoff PA. 2011. A malaria transmission-directed model of mosquito life cycle and ecology. *Malaria J* **10:** 303.

Escalante AA, Smith DL, Kim Y. 2009. The dynamics of mutations associated with anti-malarial drug resistance in *Plasmodium falciparum. Trends Parasitol* **25:** 557–563.

Ferguson HM, Maire N, Takken W, Lyimo IN, Briet O, Lindsay SW, Smith TA. 2012. Selection of mosquito life-histories: A hidden weapon against malaria? *Malaria J* **11:** 106.

Gething PW, Patil AP, Smith DL, Guerra CA, Elyazar IR, Johnston GL, Tatem AJ, Hay SI. 2011. A new world malaria map: *Plasmodium falciparum* endemicity in 2010. *Malaria J* **10:** 378.

Griffin JT, Hollingsworth TD, Okell LC, Churcher TS, White M, Hinsley W, Bousema T, Drakeley CJ, Ferguson NM, Basanez MG, et al. 2010. Reducing *Plasmodium falciparum* malaria transmission in Africa: A model-based evaluation of intervention strategies. *PLoS Med* **7:** e1000324.

Gupta S, Day KP. 1994. A theoretical framework for the immunoepidemiology of *Plasmodium falciparum* malaria. *Parasite Immunol* **16:** 361–370.

Hancock PA, Thomas MB, Godfray HC. 2008. An age-structured model to evaluate the potential of novel malaria-control interventions: A case study of fungal biopesticide sprays. *Proc Biol Sci* **276:** 71–80.

Hastings I. 2010. How artemisinin-containing combination therapies slow the spread of antimalarial drug resistance. *Trends Parasitol* **27:** 67–72.

Heffernan JM, Smith RJ, Wahl LM. 2005. Perspectives on the basic reproductive ratio. *J R Soc Interface* **2:** 281–293.

Koella JC. 1991. On the use of mathematical models of malaria transmission. *Acta Trop* **49:** 1–25.

Le Menach A, Tatem AJ, Cohen JM, Hay SI, Randell H, Patil AP, Smith DL. 2011. Travel risk, malaria importation and malaria transmission in Zanzibar. *Sci Rep* **1:** 93.

Lutambi AM, Penny MA, Smith T, Chitnis N. 2013. Mathematical modelling of mosquito dispersal in a heterogeneous environment. *Math Biosci* **241:** 198–216.

Macdonald G. 1956. Theory of the eradication of malaria. *Bull World Health Organ* **15:** 369–387.

Macdonald G, Göckel GW. 1964. The malaria parasite rate and interruption of transmission. *Bull World Health Organ* **31:** 365–377.

Mandal S, Sarkar RR, Sinha S. 2011. Mathematical models of malaria—A review. *Malaria J* **10:** 202.

Molineaux L, Diebner HH, Eichner M, Collins WE, Jeffery GM, Dietz K. 2001. *Plasmodium falciparum* parasitaemia described by a new mathematical model. *Parasitology* **122:** 379–391.

Molineaux L, Trauble M, Collins WE, Jeffery GM, Dietz K. 2002. Malaria therapy reinoculation data suggest individual variation of an innate immune response and independent acquisition of antiparasitic and antitoxic immunities. *Trans R Soc Trop Med Hyg* **96:** 205–209.

Ndiath MO, Cailleau A, Diedhiou SM, Gaye A, Boudin C, Richard V, Trape JF. 2014. Effects of the *kdr* resistance mutation on the susceptibility of wild *Anopheles gambiae* populations to *Plasmodium falciparum*: A hindrance for vector control. *Malaria J* **13:** 340.

Ngwa GA, Shu WS. 2000. A mathematical model for endemic malaria with variable human and mosquito populations. *Math Comput Model* **32:** 747–763.

Okumu FO, Govella NJ, Moore SJ, Chitnis N, Killeen GF. 2010. Potential benefits, limitations and target product-profiles of odor-baited mosquito traps for malaria control in Africa. *PLoS ONE* **5:** e11573.

Pampana E. 1963. *A textbook of malaria eradication.* Oxford University Press, London.

Penny MA, Maire N, Studer A, Schapira A, Smith TA. 2008. What should vaccine developers ask? Simulation of the effectiveness of malaria vaccines. *PLoS ONE* **3:** e3193.

Penny MA, Galactionova E, Tarantino M, Tanner M, Smith T. 2015a. The public health impact of malaria vaccine RTS,S in malaria endemic Africa: Country-specific predictions using 18 month follow-up Phase III data and simulation models. *BMC Med* **13:** 170.

Penny MA, Verity R, Bever C, Sauboin C, Galactionova E, Flasche S, White MT, Wenger EA, van der Velde N, Pemberton-Ross P, et al. 2015b. The public health impact and cost-effectiveness of malaria vaccine RTS,S/AS01: A systematic comparison of predictions and four mathematical models. *Lancet* **23:** 367–375.

Reiner RC Jr, Perkins TA, Barker CM, Niu T, Chaves LF, Ellis AM, George DB, Le MA, Pulliam JR, Bisanzio D, et al. 2013. A systematic review of mathematical models of mosquito-borne pathogen transmission: 1970-2010. *J R Soc Interface* **10:** 20120921.

Roberts L, Enserink M. 2007. Malaria. Did they really say . . . eradication? *Science* **318:** 1544–1545.

Ross R. 1911. *The prevention of malaria*, 2nd ed. John Murray, London.

Ross A, Smith T. 2010. Interpreting malaria age-prevalence and incidence curves: A simulation study of the effects of different types of heterogeneity. *Malaria J* **9:** 132.

RTS,S Clinical Trials Partnership. 2015. Efficacy and safety of RTS,S/AS01 malaria vaccine with or without a booster dose in infants and children in Africa: Final results of a phase 3, individually randomised, controlled trial. *Lancet* **386:** 31–45.

Sinden RE, Dawes EJ, Alavi Y, Waldock J, Finney O, Mendoza J, Butcher GA, Andrews L, Hill AV, Gilbert SC, et al. 2007. Progression of *Plasmodium berghei* through *Anopheles stephensi* is density-dependent. *PLoS Pathog* **3:** e195.

Smith T, Schapira A. 2012. Reproduction numbers in malaria and their implications. *Trends Parasitol* **28:** 3–8.

Smith T, Killeen GF, Maire N, Ross A, Molineaux L, Tediosi F, Hutton G, Utzinger J, Dietz K, Tanner M. 2006. Mathematical modeling of the impact of malaria vaccines on the clinical epidemiology and natural history of *Plasmodium falciparum* malaria: Overview. *Am J Trop Med Hyg* **75:** 1–10.

Smith DL, McKenzie FE, Snow RW, Hay SI. 2007. Revisiting the basic reproductive number for malaria and its implications for malaria control. *PLoS Biol* **5:** e42.

Smith T, Ross A, Maire N, Chitnis N, Studer A, Hardy D, Brooks A, Penny M, Tanner M. 2012. Ensemble modeling of the likely public health impact of a pre-erythrocytic malaria vaccine. *PLoS Med* **9:** e1001157.

Smith DL, Perkins TA, Tusting LS, Scott TW, Lindsay SW. 2013. Mosquito population regulation and larval source management in heterogeneous environments. *PLoS ONE* **8:** e71247.

Smith DL, Perkins TA, Reiner RC Jr, Barker CM, Niu T, Chaves LF, Ellis AM, George DB, Le MA, Pulliam JR, et al. 2014. Recasting the theory of mosquito-borne pathogen transmission dynamics and control. *Trans R Soc Trop Med Hyg* **108:** 185–197.

Tatem AJ. 2014. Mapping population and pathogen movements. *Int Health* **6:** 5–11.

Tatem AJ, Qiu Y, Smith DL, Sabot O, Ali AS, Moonen B. 2009. The use of mobile phone data for the estimation of the travel patterns and imported *Plasmodium falciparum* rates among Zanzibar residents. *Malaria J* **8:** 287.

Tatem AJ, Smith DL, Gething PW, Kabaria CW, Snow RW, Hay SI. 2010. Ranking of elimination feasibility between malaria-endemic countries. *Lancet* **376:** 1579–1591.

Tatem AJ, Adamo S, Bharti N, Burgert CR, Castro M, Dorelien A, Fink G, Linard C, John M, Montana L, et al. 2012. Mapping populations at risk: Improving spatial demographic data for infectious disease modeling and metric derivation. *Popul Health Metr* **10:** 8.

Walker PG, White MT, Griffin JT, Reynolds A, Ferguson NM, Ghani AC. 2015. Malaria morbidity and mortality in Ebola-affected countries caused by decreased healthcare capacity, and the potential effect of mitigation strategies: A modelling analysis. *Lancet Infect Dis* **15:** 825–832.

White MT, Griffin JT, Churcher TS, Ferguson NM, Basanez MG, Ghani AC. 2011. Modelling the impact of vector control interventions on *Anopheles gambiae* population dynamics. *Parasit Vectors* **4:** 153.

Woolhouse ME, Dye C, Etard JF, Smith T, Charlwood JD, Garnett GP, Hagan P, Hii J, Ndhlovu PD, Quinnell RJ, et al. 1997. Heterogeneities in the transmission of infectious agents: Implications for the design of control programs. *Proc Natl Acad Sci* **94:** 338–342.

WHO. 2015a. Global technical strategy for malaria 2016–2030. World Health Organization, Geneva.

WHO. 2015b. World malaria report 2014. World Health Organization, Geneva.

Index